Pain
Medicine

A COMPREHENSIVE REVIEW

Pain
Medicine
A COMPREHENSIVE REVIEW

Second Edition

P. PRITHVI RAJ, MD
Professor of Anesthesiology
Co-Director of Pain Services
International Pain Institute
Texas Tech University Health Sciences Center
Lubbock, Texas

Technical Editor
Lee Ann Paradise
Lubbock, Texas

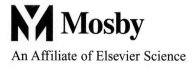
Mosby
An Affiliate of Elsevier Science

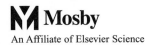

An Affiliate of Elsevier Science

11830 Westline Industrial Drive
St. Louis, Missouri 63146

NOTICE

Pain medicine is an ever-changing field. Standard safety precautions must be followed, but as new research and clinical experience broaden our knowledge, changes in treatment and drug therapy may become necessary or appropriate. Readers are advised to check the most current product information provided by the manufacturer of each drug to be administered to verify the recommended dose, the method and duration of administration, and contraindications. It is the responsibility of the treating physician, relying on experience and knowledge of the patient, to determine dosages and the best treatment for each individual patient. Neither the publisher nor the editor assumes any liability for any injury and/or damage to persons or property arising from this publication.

The Publisher

Previous edition copyrighted 1996

Library of Congress Cataloging-in-Publication Data

Pain medicine : a comprehensive review / [editedby] P. Prithvi Raj.—2nd ed.
    p. ; cm.
  Includes bibliographical references and index.
  ISBN 0-323-01470-4
  1. Pain. 2. Analgesia. I. Raj, P. Prithvi.
  [DNLM: 1. Pain. 2. Pain—therapy. WL 704 P1467 2003]
  RB127.P33248 2003
  616'.0472—dc21   2003042160

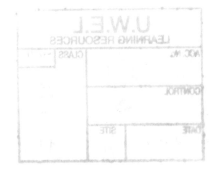

Acquisitions Editor: Allan Ross
Developmental Editor: Josh Hawkins

Printed in the United States of America

Last digit is the print number: 9   8   7   6   5   4   3   2   1

Contributors

Stephen E. Abram, MD
Professor, Department of Anesthesiology
University of New Mexico School of Medicine
Albuquerque, New Mexico

Bernard M. Abrams, BS, MD
Clinical Professor of Neurology
University of Missouri at Kansas City School of Medicine
Kansas City, Missouri

Robert G. Addison, MD
Professor of Orthopedic Surgery
Professor of Rehabilitation Medicine
Northwestern University Feinberg School of Medicine;
Consultant, Rehabilitation Institute of Chicago
Emeritus, Northwestern Memorial Hospital
Chicago, Illinois

Mahmood Ahmad, MD
Pain Management Fellow
Department of Anesthesiology
Yale Center for Pain Management
Yale University School of Medicine
New Haven, Connecticut

Michael A. Ashburn, MD, MPH
Professor of Anesthesiology
University of Utah
Salt Lake City, Utah

Solomon Batnitzky, MD
Professor and Chairman, Department of Radiology
The University of Kansas Medical Center
Kansas City, Kansas

Marshall Bedder MD, FRCP(C)
Executive Director
Neuraad Los Angeles
Beverly Hills, California
Formerly Director
University Pain Management Service
Oregon Health Sciences
Portland, Oregon

Honorio T. Benzon, MD
Professor of Anesthesiology
Chief, Division of Pain Medicine
Northwestern University Feinberg School of Medicine
Chicago, Illinois

Ira M. Bernstein, MD
Professor of Obstetrics and Gynecology
University of Vermont College of Medicine;
Attending Physician, Division of Maternal-Fetal
  Medicine
Fletcher Allen Health Care
Burlington, Vermont

George F. Blackall, Psy D, MBA
Assistant Professor of Anesthesiology, Pediatrics,
  Humanities, and Behavioral Science
Pennsylvania State University College of Medicine;
Director of Psychology, Pain Medical Center
Milton S. Hershey Medical Center
Hershey, Pennsylvania

Hemmo Bosscher, MD
Department of Anesthesiology
Texas Tech University Health Sciences Center
Lubbock, Texas

Robert J. Burton Jr, MD
Chief, Pain Management
Atlanta Georgia Anesthesia Service
Atlanta, Georgia

Terrence M Calder, MD
Chairman, Department of Anesthesiology
Hanover Hospital
Hanover, Pennsylvania

Kenneth D. Candido, MD
Associate Professor
Department of Anesthesiology
Northwestern University Feinberg School of Medicine
Chicago, Illinois

Miles Day, MD, DABPM
Assistant Professor of Anesthesiology/Pain
  Management
Co-Director Pain Services
Texas Tech University Health Sciences Center
International Pain Institute
Lubbock, Texas

Oscar A. de Leon-Casasola, MD
Vice-Chair for Clinical Affairs
Professor of Anesthesiology
University of Buffalo;
Chief, Pain Medicine
Roswell Park Cancer Institute
Buffalo, New York

Manjul D. Derasari, MD
Clinical Assistant Professor of Anesthesiology
University of South Florida College of Medicine;
Staff, Tampa General Hospital, St. Joseph's Hospital,
    University Community Hospital
Tampa, Florida

Joelle F. Desparmet, MD
Associate Professor of Anaesthesia
McGill University;
Director of Chronic Pain Center, Department of
    Anaesthesia
Montreal Children's Hospital
Montreal, Quebec, Canada

Dennis C. Doherty, DO
Adjunct Professor, Anesthesiology
Emory University School of Medicine;
Chief, Section on Pain Medicine
HealthSouth
Atlanta, Georgia

Daniel M. Doleys, PhD
Director
Pain and Rehabilitation Institute
Birmingham, Alabama

Donald Eckard, MD
Professor, Department of Radiology
University of Kansas Medical Center
Kansas City, Kansas

Valerie R. Eckard, MD
Clinical Assistant Professor
University of Kansas Medical Center
Kansas City, Kansas
North Kansas City Hospital
Kansas City, Missouri

Victor A. Filadora, MS, MD
Instructor in Anesthesia
Harvard Medical School;
Chief Resident
Brigham and Women's Hospital
Boston, Massachusetts

Marc B. Hahn, DO
Dean, Texas College of Osteopathic Medicine
University of North Texas Health Science Center
Forth Worth, Texas

Samuel Hassenbusch, MD, PhD
Professor, MD Anderson Cancer Center
University of Texas
Houston, Texas

James E. Heavner, DVM, PhD
Professor, Anesthesiology and Physiology
Director, Anesthesia Research
Texas Tech University Health Sciences Center
Lubbock, Texas

Nelson Hendler, MD, MS
Assistant Professor of Neurosurgery
Johns Hopkins University School of Medicine;
Associate Professor of Physiology
University of Maryland School of Dental Surgery
Baltimore, Maryland;
Active Staff Johns Hopkins Hospital
Clinical Director, Mensana Clinic
Stevenson, Maryland

Allen H. Hord, MD
Director, Department of Anesthesiology
Center for Pain Medicine
Emory University School of Medicine
Atlanta, Georgia

Benjamin W. Johnson, Jr., MD, MBA, DABPM
Director, Vanderbilt Pain Control Center
Associate Professor of Anesthesiology
Vanderbilt University School of Medicine
Nashville, Tennessee

Ronny Kafiluddi, MD, PhD
Staff Anesthesiologist
Genesis Medical Center
Genesis Pain Management Center
Bettendorf, Iowa

L. Douglas Kennedy, MD, DABPM
Pain Medicine Associates
Lexington, Kentucky

Mark D. Kline, MD
Medical Director, Pain Management Services
St. Luke's Hospital
Cedar Rapids, Iowa

Margaret P. Krengel, OTR/C, CHT
Consultant to Shepherd Center Upper Extremity Clinic
Atlanta, Georgia

Paul J. Kuzma, MD
Director, Pain Management Clinic
Walter Reed Army Medical Center
Washington, DC

Mark J. Lema, MS, MD, PhD
Professor and Chair, Department of Anesthesiology
University at Buffalo, State University of New York;
Chairman of Anesthesiology, Critical Care, and Pain
 Medicine
Roswell Park Cancer Institute
Buffalo, New York

Richard M. Linchitz, MD, FACPM
Medical Director of the Pain Alleviation Center
Jericho, New York

Christopher M. Loar, MD
Clinical Assistant Professor of Anesthesia, Department of
 Anesthesia
University of Texas Health Science Center at Houston
Houston, Texas

Stephen P. Long, MD
Clinical Associate Professor of Anesthesiology
Virginia Commonwealth University
Medical College of Virginia Hospital;
Medical Director, Commonwealth Pain Specialists
Richmond, Virginia

Daniel Lynch, MD
Assistant Professor of Clinical Anesthesiology
Director of Acute Pain
Jackson Memorial Hospital Pain Management Center
Miami, Florida

Donald Manning, MD, PhD
Senior Clinical Research Physician
Novartis Pharmaceuticals, Inc.
East Hanover, New Jersey

Patrick M. McQuillan, MD
Associate Professor, Anesthesiology & Pediatrics
Associate Chair for Clinical Affairs
Director, Acute Pain Management & Regional Anethesia
Penn State College of Medicine
Penn State Milton S. Hershey Medical Center
Hershey, Pennsylvania

Matthew Monsein, MD, MBA
Adjunct Clinical Professor, School of Dentistry
University of Minnesota
Medical Director, Chronic Pain Rehabilitation
Abbot Northwestern Hospital, Sister Kenny Institute
Minneapolis, Minnesota

David P. Myers, MD, CAP
Medical Director
HealthCare Connection of Tampa, Inc.
Tampa, Florida

Monica Neumann, MD
Associate Professor of Anesthesiology
Loma Linda University Health Sciences Center
Loma Linda, California

John C. Oakley, MD
Director Pain Management
Northern Rockies Pain and Palliative Rehabilitation
 Center
Billings, Montana

Judith A. Paice, PhD, RN, FAAN
Research Professor of Medicine
Northwestern University Feinberg School of Medicine
Chicago, Illinois

Winston Parris, MD
Tampa Pain Relief Center
Tampa, Florida

George Parsons, PhD
Clinical Psychologist
University of Cincinnati Physicians Pain Center

Richard B. Patt, MD
President and Chief Medical Officer
The Patt Center for Cancer Pain and Wellness
Houston, Texas

Edward T. Plata, MD
Resident, Department of Medicine
School of Medicine and Biomedical Sciences
State University of New York at Buffalo
Buffalo, New York

P. Prithvi Raj, MD
Professor of Anesthesiology
Co-Director of Pain Services
International Pain Institute
Texas Tech University Health Sciences Center
Lubbock, Texas

Somayaji Ramamurthy, MD
Professor, Department of Anesthesiology
University of Texas Health Sciences Center
San Antonio, Texas

James P. Rathmell, MD, MS
Associate Professor, Department of Anesthesiology
University of Vermont College of Medicine;
Director, Pain Management Center
Department of Anesthesia, Fletcher Allen Health Care
Burlington, Vermont

Richard Rauck, MD
Associate Professor of Anesthesia
Wake Forest University School of Medicine;
Co-Director, Pain Control Center
Wake Forest University Medical Center
Winston-Salem, North Carolina

William T. Robinson III, JD
Attorney At Law and Partner
Greenbaum, Doll, and McDonald
Covington, Kentucky

Mark E. Romanoff, MD
Southeast Anesthesiology Consultants
Charlotte, North Carolina

John C. Rowlingson, MD
Professor of Anesthesiology
Director, Pain Medicine Services
Department of Anesthesiology
University of Virginia School of Medicine
Charlottesville, Virginia

Steven Simon, MD, RPh
Professor, Department BMR
University of Kansas
Kansas City, Kansas

Paul J. Sorell III, MD, FAAPMR, Diplomat ABPMR
Medical Director
North Shore Pain Specialists
North Shore University Hospitals at Glen Cove
Long Island Jewish Medical Center
Winthrop University Hospital
Jericho, New York

Peter S. Staats, MD
Associate Professor of Anesthesiology and Critical Care
   Medicine
Director, Division of Pain Medicine
Johns Hopkins University School of Medicine
Baltimore, Maryland

Michael Stanton-Hicks, MD
Vice-Chairman, Department of Anesthesiology
The Cleveland Clinic Foundation
Cleveland, Ohio

Mark J. Stillman, MD
Section Head, Headache and Pain
Department of Neurology
Cleveland Clinic Foundation
Cleveland, Ohio

Elise A Trumble, PT, MS
Formerly, Physiotherapy Associates
Marietta, Georgia

Marc A. Valley, MD, CPE
Medical Director
River Valley Pain Clinic
Russellville, Arizona

Sridhar V. Vasudevan, MD
Clinical Professor of Physical Medicine & Rehabilitation
Medical College of Wisconsin, Milwaukee
President, Wisconsin Rehabilitation Medicine Professionals
Milwaukee, Wisconsin

Christopher M. Viscomi, MD
Associate Professor of Anesthesiology
University of Vermont;
Director of Obstetric Anesthesia
Medical Center Hospital of Vermont
Burlington, Vermont

Howard J. Waldman, MD, DO
Director, Electrodiagnostic Laboratory
Headache and Pain Center
Leawood, Kansas

Steven D. Waldman, MD, JD
Director, The Headache & Pain Center, P.A.
Clinical Professor of Anesthesiology
University Of Missouri-Kansas City School of Medicine

Nicolas E. Walsh, MD
Professor and Chairman, Department of Rehabilitation
   Medicine
University of Texas Health Science Center
San Antonio, Texas

William D. Willis Jr, MD, PhD
Professor and Chairman, Department of Anatomy and
   Neurosciences
University of Texas Medical Branch
University of Texas Medical School at Galveston;
Director, Marine Biochemical Institute
Galveston, Texas

Kevin E. Wilson, PhD
Department of Anesthesiology
Pain Control Center
Wake Forest University School of Medicine
Winston-Salem, North Carolina

Alon P. Winnie, MD
Professor of Clinical Anesthesiology
Department of Anesthesiology
Northwestern University Feinberg School of Medicine
Chicago, Illinois

To my family, friends, and future pain specialists

Preface

The editor and the publishers are encouraged by the success of the first edition of *Pain Medicine: A Comprehensive Review*. Its strength has been to provide quick review to a pain specialist who needs it to manage his or her pain patients. The book also has been popular with fellows training in pain medicine and preparing for specialty board examination.

As with the first edition, the book was developed to fill the void for a comprehensive review of theoretic knowledge and scope of pain medicine. Although the information provided is obtainable in other major texts, the format, style, and clarity of illustrations should make easy reading for the physician. Information provided is based on usual clinical practice rather than experimental data only.

The Table of Contents gently leads the reader from general issues to specifics of pain syndromes and their management. Wherever possible, mechanisms are described and appendixes are provided to further emphasize the basic knowledge required for each syndrome. A special feature of the book is a series of questions provided at the end of each chapter that help the reader to review the subject matter quickly and reliably. For those who wish to enter the examination process in the field of pain medicine, test banks are provided to help with review and preparation for the examination.

This second edition has been planned for the last two years, and the content has been updated. As the editor was preparing *Practical Management of Pain, Third Edition; Textbook of Regional Anesthesia; and Radiographic Imaging in Regional Anesthesia and Pain Management,* he felt that the contents of these books and other books could be combined to have a Table of Contents that is consistent with the objectives of the book. The selected chapters from those books are synopsized by a professional writer and edited by the authors for accuracy and simplicity. Test banks, updated text questions, new illustrations, and new chapters are provided.

The editor hopes the reader will find the book useful in his or her clinical practice.

Acknowledgements

The book would not have been possible without the tireless, unfailing support of Susan Raj. I expressly thank Marilyn Schwiers for her hard work in copyediting and Lee Ann Paradise for her manuscript editing. I am grateful to the authors for their preparation of manuscripts. I also take this opportunity to thank all editors and publishers who have given permission for publication of their works in the book.

P. Prithvi Raj

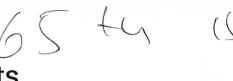 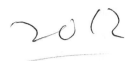

Contents

P A R T 1   General Considerations

1 The History of Pain Medicine / 3
WINSTON C. V. PARRIS

2 Education and Training of Pain Management Personnel / 7
STEPHEN E. ABRAM

3 Pain Pathways: Anatomy and Physiology / 10
JAMES E. HEAVNER AND WILLIAM D. WILLIS JR.

4 Taxonomy of Pain Syndromes / 17
MANJUL D. DERASARI

P A R T 2   Acute Pain Syndromes

5 Medical Diseases / 25
P. PRITHVI RAJ AND STEVEN D. WALDMAN

6 Trauma / 35
RICHARD L. RAUCK

7 Surgery / 43
HONORIO T. BENZON

8 Obstetrics / 49
JAMES P. RATHMELL, CHRISTOPHER M. VISCOMI, AND IRA M. BERNSTEIN

P A R T 3   Chronic Pain Syndromes

9 Nociceptive Pain / 61
NICOLAS E. WALSH, SOMAYAJI RAMAMURTY, TERRENCE M. CALDER, JOHN C. ROWLINGSON, AND ROBERT J. BURTON JR.

10 Neuropathic Pain / 77
DONALD C. MANNING, CHRISTOPHER M. LOAR, P. PRITHVI RAJ, AND ALLEN H. HORD

11 Visceral Pain / 95
P. PRITHVI RAJ AND RICHARD B. PATT

12 Caner Pain / 110
MARK J. LEMA, MILES DAY, DAVID P. MYERS, VICTOR A. FILADORA, AND EDWARD T. PLATA

13 Miscellaneous Pain Syndromes / 119
P. PRITHVI RAJ

P A R T 4   Evaluation and Investigation of Pain Patients

14 History Taking of the Patient in Pain / 127
BERNARD M. ABRAMS

15 Physical Examination / 131
STEVEN SIMON

16 Laboratory Investigation / 147
L. DOUGLAS KENNEDY

17 Psychologic Evaluation / 152
DANIEL M. DOLEYS AND DENNIS C. DOHERTY

18 Functional Evaluation / 161
ELISE A. TRUMBLE AND MARGARET P. KRENGEL

19 Disability Evaluation / 167
SRIDHAR V. VASUDEVAN AND MATTHEW MONSEIN

20 Pain Measurement / 173
MARC A. VALLEY

21 Diagnostic Tools Available for Pain Management / 182

BERNARD M. ABRAMS, HOWARD J. WALDMAN, VALERIE R. ECKARD, SOLOMON BATNITZKY, DONALD ECKARD, ALON P. WINNIE, AND KENNETH D. CANDIDO

PART 5 Modalities of Pain Management

22 Pharmacologic Techniques / 205

NELSON HENDLER

23 Interventional Techniques

SECTION 23A • Central Nerve Blocks / 212

PATRICK M. MCQUILLAN, RONNY KAFILUDDI, AND MARC B. HAHN

SECTION 23B • Somatic Nerve Blocks / 223

MARK ROMANOFF, PAUL J. KUZMA, AND MARK D. KLINE

SECTION 23C • Sympathetic Nerve Block / 250

RICHARD L. RAUCK AND OSCAR A. DE LEON-CASASOLA

SECTION 23D • Continuous Techniques / 272

P. PRITHVI RAJ

SECTION 23E • Epidural Steroid Injections / 280

HEMMO A. BOSSCHER

SECTION 23F • Facet Neurolysis Including Cryoneurolysis and Radiofrequency / 291

MONICA NEUMANN, P. PRITHVI RAJ, LLOYD JOSEPH FITZGERALD, AND MAHMOOD AHMAD

SECTION 23G • Intrathecal Implantation / 303

JOHN C. OAKLEY, PETER S. STAATS, AND SAMUEL HASSENBUSCH

24 Surgical Techniques / 309

SAMUEL HASSENBUSCH

25 Psychologic Techniques / 318

GEORGE F. BLACKALL AND KEVIN E. WILSON

26 Physical Therapy Techniques / 327

RICHARD M. LINCHITZ AND PAUL J. SORELL III

27 Home Care / 334

JUDITH A. PAICE AND MICHAEL STANTON-HICKS

28 Alternative Medicine / 340

WINSTON C. V. PARRIS

29 Palliative Medicine / 345

MARK J. STILLMAN

PART 6 Special Situations

30 Pediatric Pain / 351

JOELLE F. DESPARMET-SHERIDAN

31 Geriatric Pain / 360

DANIEL LYNCH

32 Quality Assurance and Improvement in Pain Practice / 373

MARSHALL BEDDER

33 Economics of Pain Medicine / 377

BENJAMIN W. JOHNSON JR. AND MARSHALL BEDDER

34 Regulatory Issues Affecting Pain Medicine / 385

MICHAEL A. ASHBURN AND STEPHEN P. LONG

35 Pain Medicine and the Legal System / 391

GEORGE E. PARSONS AND WILLIAM T. ROBINSON III

36 Ethical Issues in Pain Management / 398

R. G. ADDISON

Test Banks / 401

Index / 419

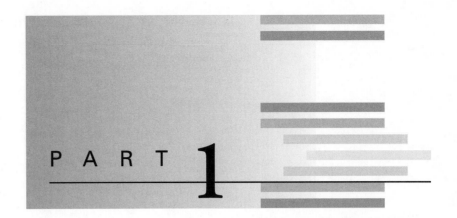

P A R T 1

General Considerations

CHAPTER 1

The History of Pain Medicine

WINSTON C. V. PARRIS

The management of pain, like the management of disease, is as old as humanity. Most diseases afflict humankind spontaneously and usually cause pain without any wrongdoing on the part of the afflicted person. In a review of history, however, there are many examples of how humans have inflicted pain on each other. The ongoing conflict in the Middle East is one example of this. Indeed, oppression, conflict, and war have been associated with untold pain, suffering, and death throughout time.

Fortunately, advances in technology and medicine have helped to bring about new concepts regarding disease and the painful states associated with disease. Focusing on some of the major historical events regarding pain and its management, this chapter highlights the important phases that led to the conceptualization of pain and its treatment as an independent specialty in modern medicine.

PAIN AND RELIGION

The early concept of pain as a form of punishment for sinful activity is as old as humankind.[1] Christians believed that pain during childbirth, for example, was a consequence of Eve's sin and was transferred to them directly by God. It was not until 1847, when Queen Victoria was administered chloroform by James Simpson[2] for obstetric pain during delivery, that Christians accepted the idea that it was not heresy to promote painless childbirth.

As epidural anesthesia has developed and techniques have been refined so that mortality and morbidity are negligible, childbirth and delivery are considered relatively painless in most developing countries. However, in many other countries the personnel and technology are still inadequate, making childbirth a painful and sometimes disastrous event.

Today, hurricanes, earthquakes, and fires, to name just a few, cause hundreds, and at times thousands, of innocent, defenseless people to die. It is sometimes hard to rationalize why seemingly good people suffer, when so many ruthless, evil-minded people seem to prosper in relative comfort.

As far back as the 1st century, many people endured suffering with the belief that they did it for the love of Christ, and they felt that their suffering identified them with Christ's suffering on the cross during his crucifixion.[3] This may be the earliest example of the value of psychotherapy as an important modality in managing pain. This concept has led to several scientifically conducted and government-sponsored studies evaluating intercessory prayer as an effective modality for controlling cancer pain.

PAIN AND THE ANCIENT CULTURES

The tribal concept of pain came from the belief that it resulted from outside sources or from an "intrusion" from outside the body. These evil spirits or "intruders" were viewed as a form of punishment sent by the gods. Because it was thought that spirits entered the body from different avenues, therapy was aimed at blocking the particular pathway chosen by the spirit.

Examples of entry points:
- In Egypt, the left nostril was considered the site of entry.[4]
- In Papua New Guinea, it was believed that evil entered a person by a spear or an arrow that produced spontaneous pain.[5]

Examples of ancient treatments:
- A shaman sucked the evil spirit from a painful wound and then neutralized it with special medicines.
- Egyptians treated some forms of pain by placing electric fish over the wounds.[6] Interestingly, it is now known that the electrical stimulation that relieved the pain actually works by a mechanism similar to transcutaneous electrical nerve stimulation (TENS), which is often used to treat pain today.

Word origins:
- Pain comes from the Latin word *poena,* meaning "punishment."
- Patient comes from the Latin word *patior,* meaning, "to endure suffering or pain."

Thus, it is easy to see that people in ancient times who experienced pain interpreted the pain as a punishment that was either given to them by the gods or should be offered up to the gods as a gift to appease them.[7]

The Chinese identified multiple points in the body where pain might originate or might be self-perpetuating.[8] Thus, attempts were made to drain the body of pain by inserting needles, a concept that may have given birth to acupuncture therapy, which is well over 2000 years old.[9]

The ancient Greeks were the first to consider pain to be a sensory function that might be derived from peripheral stimulation.[10] Although Plato believed the brain was the destination of all peripheral stimulation, Aristotle advanced the theory that the heart was the originating source or processing center for pain.

Toward the Roman Empire period, steady progress was made in understanding pain as a sensation similar to other sensations in the body. As anatomy became better understood, it was thought that the brain was indeed the center for the processing of pain.[11] In addition, other advances were taking place regarding the development of therapeutic modalities such as the use of drugs, heat, cold, and massage, to treat pain. These developments brought about the establishment of the principles of surgery for treating disease. However, throughout the Middle Ages and the Renaissance, the debate continued regarding the origin and processing center of pain.

William Harvey, known for discovering circulation, supported the heart as the pain center; however, Descartes strongly disagreed. Descartes' description of pain conduction from peripheral damage through nerves to the brain led to the first plausible pain theory called the *specificity theory.*[12]

PAIN AND PAIN THEORIES

Descartes' specificity theory was revised by Schiff[12] based on animal research; the essential theory was that each sensory modality, including pain, was transmitted along an independent pathway. Schiff, by examining the effect of incisions in the spinal cord, demonstrated that touch and pain were independent sensations.

The 18th and 19th centuries are known as the period of the Scientific Revolution because of its new discoveries and ways of thinking. Several important discoveries related to pain took place:

- The analgesic properties of nitrous oxide
- Local anesthetic agents such as cocaine
- The anatomic division of the spinal cord into sensory (dorsal) and motor (ventral) divisions

Based on Mueller's[13] theories that there was a straight-through system of specific nerve energies, in which specific energy from a given sensation was transmitted along sensory nerves to the brain, Darwin[14] proposed the intensive theory of pain. This theory maintained that the sensation of pain was not a separate modality but resulted from a sensory overload of sufficient intensity for the modality. Later the theory was modified and expanded so that by the mid-20th century, the specificity theory was universally accepted as the more plausible theory of pain.

As a result, strategies for pain therapy began to focus on identifying and interrupting pain pathways. Although this led researchers to explore surgical techniques that might relieve pain by interrupting pain pathways, it also influenced the medical community for many years to believe that pain pathways and their interruption were the total answer to the pain puzzle.

PAIN AND DISEASE

The cardinal features of disease as recognized by early philosophers included:

- Calor (heat)
- Rubor (redness)
- Tumor (swelling)
- Dolor (pain)

One of the important realizations with regard to pain medicine was the acknowledgment that although heat, redness, and swelling may disappear, pain may still exist. When pain continues long after the natural pathogenic course of the disease has ended, a chronic pain syndrome develops with the possibility of characteristic clinical features including:

- Depression
- Dependency
- Disability
- Disuse
- Drug misuse
- Drug abuse
- Doctor shopping

Throughout time, physicians and healers focused their attention on managing pain. Although many advances have been made, it has been only within the past 20 years that significant strides have been made with regard to treating chronic pain as a disease that requires specialized study, evaluation, and therapeutic interventions.

PAIN AND THE 20TH CENTURY

1846: William Morton formerly discovered general anesthesia.

1847: Simpson used chloroform to provide anesthesia for labor and delivery.

1888: Corning described the use of a local anesthetic, cocaine, for the treatment of nerve pain.

1907: Scholosser reported significant relief of neuralgic pain for long periods with an alcohol injection.

1926: Swetlow and then White in 1928 reported on the use of alcohol injections into thoracic sympathetic ganglia to treat chronic angina.

1931: Dogliotti[15] described the use of alcohol injection into the cervical subarachnoid space to treat cancer pain.

One consequence of war has been the development of new techniques and procedures to manage injuries. In World War I (1914–1918), numerous studies were associated with trauma, dismemberment, and frostbite, for example. In World War II (1936–1946), not only peripheral vascular injuries but also phantom limb phenomena causalgias and many sympathetically mediated pain syndromes occurred. Leriche developed the technique of sympathetic blocks with procaine to treat causalgic injuries of war. John Bonica, an army surgeon during World War II, proposed the concept of multidisciplinary, multimodal management for chronic pain. Considered the "father of pain," Bonica's work was the catalyst for the formation of many national and international pain organizations such as the American Pain Society and the International Association for the Study of Pain (IASP).

Anesthesia departments were considered divisions of surgery, not reaching full autonomy until after World War II. Because of morbidity associated with general anesthesia and because several new local anesthetics were being discovered, regional anesthesia and its associated techniques began to flourish in the United States. Bonica also played a major role in advancing the use of epidural anesthesia to manage the pain associated with labor and delivery.

As time passed, the general public considered pain to be unsatisfactory and unacceptable. As a result, demands were made that resulted in the development of labor and delivery anesthesia services, acute pain services, and, more recently, chronic pain clinics. The vision of Bonica was not only the development of those clinics but also the founding and maintenance of national and international pain organizations to promote research and scientific understanding in pain medicine.

An outstanding contribution in the field of research was the development and publication of the *gate control theory* by Melzack and Wall[16] in 1965. This theory, built on the pre-existing and prevalent specificity and intensive theories, provided a sound scientific basis for understanding pain mechanisms. The gate control theory emphasizes the importance of both the ascending and descending modulating systems and laid down a solid framework for the management of different pain syndromes. In essence, the gate control theory almost single-handedly legitimized pain as a scientific discipline.[17]

PAIN AND PAIN INSTITUTIONS

- The International Association for the Study of Pain and the American Pain Society
- Commission on Accreditation on Rehabilitation Facilities
- American Academy of Pain Medicine
- World Society of Pain Clinicians
- World Institute of Pain

PAIN AND THE HOSPICE MOVEMENT

The concept of *hospice*, a medieval term that represents a welcome place of rest for pilgrims of the Holy Land, dates back to the reign of Emperor Julian the Apostate when Fabiola, a Roman matron, created a place for sick and healthy travelers and cared for the dying.[18]

In 1902, The Irish Sisters of Charity founded St. Joseph's Hospice, staffed by Cecily Saunders 50 years later. Dr. Saunders was the first full-time hospice medical officer, and she was regarded as the founder and medical director of St. Christopher's Hospital in England. She later developed a keen interest in terminal cancer patients and was trained in medical school to be a physician. She emphasized the following:

- The need for taking a patient at his or her word when it came to pain assessment and scheduled doses on a time-contingent basis rather than an as-needed basis
- The importance of frequent pain assessments
- That it was unnecessary and inhumane for cancer patients to die in pain[19]

PAIN AND THE FUTURE

A review of the history of pain demonstrates that until the time of Bonica, pain management was considered to be uni-modal, unidisciplinary, and managed without any clear structural organization. Today, new drugs and creative techniques and procedures have expanded the scope of pain medicine.

Pain physicians are no longer isolated and there is a great deal of literature on the topic of pain medicine and management. Credentialing is well on the way, and two credible organizations are responsible for credentialing pain physicians in the United States: (1) the American Board of Pain Medicine, which awards a diploma, and (2) the American Board of Anesthesiology, which awards a Certificate of Added Qualification.

In addition, the training of pain specialists is given serious attention, and it is very likely that in addition to the 1-year pain fellowships now in existence, attempts will be successful in establishing pain medicine residencies. It will also be important for medical school administrators to reevaluate their educational programs to include more about pain medicine. Indeed the future of pain medicine looks very bright not only as a result of the dedicated clinicians and researchers of the past and present but also because of the new pain specialists to come.

References

1. Procacci P, Maresca M: Evolution of the concept of pain. In Sicuteri F, editor: *Advances in pain research and therapy,* vol 20. New York, Raven Press, 1984.
2. Raj PP: 1990 Labat lecture. Pain relief: Fact or fancy? *Reg Anesth* 15(4):157, 1990.
3. Caton D: The secularization of pain. *Anesthesiology* 62(4):493, 1985.
4. Todd EM: Pain: Historical perspectives. In Aronoff GM, editor: *Evaluation and treatment of chronic pain.* Baltimore, Urban and Schwarzenberg, 1985.
5. Procacci P, Maresca M: Pain concept in Western civilization: a historical review. In Benedetti C, Chapman CR, Morrica G et al, editors: *Advances in pain research and therapy, vol 7. Recent advances in the management of pain.* New York, Raven Press, 1984.
6. Castiglioni A: *A history of medicine,* ed 2. New York, Alfred A. Knopf, 1947.
7. Warfield C: A history of pain relief. *Hosp Pract* 23(12):121, 1988.
8. Lin Y: *The wisdom of India.* London, Joseph, 1949.
9. Veith I: *Huang ti ne chin su wen.* Baltimore, William & Wilkins, 1949.
10. Bonica JJ: Evolution of pain concepts and pain clinics. In Brena SF, Chapman SL, editors: *Clinics in anesthesiology: Chronic pain—management principles,* Philadelphia, Saunders, 1985.
11. Keele KD: *Anatomies of pain.* Oxford, Blackwell Science, 1957.
12. Schiff M: *Lehrbuch der physiologie, muskel, und nervenphysiologie.* Schavenberg, Germany, Lahr, 1848.
13. Mueller J (Baly W, transl): *Handbuch der physiologie des menschen.* London, Taylor and Walton, 1842.
14. Darwin E: *Zoonomia, or the laws of organic life.* London, J Johnson, 1794.
15. Dogliotti AM: Traitement des syndromes douloureux de la peripherie par alcoholisation sub-arachnoidienne. *Presse Med* 39, 1931.
16. Melzack R, Wall PD: Pain mechanisms: A new theory. *Science* 150:171, 1965.
17. Abram SE: 1992 Bonica lecture. Advances in chronic pain management since gate control. *Reg Anesth* 18(2):66, 1993.
18. Craven J, Wald FS: Hospice care for dying patients. *Am J Nurs* 75(10):1816, 1975.
19. Saunders C: The last stages of life. *Am J Nurs* 65:70, 1965.

1. In the 1st century, Christians endured suffering with what belief?

   A. To identify them with Christ's suffering
   B. To be punished for their sins
   C. To disbelieve in the teachings of Christianity
   D. To bring attention to themselves

2. Which was the first ancient civilization to consider pain as a sensory function?

   A. Ancient Pharaohs
   B. Ancient Greeks
   C. Ancient Chinese
   D. Ancient Indians

3. The "period of scientific revolution" was because of new discoveries and ways of thinking in which centuries?

   A. 1st and 2nd centuries
   B. 14th and 15th centuries
   C. 18th and 19th centuries
   D. 20th and 21st centuries

4. Gate control theory of pain by Melzack and Wall was described in

   A. 1960
   B. 1965
   C. 1970
   D. 1975

5 Cecily Saunders is considered to be the founder of

   A. Charity hospitals
   B. Pharmacy movement
   C. Hospice movement
   D. Children's hospital

ANSWERS

1. A

2. B

3. C

4. B

5. C

CHAPTER 2

Education and Training of Pain Management Personnel

STEPHEN E. ABRAM

Since 1990, subspecialty fellowship training in pain management has expanded dramatically, both in the scope of training offered and the numbers of positions. Much of this expansion has been within the subspecialty of anesthesiology, and it is in large measure attributable to the development of a process of subspecialty certification by the American Board of Anesthesiology (ABA) and fellowship training accreditation by the Accreditation Council for Graduate Education (ACGME). Although there is some effort to ensure that fellowship training programs provide comprehensive didactic and clinical teaching, there is clearly a tendency to emphasize anesthesiology-based treatments both in the scope of some fellowship programs and in the content of the ABA subspecialty certification examination.

CERTIFICATE OF ADDED QUALIFICATIONS IN PAIN MANAGEMENT

In 1993, the ABA offered the first pain management examination, which was also the first pain subspecialty examination sponsored by a specialty board approved by the American Board of Medical Specialties (ABMS). The examination system is open to ABA diplomates who have completed an ACGME-approved fellowship. The content of the Certificate of Added Qualifications (CAQ) examination is determined by the ABA. Examination questions are written by individuals within and outside the anesthesiology specialty and are then edited by a board of ABA directors and diplomates who hold a CAQ in pain management and are considered to be pain management specialists.

ESSENTIALS OF THE PAIN FELLOWSHIP

The most recent ACGME *Program Requirements for Residency Education in Pain Management* became effective in 1999 and were revised in 2002. The fellowship training program is 12 months long and begins after satisfactory completion of a core residency in anesthesiology. Subspecialty experience in pain management gained during the residency may not count toward the 1-year requirement. Most of the time in the fellowship training program must be spent managing pain patients, in contrast to working in operating room or obstetrical anesthesia.

The Association of Anesthesiology Pain Program Directors (AAPPD) has suggested that a total of 180 days of acute, chronic, and cancer pain patient care be the minimum provided during the fellowship. If this minimum cannot be met during the year because of research or other clinical work, the program should be extended for the individual.

Pain fellowship programs can be accredited only if they are administratively connected to an ACGME-approved core residency program in anesthesiology. There must also be close cooperation between the core residency program and the subspecialty program and both inpatient and outpatient experience.

A number of broad topics are provided in the recommended pain management training curriculum. In addition, a number of specific treatment techniques are listed in the program requirements. The trainee must "become familiar" with the theory, benefits, indications, and applications of these techniques. Other requirements include the opportunity to participate in research; experience in the management of a pain clinic; participation in treatment as a consultant; attendance at regularly scheduled conferences, including multidisciplinary; participation in the teaching of residents, medical students, and other health care professionals; and participation in the continuing quality improvement and utilization review processes.

ROLE OF THE RESIDENCY REVIEW COMMITTEE—FUTURE CHANGES

The Residency Review Committee (RRC) for Anesthesiology is responsible for creating the *Special Requirements for Pain Management*. This document is the basis for determining whether a given training program meets the requirements of the ACGME accreditation. The *Special Requirements for Pain Management* has recently created the additional requirement that trainees keep a log of procedures done during their fellowship training. This document is a reflection of the actual clinical experience that the fellow gains during the training period. Within core specialty training programs, there is a current movement toward requiring minimum numbers of certain procedures and types of cases.

PAIN FELLOWSHIP PROGRAM DIRECTORS

In 1995, several anesthesiology pain fellowship program directors organized a group for the purpose of deciding policy issues related to pain management fellowship training. The AAPPD, acting as an autonomous committee of the American Society of Regional Anesthesia and Pain Medicine

(ASRA), now meets twice yearly and serves as a resource for the RRC, providing information and advice regarding training program content, time allocation for clinical and research activity, and time given to duties not related to pain management. They have addressed such issues as the teaching of newer procedures that have not proved efficacious and what constitutes adequate training for procedures requiring substantial technical skill and experience. It has been decided that the AAPPD should provide hospitals with some guidelines regarding what constitutes adequate training for certain technical procedures. Other topics that have received attention of the AAPPD include the training of nonanesthesiologists in ACGME-approved anesthesiology fellowship programs, and the workforce needs for fellowship-trained pain management physicians and whether efforts should be made to regulate the number of training positions offered.

PAIN MEDICINE AS A SPECIALTY

An alternative approach to the creation of subspecialty training and credentialing in pain management has been to create a separate specialty of pain medicine. For this purpose, the American Academy of Pain Medicine (AAPM) was formed. The academy had two major objectives: (1) to obtain a seat in the American Medical Association (AMA) House of Delegates and (2) to establish a credible organization for the credentialing of pain specialists. The process of gaining ABMS recognition remains underway, with the expectation that pain medicine will be officially recognized and credentialed in the United States.

CORE CURRICULUM

The International Association for the Study of Pain (IASP) created a task force whose mission is to define a core curriculum that should be common in the training programs for physicians and perhaps all health care professionals who pursue careers in pain management. The document, entitled *Core Curriculum for Professional Education in Pain,*[1] and its bibliography are updated periodically as the scope of knowledge and the range of pain management techniques expand. The document provides a valuable study guide for pain management trainees in any discipline.

PAIN SOCIETIES AND EDUCATION

Several organizations whose primary purpose is the education of pain management professionals have been created.

The IASP was incorporated in 1974. Its purposes are to foster and encourage pain research, to promote education and training, to facilitate dissemination of information, to encourage adoption of uniform nomenclature and classification, to encourage education of the public regarding pain issues, to encourage development of an extensive data bank, and to advise political agencies on standards of pain treatment. It was the first organization to bring together physicians and nonphysicians in an educational forum regarding pain treatment and research. IASP allowed for the exchange of ideas between clinicians and basic scientists, as well as between physicians and psychologists. It also introduced specialists to the techniques and ideas of other specialties.

The American Pain Society (APS) is one of the IASP national chapters. Its purposes and membership composition reflect those of the IASP. Its annual scientific meetings are a mixture of clinical and basic science topics, and symposia often combine scientific and clinical aspects of a particular topic. The APS published the *Pain Forum* journal, which reviews clinical, ethical, and basic science topics and provides commentaries on topics offering several differing points of view. Several region sections of the APS have been organized in an effort to provide a forum for a wider range of professionals involved in pain management.

The ASRA, as it presently exists, was organized in 1976. The purpose of this resurrected society is to promote the use of regional anesthetic techniques for surgery, obstetrics, and pain management; to stimulate research on regional anesthesia and local anesthetic pharmacology; to provide an educational forum; and to stimulate the publication of scientific and educational material related to these topics. Pain control has become a major area of interest for the society, and issues beyond the realm of regional anesthetic techniques are presented at scientific and educational meetings.

The European Society of Regional Anesthesia (ESRA) has similar goals.

The World Society of Pain Clinicians is an international physician-only organization whose major focus is the dissemination of knowledge, the education of physicians, the publication of a quarterly journal *(The Pain Clinic)*, and the organization of a biannual congress on pain medicine. This organization was originally European based but is now spreading to North America, Asia, and the rest of the world so that all pain physicians may participate in the exchange of information regarding pain medicine.

Several groups have been organized to deal primarily with the management of cancer pain. Cancer pain is a major epidemiologic problem, and its management is taught poorly, if at all, in most medical school curricula. One major barrier to the delivery of appropriate analgesia to cancer patients is the inadequate or inappropriate education of health care providers. The Wisconsin Cancer Pain Initiative is an interdisciplinary effort begun in 1985 by the Wisconsin Controlled Substances Board to address the undertreatment of cancer pain.[2] A group of health care professionals, legislators, and representatives of the World Health Organization and Surgeon's General office met in 1986 to develop a strategy for the project. From that and subsequent efforts, a variety of resources were developed, including an extensive bibliography on cancer pain mechanisms and treatment, a short *Handbook of Cancer Pain Management,*[3] a compilation of resources within the state that address cancer pain problems, a listing of available cancer pain treatment techniques, a speaker's bureau, and topographic maps showing cancer mortality rates by county. Similar initiatives have been undertaken in other states, using the Wisconsin project as a model.

References

1. Fields HL: *Core curriculum for professional education in pain*, ed 2. Seattle, IASP, 1995.
2. Joranson DE, Enger D: Wisconsin initiative for improving cancer pain management: Progress report. *J Pain Symptom Manage* 1(3):180, 1986.
3. Weissman DE, Burchman SL, Dinnorf PA, et al: *Handbook of cancer pain management.* Madison: Wisconsin Cancer Pain Initiative, 1988.

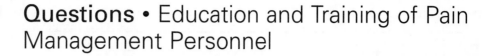

1. The first pain management subspecialty examination approved by the American Board of Medical Specialties is a "Certificate of Added Qualifications" from the

   A. International Association for the Study of Pain
   B. American Academy of Pain Medicine
   C. American Society of Regional Anesthesia
   D. American Board of Anesthesiology

2. The American College of Graduate Medical Education requirements for residency in pain management as published in 1992 consist of

   A. 6 months training in pain management after satisfactory completion of a core residency in anesthesiology
   B. 12 months training in pain management after satisfactory completion of a core residency in anesthesiology
   C. 18 months training in pain management after satisfactory completion of a core residency in anesthesiology
   D. 24 months training in pain management after satisfactory completion of a core residency in anesthesiology

3. In 1995, pain fellowship program directors organized a group for the deciding policy issues related to pain management fellowship training. This group is an autonomous committee of

   A. American Board of Medical Specialties
   B. American Society of Anesthesiology
   C. American Society of Regional Anesthesia
   D. American Board of Pain Medicine

4. The core curriculum for training programs for the physicians who pursue careers in pain management was created by

   A. Task force of the International Association for the Study of Pain
   B. Task force of the American Society of Regional Anesthesia
   C. Task force of the American Board of Pain Medicine
   D. Task force of the American Society of Regional Anesthesiology

5. The American Academy of Pain Medicine was formed for all of these except

   A. To obtain a seat in the American Medical Association House of Delegates
   B. To establish a credible organization for the credentialing of pain specialists
   C. To create a body for certification in the practice of pain management
   D. To be an alternative to the secondary board certification granted by the American Board of Medical Specialties

ANSWERS

1. D
2. B
3. C
4. A
5. D

CHAPTER 3

Pain Pathways: Anatomy and Physiology

JAMES E. HEAVNER AND WILLIAM D. WILLIS JR.

The *pain system* is analogous to other sensory systems such as the visual or auditory systems.[1] It consists of specialized nerve endings called nociceptors attached to axons (A-delta or C fibers) that project to the spinal cord or brainstem nuclei in an ordered fashion. Nociceptive information is then distributed to the various spinal targets and to supraspinal targets via identifiable routes. The information is ultimately passed on to various subcortical and cortical structures of the brain, resulting in conscious perception; subconscious activities; and consciously and unconsciously initiated neuromodulatory, effector (motor), endocrine, and emotional responses (Fig. 3–1).

In normal healthy individuals the pain system responds to controlled stimuli in a predictable and reproducible fashion. This does not imply that the "normal" functioning of the pain system is fully understood.

Like other sensory systems, the pain system may be altered by injury, disease, or heritable influences that cause pathophysiologic functioning of the system. Changes may include processes in pain perception that are not normally involved in generating this sensation.

Complete understanding of normal physiologic processes is an important step to appreciating and treating pathologic states.

NOCICEPTORS AND ASSOCIATED AXONS

Nociceptors

Morphologically unique structures at the distal end of primary afferent axons that are depolarized by stimuli that threaten or produce damage are classified as nociceptors.[2] Nociceptors supply skin, subcutaneous tissue, periosteum, joints, muscles, and visceral tissue (Fig. 3–2).[3] They are depolarized (activated) by noxious thermal, mechanical, or chemical stimuli.

A "silent nociceptor" exists that is very difficult to activate under normal circumstances but becomes very easy to activate when sensitized by influences such as inflammation.[4–7]

The sensation aroused by adequate stimulation of cutaneous nociceptors is either pricking pain or burning or dull pain.[8,9] Muscle nociceptors evoke aching pain,[10] as do nociceptors that supply other deep tissues, such as joints, tendons, and periosteum.

A-Delta and C Fibers

Axons in peripheral nerves were classified by Erlanger and Gasser[11] as A, B, and C with A fibers subgroups of alpha, beta, gamma, and delta. A and B fibers are myelinated; C fibers are not.

According to Hagbarth,[12] 10% of all myelinated fibers in human cutaneous nerves carry nociceptive information; more than 90% of all unmyelinated fibers carry nociceptive information (Fig. 3–3).

SPINAL CORD DORAL HORN NEURONS AND ASCENDING SPINAL TRACTS

Rexed Laminae

Primary afferent axons carrying nociceptive information form synaptic contacts with neurons in the spinal cord gray matter (or equivalent brainstem nuclei for cranial nerves). The neurons distribute the information locally and into centrally projecting pathways. A landmark for contemporary studies of nociceptive information processing was the description of a cytoarchitectural organization pattern of the spinal cord gray matter by Rexed in 1952.[13]

Nociceptive afferent fibers from the skin terminate in laminae I, II, and V of the dorsal horn, with a few around the central canal. Fine afferents from viscera, muscle, and other deep tissues tend to avoid lamina II but end in laminae I, V, and X.[14–17]

Depending on their responses to peripheral stimuli, central neurons that receive nociceptive information are classified as nociceptive-specific or wide dynamic range (WDR) neurons (Fig. 3–4).[18]

ASCENDING SPINAL NOCICEPTIVE PATHWAYS

The following ascending spinal cord pathways have been implicated as routes for processing nociceptive information:

- The spinothalamic tract (STT)
- The spinoreticular tract (SRT)
- The spinomesencephalic tract (SMT)
- The postsynaptic dorsal column tract (PSDCT)

Pathways ascending by the anterolateral route apparently play a major role in signaling pain, because cordotomies

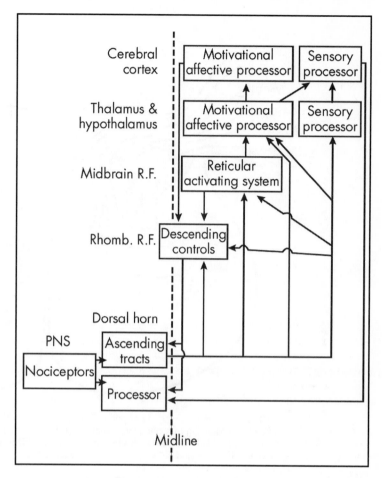

FIG. 3–1 Pathways of the pain system. The primary afferent nociceptors in the peripheral nervous system convey nociceptive information to the dorsal horn, where the information is processed by interneurons and ascending-tract cells. Nociceptive information is then signaled to the reticular activating system and other parts of the brain, including the thalamus and cerebral cortex, responsible for sensory and for motivational-affective processing. Descending controls originate at all levels and influence the processing of nociceptive information in the dorsal horn. *(Redrawn from Willis WD: Physiology of pain perception. In Takagi H, Oomura Y, Ito M, Otsuka M, editors:* Biowarning system in the brain. *Tokyo, University of Tokyo Press, 1988).*

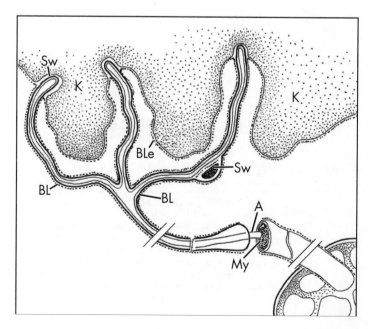

FIG. 3–2 Schematic drawing showing termination in the skin of nerve fiber of a mechanical nociceptor. This schema was established for the cat by determining the nature of neural structures consistently present under the small spot-like areas of marked, receptive fields of mechanical nociceptors with myelinated fibers. A single thin myelinated fiber (A) separates from a nerve bundle and in continuing superficially branches and loses the myelin (My) covering but remains surrounded by a Schwann cell (Sw) and its basal lamina (BL). The Schwann cell-neurite complex fuses its basal lamina with that of the epidermis as the complex penetrates the epidermis. The epidermal nerve terminal remains largely or completely covered by extension of the Schwann cell. *(Redrawn from Perl ER: Characterization of nociceptors and their activation of neurons in the superficial dorsal horn: First steps for the sensation of pain. In Kruger L, Liebeskind JC, editors:* Advances in pain research and therapy, vol 6. *New York, Raven Press, 1984.)*

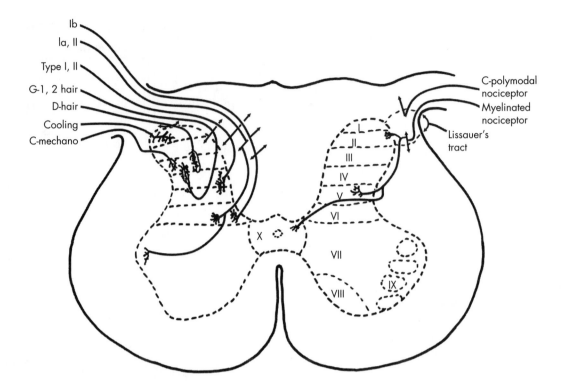

FIG. 3–3 Termination zones of primary afferent fibers in the spinal cord gray matter. The dotted lines in the drawing of a transverse section of the spinal cord show the boundaries of the gray matter and of laminae I through VI of the dorsal horn. The characteristic lines of termination of large somatic afferents and cutaneous mechanoreceptors and of thermoreceptors are shown on the left and those of cutaneous nociceptors are shown on the right. *(Redrawn from Light AR: The initial processing of pain and its descending control: Spinal and trigeminal systems. In Gildenberg PL, editor: Pain and headache. Basel, Karger, 1992.)*

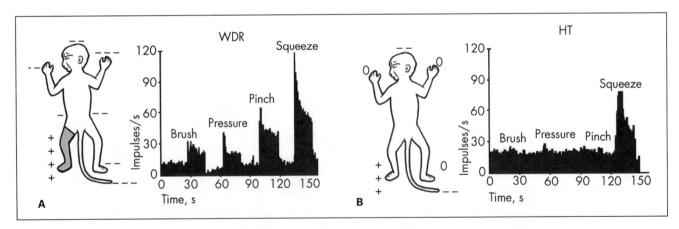

FIG. 3–4 The responses of a "wide dynamic range" or multireceptive spinothalamic tract cell are shown in *A* and of a high-threshold spinothalamic tract cell in *B*. The figurines indicate the excitatory (plus signs) and inhibitory (minus signs) receptive fields. The graphs show the responses to graded intensities of mechanical stimulation. Brush is with a camel's hair brush repeatedly stroked across the receptive field. Pressure is applied by attachment of an arterial clip to the skin. This is a marginally painful stimulus to a human. Pinch is by attachment of a stiff arterial clip to the skin and is distinctly painful. Squeeze is by compressing a fold of skin with forceps and is damaging to the skin. *(Redrawn from Willis WD: Ascending pathways from the dorsal horn. In Brown AG, Rethelyi M, editors: Spinal cord sensation: Sensory processing in the dorsal horn. Edinburgh, Scottish Academic Press, 1981.)*

interrupting this part of the spinal cord produce analgesia in humans[19] (Fig. 3–5; Table 3–1).

According to Willis,[20] a potential additional role in pain sensation for ipsilaterally projecting systems, such as uncrossed components of the STT, SRT, and SMT and the postsynaptic dorsal column pathway, should not be overlooked.

Spinothalamic Tract

The STT should not be equated with the anterolateral quadrants (ALQs) of the spinal cord, as is often done. Also, the ALQ must not be considered as a system exclusively conveying nociceptive messages.

TABLE 3–1 Distribution in the Spinal Cord Gray Matter Lamina of Neurons Giving Origin to Ascending Nociceptive Pathways

Spinal Tract	Laminae
Spinothalamic	All, most concentrated in LI and LV
Spinoreticular	LVII, a few in the posterior horn
Spinomesencephalic	Anterior and posterior horns
Postsynaptic dorsal column	LIII, LIV, LVII, LX

According to Willis,[20] the STT is the best characterized of the ascending nociceptive tracts. STT neurons are located in all of Rexed's laminae,[21] but they are most concentrated in laminae I and V. According to Besson and Chaouch,[22] there are three main zones of origin of spinothalamic fibers—the marginal zone; laminae IV to VI; and a medial deeper zone composing the base of the dorsal horn, the intermediate zone (laminae VII), and the ventral horn (lamina VIII).

In an attempt to classify STT neurons in the lumbosacral dorsal horn of a monkey spinal cord in a more objective fashion, Willis and colleagues[23,24] subdivided the neurons into four classes based on normalized responses of each neuron. Two classes of neurons were considered minor classes, one of which consisted chiefly of tactile neurons; the other two classes of cells (74% of the cells sampled) were clearly nociceptive. Of the latter classes, cells in one responded to brushing the skin or to compressing the skin with a stimulus that was just above the threshold of pain in a human observer, but they responded maximally to two different intensities of very painful compressive stimuli. The other major class of STT neurons responded maximally only when the most intense compressive stimulus was used, squeezing a fold of skin with serrated forceps.

Data from studies reviewed by Besson and Chaouch[22] demonstrate that (1) at lumbar and thoracic levels, the STT projections are mainly contralateral (90% to 95% at the lumbar enlargement) in the anterior commissure but (2) at the sacral and second cervical levels, ipsilateral contributions are not significant.

Spinoreticular Tract

Although studies favor involvement of the reticular formation of the brainstem in nociception, data on the SRT are much more difficult to interpret than data on the STT.[22] Reasons for this include:

1. SRT projections arrive at difficult levels of the brainstem, extending between the medulla and mesencephalon.
2. The nociceptive role of certain components such as those projections to the lateral reticular nucleus usually implicated in cerebellar function is still little understood.
3. SRT axons that travel in the ventral part of the lateral or ventral quadrant of the cord are intermingled with STT and spinocerebellar axons.
4. STT axons can send collaterals toward bulbar and mesencephalic reticular regions.
5. Laterality of SRT neuron projections is variable.[22]

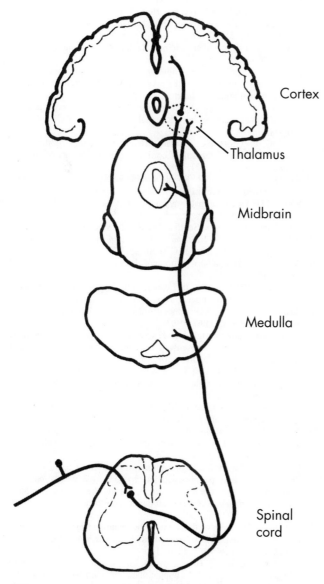

FIG. 3–5 Transmission along the nociceptive pathway with illustration of mechanisms for neuropathic pain, processing nociceptive information at the "first" synapse and functional mapping of pain at the level of the cortex. *(Modified from Levine JD: New directions in pain research: Molecules to maladies. Neuron 20:649, 1998.)*

Spinomesencephalic Tract

Electrophysiologic and anatomic studies defining this pathway and its characteristics have been carried out in zones making up the mesencephalic tegmentum, periaqueductal gray (PAG), cuneiform area, and deep laminae of the superior colliculus and adjacent regions.

SMT neurons originate in the posterior horn and deeper in the spinal cord gray matter. SMT projections are more often contralateral, but both ipsilateral and bilateral projections have also been reported.[22]

Postsynaptic Dorsal Column Fibers

The existence of postsynaptic dorsal column fibers (PSDCFs) was first described in 1968.[25] Angaut-Petit[26] found that most of the PSDCFs were excited by nociceptive stimuli (77% nociceptive-nonspecific; 6.7% nociceptive-specific). The destination of messages sent by PSDCF is not known. Most studies using a section of the dorsal column do not report changes in the nociceptive threshold.[22] However, interruption of this pathway likely accounts for pain relief afforded by commissural myelotomy.[27]

Cerebral Nociceptive Processing

Collective evidence, including recent functional imaging studies such as human positron emission tomography studies, suggests that the following brain structures are involved in processing nociceptive information: cingulate cortex, PAG, thalamus, lentiform nucleus, insula, anterior cingulate (areas 24, 25, 32, and 24[1]), prefrontal cortex (areas 9, 11, and 14), inferior parietal cortex (area 30/40), and—somewhat variably—primary and secondary somatosensory cortices.[27]

Nociceptive responses have been recorded from neurons in the lateral thalamus of experimental animals.[28]

Lateral thalamic nuclei in human patients have also been shown to contain nociceptive neurons. Nociceptive neurons were occasionally observed in the somatosensory thalamus, and microstimulation sometimes evoked a sensation of pain.[29–33]

Nociceptive responses have been reported not only in the lateral thalamus of monkeys and humans but also in the medial thalamic nuclei of the intralaminar complex in awake, behaving monkeys[34] and in the ventral medial nucleus (VMpo).[35]

Thalamic responses to nociceptive information are relayed to the appropriate regions of the cerebral cortex. Nociceptive responses have been recorded from cortical neurons in SI and SII regions in monkeys,[36–40] as would be expected from observations of nociceptive neurons in the ventral posterolateral and ventral posterolateral nuclei. However, a number of other cortical areas are likely to participate in the processing of nociceptive information at a cortical level and to contribute to different aspects of the pain experience.

References

1. Perl ER: Is pain a specific sensation? *J Psychiatr Res* 8(3):273, 1971.
2. Sherrington CS: *The integrative action of the nervous system,* ed 2. New Haven, Conn, Yale University Press, 1906.
3. Perl ER: Characterization of nociceptors and their activation of neurons in the superficial dorsal horn: First steps for the sensation of pain. In Kruger L, Liebeskind JC, editors: *Advances in pain research and therapy,* vol 6. New York, Raven Press, 1984.
4. Schaible HC, Schmidt RF: Time course of mechanosensitivity changes in articular afferents during a developing experimental arthritis. *J Neurophysiol* 60(6):2180, 1988.
5. Häbler HJ, Jänig W, Koltzenburg M: Activation of unmyelinated afferent fibers by mechanical stimuli and inflammation of the urinary bladder in the cat. *J Physiol* 425:545, 1990.
6. Handwerker HO, Kilo S, Reech PW: Unresponsive afferent nerve fibers in the sural nerve of the rat. *J Physiol* 435:229, 1991.
7. Davis KD, Meyer RA, Campbell JN: Chemosensitivity and sensitization of nociceptive afferents that innervate the hairy skin of monkey. *J Neurophysiol* 69(4):1071, 1993.
8. Konietzny F, Perl ER, Trevino D, et al: Sensory experiences in man evoked by intraneural electrical stimulation of intact cutaneous afferent fibers. *Exp Brain Res* 42(2):219, 1981.
9. Ochoa J, Torebjörk E: Sensations evoked by intraneural microstimulation of C nociceptor fibers in human skin nerves. *J Physiol* 415:583, 1989.
10. Lewis T: *Pain.* New York, MacMillan, 1942.
11. Erlanger J, Gasser HS: *Electrical signs of nervous activity.* Philadelphia, University of Pennsylvania Press, 1937.
12. Hagbarth KE: Exteroceptive, proprioceptive, and sympathetic activity recorded with microelectrodes from human peripheral nerves. *Mayo Clin Proc* 54(6):353, 1979.
13. Rexed B: The cytoarchitectonic organization of the spinal cord of cat. *J Comp Neurol* 96:415, 1952.
14. Craig AD, Mense S: The distribution of afferent fibers from the gastrocnemius-soleus muscle in the dorsal horn of the cat, as revealed by the transport of horseradish peroxidase. *Neurosci Lett* 41(3):233, 1983.
15. Cervero F, Connell LA: Distribution of somatic and visceral primary afferent fibres within the thoracic spinal cord of the cat. *J Comp Neurol* 230(1):88, 1984.
16. Kuo DC, de Groat WC: Primary afferent projections of the major splanchnic nerve to the spinal cord and gracile nucleus of the cat. *J Comp Neurol* 231(4):421, 1985.
17. Mense S, Prabhakar NR: Spinal termination of nociceptive afferent fibres from deep tissues in the cat. *Neurosci Lett* 66(2):169, 1986.
18. Willis WD: Ascending pathways from the dorsal horn. In Brown AG, Rethelyi M, editors: *Spinal cord sensation: Sensory processing in the dorsal horn.* Edinburgh, Scottish Academic Press, 1981.
19. White JC, Sweet WH: *Pain and the neurosurgeon: A forty year experience.* Springfield, Ill, Charles C Thomas, 1969.
20. Willis WD Jr: Dorsal horn neurophysiology of pain. *Ann N Y Acad Sci* 531:76, 1988.
21. Willis WD, Kenshalo DR Jr, Leonard RB: The cells of origin of the primate spinothalamic tract. *J Comp Neurol* 188(4):543, 1979.
22. Besson JM, Chaouch A: Peripheral and spinal mechanisms of nociception. *Physiol Rev* 67(1):67, 1987.
23. Chung JM, Surmeier DJ, Lee KA, et al: Classification of primate spinothalamic and somatosensory thalamic neurons based on cluster analysis. *J Neurophysiol* 56(2):308, 1986.
24. Surmeier DJ, Honda CN, Willis WD: Natural groupings of primate spinothalamic neurons based on cutaneous stimulation. Physiological and anatomical features. *J Neurophysiol* 59(3):833, 1988.
25. Uddenberg N: Functional organization of long, second-order afferents in the dorsal funiculus. *Exp Brain Res* 4(4):377, 1968.
26. Angaut-Petit D: The dorsal column system: II. Functional properties and bulbar relay of the postsynaptic fibres of the cat's fasciculus gracilis. *Exp Brain Res* 22(5):471, 1975.
27. Gybels JM, Sweet WH: Neurosurgical treatment of persistent pain: Physiological and pathological mechanisms of human pain. In Gildenberg PL, ed: *Pain and headache,* vol 11. Basel, Karger, 1985.
28. Jones A: The pain matrix and neuropathic pain. *Brain* 121(part 5):783, 1998.
29. Willis WD: Nociceptive functions of the thalamic neurons. In Steriade M, Jones EG, McCormick DA, editors: *Thalamus, vol II. Experimental and clinical aspects.* Amsterdam, Elsevier, 1997.
30. Lenz FA, Gracely RH, Hope EJ, et al: The sensation of angina can be evoked by stimulation of the human thalamus. *Pain* 59(1):119, 1994.
31. Lenz FA, Dougherty PM: Pain processing in the human thalamus. In Steriade M, Jones EG, McCormick DA, editors: *Thalamus, vol II.* Amsterdam, Elsevier, 1997.
32. Lenz FA, Gracely RH, Rowland LH, et al: A population of cells in the human thalamic principal sensory nucleus respond to painful mechanical stimuli. *Neurosci Lett* 180(1):46, 1994.

33. Lenz FA, Seike M, Lin YC, et al: Neurons in the area of human thalamic nucleus ventralis caudalis respond to painful heat stimuli. *Brain Res* 623(2):235, 1993.
34. Lenz FA, Seike M, Richardson RT, et al: Thermal and pain sensations evoked by microstimulation in the area of human ventrocaudal nucleus. *J Neurophysiol* 70(1):200, 1993.
35. Bushnell MC, Duncan GH: Sensory and affective aspects of pain perception: Is medical thalamus restricted to emotional issues? *Exp Brain Res* 78(2):415, 1989.
36. Craig AD, Bushnell MC, Zhang ET, et al: A thalamic nucleus specific for pain and temperature sensation. *Nature* 372(6508):770, 1994.
37. Robinson CJ, Burton H: Somatic submodality distribution within the second somatosensory (SII), 7b, retroinsular, postauditory, and granular insular cortical areas of M. fascicularis. *J Comp Neurol* 192(1):93, 1980.

38. Kenshalo DR Jr, Isensee O: Responses of primate SI cortical neurons to noxious stimuli. *J Neurophysiol* 50(6):1479, 1983.
39. Kenshalo DR Jr, Chudler EH, Anton F, et al: SI cortical nociceptive neurons participate in the encoding process by which monkeys perceive the intensity of noxious thermal stimulation. *Brain Res* 454(1-2):378, 1988.
40. Dong WK, Salonen LD, Kawakami Y, et al: Nociceptive responses of trigeminal neurons in SII-7b cortex of awake monkeys. *Brain Res* 484(1-2):314, 1989.
41. Chudler EH, Anton F, Dubner R, et al: Responses of nociceptive SI neurons in monkeys and pain sensation in humans elicited by noxious thermal stimulation: Effect of interstimulus interval. *J Neurophysiol* 63(3):559, 1990.

Questions • Pain Pathways: Anatomy and Physiology

1. Morphologically unique structures at the distal end of primary efferents that are depolarized by stimuli that produce damage to the body tissue are

   A. Pressure receptors
   B. Nociceptors
   C. Touch receptors
   D. Temperature receptors

2. Axons in peripheral nerves classified by Erlanger and Gasser are all of the following except

   A. Nonmyelinated C fibers
   B. Myelinated A fibers
   C. I, II, or III fibers
   D. Alpha, beta, gamma, and delta fibers

3. Nociceptive afferent fibers from the skin terminate in

   A. Laminae I
   B. Laminae I, II, and V
   C. Laminae V
   D. Laminae II and V

4. Recent functional imaging positron emission tomography studies suggest the following brain structures are involved in processing nociceptive information except

   A. Cingulate cortex
   B. Thalamus
   C. Periaqueductal grey
   D. Cerebellum

5. Thalamic responses to nociceptive information are relayed to

   A. S I and S II cortical region
   B. Insula
   C. Cerebellum
   D. Frontal cortex

ANSWERS

1. B
2. C
3. B
4. D
5. A

CHAPTER 4

Taxonomy of Pain Syndromes

MANJUL D. DERASARI

Taxonomy is defined as the classification of living and extinct organisms or, in a broader sense, the theory and practice, or science, of classification. Its basic methodology requires the comparison of characteristics of an organism's structure by using comparative anatomy methods and then interpreting these differences and similarities in light of genetics, biochemistry, physiology, embryology, behavior, etiology, and geography. Classification systems are used to sort the complex elements into reasonable and logical entities. Swedish botanist Carolus Linnaeus, considered the father of modern taxonomy, is credited for creating the binomial method of classification by which plants are categorized.

Taxonomy is no longer limited to just plants and animals and is now used in information classification for all branches of medicine. Its major uses today are (1) to predict outcome and responses to specific therapies and (2) to communicate experiences to others who are doing research.[1]

THE NEED FOR TAXONOMY

Pain remains one of the most common reasons for patients to seek professional health care. Often this pain is identified and treated, although for a significant number of patients it never disappears. Some persistent pains have identifiable causes, but in many cases the cause is unknown. These difficult pain syndromes are managed daily by almost all medical specialists, who treat problems in different ways depending on their particular discipline.

Thus, a common body of knowledge about pain is required to help define the problem, standardize or verify different treatments, allow measurements, and compare treatment outcomes for both clinicians and clinical researchers. Pain research may also be assisted by a common terminology for research protocol development and the storage and retrieval of data. An effective taxonomy would provide a vehicle by which pain practitioners and researchers could communicate regarding patient diagnoses.

With the current widespread use of the Internet and the penetration of managed care and the need for outcome data, this necessity of pain classification has taken on a new meaning. Classification systems for finding solutions to pain problems are undergoing constant review by various agencies and professionals involved in pain management. Well-defined terminology and clearly stated categories of pain syndrome help considerably. Moreover, classifications are an essential part of the "language of health" that is being created for the electronic clinical record.[2]

CLASSIFICATIONS IN MEDICAL DISCIPLINES

In 1676, Syndenham was credited with the introduction of classification in medicine. His objective was to identify the disease to predict the prognosis. Later, with the progress in clinical pathology and technology, the framework of classification changed, but the main purpose remained the same. Classes of a satisfactory taxonomy must be mutually exclusive and jointly exhaustive, although complete consistency is beyond the hope of any medical system of classification.[3] In clinical practice and in planning services, disease-specific classification is needed.[4]

The historical fluxes in medical understanding are reflected by the inconsistency in taxonomies. In medical classification, one finds diagnostic categories based on pathology, pathophysiology, nosology, functional complaints, symptom diagnosis, and problem behaviors.[5] Malterud and Hollnagel[1] described this unstructured approach as a sign of the pragmatic attitudes in clinical medicine, which is not always compatible with the image of medicine as a scientific and strictly logical discipline.

INTERNATIONAL CLASSIFICATION OF DISEASES

The International Classification of Diseases (ICD) is published by the World Health Organization (WHO) and is used primarily for documenting mortality and morbidity worldwide.[6] Although the 10th revision (ICD-10) was published in 1992,[7] the ICD-9CM (CM implies "clinical modification") is still widely used in the United States. Published by the United States Department of Health and Human Services, Public Health Services–Health Care Financing Administration, the ICD-9CM's coding system consists of:

- Volume 1: a tabular list of numeric codes
- Volume 2: an alphabetical index of diseases
- Volume 3: a list of procedural codes

Volumes 1 and 2 are needed to determine the appropriate code for the patient's condition, whereas Volume 3 is used mainly by hospitals.[8]

DIAGNOSTIC AND STATISTICAL MANUAL OF MENTAL DISORDERS

The initial impetus for developing a classification of mental disorders was the need to collect statistical information for a general census. The *Diagnostic and Statistical Manual of Mental Disorders* (DSM), published by the American Psychiatric Association,[9] attempts to fulfill this need. DSM-I was developed as a variant of the ICD-6 in 1952. The codes and terms provided in the latest version, DSM-IV (1994), are fully compatible with ICD-9CM and ICD-10.

The basic divisions of the DSM-IV are as follows:

- Axis I: clinical psychiatric diagnoses
- Axis II: personality disorders/mental retardation
- Axis III: general medical conditions
- Axis IV: psychosocial and environmental problems
- Axis V: global assessment of functioning

An attractive feature of DSM-IV classification is its usefulness in multiaxial assessment, which allows for evaluation on several axes, each referring to different domains of information that may help the clinician plan treatment and predict outcome.

A drawback to DSM-IV is that it emphasizes the assessment of mental functioning and psychopathology, which often is not suitable for most patients with chronic pain.[10]

CLASSIFICATION IN PAIN MEDICINE

Classifying pain, especially chronic pain, is difficult because of its subjective nature. Turk and Rudy[11] address classification strategies in chronic pain, saying two important considerations are (1) approach to classification and (2) dimensions of a classification (Fig. 4–1).

The theoretical approach involves testing predetermined theoretical formulations in the classification, whereas the empirical approach is inductive and tries to identify naturally occurring sets of variables that characterize various subgroups. The other important consideration in classification systems is dimension, the nature of the information used in assigning categories.

Various attempts have been made to classify pain, but many pertain to a particular category only. Some of the most common categories are described in Table 4–1. Pain classifications are listed in Table 4–2.

Nociceptive Category

The nociceptive category describes a laboratory prototype pain and can be seen as an unpleasant sensation. Nociceptors, identified in all tissues and organs except the nervous system, are stimulated by noxious stimuli transmitted via pain fibers to the spinal cord, then to the thalamus, and ultimately perceived as pain by the cerebral cortex.

TABLE 4–1 Some Commonly Used Categories of Pain

1. Neurophysiologic mechanism
   a. Nociceptive
      (1) Somatic
      (2) Visceral
   b. Neuropathic (non-nociceptive)
      (1) Neuropathic
         (I) Central
         (II) Peripheral
      (2) Psychogenic
2. Temporal (time-related)
   a. Acute
   b. Chronic
3. Etiologic
   a. Cancer pain
   b. Postherpetic neuralgia
   c. Pain of sickle cell disease
   d. Pain of arthritis
4. Regional pain
   a. Headache
   b. Orofacial pain
   c. Low back pain
   d. Pelvic pain

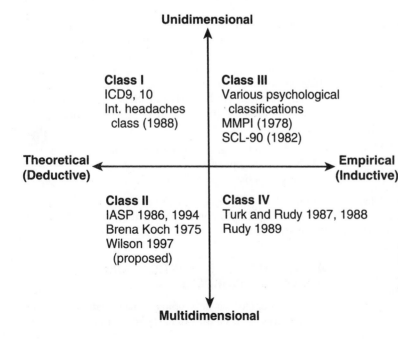

FIG. 4–1 A pain classification may be approached from a theoretical or from an evidence-based (empirical) basis. In addition, dimension is an important factor. By crossing these two concepts, pain classifications are grouped in four cells: ICD, International Classification of Disease; MMPI, Minnesota Multiphasic Personality Inventory; SCL, Symptoms Check List; IASP, International Association for the Study of Pain. *(Modified from Turk DC, Rudy TE: Classification logic and strategies in chronic pain. In Turk DC, Melzack R, editors: Handbook of pain assessment. New York, Guilford Press, 1992.)*

The nociceptive category includes *somatic* pain (carried along the sensory fibers) and *visceral* pain (carried by autonomic [sympathetic] fibers).

It is likely that there is an automatic component to every pain.[25] Somatic pain is more intense and discrete, whereas visceral pain is diffuse and poorly localized. Although the phenomenon of *referred pain* can cause difficulty in evaluation, overall nociceptive pain is relatively easy to diagnose and manage.

Neuropathic Category

Non-nociceptive pain is commonly called neuropathic pain, defined as pain produced by an alteration of neurologic structure and/or function (Table 4–3). The main difference between neuropathic and nociceptive pain is the absence of a continuous nociceptive input. Wall[26] described four possible mechanisms of peripheral neuropathic pain:

1. The "gate" might be caused to malfunction.
2. The nerve might become mechanically sensitive and generate an ectopic impulse.
3. Crosstalk might be occurring between large and small fibers.
4. The central processing function might be damaged.

CENTRAL NEUROPATHIC PAIN CATEGORY:

Lesions in the central nervous system causing pain (such as thalamic, poststroke, postparaplegia, or postquadriplegia pain) are among the most therapeutically challenging categories to manage.

PERIPHERAL NEUROPATHIC PAIN CATEGORY:

Peripheral neuropathic pain is categorized by lesions in the peripheral nervous system responsible for a persistent pain state (such as complex regional pain syndrome [CRPS] II [causalgia], postherpetic neuralgia, or painful neuropathies).

Psychogenic Pain Category

Before psychogenic pain is diagnosed, a careful search to exclude all somatic pathology and a thorough assessment by a psychiatrist are essential. The diagnosis should not be made solely on the basis of a diagnostic or differential nerve block. DSM-IV (Table 4–4) lists a number of psychologic or psychiatric conditions in which pain may be a significant factor.

Temporal (Time-Related) Acute Pain Category

Acute pain caused by internal disease serves a biologic purpose by prompting an individual to seek help to relieve or remedy it. Often, acute pain and its associated psychologic, autonomous, and behavioral responses are provoked by noxious stimulation of injury or disease that does not produce actual tissue damage[27] (Table 4–5). Effective treatment may abolish it in days or weeks, but improper or ineffective therapy may result in persistent or chronic pain.

Chronic Pain Category

The essential criterion of chronic pain is related to the cognitive-behavioral aspects, not duration or any nociceptive components. Although it does not serve a biologic function, chronic pain may impose several physical, emotional,

---

TABLE 4–2   Pain Classifications

Taxonomy of pain[12]
Taxonomy for diagnosis and information storage in chronic pain[13]
Chronic pain state[14]
International Headache Society—classification and diagnostic criteria for headache disorders, cranial neuralgias, and facial pain[15]
Chronic pain[3]
Cancer pain[16]
Advanced cancer pain[17]
Chronic pain patients: a multiaxial approach[18]
Spinal cord injury[19]
Numerical approach—topology for facial pain[20]
Widespread pain[21]
Tumor pain[22]
Chronic pain: empirically derived patient profiles[10]
Reflex sympathetic dystrophy[23]
Neuropathic pain[24]

TABLE 4–3   Neuropathic Pain

Pathophysiologic Factors
- Biology not useful
- Well-defined neurologic damage—central or peripheral
- Poorly defined nociceptive mechanisms
- Poorly defined central pathways
- Poorly defined inhibitory mechanisms
- Pain possibly felt in the region of sensory deficit (anesthesia dolorosa)

Psychologic Factors
- Severe adverse psychologic consequences
- Little interaction with social, cultural, or personality factors
- No predisposition of social, cultural, or personality factors

---

TABLE 4–4   Guidelines for the Diagnosis of Pain Disorders*

1. Pain is the predominant focus of the clinical presentation and is of sufficient severity to warrant clinical attention.
2. The pain causes significant distress or impairment in social, occupational, or other important areas of functioning.
3. Psychologic factors are judged to play a significant role in the onset, severity, exacerbation, or maintenance of pain.
4. The pain is not intentionally produced or feigned, as in factitious disorder or malingering.
5. Pain disorder is not the diagnosis if the pain is better accounted for by a mood, anxiety, or psychotic disorder or if the pain presentation meets the criteria for dyspareunia.

*Adapted from American Psychiatric Association (APA): *Diagnostic and statistical manual,* 4th revised edition (DSM-IV). Washington DC, APA, 1994.

TABLE 4–5   Acute Pain

Pathophysiologic Factors
- Biologically useful, warning of impending tissue damage
- Well-defined, with peripheral nociceptive mechanisms
- Stress response (fight or flight) valuable

Psychosocial Factors
- Expectation of occurrence and resolution
- Social, cultural, and personality factors interact
- Anxiety increases perception
- Economic and domestic factors may be involved
- Secondary gain usually not a factor

or socioeconomic stresses on the patient, family, and society (Table 4–6). This type of pain is prevalent and very difficult to treat and classify.

Etiologic Category

The most important etiologic category in pain is pain associated with cancer. Usually, the pain is caused directly by the cancer or its treatment, but it may also result from a preexisting or coexisting noncancerous condition.

INTERNATIONAL ASSOCIATION FOR THE STUDY OF PAIN CLASSIFICATION

The classification of chronic pain developed by the International Association for the Study of Pain (IASP) is the most detailed classification to date. It is a theoretically based, multiaxial classification of chronic pain syndromes designed to standardize the descriptions of pain syndromes and to codify them. Hempel[28] notes that description and theoretical systemization are two basic functions of scientific concepts and, therefore, of taxonomic systems. The first classification was published in 1986; a revised version was published in 1994.

The five-axial system focuses primarily on physical manifestations of pain, as follows:

Axis I: anatomical region
Axis II: organ system
Axis III: temporal characteristics
Axis IV: patient's statement of intensity and time of onset
Axis V: etiology

Usually, the physician describes the pain mentioned in the patient's complaint, first in terms of region and later in terms of etiology. Using this classification is not an assessment procedure but rather a multiaxial grid detailing symptoms of various pain conditions. With this coding system, relatively generalized syndromes are presented first, followed by the regional ones. The detailed descriptions of pain syndromes that follow were compiled using systematic input from various pain specialists.

The IASP's definition of pain and other pain-related terms are widely accepted by the general medical community, but the coding system is infrequently used.

In 1988, Vervest and Schimmer[29] reported numerous overlap problems with the first classification. In the second edition, they helped correct them.[3] Turk and Rudy,[30] in a pre-

liminary assessment of reliability of IASP taxonomy, found overall Axis I reliability to be excellent, although several subcategories were not very reliable. Siddall and coworkers[19] noted that no attempt was made in the revised (1994) edition to define or categorize pain that occurs after spinal injury. Despite these limitations, criticisms, or even omissions,[19] the IASP classification remains a monumental international effort that could be used more extensively.

EMORY PAIN ESTIMATE MODEL

Probably the first attempt at evidence-based integration of the multiaxial assessment of pain was proposed by Brena and Koch[31] in the form of the Emory Pain Estimate Model (EPEM).[14] Brena developed a two-dimensional strategy in which the presence of pathology and behavior was the axis. Then, with the median division of these dimensions, four classes of chronic pain were created. These classes have proved useful in establishing triage and prognosis in certain groups of pain patients, specifically those with chronic lower back pain and chronic headache (Fig. 4–2).

MULTIAXIAL ASSESSMENT OF PAIN

Psychologists play an important role in the delivery of clinical services to patients with chronic pain. Their involvement is based on evidence supporting the important contributions of cognitive,[32] affective,[33] and behavioral[34] contributions to the perception and reporting of pain. To address this aspect, in 1987 Turk and Rudy[18] proposed a classification system (the Multiaxial Assessment of Pain [MAP]) for such patients based on the empirical integration of psychosocial and behavioral data. These investigators[35] identified three unique subgroups of chronic pain patients:

1. Dysfunctional
2. Interpersonally distressed
3. Minimizers or adaptive copers

=== **TABLE 4–6**   Chronic Pain

Pathophysiologic Factors
- Not biologically useful
- Poorly defined:
  - Peripheral nociceptive mechanisms
  - Peripheral neural transmission, central
  - Connections, central pathways
- Stress response not present

Psychological Factors
- Premorbid personality significant
- May be an expression of psychosis or neurosis
- Depression common
- Secondary gain present
- Sick role present
- Abnormal illness behavior often present

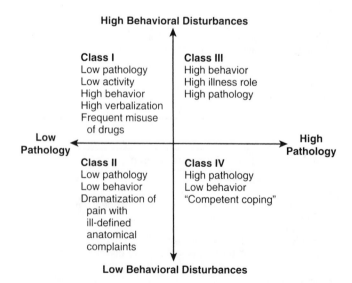

FIG. 4–2   The Emory Pain Estimate Model offers a practical guide to classify commonly encountered pain problems. *(Modified from Brena SF, Chapman SL: Management of patients with chronic pain. New York, Spectrum Publications, 1983.)*

Their primary hypothesis was that certain modal psychosocial and behavioral response patterns recur in these patients and represent somewhat homogeneous subgroups of chronic pain patients, independent of medical diagnosis. In their study, they cross-validated and confirmed the uniqueness and accuracy of taxonomy.

The instrument used to collect the data, the Multidimensional Pain Inventory (MPI),[35] has the advantage of having been standardized on a population of patients with chronic pain. Its robustness was tested on three common, but diverse, groups of chronic pain patients. The data suggested that, despite differences in demographic and medical diagnosis among disorders, the psychosocial and behavioral responses associated with chronic pain are common.[36]

SUMMARY

Chronic pain is recognized as a complex condition influenced by various factors, including biologic, physiologic, behavioral, environmental, and social aspects.[26] Classification systems are devices for sorting the complex elements of reality into logical entities.[1] The IASP classification provides a deductive multiaxial approach to pain when physical descriptions of pain are detailed but operates to some extent at the expense of psychosocial and behavioral aspects of chronic pain. The MAP provides good reliability and external validity and has the advantage of having been tested on diverse groups of chronic pain patients. A polydiagnostic approach, as proposed by Turk and Rudy, may prove complementary. Currently existing pain classifications, after refinement, modification, and improvement, may lead to their acceptance for wider use.

References

1. Malterud K, Hollnagel H: The magic influence of classification systems in clinical practice. *Scand J Primary Health Care* 15(1):26–9, 1997.
2. Stuart-Buttle C, Read J, Sanderson H: *A language of health in action: Read codes, classifications, and groupings.* Proceedings AMIA Annual Fall Symposium, NHS Centre for Coding and Classification, England, 1992.
3. Merskey H, Bogduk N: *Classification of chronic pain,* ed 2. Seattle, IASP Press, 1994.
4. Harper A: Symptoms of impairment, disability, and handicap in low back pain: A taxonomy. *Pain* 50:189, 1992.
5. Lamberts H, Woods M: International primary care classifications: The effect of fifteen years' evolution. *Fam Pract* 9:330, 1992.
6. World Health Organization (WHO): *International classification of diseases,* 9th revision. Geneva, WHO, 1992.
7. World Health Organization (WHO): *International statistical classification of disease and related health problems,* 10th revision (ICD-10), vol 1. Geneva, WHO, 1992.
8. Merskey H: *Development of a universal language of pain syndromes: Advances in pain research and therapy,* vol 5. New York, Raven Press, 1983.
9. American Psychiatric Association (APA): *DSM-IV: Diagnostic and statistical manual of mental disorders,* revised ed 4. Washington DC, APA, 1994.
10. Jamison RN, Rudy TE, Penzien DB, Mosley TH: Cognitive and behavioral classifications of chronic pain: Replication and extension of empirically derived patients profiles. *Pain* 57:277, 1994.
11. Turk DC, Rudy TE: Classification logic and strategies in chronic pain. In Turk DC, Melzack R, editors: *Handbook of pain assessment.* New York, Guilford Press, 1992.
12. Loser J: A taxonomy of pain. *Pain* 1:81, 1975.
13. Agnew D: A taxonomy for diagnosis and information storage in chronic pain. *Bull Los Angeles Neurol Soc* 44:84, 1976.
14. Brena SF: Chronic pain states: A model classification. *Psychiatr Ann* 14:778, 1984.
15. Oleson J: International Headache Society classification and diagnosis criteria for headache disorders, cranial neuralgias, and facial pain. *Cephalalgia* 8:S7, 1988.
16. Twycross R: Cancer pain classification. *Acta Anaesthesiol Scand* 41:141, 1997.
17. Cherny N, Coyle N, Foley K: Suffering in the advanced cancer patient: A definition and taxonomy. *J Palliat Care* 10:2, 1994.
18. Turk DC, Rudy TE: Towards a comprehensive assessment of chronic pain patients: A multiaxial approach. *Behav Res Ther* 25:237, 1987.
19. Siddall PJ, Taylor DA, Cousins MJ: Classification of pain following spinal cord injury. *Spinal Cord* 35:69, 1997.
20. Wastell D, Gray R: The numerical approach to classification: A medical application to develop a typology for facial pain. *Stat Med* 6:137, 1987.
21. MacFarlane GJ, Croft PR, Schollum J, Silman AJ: Widespread pain: Is an improved classification possible? *J Rheumatol* 23:1628, 1996.
22. Weber F, Rust M: Diagnosis and therapy of tumor pain: 1. Classification of tumor pain (German). *Fortschr Med* 112:429, 1994.
23. Stanton-Hickson M, Janig W, Hassenbusch S et al: Reflex sympathetic dystrophy: Changing concepts and taxonomy. *Pain* 63:127, 1995.
24. Elliott K: Taxonomy and mechanism of neuropathic pain. *Semin Neurol* 14:195, 1994.
25. Wilson PR: Sympathetically maintained pain. In Stanton-Hicks M, editor: *Pain and sympathetic nervous system.* Boston, Kluwer Academic Publishers, 1990.
26. Wall PD: Introduction. In Wall PD, Melzack R, editors: *Textbook of pain,* ed 2. Edinburgh, Churchill Livingstone, 1989.
27. Bonica JJ: *The management of pain,* ed 2. Philadelphia, Lea & Febiger, 1990.
28. Hempel C: Introduction to the problem of taxonomy. In Zubin J, editor: *Field studies in the mental disorders.* New York, Grune & Stratton, 1961.
29. Vervest A, Schimmer G: Taxonomy of pain of the IASP. *Pain* 34:318, 1988.
30. Turk DC, Rudy TE: IASP taxonomy of chronic pain syndromes: Preliminary assessment of reliability. *Pain* 30:177, 1987.
31. Brena SF, Koch DL: The pain estimate model for the quantification of classification of chronic pain states. *Anesthesiol Rev* 2:8, 1975.
32. Turk DC, Rudy TE: Assessment of cognitive factors in chronic pain: A worthwhile enterprise. *J Consult Clin Psychol* 54:760, 1986.
33. Melzack R, Casey KL: Sensory, motivation and central control determinants in pain: A new conceptual model. In Kenshalo D, editor: *The skin senses.* Springfield, Ill, Charles C Thomas, 1968.
34. Fordyce WE: *Behavioral methods for chronic pain and illness.* St. Louis, Mosby, 1976.
35. Turk DC, Rudy TE: Towards an empirically derived taxonomy of chronic pain patients: Integration of psychological assessment data. *J Consult Clin Psychol* 56:233, 1988.
36. Kern RD, Turk DC, Rudy TE: The West Haven-Yale Multidimensional Plan Inventory (WHYMPI). *Pain* 23:345, 1985.

1. Taxonomy is defined in a broader sense as a theory and practice of

   A. Classification
   B. Outcomes of treatment
   C. Mortality rates
   D. Birth rates

2. The International Classification of Diseases (ICD) is published by the

   A. Library of Congress
   B. United States Congress
   C. World Health Organization
   D. American Medical Association

3. ICD-9CM coding system consists of Volume 1—a tabular list of numeric codes, Volume 2—an alphabetical index of diseases, and Volume 3—a list of procedure codes. Which volume is mainly used by hospitals?

   A. Volume 1
   B. Volume 2
   C. Volume 3
   D. Volumes 1, 2, and 3

4. The classification of chronic pain developed by the IASP focused primarily on physical magnification of pain and has a

   A. One-axial system
   B. Two-axial systems
   C. Three-axial systems
   D. Five-axial systems

5. Brena and Koch devised a multiaxial assessment of pain called the

   A. International Association for the Study of Pain (IASP) taxonomy
   B. Emory Pain Estimate Model
   C. Psychogenic pain category
   D. Neuropathic category

ANSWERS

1. A
2. C
3. C
4. D
5. B

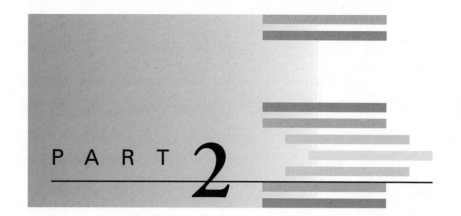

P A R T 2

Acute Pain Syndromes

CHAPTER 5

Medical Diseases

P. PRITHVI RAJ AND STEVEN D. WALDMAN

This chapter provides physicians with a practical approach to evaluating and treating headache and facial pain and various forms of pain caused by acute medical diseases. By understanding these conditions, physicians can ease anxiety while evaluating and treating patients suffering from these ailments.

HEADACHE AND FACIAL PAIN

Headache is the most common medical complaint encountered in medical practice. It is estimated that more than 40 million Americans have headaches severe enough to require medical care.

Targeted History

The most important portion of evaluating a patient suffering from headache and facial pain syndromes is obtaining a targeted history. From responses to targeted questions, a specific constellation of symptoms should emerge, allowing the physician to make an accurate diagnosis. Failing to obtain a targeted history can lead to ill-advised treatment and, in some cases, failure to recognize life-threatening disease.

The following areas of historical information should be explored not only to distinguish sick patients but also to try to ascertain the specific diagnosis:

1. **Chronicity**—The length of the illness sets the direction of the initial history and carries much weight in determining sick from well. For this reason, it serves as the starting point of the targeted history (Table 5–1).
2. **Age at onset**—Knowing when headaches and facial pain begin, that is, in childhood or later in life, helps determine the nature of pain.[1,2]
3. **Duration and frequency of pain**—Duration and frequency of pain provide the best clues to classification and diagnosis.

4. **Onset-to-peak time**—When combined with information obtained in the duration and frequency portion of the targeted history, the onset-to-peak time may help narrow the diagnostic possibilities (Fig. 5–1, see Table 5–1).
5. **Location**—The location of headache or facial pain may provide additional information about the classification and diagnosis of the patient's pain syndrome. Pain localized to an anatomic structure should be evaluated in the context of common disease entities for that structure.
6. **Character and severity of pain**—Although there is considerable overlap in character and severity of pain, some generalizations can be made when taking a target history.
7. **Premonitory symptoms and aura**—Premonitory symptoms (which usually precede the attack by 2 to 48 hours) and aura are usually associated with vascular headaches, specifically migraine. Aurae are manifested by focal cerebral dysfunction (Table 5–2).
8. **Associated symptoms**—The targeted history should include questions regarding symptoms associated with the painful conditions reported (such as photophobia, sonophobia, nausea, and focal neurologic changes).[3]
9. **Precipitating factors**—Various factors (such as change in diet or sleeping patterns, stress, depression, etc.) may act as triggers for different forms of headaches and must be examined.
10. **Environmental factors**—Changes in environmental conditions, both physical and psychologic, may be precipitating factors for headaches.
11. **Family history**—Migraine is a familial disease. Thus, if parents have them, there is an increased chance of their children suffering from them as well.[2]

TABLE 5–1   Factors that Cause Concern

New headache of recent onset ("the first")
New headache of unusual severity ("the worst")
Headache associated with neurologic dysfunction
Headache associated with systemic illness (especially infection)
Headache that peaks rapidly
Headache associated with exertion
Focal headache
Sudden change in a previously stable headache pattern
Headache associated with Valsalva's maneuver
Nocturnal headache

TABLE 5–2   Commonly Occurring Aurae

Ocular Symptoms
Fortification spectra (teichopsia)
Flashing lights (photopsia)
Scotomata
Hemianopia
Visual hallucinations

Auditory Symptoms
Auditory hallucinations

Olfactory Symptoms
Olfactory hallucinations

Motor and Sensory Symptoms
Weakness
Paresthesia

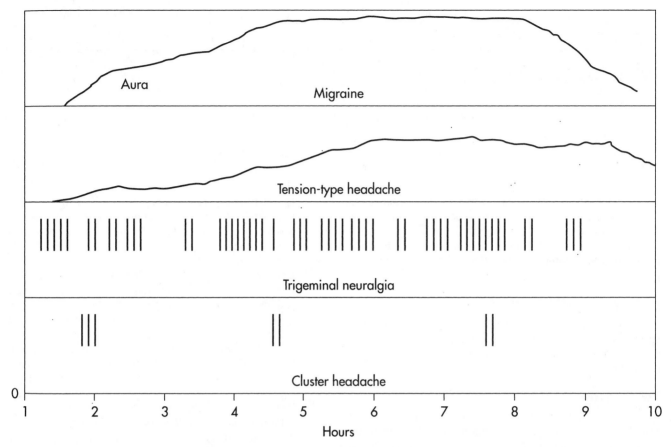

FIG. 5–1 Peak-to-onset profile in headache and facial pain syndromes.

12. **Pregnancy and menstruation**—Migraine may commonly occur with the onset of menses. Pregnancy after the first trimester and menopause may provide some amelioration of migraine.[4] Some migraine headaches worsen with the initiation of oral contraceptives.

13. **Medical/surgical history**—Headache can be a symptom of most systemic illnesses, and answers to medical/surgical history–oriented questions may provide valuable clues.

14. **Past treatments**—A physician must consider the success or failure of previous treatment modalities when diagnosing pain syndromes and when determining what type of treatment would be currently beneficial.

15. **Previous diagnostic tests**—Physicians must evaluate adequacy, validity, age, and quality of previous testing when deciding whether additional tests are required.

Targeted Physical Examination

In the physical examination, the patient's history helps direct the pain management specialist to look for physical findings that may be associated with the pain syndrome being considered. A careful examination for findings related to the pain problem or other systemic illness is mandatory for every patient. Failure to examine the patient or relying solely on history, laboratory, and radiographic findings puts the patient at extreme risk.

The following are the factors to be considered during a physical examination:

1. **General appearance**—Evaluating the patient for depression, anxiety, and general appearance may yield valuable information about possible underlying psychopathology.

2. **Examination of the head**—Careful examination of the head for various factors (such as scars, trigger points, tumors, infections, etc.) may reveal important clues.

3. **Cervical spine**—Abnormality of the cervical spine is probably a much more common etiologic factor in headache and facial pain than is recognized and should be investigated properly.

4. **Cranial nerve evaluation**—Examination of all cranial nerves helps rule out neurologic dysfunction in all patients suffering from headache and facial pain.[5]

5. **Sensory examination**—The presence of local numbness after a radicular distribution in the upper extremity may suggest cervical spine disease that may be wholly or partly responsible for some headache syndromes.[1]

6. **Motor examination**—A motor deficit in the upper extremity after a radicular distribution suggests cervical spine disease that may be wholly or partly responsible for some headache syndromes.[6]

7. **Reflexes**—Reflex abnormalities may indicate radiculopathy, neuropathy, myelopathy, and demyelinating disease.

Diagnostic Testing

The headache and facial pain patient may represent the most overtested group of patients in medicine today. Three important points must be stressed regarding testing in this group of patients:

1. Explain negative test results to the patient, because they are helpful in ruling out life-threatening disease.
2. Negative test results do not mean that the patient is not suffering from real pain.
3. Negative test results simply indicate that at the time of the test, the findings were reported as negative. The pain management specialist must understand this and retest immediately when new headache or facial pain symptoms occur in acute systemic illness (especially infection) or in changing or deteriorating neurologic findings.

Laboratory Testing

Laboratory testing is generally ordered to rule out unsuspected systemic illness in which headache or facial pain may be featured (such as anemia, infection, diabetes, etc.).

Radiographic Testing

Plain skull radiographs can provide limited, but useful, information to evaluate the patient suffering from headache and facial pain.

Computed Tomography

The computed tomography (CT) scan can rapidly identify a wide variety of life-threatening conditions that previously could be demonstrated only by risky and highly invasive procedures or conditions that could be diagnosed only after significant central nervous system compromise had occurred.[5]

Magnetic Resonance Imaging

Although the indications for magnetic resonance imaging (MRI) in headache and facial pain closely parallel the indications for CT scanning, it should be the test of choice when evaluating cervicogenic headache.[5]

Electroencephalogram and Evoked Potential Testing

The electroencephalogram (EEG) and evoked potential are neurophysiologic tests that are useful in the evaluation of selected headache and facial pain patients. An EEG can evaluate the rare headache patient whose headaches appear to be related to seizure disorder; it is also indicated if an infectious cause is being considered.[7] Evoked potential testing is indicated as a confirmatory test in the patient with facial pain in whom multiple sclerosis is suspected.[5] Brainstem-evoked, somatosensory-evoked, and visual-evoked potentials may also be useful in determining other difficulties or abnormalities.

Lumbar Puncture

Lumbar puncture to obtain spinal fluid for analysis is indicated as an emergency diagnostic procedure in all patients with the acute onset of headache or facial pain in whom an infectious cause is considered likely.[5] It is also indicated to ascertain if blood is present in the spinal fluid if a cerebral vascular accident is suspected.[7] However, lumbar puncture should not be performed in the presence of increased intracranial pressure evidenced by papilledema on funduscopic examination or findings on CT or MRI scanning.[7,8]

Arteriography and Digital Subtraction Angiography

Arteriography and digital subtraction angiography are neuroanatomic diagnostic tests indicated in patients suspected of having aneurysms, angiomas, arteriovenous malformations, and vascular tumors responsible for their headache and facial pain symptomatology.[5]

Specific Headache and Pain Syndromes

Tension-Type Headache

The term *tension-type headache* refers to nonvascular headaches that can be episodic or chronic.

Patient Profile

1. Usually bilateral, but can be unilateral
2. Possible bandlike nonpulsatile ache or tightness in the frontal, temporal, and occipital regions[9]
3. Often has associated neck symptomatology
4. Evolves over a period of hours or days, then tends to remain constant without progressive symptomatology
5. No aura
6. Significant sleep disturbance usually present
7. Frequently occur between 4 AM to 8 AM and 4 PM to 8 PM[1]
8. Women predominate
9. No hereditary pattern

Triggering Factors

The triggering event for acute episodic tension-type headache is invariably either physical or psychologic stress. A worsening of preexisting degenerative cervical spine conditions or the existence of temporomandibular joint (TMJ) dysfunction can also trigger a headache.[10]

Therapy

Episodic Treatment. If the patient suffers from tension-type headache once every 1 or 2 months, the condition can be managed through teaching the patient to reduce or avoid stress. Analgesics or nonsteroidal anti-inflammatory drugs can provide symptomatic relief during acute attacks.[11]

Prophylactic Treatment. If the headaches occur more frequently than once every 1 or 2 months or are so severe that the patient's social and work life are repeatedly hindered, then prophylactic treatment is indicated. Antidepressants are generally the drugs of choice for this form of headache treatment.[1] Monitored relaxation training combined with patient education about coping strategies and stress-management techniques may be valuable in the motivated tension-type headache sufferer.[12] Finally, Cronen and Waldman[13,14] have demonstrated the efficacy of cervical steroid epidural *nerve blocks* in providing long-term relief for patients who failed to respond to all other modalities.

Migraine Headache

Migraine headache is defined as a periodic unilateral headache that may begin in childhood but also almost always develops before age 30.[15] Attacks may occur every few days or only every 5 or 6 months. The headache may become generalized as the attack occurs. The pain is usually described as throbbing or pounding and may "settle" behind one eye. Attacks usually last for more than 4 hours and frequently persist for 24 hours or more. The sufferers are often female (60% to 70%), and many report a family history of the disorder.

Special Forms of Migraine

Migraine without aura is simply called the *common migraine.* If the patient experiences painless preheadache focal neurologic symptoms (i.e., aura), it is *migraine with aura.* If the focal neurologic symptoms persist beyond the immediate headache period, this syndrome is termed *migraine with prolonged aura,* which was previously called *complicated migraine.*[3]

Therapy

If the patient's attacks occur only once every 1 or 2 months, a trial of *abortive therapy* to provide symptomatic relief of the acute attack may be warranted. In order for abortive therapy to be effective, it must be initiated at the first sign of headache.

Isometheptene mucate should be considered first-line abortive therapy, because of its extremely favorable risk-to-benefit ratio without the side effects seen in ergot alkaloids.[8]

Ergot alkaloids were among the first group of abortive agents used to treat migraine headaches.[1] However, they have significant side effects, including nausea, vomiting, rebound, or dependence.

Oxygen inhalation may abort or ameliorate migraine headache and can be combined with other abortive drugs and treatment.

The *sphenopalatine ganglion block* can abort the acute attack, and its simplicity makes it useful in the pain center or emergency department.[16,17] It can be safely used with oxygen and various other abortive treatments.

Biofeedback combined with autogenic training has enabled some patients to abort or prevent attacks of migraine.

Several recent studies have reported that *intravenous (IV) lidocaine* alone or combined with antiemetics such as droperidol or promethazine relieved acute migraine attacks.[18] Other recent studies describe using *naproxen sodium* as an abortive agent, although nausea and vomiting associated with acute migraine have limited the effectiveness of this approach in many patients.[19]

Finally, recent studies have demonstrated the efficacy of *subcutaneous sumatriptan* in the palliation of acute migraine. However, this drug should be used with care in patients with coronary artery disease and peripheral vascular insufficiency.[20]

Prophylactic treatment is indicated if headaches occur with greater frequency or cause the patient to miss work or be hospitalized.

Beta blockers are now viewed as the first-line therapy for migraine prophylaxis, because of their ability to decrease the frequency and severity of migraine attacks.[21]

The use of *antidepressants* to control the onset of migraines, although controversial, has decreased the fre-

quency and severity of episodic migraine headaches in some patients.[1]

Some migraine sufferers who do not experience diminution of headaches with beta blockers find the *calcium channel blockers* to be of value.[15]

Methysergide is an antiserotonergic compound closely related to the ergot alkaloids.[8] It is useful in the prophylaxis of intractable migraine headaches that fail to respond to the previously mentioned therapies.

Coexisting Migraine and Tension-Type Headache

The coexisting migraine and tension-type headache occurs more often than commonly recognized.[8] Careful questioning helps identify this subset of patients. Occasionally it is necessary to use medications for both types of headaches to control the symptoms. The physician must be aware that analgesic rebound may trigger both migraine and tension-type headache, and discontinuation of abortive headache medications and analgesics may be necessary to relieve the patient's headache symptomatology.

Cluster Headache

Characteristics

Cluster headache derives its name from its occurrence in time "clusters," which are followed by headache-free remission periods. The condition is often confused with migraine, but there are several differences:

1. Male predominance (M/F = 8:1)
2. Unilateral distribution of pain
3. Pain duration usually 30 to 120 minutes
4. No family history in most cases
5. Headache occurs in daily attacks for 4 to 12 weeks
6. One to three attacks occur per day, often during sleep
7. Total remission after a cluster, often 6 to 18 months.[22] Sometimes this remission period is markedly diminished, and the frequency increases up to 10-fold—termed *chronic cluster headache*[22,23]

Physiologic and Psychologic Effects

Cluster headache pain is characterized as unilateral, retro-orbital, and temporal in location, with a deep burning or drilling quality. Horner's syndrome, consisting of ptosis, abnormal pupil contraction, facial flushing, conjunctival injection, and profuse lacrimation and rhinorrhea, is often present. Suicides have been associated with prolonged, unrelieved attacks of cluster headaches, so hospitalization is recommended in cases of uncontrollable pain.[1]

Therapy

Although prophylaxis and evaluation of treatment are difficult because of this disease's unpredictable nature, the physician must recognize that this disorder should be viewed as a true pain emergency and treated actively and aggressively. The following are accepted treatments for cluster headache.

Oxygen inhalation remains the safest and most effective means to abort the acute cluster headache.[1]

Methysergide, an antiserotonergic compound, is the medication of choice for episodic cluster headache. It may be used in combination with oxygen inhalation and sphenopalatine ganglion block.[1]

A short, tapering course of *steroids* may be effective in patients that fail to respond to the previously mentioned treatment modalities.[24]

Lithium carbonate is the treatment of choice for chronic cluster headache and can be useful in a small number of episodic cluster patients who fail to respond to methysergide or steriods.[22]

In rare instances, cluster headaches may become refractory to all treatment modalities. In this case, consideration may be given to destruction of the gasserian ganglion either by retrogasserian injection of glycerol or by radiofrequency lesion.[17,25]

Trigeminal Neuralgia

Trigeminal neuralgia occurs in many patients because tortuous or aberrant blood vessels compress the trigeminal root.[23] Acoustic neuromas, cholesteatomas, aneurysms, angiomas, and bony abnormalities may also lead to the compression of nerve roots.

Characteristics

Trigeminal neuralgia is an episodic pain afflicting the areas of the face supplied by the trigeminal nerve.

1. Pain is unilateral in 97% of reported cases.[26]
2. The second or third division of the nerve is affected in most patients.[26]
3. Pain develops on the right side of face in unilateral disease 57% of the time.[27,28]
4. Pain is characterized by paroxysms of electric shock–like pain lasting several seconds to less than 2 minutes.
5. Progression from onset to peak is essentially instantaneous.
6. Daily activities involving contact with trigger areas often provoke attacks.
7. Pain usually causes spasms of the facial muscles on affected side; hence the condition is also called *tic douloureux.*
8. Between attacks the patient is relatively pain free.

Drug Therapy

Carbamazepine is considered first-line treatment for trigeminal neuralgia. In fact, rapid response to this drug confirms a clinical diagnosis of trigeminal neuralgia. Baseline blood tests should be obtained before therapy.

In the uncommon event that carbamazepine does not adequately control a patient's pain, *phenytoin* may be considered.[23] As with carbamazepine, obtain baseline blood tests before starting therapy.

Baclofen has been reported to be of value to some patient who fail to respond to the aforementioned medications.[29]

Invasive Therapy

The use of *trigeminal nerve block* with local anesthetic and a steroid serves as an excellent adjunct to drug treatment of trigeminal neuralgia.[17,25] This technique rapidly relieves pain while oral medications are being titrated to effective levels.

The injection of small quantities of glycerol into the area of the gasserian ganglion provides long-term relief for patients suffering from trigeminal neuralgia who have not responded to optimal trials of the previously mentioned therapies.[25]

The destruction of the gasserian ganglion can be carried out by creating a radiofrequency lesion under biplanar fluoroscopic guidance.[30] This procedure is reserved for patients who have failed all of the previously mentioned treatments for intractable trigeminal neuralgia.

Microvascular decompression of the trigeminal root, or *Jannetta's procedure,* is the major neurosurgical procedure of choice for intractable trigeminal neuralgia.[31] It is based on the theory that trigeminal neuralgia is in fact a compressive mononeuropathy. By relieving that compression, the pain is relieved.

ACUTE VASCULAR DISORDERS

In patients who develop rather sudden, severe circulatory insufficiency of the limb from trauma, embolism, thrombosis, or chemical irritation, the local lesion initiates reflex spasm of the collateral vessels. The spasm aggravates the circulatory insufficiency, which becomes much greater than if the collateral vessels were not so affected. Sympathetic block should be promptly initiated before changes occur that favor thrombosis in the endothelium of the vasospastic collateral vessels. The block reestablishes normal blood flow through the collaterals and thus decreases or totally prevents tissue damage that might otherwise progress to gangrene.

After acute single injuries or repeated trauma, some patients develop segmentary vasospasm, which is manifested by a cold, cyanotic, painful, and edematous extremity. Although the vessels are not grossly injured, the degree of vasospasm may be so severe that it produces ischemia and consequent gangrene comparable with the results of intraluminal obstruction or section of the vessels. In such cases, sympathetic blocks may determine whether the severe ischemia is a result of organic obstruction or actual division of the blood vessels or merely because of severe spasm.

Interarterial injection of thiopental (Pentothal) or other very irritable agents often provokes very severe, intense spasm of the arteries and arterioles, which produces excruciating pain and often threatens the viability of the limb. In such patients, sympathetic interruption by intravenous infusion of guanethidine may be more effective than regional sympathetic block, but often even this does not relieve pain. Pain relief may be achieved only with a block of the brachial plexus.[32,33]

Acute Arterial Occlusion

Thrombosis, embolism, or direct injury may cause acute arterial occlusion. The clinical picture varies depending on location of the obstruction, functional capability of the existent collateral circulation, and general condition of the patient. Pain develops rapidly as a result of tissue ischemia, which may be the product of the primary obstruction and reflex collateral vasospasm.[32,34] Treatment of an embolism consists of embolectomy, anticoagulant therapy, and concomitant sympathetic interruption to relieve the reflex spasm.

Acute Venous Thrombosis

Acute venous thrombosis encompasses a spectrum of symptoms and signs usually considered under the diagnostic category of thrombophlebitis. Acute venous thrombosis is characterized by severe pain, marked edema, and excessive perspiration that is probably due to sympathetic hyperactivity with consequent reflex spasm of the arterioles and venules and increased sudomotor function.[32,34] Treatment should be largely supportive; one should apply heat and elevate to minimize swelling. If the thrombosis is localized to the superficial system, anticoagulants are not needed. However, if the deep venous system is also occluded, anticoagulants are definitely required.[35] In addition, sympathetic interruption may prove effective in decreasing the pain and edema.

Cold Injuries

Peripheral vascular disorders resulting from exposure to cold, such as trench foot and frostbite, are often characterized by initial and late vasospastic phases and an intermediate hyperemic phase.[34,35] Prompt institution of a continuous sympathetic block probably relieves the symptoms of the first phase and may decrease the degree of tissue damage. In the late phase, vasospasm and the consequent coldness, pain, paresthesia, hyperhidrosis, and stiffness are chronic. Therefore, although transient blocks are of diagnostic-prognostic value, the best therapeutic effects are produced by sympathectomy. However, even sympathectomy does not obviate amputation in severe cases with gangrene.

CHRONIC VASOSPASTIC DISORDERS

Raynaud's Disease

Raynaud's disease is a relatively common clinical problem characterized by vasospasm of the microcirculation of the fingers unassociated with any other pathologic process.[32–35] The condition involves the digits of the upper extremity bilaterally, but there are patients who have all digits of all four extremities involved. The condition is manifested by intense whiteness of the fingers, which then turn blue and finally red during the rewarming process. With continuous precaution against exposure to cold, most of these patients can avoid tissue ischemia, which eventually causes necrosis of the skin of the fingertips.

In Raynaud's disease and other chronic spastic disorders involving small arteries of the microcirculation, sympathetic blocks may be used as diagnostic and prognostic procedures (Fig. 5–2).

Raynaud's Phenomenon

Raynaud's phenomenon is characterized by the same symptomatology as Raynaud's disease but is caused by different underlying disorders. The condition is usually not bilateral, and primary therapy is directed toward elimination of the underlying cause. If this is not possible and the vasospasm is intense and causes tissue necrosis, the patient should be treated with diagnostic sympathetic blocks. If these blocks produce adequate vasodilation and decrease or eliminate existing pain, then prolonged sympathetic interruption by chemical or surgical sympathectomy or vasodilative drugs should be considered.

Other Disorders of Microcirculation

Acrocyanosis is a vasospastic disorder manifested by persistent coldness, intense cyanosis, and often edema and hyperhidrosis.

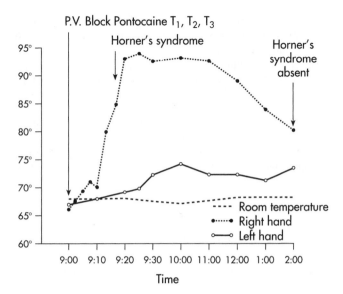

FIG. 5–2 Graph of skin temperature in a patient with Raynaud's disease in response to paravertebral sympathetic block. After the injection of 5 ml of 0.2% tetracaine (Pontocaine) through a needle placed at T2 vertebral level, the patient developed Horner's syndrome and a maximal increase in skin temperature of the upper limb, which persisted for nearly 6 hours (indicating block of T1-T3).

Livedo reticularis is characterized by marble-like mottling of the skin, which is aggravated by exposure to cold.

Erythromelalgia is almost the exact antithesis of Raynaud's disease and acrocyanosis. It is characterized by redness and burning pain in the extremities caused by abnormal vasodilation.

Thromboangiitis Obliterans

Thromboangiitis obliterans is described as a specific nonarteriosclerotic lesion involving arteries, veins, and nerves. This disease often leads to gangrene and tends to be limited to medium-sized arteries of the distal leg or arm. The condition occurs almost exclusively in young, cigarette-smoking males. It is usually bilateral and symmetric in involvement and is manifested by instep claudication if the condition involves distal arteries of the arm and digits. Also, at least half of the patients manifest sensitivity to cold. The most bothersome and most common pain problems are instep claudication and ischemic rest pain. The best therapy is total cessation of smoking.

Arteriosclerosis Obliterans

Occlusive arteriosclerotic disease of the lower limb vessels is the most common problem for vascular insufficiency. This process produces a progressive decrease in tissue blood flow with consequent claudication, rest pain, incipient gangrene, or ulceration. In general, this condition is best treated by medical and surgical therapy. Vascular grafts that can bypass the obstruction of large- or medium-sized vessels in the limb have become important and widely used procedures and have decreased or postponed amputation. However, in patients for whom bypass graft surgery cannot be used because the obliterating vascular disorder is too extensive,

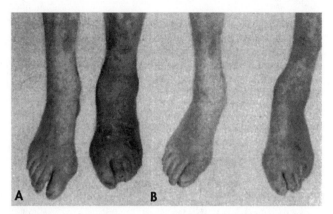

FIG. 5–3 Feet of a patient with arteriosclerosis obliterans and diabetes. *A,* Lesions of the left foot. *B,* Four months after left lumbar sympathetic block with aqueous phenol. *(From Bonica JJ: The management of pain, ed 2. Philadelphia, Lea & Febiger, 1990).*

sympathectomy is effective in relieving some of the symptomatology and postponing amputation (Fig. 5–3).

SICKLE CELL DISEASE

Hemoglobin A, the predominant form of hemoglobin in red blood cells (RBCs), is composed of two α and two β subunits. Abnormal hemoglobins (Hb S) may result from an amino acid substitution in one of the β chains. These hemoglobins can result in the formation of sickled RBCs under conditions of decreased oxygen tension. Homozygosity for Hb S occurs in 0.15% of black children and results clinically in sickle cell anemia.[36]

Patients with sickle cell anemia often manifest vasoocclusive phenomena, which are due to sludging in the microcirculation, with tissue hypoxia and infarction. These patients may experience episodic crises. The frequency and intensity of crises vary between patients with sickle cell disease and in the same patient.[37] Factors with sickle crises include hypothermia, dehydration, exertion, hypoxemia, acidosis, and bacterial or viral infections.[36]

Acute pain may occur at multiple locations, including abdominal pain, pleuritic chest pain, acute arthritis with synovial effusion, and bone pain.[36] Rarely, males develop painful priapism. Patients may also experience chronic pain, often related to recurrent vasoocclusive episodes.[36]

Pain management of sickle cell disease can be difficult. Unfortunately, there is no specific treatment, and the lack of objective means to quantify disease activity requires the physician to treat the pain solely on the patient's report.[37]

Acute pain crises often require hospitalization. Parenteral narcotics via intramuscular (IM) or subcutaneous routes should be given as need, in addition to intravenous (IV) fluids, oxygen, and keeping the patient warm.[37] Continuous IV infusions of narcotics have also been successful, although close adjustment of the narcotic dose is necessary to decrease the incidence of problems.[38] Patient-controlled analgesia with narcotics can be effective and, in the future, may become standard therapy.[39]

Chronic pain, if not severe, can be managed with acetaminophen or nonsteroidal anti-inflammatory drugs. Nonsteroidal anti-inflammatory drugs, however, may cause renal failure in patients with borderline renal function. For more severe pain, narcotic analgesics are often necessary.[38]

HEMOPHILIA

Hemophilia is a congenital bleeding disorder. *Hemophilia A,* also known as classic hemophilia, is associated with a deficiency or abnormality of factor VIII, whereas *hemophilia B* is related to a deficient or dysfunctional factor IX. Both of these disorders are X-linked and, therefore, occur almost exclusively in males. The incidence of classic hemophilia is one in 10,000 men.[40]

Hemophiliacs experience hemorrhages that can occur hours or days after trauma, may involve any organ, and may persist for weeks. Patients often develop pain in a weight-bearing joint followed by swelling caused by hemarthrosis.[40] Recurrent bleeding into the joint can lead to chronic hemophiliac arthropathy, which is characterized by osteoarthritis, articular fibrosis, joint ankylosis, and muscular atrophy.[40,41] Pain from an acute hemarthrosis can be severe but is otherwise similar to the pain associated with chronic arthropathy, and it can be difficult for adult hemophiliacs to distinguish.[41] Other sources of pain include soft tissue and muscle hemorrhages that can result in compartment syndromes, pseudophlebitis, and ischemic neuropathy.

Primary therapy consists of administering highly purified factor VIII concentrates for classic hemophiliacs. *Desmopressin* can sometimes be helpful in hemophiliacs with mild disease because it elevates factor VIII levels.[40] Narcotics may be necessary but should not be administered IM. *Acetaminophen* may be helpful, but nonsteroidal anti-inflammatory drugs should be avoided because of antiplatelet effects that may increase bleeding. Other therapies demonstrated to reduce pain in hemophiliacs include transcutaneous electrical nerve stimulation and relaxation techniques.[42,43]

RHEUMATOID ARTHRITIS

Rheumatoid arthritis is a systemic illness that afflicts approximately 1% of the population.[44] It is usually insidious in onset but may occur with an acute presentation.[45] Onset of rheumatoid arthritis is more frequent in winter than in summer. Most patients develop their initial symptoms between ages 30 and 50, and there appears to be an association between rheumatoid arthritis and the major histocompatibility antigen HLA-DR4.[44] Many patients tend to have a progressive, disabling, and destructive form of the disease, although some have an intermittent disease form, and rarely there are long remissions.[44]

Diagnosis of rheumatoid arthritis is made on the basis of having four out of seven of the following clinical criteria.[46]

1. Morning stiffness
2. Arthritis of three or more joint areas
3. Arthritis of hand joints
4. Symmetric arthritis
5. Rheumatoid nodules
6. Serum rheumatoid factor
7. Radiographic changes

The cause of rheumatoid arthritis remains unknown.[45] Nevertheless, on pathologic examination, microvascular injury and an increase in the number of synovial lining cells appear early in rheumatoid arthritis. There is evidence of ongoing inflammation and immune activation. As the disease progresses, the synovium swells and villous projections protrude into the joint space. In time, the synovium erodes into bone and invades periarticular structures such as tendons and fascia.[47]

Patients with rheumatoid arthritis often have pain and stiffness involving multiple joints.[44] Pain appears to be due to stretching of the joint capsule from the accumulation of synovial fluid, hypertrophy of the synovium, and thickening of the joint capsule.[45] Pain in the affected joints typically worsens with movement, and the amount of pain from a given joint may not correlate with the degree of active inflammation.

The treatment of rheumatoid arthritis aims to relieve pain, reduce inflammation, preserve functional capacity, resolve the pathologic process, and facilitate healing.[45] A number of modalities besides drug therapy may be beneficial:

1. Rest and splinting
2. Exercise to maintain muscle strength and joint mobility
3. Orthotic devices to decrease joint stress and therefore pain

First-line drug therapy consists of using salicylates and other nonsteroidal anti-inflammatory drugs.[48] These agents can decrease pain and, thus, improve function; however, they do not interrupt disease progression. They should be taken in maximal doses.

Patients with refractory disease may be candidates for immunosuppressive therapy.[45] Drugs that have been used include methotrexate, cyclophosphamide, and azathioprine.

Surgery may be a last resort for rheumatoid arthritis patients, with total joint replacement for structural joint damage.[49] Major indications include intolerable pain or prohibitive limitation of function, and the goals are to relieve pain, correct deformity, and improve function.[44,49]

PANCREATITIS

Acute pancreatitis is associated with multiple causes (Table 5–3), but alcohol abuse and cholelithiasis account for most cases.[50] It is characterized by poorly localized, steady, dull or drilling epigastric or upper left quadrant pain that may radiate to the back and appears to lessen when sitting up and/or flexing the spine.[50,51] The pain reaches maximum intensity within 15 minutes to an hour and usually lasts 3 to 7 days.

Diagnosis of acute pancreatitis is based on clinical history and examination and possible elevated serum amylase and/or lipase levels.

Acute pancreatitis is due to autodigestion by premature release of activated proteolytic pancreatic enzymes.[50] What causes the activation of these enzymes currently remains unknown.

Therapy for acute pancreatitis is largely supportive, because randomized, controlled trials have not demonstrated a decrease in morbidity or mortality for any specific type of therapy.[50]

TABLE 5–3 Conditions Associated with Acute Pancreatitis[25]

Cholelithiasis
Ethanol abuse
Idiopathic conditions
Medication
Abdominal operations
Hyperlipidemia
Injection into pancreatic duct
Trauma
Hypercalcemia
Pregnancy
Peptic ulcer
Outflow obstruction
Pancreas divisum
Organ transplantation
End-stage renal failure
Hereditary conditions (e.g., familial pancreatitis)
Scorpion bite
Miscellaneous: hypoperfusion, viral infections, Mycoplasma pneumoniae infection, intraductal parasites

References

1. Diamond S, Dalessio DJ: *The practicing physician's approach to headache,* ed 3. Baltimore, Williams & Wilkins, 1982.
2. Russell RW, Graham EM: Trigeminal neuralgia. In Hopkins A, editor: *Headache.* Philadelphia, WB Saunders, 1988.
3. Freitag FG: Migraine headache variants. *Clin J Pain* 5:11, 1989.
4. Epstein MT, Hockaday JM, Hockaday TDR: Migraine and reproductive hormones throughout the menstrual cycle. *Lancet* 1(7906):543, 1975.
5. Bannister R: The examination of the patient. In *Brain's clinical neurology.* New York, Oxford University Press, 1985.
6. Robinson CA: Cervical spondylosis and muscle contraction headache. In Dalessio DJ, editor: *Wolff's headache.* New York, Oxford University Press, 1980.
7. Bannister R: Ancillary investigations. In *Brain's clinical neurology.* New York, Oxford University Press, 1985.
8. Saper JR: *Headache disorders: Current concepts and treatment strategies.* Boston, John Wright, 1983.
9. Headache Classification Committee of the International Headache Society: Classification and diagnostic criteria for headache disorders, cranial neuralgias and facial pain. *Cephalalgia* 8(Suppl 7):19, 1988.
10. Dalessio D: *Wolff's headache.* New York, Oxford University Press, 1980.
11. Miller DS, Talbot CA, Simpson W et al: A comparison of naproxen sodium, acetaminophen, and placebo in the treatment of muscle contraction headache. *Headache* 27:392, 1987.
12. Marcer D: Biofeedback and pain. In Marcer D, editor: *Biofeedback and related therapies in clinical practice.* Rockville, Md, Aspen, 1986.
13. Cronen MC, Waldman SD: Cervical epidural blocks in the treatment of tension-type headache. *Headache* 28:314, 1988.
14. Cronen MC, Waldman SD: Cervical steroid epidural nerve block in the palliation of pain secondary to intractable tension-type headache. *J Pain Symptom Manage* 5:379, 1990.
15. Diamond S: Diagnosis and treatment of migraine. *Clin J Pain* 5:3, 1989.
16. Phero J, Robbins G: Sphenopalatine ganglion block. In Raj PP, editor: *Handbook of regional anesthesia.* New York, Churchill Livingstone, 1985.
17. Waldman SD: The role of neural blockade in pain management. In Weiner RS, editor: *Innovations in pain management.* Winter Park, Fla, PMD Publishers Group, 1990.
18. Saper JR: Emergency management of headache. *Top Pain Manag* 4:29, 1989.
19. Ziegler DK, Ellis DJ: Naproxen in the prophylaxis of migraine. *Arch Neurol* 42:582, 1985.
20. Waldman SD: Sumatriptan. *Pain Digest* 3:260, 1993.
21. Diamond S, Medina JL: The treatment of migraine headaches. *Headache* 16:24, 1976.

22. Pearce JMS: Cluster headache and its variants. *Headache Q* 2:187, 1991.
23. Graham JG: Cluster headache and pain in the face. In Hopkins A, editor: *Headache.* Philadelphia, WB Saunders, 1988.
24. Jammes JL: The treatment of cluster headache with prednisone. *Dis Nerv Syst* 12:275, 1975.
25. Feldstein GS: Percutaneous retrogasserian glycerol rhizotomy in the treatment of trigeminal neuralgia. In Racz GB, editor: *Techniques of neurolysis.* Boston, Academic Publishers, 1989.
26. Waldman SD: Evaluation of common headaches and facial pain syndromes. In Raj PP, editor: *Practical management of pain.* St. Louis, Mosby, 1992.
27. Dalessio DJ: Management of the cranial neuralgias and atypical facial pain. *Clin J Pain* 5:55, 1989.
28. Kitrell JP, Grouse DS, Seybold M: Cluster headache: Local anesthetic abortive agents. *Arch Neurol* 42:496, 1985.
29. Fromm GH, Terrence CF, Chatta AS: Baclofen in the treatment of face pain. *Ann Neurol* 15:240, 1984.
30. Sweet WH: The treatment of trigeminal neuralgia. *N Engl J Med* 315:174, 1986.
31. Jannetta PJ: Trigeminal neuralgia: Treatment by microvascular decompression. In Wilkins RH, Rengachary SS, editors: *Neurosurgery.* New York, McGraw-Hill, 1985.
32. Bonica JJ: *The management of pain.* Philadelphia, Lea & Febiger, 1953.
33. Loh L, Nathan PW: Painful peripheral states and sympathetic blocks. *J Neurol Neurosurg Psychiatry* 41:664, 1978.
34. Bonica JJ: *Clinical applications of diagnostic and therapeutic nerve blocks.* Springfield, Ill, Charles C Thomas, 1959.
35. Strandness DE Jr: *Peripheral arterial disease: A physiologic approach.* Boston, Little, Brown, 1969.
36. Bunn HF: Disorders of hemoglobin. In Wilson JD, Braunwald E, Isselbacher KJ et al, editors: *Harrison's principles of internal medicine,* ed 12. New York, McGraw-Hill, 1991.
37. Benjamin LJ: Pain in sickle cell disease. In Foley KM, Payne RM, editors: *Current therapy of pain.* Philadelphia, BC Decker, 1989.
38. Cole TB et al: Intravenous narcotic therapy for children with severe sickle cell pain crises. *Am J Dis Child* 140:1255, 1986.
39. Schecter NL, Berrien FB, Katz SM: The use of patient-controlled analgesia in adolescents with sickle cell pain crisis: A preliminary report. *J Pain Symptom Manage* 3:109, 1988.
40. Handin RI: Disorders of coagulation and thrombosis. In Wilson JD, Braunwald E, Isselbacher KJ et al, editors: *Harrison's principles of internal medicine,* ed 12. New York, McGraw-Hill, 1991.
41. Choiniere M, Melzack R: Acute and chronic pain in hemophilia. *Pain* 31:317, 1987.
42. Roche PA, Gijsbers K, Belch JJ et al: Modification of haemophiliac haemorrhage pain by transcutaneous electrical nerve stimulation. *Pain* 21:43, 1985.
43. Varni JW: Behavioral medicine in hemophilia arthritis pain management: Two case studies. *Arch Phys Med Rehabil* 62:183, 1981.
44. Harris ED: The clinical features of rheumatoid arthritis. In Kelley WN, Harris ED, Ruddy S et al, editors: *Textbook of rheumatology,* ed 3. Philadelphia, WB Saunders, 1989.
45. Lipsky PE: Rheumatoid arthritis. In Wilson JD, Braunwald E, Isselbacher KJ et al, editors: *Harrison's principles of internal medicine,* ed 12. New York, McGraw-Hill, 1991.
46. Lewis MS, Hill S Jr, Warfield C: Medical diseases causing pain. In Raj PP, editor: *Practical management of pain,* ed 2. St. Louis, Mosby, 1992.
47. Bennet JC: Rheumatoid arthritis. In Wyndgaarden JB, Smith LH, editors: *Cecil textbook of medicine,* ed 17. Philadelphia, WB Saunders, 1985.
48. Harris ED: Management of rheumatoid arthritis. In Kelley WN et al, editors: *Textbook of rheumatology,* ed 3. Philadelphia, WB Saunders, 1989.
49. Docken WP, Warfield CA: Rheumatologic causes of pain: Rheumatoid arthritis. *Hosp Prac (Off Ed)* 23:57, 1988.
50. Soergel KH: Acute pancreatitis. In Sleisinger M, Fordtran JS, editors: *Gastrointestinal disease: Pathophysiology, diagnosis, management,* ed 4. Philadelphia, WB Saunders, 1989.
51. Lankisch PG: Diagnosis of abdominal pain: How to distinguish between pancreatic and extrapancreatic causes. *Eur J Surg* 156:273, 1990.

Questions • Medical Diseases

1. In the United States, it is estimated that headaches severe enough to require medical care are

   A. More than 10 million
   B. More than 20 million
   C. More than 40 million
   D. More than 80 million

2. To ascertain targeted history of headache and facial pain, all of the following is important except one

   A. Location
   B. Chronicity
   C. Addiction to sports
   D. Age at onset

3. The following signs and symptoms allow the physician to categorize the headache as

   - Headache is usually bilateral
   - Not bandlike
   - Tightness in frontal temporal or occipital region
   - No aura
   - Significant sleep disturbance
   - Predominates in women
   - No hereditary pattern

   A. Migraine headaches
   B. Tension-type headache
   C. Cluster headaches
   D. Organic headaches

4. Raynaud's disease or phenomenon is a clinical problem, characterized by all except one

   A. Usually involves digits of the upper extremity first
   B. Intense whiteness of fingers
   C. Pain and symptoms exaggerated by exposure to cold
   D. Vasodilation of the microcirculation of the fingers

5. Hemophilia is a congenital bleeding disorder. Hemophilia B is related to a deficient or dysfunctional

   A. Factor IX
   B. Factor VIII
   C. Factor X
   D. Factor III

ANSWERS

1. C
2. C
3. B
4. D
5. A

CHAPTER 6

Trauma

RICHARD L. RAUCK

Traumatic injuries rank as the leading cause of death in the United States for persons younger than the age of 40 years.[1,2] Overall, trauma ranks third in the listed causes of mortality.[3] Two major causes contribute to the high mortality associated with trauma in this country. First, the advent of the high-speed automobile, coupled with an increasing population, has resulted in a steady and dramatic rise in automobile-related deaths over the past 50 years. Second, the rapid and continuing escalation of violent crimes in the past decade has produced many trauma victims.

Management of trauma victims requires a multidisciplinary team.[4–7] Pain and the associated stress response observed in trauma patients should always be viewed as detrimental, and attempts at alleviating the pain need high priority. However, other issues such as monitoring cerebral function can sometimes be viewed as conflicting with pain management. In reality, effective optimal pain management should consider the entire clinical condition and be tailored to address all concerns.

Pain management in trauma victims has focused on the acute setting. Unfortunately, too many trauma patients develop chronic pain syndromes. More focus in the acute period should center on prevention of long-term pain syndromes. The costs of long-term pain management of both treatment and disability far outweigh the short-term cost of acute pain management in trauma care.

Fortunately understanding of pain management techniques is slowly evolving for patients with chest trauma; however, less enlightenment is often witnessed for patients with other trauma. Multitrauma patients always require resuscitative efforts as the utmost priority. However, once the initial resuscitation has occurred and patients have stabilized, attention to pain management should be viewed as more than a luxury. Pain relief should be one goal, because the benefits of effective pain management extend well beyond initial relief. Earlier, more effective rehabilitation occurs in patients who are optimally pain managed.

PATHOPHYSIOLOGY

It is beyond the scope of this chapter to describe all the pathophysiologic events involved in different types of traumatic injuries. However, the pain physician should have a working knowledge of the important processes involved and their relationship to pain management techniques.

Chest Wall Lesion

The role of pain management in the trauma patient depends on the injuries involved and the underlying pathophysiology. Uncontrolled pain should never be considered beneficial in any trauma patient. Circulating catecholamines and other neuroendocrine peptides have repeatedly been shown to be deleterious in animals and humans.[8,9] All trauma patients should be provided with optimal pain management that is tailored to the injuries sustained.

A commonly injured area in trauma is the chest region. Injuries to the chest can be classified as either nonpenetrating or penetrating, which is an important distinction because survival for nonpenetrating injuries has not shown the dramatic improvement recorded for penetrating injuries.[10–12] This reflects the increasing severity of nonpenetrating injuries, most commonly the automobile accident, in which kinetic energy from deceleration injuries transmits tremendous force and ultimate disruption of the bony thorax and underlying tissues, in particular to the pulmonary parenchymal tissue.[13]

Rib fractures are the most common injury to the bony thorax.[11] In severely compromised pulmonary patients a rib fracture can prevent them from breathing effectively or clearing secretions adequately. Elderly or compromised patients must be watched very carefully and their pain effectively managed to prevent atelectasis or pneumonia.

When more than one rib has been fractured in two locations, a flail chest segment can result.[14–18] The flail segment enlarges with the number of ribs involved. With a flail segment the chest wall becomes unstable and ventilation is impaired. Mortality for patients with greater than six fractured ribs is twice that of patients with fewer fractures.[10,19–21] Sometimes flailed segments can be difficult to detect; however, it is especially important to find them when the upper four ribs are involved, because the integrity of the upper rib cage is essential for adequate ventilation.[22]

Controlling pain in patients with underlying derangements to the pulmonary parenchyma has proved to be challenging.[23-27] Pulmonary contusion describes the physiologic and anatomic lesion, which occurs most often after nonpenetrating, compression-depression injuries. Pain does not represent a major limiting problem in this setting, because lung tissue has few primary nociceptive afferents.

Trauma to the lung causes a disruption at the alveolar capillary interface, resulting in both hemorrhage and edema in the alveolar and interstitial spaces.[28,29] Alveolar tissue may also shear from the bronchial tree, secondary to interstitial forces and airway distention from sudden pressure changes.

35

Associated Thoracic Injuries

Common thoracic injuries associated with patients sustaining rib fractures are:

- Pulmonary contusion
- Cardiac contusion
- Aortic disruption
- Pneumo/hemothorax
- Other great vessel disruption
- Neural injury
  Intercostal
  Long thoracic
  Thoracodorsal
  Brachial plexus disruption
- Orthopedic injuries
  Clavicular fracture
  Scapular fracture
  Sternal fracture: displaced or nondisplaced
- Bronchial/tracheal disruption
- Esophageal perforation
- Diaphragmatic rupture

Enhanced morbidity should be feared with the coexistence of the previously listed injuries.[30–33] Sternal fractures are often associated with other thoracic trauma including cardiac injuries, tamponade, and disruption of the great vessels in the thorax.[34] Patients with fractured clavicles must be evaluated for any compromise to the subclavian vessels or brachial plexus.[31] Scapular fractures occur more infrequently but must be considered serious.[32]

Nonthoracic Trauma

Injuries to the extremities can often benefit from pain management techniques. Because of the differences in severity of these injuries, the need for specific pain management techniques may not always be considered when deciding on the importance and relevance of any technique.[4,35]

Patients who have brachial plexus injuries often suffer from multisystem trauma.[36] Patients who have demonstrated injury to a major nerve of an extremity are vulnerable to the development of causalgia. Causalgia should be considered in any patient with a partial nerve injury to a major somatic nerve, particularly the sciatic nerve or brachial plexus.[37] Primary symptoms include exquisite burning pain and intense allodynia. These symptoms appear out of proportion to the injury and may not be readily apparent immediately after the injury. They can occur several days or, uncommonly, weeks after the injury. The practitioner must be prepared to reexamine the patient frequently for the development of the syndrome.

Sympathetic hyperactivity occurs reflexively in patients with vascular disruption. With vascular reanastomosis, the sympathetic activity may remain elevated, which further compromises flow. Techniques to diminish sympathetic overactivity and provide pain relief augment blood flow to the extremity in question.[37]

Patients who suffer traumatic amputations are at risk of developing phantom limb pain. Traumatic amputations elicit a barrage of nociceptive activity, which cannot be turned off easily in the post-traumatic period. The increased afferent activity makes the patient susceptible to more permanent changes in the dorsal horn of the spinal cord.

Epidural anesthesia or analgesia can minimize the severity and decrease the incidence of phantom limb pain.[38,39] In a trauma setting, a catheter cannot be placed preemptively, but theoretically it may still provide excellent analgesia and prevent the N-methyl-D-aspartate receptor or other receptors from producing chronic intraspinous changes that lead to chronic pain and long-term phantom pain. If no contraindications exist, these catheters should be placed as soon as the patient has stabilized either preoperatively, postoperatively, or in the intensive care unit. Epidural catheters can be managed for 5 to 7 days with local anesthetic and low-dose opiates. Early psychologic intervention, teaching imagery, and telescoping techniques can also aid in pain relief.

Soft-tissue injuries occur with all penetrating lesions and most nonpenetrating or blunt trauma. Whether the acutely injured person will develop a chronic pain syndrome is often determined by:

1. The degree of the injury
2. The treatment rendered
3. The patient characteristics

Traumatic injuries do not always occur as a single event. Cumulative trauma disorders account for 50% of all occupational illnesses in the United States.[40] These result from the performance of repetitive tasks and the risk factors include:

- Repetition
- High force
- Awkward joint posture
- Direct pressure
- Vibration
- Prolonged constrained posture[40]

Rest, job alterations, physical therapy, nonsteroidal anti-inflammatory drugs and/or other adjunct medications, and nerve blocks may be indicated. Early detection and treatment help prevent long-term derangement and chronic pain syndromes.

The incidence of head trauma is more frequent in children than adults. Rib fractures and flail chest occur less often in children because of increased elasticity in the incompletely ossified bony structure.[41] Pain management techniques used with adults that can also be used with children are as follows:

- Epidural analgesia
- Intercostal nerve blocks
- Interpleural catheters
- Brachial plexus blocks
- Stellate ganglion blocks[42]

An age of 5 or 6 years is required for patient-controlled analgesia (PCA).

Delayed Sequelae

With the advent of trauma centers and specialized trauma teams, more patients survive the immediate effects of severe multitrauma. As a result a larger group of patients have emerged with long-term sequelae from their trauma.[43,44] In a review of patients who sustained flail chest injuries, only 12 of 32 questioned were employed full time, 1 year after their injury. Abnormal spirometry was observed in 57% of the patients.[45]

Associated trauma and long-term morbidity are often observed with rib fractures. Intercostal nerves are often implicated. Damage can occur secondary to entrapment from the caudal edges of the rib fragments, hematoma, or direct laceration.[30] During the healing process, the rib forms a callus, which can either engulf the nerve or distend the nerve. Neuromas can also develop if the intercostal nerve has been completely transected.[30] Iatrogenic intercostal nerve damage can also occur during thoracostomy tube placement or during surgery from retractors. The pain is neuralgic in origin and follows the dermatomal pattern of the injured nerve. Numbness may or may not be present.

Long-term sequelae from peripheral somatic nerve injuries often result and can be particularly difficult to treat. Whenever possible, these pain syndromes should be recognized during the acute injury phase and treatment should take place early.

Myofascial pain as well as whiplash injuries and post-traumatic headaches represent major long-term problems in trauma patients.[46,47] Whiplash injuries most commonly involve the muscular and ligament tissues of the posterior neck. In the acute phase, symptomatic treatment suffices such as anti-inflammatory drugs, ice, or a short course of physical therapy, when indicated. Chronic pain and prolonged treatment can result when a patient is susceptible or when the acute injury is not properly managed. Whiplash injuries can often produce headaches, which are commonly posterior in location and are in contradistinction to other post-traumatic headaches.[48,49] Post-traumatic headaches have been classified into three types:

1. Type I results from excessive muscle contraction.
2. Type II occurs after scarring of scalp tissue with entrapment of sensory nerves at the site of the injury.
3. Type III is vasodilatory in nature.

These headaches can become chronic and difficult to treat. Studies suggest that post-traumatic headaches continue to improve over the initial 6 months of the trauma but tend to plateau.[50]

Another sequela of head and face trauma includes disorders of the temporomandibular joint.[51] Unless Le Fort fractures are also present, many chronic temporomandibular disorders are not readily apparent at the initial injury. Chronic degenerative temporomandibular disorders often arise from traumatic injuries, although the inciting event may be temporally removed from the development of the symptoms.

Several orthopedic injuries can require many months to heal. Many of these patients can be expected to have significant pain during the process. External fixators in place for prolonged periods can provide ongoing afferent nociception for some patients. These patients should be viewed as having subacute pain rather than chronic pain, if the healing process is continuing. Many do not require further treatment after the offending device has been removed and the lesions have healed. Other patients develop chronic pain syndromes from these severe orthopedic injuries, in part as a result of the anatomic abnormality that alters gait and/or function. The compensatory mechanism of the body can either be incomplete or lead to their own pain problems.

PAIN MANAGEMENT

Early evaluation of the trauma victim by the pain management team allows an individual treatment regimen tailored to the specific injuries of each patient. Full assessments may not always be feasible in the more seriously injured patient. However, awareness of the injuries sustained and knowledge of the common acute and chronic pain syndromes that can result leads to a more proactive course of pain therapy. Timing of therapies is also important and must be coordinated with all aspects of the patient's care.

Regional Techniques

Excellent analgesia can be provided through the use of regional anesthetic techniques. The decision to employ these techniques must involve the trauma team, the pain management team, and the patient's family. Different specialists working in concert also minimize any legal risk that may exist in this group of sick patients.

Management of Thoracic Injury

Intercostal nerve blocks have been used for many years to treat rib fractures.[52] They can be combined with parenteral opiates to improve deep breathing and coughing. When the fractured ribs are unilateral, the patient can be positioned with the affected side up.

Because of the overlap in innervation of the intercostal nerves, one level above and below the fractured ribs should be blocked whenever possible.[37,53] The interspace should be marked before starting the procedure. The location for blockage depends on the fracture site; success necessitates blocking the nerve proximal to the fracture site.

A different approach to the intercostal nerve is through the interpleural space. Unlike placing catheters at the T7-T8 interspace, an interpleural catheter placed for thoracic pain performs better when positioned at the midpoint of the fractured ribs. Alternatively, it has been recommended to place these catheters close to the apex of the lung.[54]

Much like an intercostal nerve block, the catheter works best when positioned proximal to the fracture site. When thoracostomy tubes are present, the risk of having substantial amounts of local anesthetic sucked from the site of action exists and must be guarded against.[55] This can be best achieved by either placing the catheter distant from the thoracostomy tube or delaying suction for 15 to 20 minutes after instillation of the drug. The decision to do the latter should only be made after a surgical consult and with appropriate monitoring of the patient.

Intermittent injections or continuous infusions through an interpleural catheter can be used. Some patients respond better to intermittent injections, although continuous infusions appear to work well later in the course of the healing process. Intermittent doses that provide adequate analgesia range from 20 to 30 ml of 0.5% bupivacaine. If bilateral catheters are employed, the concentration of bupivacaine should be halved to prevent toxicity from the local anesthetic.

Excessively high plasma levels of local anesthesia must be watched for when patients have bilateral catheters. A damaged pleura can result in altered pharmacokinetics and uptake of the drug from pleura into plasma.[56]

Epidural Analgesia

Epidural analgesia for traumatic injuries has been used for several decades. Its use was sporadic until physicians became aware that many trauma victims could be managed conservatively if their pain was adequately controlled.

The last two decades have greatly enhanced our understanding of the pathophysiology of thoracic trauma and, consequently, the outcome of seriously injured patients. The heterogeneity of the trauma patient can make it difficult to compare the results of different studies.

To successfully manage this group of patients, several key points must always be remembered:

1. It is important to recognize and treat the underlying pulmonary contusion.
2. Conservative, nonventilatory management should be used whenever clinically possible.
3. Aggressive pain management should be attempted to facilitate deep breathing, coughing, and respiratory physiotherapy and to avoid splinting, atelectasis, and respiratory failure.[57]

Pain Management of Intra-abdominal Injuries

Blunt or penetrating injuries of the abdominal cavity often require surgical intra-abdominal exploration and repair. Splenic rupture, liver lacerations, and great vessel lacerations are some of the injuries that require intervention. It is well known from the surgical literature that patients undergoing upper abdominal procedures splint; guard; and show decreases in functional respiratory capacity, vital capacity, and maximum inspiratory pressure.[58]

The surgical literature indicates that trauma patients who have required upper abdominal surgical exploration can benefit from aggressive pain management techniques. The treatment of choice for trauma victims who require abdominal operations should be low or midthoracic epidurals, dependent on the procedure performed. As with the thoracic patient, some factors may preclude the use of this technique, including:

1. Emergent or unstable presentation, which may not allow sufficient time for placement before surgery.
2. Spinal cord injuries, which in most situations are considered a contraindication to epidural placement.
3. Impending disseminated intravascular coagulation, which may be impossible to predict. However, clinical indices such as massive intraoperative transfusions can alert a physician to its probability. The total patient must be assessed and discussed with the trauma team before proceeding with any epidural instrumentation.

Compression fractures and other vertebral abnormalities may not preclude the use of an epidural, but a consultation with the trauma team and sometimes a neurosurgeon is required before placement.

When epidural analgesia is contraindicated, blockade of the intercostal nerves, either by intercostal nerve block or interpleural analgesia, can often provide excellent analgesia, improved pulmonary dynamics, and probably many of the other benefits that are found with an epidural technique.

Pain Management of Extremity Injuries

Extremity injuries can involve:

- Bony disruption
- Major somatic nerve injury
- Vascular injury
- Extensive soft-tissue injury as seen in crush injuries[59]

Injuries can be classified as either blunt or penetrating and can disrupt a variety of systems. Sympathetic denervation during and after extremity reanastomosis can greatly benefit blood flow to the involved extremity. Whenever possible, this should be provided in a continuous manner. Brachial plexus catheters are particularly well suited for this situation and can be left in place for a week or longer if necessary.[57] If prolonged catheterization is used, closely watch for signs and symptoms of infection.

Dilute solutions of local anesthetics (0.076% to 0.15% bupivacaine) usually suffice. The application of narcotics is not indicated because opiate receptors have not been shown to exist along axonal sheaths of somatic nerves.

Brachial plexus catheters may be contraindicated most commonly when the surgeon wishes to monitor neurologic recovery and feels the potential for prolonged somatic blockade should be avoided. In these situations, a stellate ganglion block can be performed for upper-extremity situations. For lower-extremity situations, a lumbar sympathetic catheter can be placed.

Crush injuries are particularly prone to developing reflex sympathetic dystrophy. Because this will not happen in most patients, when a patient feels pain that is out of proportion to the injury or does not respond well to standard opiates, the patient should be checked for reflex sympathetic dystrophy. Sympathetic blockade remains the treatment of choice in early, post-traumatic reflex sympathetic dystrophy.

Neurologic injuries to peripheral somatic nerves almost always produce significant pain.[59] A partial nerve injury to a major somatic nerve with resulting burning pain should be considered causalgia and treated as such until proven otherwise. Sympathetic interruption should be obtained and maintained continuously. Catheters that can be considered appropriate for causalgia or other nerve injuries include:

- Epidural (lumbar, thoracic, or cervical)
- Brachial plexus (predominantly axillary or infraclavicular)
- Sciatic
- Lumbar sympathetic

Head-Injured Patients and Pain Management

The head-injured patient can pose significant and unique problems for appropriate and aggressive pain management. In severe head injuries, pain management that interferes with neurologic monitoring should be avoided. The fear of neurologic side effects with opiates has classically led to the underuse of opiates in patients with head injuries. Epidural administration can decrease the total amount of drug necessary and may be preferred in some situations.

Pain Management Paradigm for the Trauma Patient

Whenever possible, a member of the acute pain management team should be available 24 hours a day as part of the trauma team. Deciding on what type of pain relief technique is needed must be based on a complete knowledge of the patient. Figures 6–1 and 6–2 illustrate a paradigm to use when deciding on how to manage a trauma patient's pain.

Patients discharged from the emergency department are most commonly treated with oral analgesics. Patients who require early intubation and mechanical ventilation should be evaluated for the long-term necessity of such assistance. Because it can often be difficult to initially judge how long

a patient will need ventilation assistance, it is best to wait until the patient stabilizes and then wean him or her off the ventilator.

Contraindications to epidurals in trauma patients are clotting abnormalities, septicemia, and/or severe mental status changes. Clotting abnormalities can be easily determined with prothrombin, partial thromboplastin, and platelet determinations.

Early bacteremia is common in many of these patients. Whenever possible, it is best to place epidurals before any temperature elevation. It is a sound policy not to remove epidural catheters early in a patient's fever course if there is a known cause of the fever and the epidural catheter is

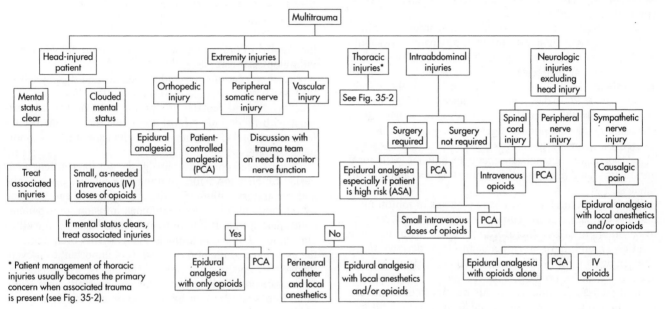

FIG. 6–1 Flow chart illustrating management of trauma patients.

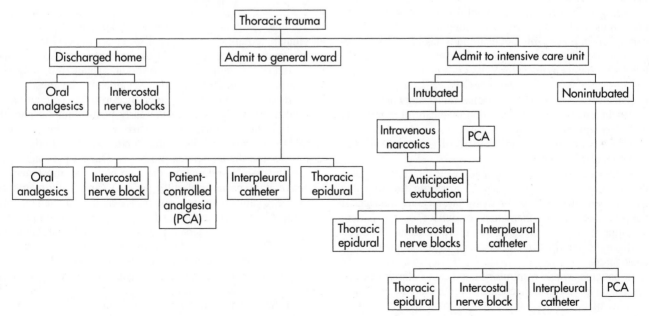

FIG. 6–2 Flow chart illustrating pain management techniques for thoracic trauma patients.

deemed necessary by the trauma team. The epidural site must be monitored carefully for signs of infection and of epidural abscess or meningitis. A decision to leave a catheter in a patient who is at relative high risk should be a joint one with the trauma team, and the trauma team should document that the benefits outweigh the risks.

Patients with severe impairment in mental status will most likely be intubated, and an epidural catheter may be contraindicated. Head-injured patients who are extubated have associated painful lesions and require frequent mental status checks. These patients need not be excluded from epidural analgesia; lower-dose opiates are required through the epidural catheter to allow the patient clearer mental activity, if other factors are equal. Sometimes the opiates can be completely removed with the patient managing solely on epidural local anesthetics.

Patients who have not sustained thoracic injuries but have abdominal, pelvic, or significant extremity pathology should be considered for pain management techniques. The options include epidural analgesia, peripheral nerve catheters, or sympathetic nerve blocks. The decision to use these techniques versus PCA depends on the severity of the lesions and the goal of the team. PCA is less invasive to the patient and can provide very good analgesia when pain relief is considered the primary goal. However, PCA cannot improve blood flow like regional anesthetic techniques with local anesthetics and also usually requires larger amounts of opiates.

Deciding on the location of the catheter in multitrauma patients can be difficult. Thoracic lesion takes precedence over other injuries; therefore, patients with thoracic injuries should have a catheter inserted dermatomally, appropriate to the thoracic lesions. Other injuries may require systemic opiates to cover pain that cannot be controlled with the epidural. If this becomes necessary, the clinician should remove the opiate from the epidural and use local anesthetics alone. The patient should be supplemented with systemic opiates by PCA or intermittent intravenous bolus.

During placement of the epidural catheter, sterile technique must have top priority. How long an epidural catheter can be left in place without changing it has never been adequately addressed. If no signs of septicemia are present, leaving catheters in place for 7 days is a good policy. In rare cases when a specific indication exists, catheters can be left in place for up to 14 days because reinstrumentation may represent a greater risk of infection than careful monitoring of the patient. Fortunately, few catheters need to be kept in place for more than 5 days and most are removed after 72 hours (Table 6-1).

Regardless of how long an epidural catheter is in place, the site must be monitored daily. Clear sterile dressings that can be examined without breaking sterility are advised. If the site becomes erythematous or tender or the patient develops an ongoing fever with an elevated white blood cell count, replacing the catheter or changing technique must be considered.

In patients whose respiratory condition deteriorates and for whom prolonged mechanical ventilation is predicted, removal of the catheter is often advocated with reinsertion later after the patient is actively weaned. This helps to keep

TABLE 6-1 Data on Trauma Patients Receiving Epidural Catheters*

Duration of epidural catheter (n = 74)	43 days (1 to 9 days)[†]
Intensive care unit stay	5.7 days (0 to 19 days)[†]
Associated Injuries	
Rib fractures (number)	7 (2 to 12)[†]
Pulmonary contusion	46
Pneumothorax	24
Hemothorax	14
Flail symptoms	19
Other fractures	1.3 (0 to 6)[†]

*Based on personal experience; [†]range.

the number of prolonged catheters to a minimum while providing optimal care.

Recommendations for epidural agents and dosing schedules are patient specific. Morphine sulfate has been used successfully and remains the prototypical opiate. Meperidine, with its definitive local anesthetic action, has been a frequent second choice in patients who cannot tolerate morphine sulfate.

Patients need continuous analgesia, not intermittent analgesia, which allows for splinting, atelectasis, pneumonia, and respiratory failure. Continuous analgesia can be done by intermittent injection, continuous infusion, or a patient-controlled design. If intermittent injection is used, the clinician should reinject in a timely manner. This often requires the assistance of the nursing staff. It is important to prevent inadvertent injections of other medications, which is a circumstance potentially catastrophic and possibly more likely in an intensive care unit because so much activity is going on at the bedside.

SUMMARY

Trauma patients, particularly complex multitrauma individuals, require a highly specialized team to provide optimal care and outcome. The pain management team should work as part of the trauma team and should manage the analgesic requirements in these patients. Specifically, the anesthesiologist has the training and experience to offer regional techniques often necessary in the early post-traumatic period. Pain physicians must assume active roles in trauma patient therapy because they know the pain to expect from different lesions and the associated morbidity. Once a pain management course is undertaken, the pain physician must stay an active, daily participant in the patient's care. Other members of the trauma team are not in a position to manage the complex pain-relieving techniques presently employed. Monitoring the patient's progress demands attention to detail. Flexibility should be available in any plan to accommodate changes in the initial situation. With the present emphasis on conservative management for many trauma patients, providing optimal analgesia becomes even more important. That ability exists and should be afforded to the trauma patient whenever possible.

References

1. National Safety Council: *Accident facts: Preliminary condensed edition,* Itasca, Ill, NSC, 1983.
2. Mackersie RC, Karagianes TG: Pain management following trauma and pain. *Crit Care Clin* 6:433, 1990.
3. Asburn MA, Fine PG: Persistent pain following trauma. *Mil Med* 154:86, 1989.
4. Baker SP, O'Neill B, Haddon W Jr et al: The injury severity score: A method for describing patients with multiple injuries and evaluating emergency care. *J Trauma* 14:187, 1974.
5. Williams WG, Smith RE: Trauma of the chest. *The Coventry Conference.* Bristol, England, John Wright & Sons, 1977.
6. Kaiser KS: Assessment and management of pain in the critically ill trauma patient. *Crit Care Nursing* 15:14, 1992.
7. Mlynczak B: Assessment and management of the trauma patients in pain. *Crit Care Nursing Clin North Am* 1:55, 1989.
8. Davis RF, DeBoer LWV, Maroko PR: Thoracic epidural anesthesia reduces myocardial infarct size after coronary artery occlusion in dogs. *Anesth Analg* 65:711, 1986.
9. Klassen GA, Bramwell RS, Bromage PR et al: Effect of acute sympathectomy by epidural anesthesia on the canine coronary circulation. *Anesthesiology* 52:8, 1980.
10. Conn JH, Hardy JD, Chavez CM, et al: Thoracic trauma: Analysis of 1022 cases. *J Trauma* 3:22, 1963.
11. Trinkle JK: Management of major thoracic wall trauma. *Curr Surg* 42:181, 1985.
12. Moseley RV, Vernick JJ, Doty DB: Responses to blunt chest injury: A new experimental model. *J Trauma* 10:673, 1970.
13. Newman RJ, Jones IS: A prospective study of 413 consecutive car occupants with chest injuries. *J Trauma* 24:129, 1984.
14. Duff JH, Goldstein M, McLean AP et al: Flail chest: A clinical review and physiological study. *J Trauma* 8:63, 1968.
15. Lewis F, Thomas AN, Schlobohm RM: Control of respiratory therapy in flail chest. *Ann Thorac Surg* 20:170, 1975.
16. Parham AM, Yarbrough DR, Redding JS: Flail chest syndrome and pulmonary contusion. *Arch Surg* 113:900, 1978.
17. Sankaran S, Wilson RF: Factors affecting prognosis in patients with flail chest. *J Thorac Cardiovasc Surg* 60:402, 1970.
18. Shackford SR, Smith DE, Zarins CK et al: The management of flail chest. A comparison of ventilatory and nonventilatory treatment. *Am J Surg* 132:759, 1976.
19. Howell JF, Crawford ES, Jordan GL: The flail chest. *Am J Surg* 106:628, 1963.
20. Dougall AM, Paul ME, Finely RJ et al: Chest trauma—Current morbidity and mortality. *J Trauma* 17:547, 1977.
21. Mulder DS: Chest trauma: Current concepts. *Can J Surg* 23:340, 1980.
22. Perry JF, Galway CF: Factors influencing survival after fail chest injuries. *Arch Surg* 91:216, 1965.
23. Daughtry DC: *Thoracic trauma.* Boston, Little, Brown, 1980.
24. Hankins JR, Attar S, Turney SZ et al: Differential diagnosis of pulmonary parenchymal changes in thoracic trauma. *Am Surg* 39:309, 1973.
25. Johnson JA, Cogbill TH, Winga ER: Determinants of outcome after pulmonary contusion. *J Trauma* 26:695, 1986.
26. Keen G: *Chest injuries.* Bristol, England, John Wright & Sons, 1975.
27. Kirsh MM, Sloan H: *Blunt chest trauma.* Boston, Little, Brown, 1977.
28. Rutherford RB, Valentia J: An experimental study of "traumatic wet lung." *J Trauma* 11:146, 1971.
29. Schaal MA, Fischer RP, Perry JF: The unchanged mortality of flail chest injuries. *J Trauma* 19:492, 1979.
30. Hix WR, Aaron BL: *Residual of thoracic trauma.* New York, Futura Publishing, 1987.
31. Howard FM, Shafer HJ: Injuries to the clavicle with neurovascular complications: A study of fourteen cases. *J Bone Joint Surg Am* 47A:2335, 1965.
32. Imatini RJ: Fractures of the scapula: A review of 53 fractures. *J Trauma* 15:473, 1975.
33. Iverson LI , Mittal A, Dugan DJ et al: Injury to the phrenic nerve resulting in diaphragmatic paralysis with special reference to skeletal trauma. *Am J Surg* 132:263, 1976.
34. Hills MW, Deprado AM, Deane SA: Sternal fractures: Associated injuries and management. *J Trauma* 35:55, 1993.
35. Greenspan L, McLelan BA, Greig H: Abbreviated injury scale and injury severity score: A scoring chart. *J Trauma* 25:60, 1985.
36. Werken C, de Vries LS: Brachial plexus injury in multitraumatized patients. *Clin Neurol Neurosurg* 95:S30, 1993.
37. Hartrick C: Pain due to trauma, including sports. In Raj PP, editor: *Practical management of pain.* St. Louis, Mosby, 1986.
38. Wesolowski JA, Lema MJ: Phantom limb pain. *Reg Anesth* 18:121, 1993.
39. Bach S, Noreng MF, Tjellen NU: Phantom limb pain in amputees during the first 12 months following amputation, after preoperative lumbar epidural blocks. *Pain* 33:297, 1988.
40. Rempel DM, Harrison RJ, Barnhart S: Work-related cumulative trauma disorders of the upper extremity. *JAMA* 267:838, 1992.
41. Dickenson CM: Thoracic trauma in children. *Crit Care Nursing Clin North Am* 3:423, 1991.
42. Tobias JD: Indications and application of epidural anesthesia in a pediatric population outside the perioperative period. *Clin Pediatr* 32:81, 1993.
43. Christensson P, Gisselsson L, Lecerof H et al: Early and late results of controlled ventilation in flail chest. *Chest* 75:456, 1979.
44. Hanning CD, Ledingham E, Ledingham I: Late respiratory sequelae of blunt chest injury: A preliminary report. *Thorax* 36:204, 1981.
45. Landercasper J, Cogbill TH, Lindesmith LA: Long-term disability after flail chest injury. *J Trauma* 34:410, 1984.
46. Evans RW: Some observations on whiplash injuries. *Neurol Clin* 10:975, 1992.
47. Radanov BP, di Stefano G, Schnidrig A et al: Role of psychosocial stress recovery from common whiplash. *Lancet* 338:712, 1991.
48. Vijayan N, Watson C: Site of injury headache. *Headache* 29(8):502, 1989.
49. Packard RC, Ham LP: Impairment ratings for post-traumatic headache. *Headache* 33:359, 1993.
50. Packard RC, Ham LP: Post-traumatic headache: Determining chronicity. *Headache* 33:133, 1993.
51. Pullinger AG, Seligman DA: Trauma history in diagnostic groups of temporomandibular disorders. *Oral Surg Oral Med Oral Pathol* 71:529, 1991.
52. Pedersen VM, Schulze S, Hoier-Madsen K et al: Air-flow meter assessment of the effect of intercostal nerve blockade on respiratory function in rib fractures. *Eur J Surg* 149:119, 1983.
53. Cousins MJ, Bridenbaugh PO: Neural blockade. In Cousins MJ, Bridenbaugh PO, editors: *Clinical anesthesia and management of pain.* Philadelphia, JB Lippincott, 1988.
54. Iwana H, Kawamae K, Katsumi A, et al: Intrapleural regional anesthesia in pain management after chest trauma. *Masui* 42:669, 1993.
55. Knottenbelt JD, James MF, Bloomfield M: Intrapleural bupivacaine analgesia in chest trauma: A randomized double-blind controlled trial. *Injury* 22:114, 1991.
56. Wulf H, Jeckstrom W, Maier C et al: Intrapleural catheter analgesia in patients with multiple rib fractures. *Anaesthetist* 40:19, 1991.
57. Trinkle JK, Furman RW, Hinshaw MA et al: Pulmonary contusion: pathogenesis and effect of various resuscitative measures. *Ann Thorac Surg* 16:568, 1973.
58. Rauck RK et al: Comparison of the efficacy of epidural morphine given by intermittent injection or continuous infusion for the management of postoperative pain. *Reg Anesth* 19:316, 1994.
59. Nulsen F, Klein DG: Acute injuries of peripheral nerves. In Yomans JR editor: *Neurologic surgery.* Philadelphia, WB Saunders, 1973.

1. Two major causes contribute to the high immortality associated with trauma in the United States. They are

   A. Advent of high-speed automobiles and increase in violent crimes
   B. Rapid growth in young population and watching television
   C. Increase in survival of geriatric population and increase in motor vehicle licenses in this group
   D. Lack of education of general population in defensive driving and decrease in morality

2. Contraindications to epidural procedure in trauma patients include all but one of the following

   A. Normal clotting mechanism
   B. Septicemia
   C. Severe mental status changes
   D. Severe hemorrhage

3. Extremity injuries commonly do not involve

   A. Vital organs
   B. Bony disruption
   C. Major somatic nerves
   D. Crush injuries

4. Neurologic injuries to peripheral somatic nerves almost always produce

   A. Increased reflexes
   B. Significant pain
   C. Increased motor strength
   D. Increased vascular access to the extremity

5. To successfully manage thoracic trauma patients these key points should be recommended except one

   A. Recognize and treat underlying pulmonary conditions
   B. Internal defense mechanisms will heal themselves
   C. Conservative nonventilatory management should be attempted first
   D. Aggressive pain management is directed to facilitate deep breathing and to avoid atelectasis respiratory failure

ANSWERS

1. A

2. A

3. A

4. B

5. B

CHAPTER 7

Surgery

HONORIO T. BENZON

VARIABILITY OF BLOOD LEVELS AND ANALGESIC RESPONSES FROM MULTIPLE INTRAMUSCULAR OPIOID INJECTIONS

The traditional technique of intramuscular (IM) opioid injections at fixed intervals is associated with variable blood levels and inconsistent analgesic responses. This variability, secondary to unpredictable absorption from the site of injection, resulted in inadequate or transient analgesia. Erratic absorption and the relationship between variations in blood meperidine concentration and analgesic response[1] are the major reasons for the variable control after IM injections.

PREEMPTIVE ANALGESIA

Injury to nociceptive nerve fibers induces neural and behavioral changes that persist long after the injury has healed or the offending stimulus has been removed. This post-injury pain hypersensitivity can be due to post-traumatic changes in the peripheral nervous system (hyperalgesia) or in the central nervous system (CNS) (hyperexcitability). The noxious stimulus-induced neuroplasticity can be preempted by administration of analgesic agents or by regional nerve blockade.[2] These treatments are less effective when administered after the injury or when the prolonged central excitability has already been established.[3] Some clinical studies have supported preemptive analgesia, while other studies have not.

PATIENT-CONTROLLED ANALGESIA

Patient-controlled analgesia (PCA) eliminates the variable absorption of the opioid from the injection site and bypasses the unavoidable delays that occur when an opioid is requested. These delays include the response of a very busy nurse; screening by the nurse regarding the appropriateness of the request; signing out and preparation of the drug; and, finally, injection of the opioid.[4] PCA is unique in that patients titrate their analgesic needs against sedation and other side effects of the opioid.

The attributes of an ideal analgesic for PCA use include a rapid onset of analgesic action, high analgesic efficacy (i.e., no ceiling effect), and an intermediate duration of the effect for better controllability.[5] Morphine and meperidine satisfy most of these characteristics and are, therefore, the most widely used drugs (Table 7–1).

Studies that compared different analgesics for PCA use showed that movement-associated pain is least with morphine[6,7] and highest with meperidine.[7]

The use of basal morphine infusion to the PCA, which was recommended to decrease the trough in morphine plasma concentrations during PCA, was found not to decrease resting pain but to reduce movement-associated pain scores.[8] The addition of a basal oxymorphone infusion to the oxymorphone PCA significantly reduced the visual analogue scores (VAS) associated with rest and movement

---

TABLE 7–1 Guidelines When Using a Patient-Controlled Analgesia (PCA) System

Drug	Bolus Dose (mg)	Lockout Interval (min)	Continuous Infusion (mg/hr⁻¹)
Agonists			
Fentanyl citrate	0.015–0.05	3–10	0.02–0.1
Hydromorphone hydrochloride	0.10–0.5	5–15	0.2–0.5
Meperidine hydrochloride	5–15	5–15	5–40
Methadone hydrochloride	0.50–3.0	10–20	—
Morphine sulfate	0.50–3.0	5–20	1–10
Oxymorphone hydrochloride	0.20–0.8	5–15	0.1–1
Sufentanil citrate	0.003–0.015	3–10	0.004–0.03
Agonist-Antagonists			
Buprenorphine hydrochloride	0.03–0.2	10–20	—
Nalbuphine hydrochloride	1–5	5–15	1–8
Pentazocine hydrochloride	5–30	5–15	6–40

Note: The addition of a basal infusion to the PCA is controversial (see text). Adapted from Lubenow TR, McCarthy RJ, Ivankovich AD: Management of acute postoperative pain. In Barash PG, Culen BF, Stoelting RD, editors: *Clinical anesthesia,* ed. 2. Philadelphia, JB Lippincott, 1992.

but resulted in a significantly higher incidence of nausea and vomiting.[8]

The addition of a nighttime basal opioid infusion did not improve the patients' ability to sleep or rest comfortably. Their postoperative scores for pain, sedation, fatigue, discomfort, and anxiety were the same whether a nighttime basal infusion was added or not.[9]

The VAS of patients who used PCA was found to be similar to those who had IM injections. The incidence of sedation, however, was significantly lower in the PCA group.[10] The decreased sedation, together with the control that patients have over their analgesic needs, explains why more patients rate their pain relief to be superior with PCA and preferable over the IM route.

Studies that directly compared PCA with the IM and epidural routes of opioid administration showed significantly lower VAS with the epidural technique.[11,12] However, the significantly higher incidence of pruritus with epidural morphine made several patients prefer other modes of analgesic therapy for their next surgery.[11]

EPIDURAL OPIOID INJECTIONS

Intraspinal opioid injections are based on the existence and pharmacology of spinal opiate receptors that provide an attractive means to achieve regional anesthesia with minimal central effects. Initially, the opioid was injected intrathecally; but the higher incidence of respiratory depression with this approach led to the popularity of the epidural technique.

The latency and duration of postoperative analgesia with the different epidural opioids are listed in Table 7–2.[13]

Morphine was the opioid initially employed, and Ready and coworkers established their safety and efficacy. In their two-year experience with 11,089 individual morphine injections in 1106 patients, they had no death, neurologic injury, or infection.[14] Catheter-related problems occurred in 5% of their patients. Their treatment, including morphine strength, interval between injections, and duration of treatment, is shown in Table 7–3.

Complications of intraspinal opioid administration include pruritus, nausea and vomiting, urinary retention, and respiratory depression (Table 7–4).[15]

Randomized, double-blind studies showed the superiority of intermittent epidural morphine injections over IM or intravenous (IV) morphine injections. In a study of patients who underwent gastroplasty, the use of epidural morphine resulted in earlier ambulation, earlier recovery of pulmonary and bowel function, and a shorter hospital stay.[16] In patients who had thoracotomy, epidural morphine provided significantly better analgesia and better pulmonary function than IV morphine.[17] This advantage of the epidural over the IV route was not seen after cesarean section,[18] a less painful operation than thoracotomy or gastroplasty.

Continuous infusions of epidural morphine, in contrast to intermittent epidural morphine injections, effectively reduce postoperative pain with minimal side effects.[19] Epidural fentanyl infusions, compared with morphine infusions, provide comparable analgesia with a lower incidence of nausea and pruritus.[20]

Inordinately high infusion rates of epidural fentanyl maintained adequate pain relief. Some have theorized that the predominant mechanism of analgesic effect of the fentanyl infusion is systemic in nature. Studies with cesarean section,

TABLE 7–2 Epidural Opioids: Latency and Duration of Postoperative Analgesia

| Agent | Bolus Done | Analgesic Effect | | | Continuous Infusion | |
		Onset (min)	Peak (min)	Duration (hr)	Concentration	Rate (ml/hr^{-1})
Meperidine	30–100 mg	5–10	12–30	4–6	—	—
Morphine	3–5 mg	24 ± 6	30–60	12–24	0.005%	3–8
Methadone	5 mg	12 ± 2	17 ± 3	7 ± 5	—	—
Hydromorphone	0.5–1 mg	13 ± 4	23 ± 8	11 ± 6	0.001%	6–8
Fentanyl	50–100 µg	4–10	20	3 ± 6	0.0005%	4–12
Diamorphine	5 mg	5	9–15	12 ± 6	—	—
Sufentanil	30–50 µg	7 ± 6	26 ± 8	4 ± 7	0.0001%	10
Alfentanil	15 µg/kg^{-1}	15	—	1–2	—	—

Adapted from Cousins MJ, Mather LE: Intrathecal and epidural administration of opioids. *Anesthesiology* 61:276, 1984.

TABLE 7–3 Treatment of Postoperative Pain with Intermittent Epidural Morphine

| | Surgical Site | | | |
	Thorax	Abdomen	Lower Extremity	Perineum
Patients (number)	146	584	322	54
Morphine (mg)	4 ± 1	4 ± 1	4 ± 1	3 ± 1
Injection interval (hr)	8 ± 3	9 ± 3	11 ± 5	12 ± 6
Morphine (total mg/24 hr) (calculated)	13	10	8	7
Rest pain	1(3)	1(2)	1(3)	0(1)
Incident pain	5(4)	4(4)	4(4)	3(6)
Duration of treatment (days)	5 ± 3	4 ± 3	3 ± 2	2 ± 1

Morphine, injection interval, and duration of treatment, mean ± standard deviation.
Rest pain and incident pain, median and interquartile range (in parentheses).
Adapted from Ready LB et al: Postoperative epidural morphine is safe on surgical wards. *Anesthesiology* 75:452, 1991.

TABLE 7–4 Complications of the Use of Intraspinal Narcotics

Complications	Reported Incidence (%)*		Treatment
	Spinal	Epidural	
Respiratory depression	5–7	0.1–2	Support ventilation; naloxone
Pruritus	60	1–100	Antihistamine; naloxone
Nausea and vomiting	20–50	20–30	Antiemetic; transdermal scopolamine; naloxone
Urinary retention	50	15–25	Catheterize; naloxone

*Reported incidences vary widely, appear to be related to dose, and are higher with spinal than epidural administration. From Ready LB: Regional anesthesia with intraspinal opioids. In Bonica JJ, editor: *The management of pain,* ed 2. Philadelphia, Lea & Febiger, 1990.

hysterectomy, and knee surgery have supported this impression. Other studies, dealing with more painful surgical procedures, showed the epidural route to be more effective than the parenteral route (Table 7–5). Infusion rates may be related to the vertebral placement level of the epidural (Table 7–6).

Outcome Studies on Epidural Opioid Injections

Most studies showed improved pain relief, decreased postoperative morbidity, and a shortened hospital stay after the postoperative administration of epidural opioids. Epidural morphine, compared with IM morphine, decreased the hospitalization stay after gastroplasty from 9 to 7 days.[16] A shorter hospital stay was also noted after thoracotomy when a thoracic epidural fentanyl infusion was used.[21] Two outcome studies showed significantly lower complication rates after epidural anesthesia and postoperative epidural analgesia in high-risk patients[22] and in patients undergoing major vascular surgery.[23] A recent outcome study confirmed better pain relief and postoperative pulmonary function with operative epidural opioid analgesia but showed no reduction of pulmonary complications or diminution of hospital stays.[24]

TRANSDERMAL FENTANYL

Transdermal fentanyl can be administered in doses of 25, 50, 75, and 100 μg/hr. Doses of 75 and 100 μg/hr are the most commonly used dosages for postoperative analgesia. In a double-blind, placebo-controlled study, the analgesia from a 75 μg/hr transdermal therapeutic system of fentanyl was found to be significantly better than placebo.[25] Patients in the fentanyl group required significantly less morphine during the 24 hours that the systems were in place and for the first 12 hours after removal of the patch.[25] Transdermal fentanyl is not recommended for postoperative pain because there is a delay of 13 ± 10 hours before effective blood fentanyl concentrations are reached. There is also a decay time of 16 ± 7 hours after the patch is removed for blood fentanyl concentrations to decrease below the mean minimum effective analgesic concentration.

INTRA-ARTICULAR MORPHINE

The existence of opiate receptors in the periphery led to clinical trials testing the analgesic effect of opioids injected in the vicinity of peripheral sensory nerve terminals. Stein and coworkers[26] showed that 1 mg of morphine injected intra-articularly after knee arthroscopy lowered postopera-

tive VAS and reduced analgesic consumption. They also found that the concurrent administration of naloxone reversed the analgesic effect of intra-articular morphine.

Studies that compared intra-articular morphine with intra-articular bupivacaine showed slightly different results, depending on the dose of morphine.

AGENCY FOR HEALTH CARE POLICY AND RESEARCH CLINICAL PRACTICE GUIDELINES

The Agency for Health Care Policy and Research (AHCPR) of the U.S. Department of Health and Human Services published clinical practice guidelines for the management of acute pain.[27] They stated that, unless contraindicated, pharmacologic management of mild-to-moderate postoperative pain should begin with a nonsteroidal anti-inflammatory drug. Nonsteroidal anti-inflammatory drugs decrease levels of inflammatory mediators at the site of tissue injury, do not cause sedation or respiratory depression, and do not interfere with bowel or bladder function. These drugs also have an opioid dose-sparing effect.

Moderately severe to severe pain should be treated initially with an opioid. The opioid should be withheld if the patient is sedated or when the respiratory rate is less than 10 breaths per minute. As soon as the patient tolerates oral intake, he or she should be switched to the oral route.

For patients who are known or suspected drug abusers, the AHCPR recommended the following[27]:

1. The mechanism of the pain should be defined and treated. Infection, ischemia, or a new surgical diagnosis should be treated accordingly.
2. Clinicians should distinguish between the temporal characteristics of abuse behavior. A history of drug abuse behavior may predispose to reemergence of the abuse behavior but does not require treatment approaches different from nonaddicted patients.
3. Pharmacologic principles of opioid use should be followed.
4. Nonopioid treatments such as nonsteroidal anti-inflammatory drugs, nerve blocks, or transcutaneous electrical nerve stimulation should be given concomitantly with or to replace opioids.
5. Drug abuse behavior should be recognized and dealt with firmly.
6. Limits should be set to avoid excessive negotiations about drug selections or choices.

TABLE 7–5 Comparison of Epidural with Parenteral Opioids for Postoperative Pain

Authors	Type of Study	Type of Surgery	Routes Compared	Drugs Used	Superior Technique
Rawal et al[a]	R, DB	Gastroplasty	TE vs. IM	Morphine	Epidural
Shulman et al[b]	R, DB	Thoracotomy	LE vs. IV	Morphine	Epidural
Camann et al[c]	R, DB	Cesarian section	LE vs. IV	Butorphanol	Equal
Loper et al[d]	R, DB	Knee surgery	LE vs. IV	Fentanyl	Equal
Ellis et al[e]	R, DB	Cesarian section	LE vs. IV	Fentanyl	Equal
Camu et al[f]	R	Hysterectomy	LE vs. IV	Alfentanil	Equal
Geller et al[g]	R, DB	Abdominal	LE vs. IV	Sufentanil (LE,IV) Fentanyl (LE)	Epidural
Sandler et al[h]	R, DB	Thoracotomy	LE vs. IV	Fentanyl	Equal
Salomaki et al[i]	R, DB	Thoracotomy	TE vs. IV	Fentanyl	Epidural
Guinard et al[j]	R	Thoracotomy	LE vs. TE vs IV	Fentanyl	TE
Grant et al[k]	R, DB	Thoracotomy	LE vs. PCA	Fentanyl	Epidural
Benzon et al[l]	R, DB	Thoracotomy	TE vs. PCA	Fentanyl (TE) Morphine (PCA)	Epidural
Allaire et al[m]	R	RRP	LE vs. PCA	Fentanyl (LE) Morphine (PCA)	Epidural
Chauvin et al[n]	R	Abdominal	LE PCA vs. IV PCA	Alfentanil	Equal[o]
Glass et al[p]	R, DB, C	Lower extremity, abdominal	LE PCA vs. IV PCA	Fentanyl	Equal

C, Cross over; DB, double-blind; IM, intramuscular; IV, intravenous; LE, lumbar epidural; PCA, patient-controlled analgesia; R, randomized; RRP, radical retropubic prostatectomy; TE, thoracic epidural.

[a]Rawal N et al: Comparison of intramuscular and epidural morphine for postoperative analgesia in the grossly obese: Influence on postoperative ambulation and pulmonary function. *Anesth Analg* 63:583, 1984.

[b]Shulman M et al: Postthoracotomy pain and pulmonary function following epidural and systemic morphine. *Anesthesiology* 61:569, 1984.

[c]Camann WR, Loferski BL, Fanciullo GJ: Does epidural administration of butorphanol offer any clinical advantage over intravenous route? *Anesthesiology* 76:216, 1992.

[d]Loper KA et al: Epidural and intravenous fentanyl infusions are clinically equivalent after knee surgery. *Anesth Analg* 70:72, 1990.

[e]Ellis DJ, Millar WA, Reisner LS: A randomized double-blind comparison of epidural versus intravenous fentanyl infusion for analgesia after cesarean section. *Anesthesiology* 72:981, 1990.

[f]Camu F, Debucquoy F: Alfentanil infusion for postoperative pain: A comparison of epidural and intravenous routes. *Anesthesiology* 75:171, 1991.

[g]Geller E et al: A randomized, double-blind comparison of epidural sufentanil versus intravenous sufentanil or epidural fentanyl analgesia after major abdominal surgery. *Anesth Analg* 76:1243, 1993.

[h]Sandler AN et al: A randomized, double-blind comparison of lumbar epidural and intravenous fentanyl infusions for postthoracotomy pain relief. *Anesthesiology* 77:626, 1992.

[i]Salomaki TE, Laitinen JO, Nuutinen LS: A randomized double-blind comparison of epidural versus intravenous fentanyl infusion for analgesia after thoracotomy. *Anesthesiology* 75:790, 1991.

[j]Guinard JP et al: A randomized comparison of intravenous versus lumbar and thoracic epidural fentanyl for analgesia after thoracotomy. *Anesthesiology* 77:1108, 1992.

[k]Grant RP et al: Patient-controlled lumbar epidural fentanyl compared with patient-controlled intravenous fentanyl for postthoracotomy pain relief. *Can J Anaesth* 39:214, 1992.

[l]Benzon HT et al: A randomized double-blind comparison of epidural fentanyl infusion versus patient-controlled analgesia with morphine for postthoracotomy pain. *Anesth Analg* 76:316, 1993.

[m]Allaire PH et al: A prospective randomized comparison of epidural infusion of fentanyl and intravenous administration of morphine by patient-controlled analgesia after radical retropubic prostatectomy. *Mayo Clin Proc* 67:1031, 1992.

[n]Chauvin M, Hongnat JM, Mourgeon E: Equivalence of postoperative analgesia with patient-controlled intravenous or epidural alfentanil. *Anesth Analg* 76:1251, 1993.

[o]Total alfentanil dose was higher in the IV PCA group.

[p]Glass PSA et al: Use of patient-controlled analgesia to compare the efficacy of epidural to intravenous fentanyl administration. *Anesth Analg* 74:345, 1992.

TABLE 7–6 Lumbar versus Thoracic Epidural Placement for Post-thoracotomy Epidural Analgesia

Type of Study	Drug Used	Comparative Efficacy
Retrospective[a]	Morphine, intermittent	Equal
Randomized, blind[b]	Fentanyl, infusion	Equal[c]
Randomized[d]	Fentanyl, infusion	Equal[e]
Randomized[f]	Fentanyl with bupivacaine, infusion	Equal[g]

[a]Fromme GA, Steidl LJ, Danielson DR: Comparison of lumbar and thoracic epidural morphine for relief of postthoracotomy pain. *Anesth Analg* 64:454, 1985.
[b]Coe A et al: Pain following thoracotomy: A randomized, double-blind comparison of lumbar versus thoracic epidural fentanyl. *Anaesthesia* 46:918, 1991.
[c]Total fentanyl requirement was higher in the lumbar group.
[d]Guinard JP et al: A randomized comparison of intravenous versus lumbar and thoracic epidural fentanyl for analgesia after thoracotomy. *Anesthesiology* 77:1108, 1992.
[e]Patients in the thoracic group had earlier recovery of gastrointestinal and pulmonary functions and had shorter hospital stay.
[f]Hurford WE et al: Comparison of thoracic and lumbar epidural infusions of bupivacaine and fentanyl for postthoracotomy analgesia. *J Cardiothorac Vasc Anesth* 7:521, 1993.
[g]Higher infusion rates were needed in the lumbar group to attain comparable analgesia.

References

1. Austin KI, Stapleton JV, Mather LE: Relationship between blood meperidine concentrations and analgesic response. A preliminary report. *Anesthesiology* 53:460, 1980.
2. Gonzalez-Darder JM, Barbera J, Abellan MJ: Effects of prior anaesthesia on autonomy following sciatic transection in rats. *Pain* 24:87, 1986.
3. Woolf CJ, Wall PD: Morphine sensitive and morphine-insensitive actions of C-fibre input on the rat spinal cord. *Neurosci Lett* 64:221, 1986.
4. Graves DA, Foster TS, Batenhorst RL et al: Patient-controlled analgesia. *Ann Intern Med* 99:360, 1983.
5. White PD: Patient-controlled analgesia: A new approach to the management of post-operative pain. *Sem Anesth* 4:255, 1985.
6. Bahar M, Rosen M, Vickers MD: Self-administered nalbuphine morphine and pethidine. Comparison by intravenous route, following cholecystectomy. *Anaesthesia* 40:529, 1985.
7. Sinatra RS, Lodge K, Sibert K et al: A comparison of morphine, meperidine, and oxymorphone as utilized in patient-controlled analgesia following cesarean delivery. *Anesthesiology* 70:585, 1989.
8. Sinatra R, Chung KS, Silverman DG et al: An evaluation of morphine and oxymorphone administered via patient-controlled analgesia (PCA) or PCA plus basal infusion in post-cesarean-delivery. *Anesthesiology* 71:502, 1989.
9. Parker RK, Holtmann B, White PF: Effects of a nighttime opioid infusion with PCA therapy on patient comfort and analgesic requirements after abdominal hysterectomy. *Anesthesiology* 76:362, 1992.
10. Ferrante FM, Orav EJ, Rocco AG et al: A statistical model for pain in patient-controlled analgesia and conventional intramuscular opioid regimens. *Anesth Analg* 67:457, 1988.
11. Eisenach JC, Grice SC, Dewan DM: Patient-controlled analgesia following cesarean section: A comparison between epidural and intramuscular narcotics. *Anesthesiology* 68:444, 1988.
12. Harrison DM, Sinatra R, Morgese L et al: Epidural narcotics and patient-controlled analgesia for post-cesarean section pain relief. *Anesthesiology* 68:454, 1988.
13. Cousins MJ, Mather LE: Intrathecal and epidural administration of opioids. *Anesthesiology* 61:276, 1984.
14. Ready LB, Loper KA, Nessly M et al: Postoperative epidural morphine is safe on surgical wards. *Anesthesiology* 75:452, 1991.
15. Ready LB: Regional anesthesia with intraspinal opioids. In Bonica JJ, editor: *The Management of Pain*, ed 2. Philadelphia, Lea & Febiger, 1990.
16. Rawal N, Sjostrand U, Christoffersson E et al: Comparison of intramuscular and epidural morphine for post-operative analgesia in the grossly obese: Influence on post-operative ambulation and pulmonary function. *Anesth Analg* 63:583, 1984.
17. Shulman M, Sandler AN, Bradley JW et al: Post-thoracotomy pain and pulmonary function following epidural and systemic morphine. *Anesthesiology* 61:569, 1984.
18. Camann WR, Loferski BL, Fanciullo GJ: Does epidural administration of butorphanol offer any clinical advantage over intravenous route? *Anesthesiology* 76:216, 1992.
19. El-Baz NM, Faber P, Jensik RJ: Continuous epidural infusion of morphine for treatment of pain after thoracic surgery: A new technique. *Anesth Analg* 63:757, 1984.
20. Fischer RL, Lubenow TR, Liceaga A et al: Comparison of continuous epidural infusion of fentanyl-bupivacaine and morphine-bupivacaine in management of post-operative pain. *Anesth Analg* 67:559, 1988.
21. Guinard JP, Mavrocordatos P, Chiolero R et al: A randomized comparison of intravenous versus lumbar and thoracic epidural fentanyl for analgesia after thoracotomy. *Anesthesiology* 77:1108, 1992.
22. Yeager MP, Glass DD, Neff RK et al: Epidural anesthesia and analgesia in high-risk surgical patients. *Anesthesiology* 66:729, 1987.
23. Tuman KJ, McCarthy RJ, March RJ et al: Effects of epidural anesthesia and analgesia on coagulation and outcome after major vascular surgery. *Anesth Analg* 73:696, 1991.
24. Jayr C, Thomas H, Rey A et al: Postoperative pulmonary complications: Epidural analgesia using bupivacaine and opioids versus parenteral opioids. *Anesthesiology* 78:666, 1993.
25. Caplan RA, Ready LB, Oden RV et al: Transdermal fentanyl for postoperative pain management: A double-blind placebo study. *JAMA* 261:1036, 1989.
26. Stein C, Comisel K, Haimerl E et al: Analgesic effect of intraarticular morphine after arthroscopic knee surgery. *N Engl J Med* 235:1123, 1991.
27. Clinical Practice Guidelines. Acute pain management: Operative or medical procedures and trauma. Washington, DC, US Department of Health and Human Services Agency for Health Care Policy and Research, 1992.

Questions • Surgery

1. The traditional technique of IM opioid injections at periodic intervals is associated with
   A. High blood levels and effective analgesia
   B. Variable blood levels and inconsistent analgesic responses
   C. Low blood levels and effective analgesia
   D. Low blood levels and ineffective analgesia

2. The attributes of ideal analgesic for PCA include
   A. Slow onset of action and high analgesic efficacy
   B. Rapid onset of action and high analgesic efficacy
   C. Rapid onset of action and low analgesic efficacy
   D. Slow onset of action and low analgesic efficacy

3. Effective postoperative pain control with minimal side effects can be produced by
   A. Intermittent epidural morphine
   B. Continuous epidural morphine
   C. Intermittent IV morphine
   D. Intermittent IM morphine

4. Intra-articular morphine (1 mg) can reduce postoperative VAS score and analgesic consumption because there are
   A. Nociceptors in the periphery
   B. Opioid receptors in the periphery
   C. Opioid receptors in the dorsal horn of spinal cord
   D. Opioid receptors in the cranial segment of CNS

5. The Agency for Health Care Policy and Research (AHCPR) in producing clinical practice guidelines for the management of acute pain state that pharmacological management of mild-to-moderate postoperative pain should start with
   A. Low potency opioids
   B. Epidural local anesthetics
   C. Nonsteroidal anti-inflammatory drugs
   D. Epidural narcotics

ANSWERS

1. B

2. B

3. B

4. B

5. C

CHAPTER 8

Obstetrics

JAMES P. RATHMELL, CHRISTOPHER M. VISCOMI, AND IRA M. BERNSTEIN

Pain occurs at some point in nearly all pregnant women. This chapter reviews the potential toxicities associated with medications used in treating pain in the pregnant or breast-feeding mother, discusses many of the conditions that occur with pain during pregnancy, and describes an approach to the evaluation and management of several chronic pain conditions in the pregnant patient.

USE OF MEDICATIONS DURING PREGNANCY

The first tenet in the medical management of the pregnant patient is to minimize the use of all medications and use nonpharmacologic therapies whenever possible. When drug therapy is necessary, the clinician should begin by considering any potential harm to the mother, the fetus, and the course of the pregnancy. With the exception of large polar molecules (such as heparin and insulin), nearly all medications reach the fetus to some degree. The following affect the placental transfer of medications from maternal to fetal circulations:

1. The degree of protein binding and lipid solubility of the medicine
2. The speed of the maternal metabolism
3. The molecular weight

One of the major limitations in evaluating a medication's potential for causing harm to a developing fetus is the degree of species specificity for congenital defects.

The most critical period for minimizing maternal drug exposure is during early development. Drug exposure before organogenesis (before the fourth menstrual week) usually causes an all-or-none effect; either the embryo does not survive or it develops without abnormalities.[1] Drug effects later in pregnancy typically lead to single-organ or multiple-organ involvement, developmental syndromes, or intrauterine growth retardation.[2] Certain medications may not directly influence fetal organ development, but they have the potential to adversely influence the physiology of pregnancy. The present knowledge about the adverse effects of uncontrolled pain and the risks of administering medications during pregnancy remains incomplete, leaving the practitioner to weigh the risks against the benefits of drug therapy with each person.

USE OF MEDICATIONS IN THE BREAST-FEEDING MOTHER

High lipid solubility, low molecular weight, minimal protein binding, and the deionized state all facilitate the excretion of medications into breast milk. The neonatal dose of most medications obtained through breast-feeding is 1% to 2% of the maternal dose.[3] Even with minimal exposure via breast milk, neonatal drug allergy and slower infant drug metabolism must be considered.[4]

Most breast milk is synthesized and excreted during and immediately following breast-feeding. Taking medications after breast-feeding or during times when the infant has the longest interval between feedings and avoiding any long-acting medications minimize drug transfer via breast milk.[5] However, the effective treatment of pain often requires the use of long-acting medications. The American Academy of Pediatrics has categorized medications in relation to the safety of ingestion by breast-feeding mothers[6] (see Table 8–1).

MEDICATIONS COMMONLY USED IN PAIN MANAGEMENT

Nonsteroidal Anti-inflammatory Drugs (NSAIDs)

Aspirin remains the prototypical NSAID and is the most thoroughly studied of this class of medications. The results of the Collaborative Perinatal Project suggest that first-trimester exposure to aspirin does not pose appreciable teratogenic risk.[7] Prostaglandins appear to trigger labor, and the aspirin-induced inhibition of prostaglandin synthesis may result in prolonged gestation and protracted labor.[2]

Aspirin has well-known platelet-inhibiting properties and, theoretically, may increase the risk of peripartum hemorrhage. Neonatal platelet function is inhibited for up to 5 days after delivery in aspirin-treated mothers.[8] Although low-dose aspirin therapy (60 to 150 mg/day) has not been associated with maternal or neonatal complications, higher doses appear to increase the risk of intracranial hemorrhage in neonates born before 35 weeks' gestation.[9]

Circulating prostaglandins modulate the patency of the fetus ductus arteriosus. NSAIDs have been used therapeutically in neonates with persistent fetal circulation to induce closure of the ductus arteriosus via inhibition of

TABLE 8–1 Classification of Maternal Medication Use During Breast Feeding

	Definition	Examples
Category 1	These medications should not be consumed during lactation. Strong evidence exists that serious adverse effects on the infant are likely with maternal ingestion of these medications during lactation.	Ergotamine.
Category 2	The pharmacologic effects in human infants are unknown, but caution is urged.	Amitriptyline, desipramine, doxepin, fluoxetine, imipramine, trazodone.
Category 3	These medications are compatible with breast-feeding.	Carbamazepine, phenytoin, valproate. Atenolol, propranolol, diltiazem. Codeine, fentanyl, methadone morphine, propoxyphene. Butorphanol. Lidocaine, mexiletine. Acetaminophen. Ibuprofen, indomethacin, ketorolac, naproxen. Caffeine.

prostaglandin synthesis. Patency of the ductus arteriosus *in utero* is essential for normal fetal circulation. Indomethacin has shown promise for the treatment of premature labor,[10] but its use has been linked to antenatal narrowing[11] and closure of the fetal ductus arteriosus.[12]

Ibuprofen has not been linked to congenital defects. The use of ibuprofen during pregnancy may result in reversible oligohydramnios (reflecting diminished fetal urine output) and mild constriction of the fetal ductus arteriosus.[13] Similarly, no data exist to support any association between naproxen administration and congenital defects. Because it shares the renal and vascular effects of ibuprofen, naproxen should be considered to have the potential to diminish ductus arteriosus diameter and to cause oligohydramnios.[9]

Ketorolac is a relatively new NSAID. According to the manufacturer's prescribing information,[14] ketorolac did not cause birth defects in the offspring of pregnant rabbits; however, when administered during labor it did lead to dystocia in rodents. Ketorolac shares the platelet-inhibiting properties of other NSAIDs.[15] Until more information is available, it may be prudent to choose more extensively studied NSAIDs for use during pregnancy.

The use of indomethacin during pregnancy for the treatment of preterm labor has raised concerns regarding potentially serious fetal risks of prolonged prenatal maternal ingestion of NSAIDs. Indomethacin when used for courses as short as two weeks has been associated with neonatal renal failure, persistent pulmonary hypertension of the newborn (PPHN) and neonatal death.[16,17] Even shorter courses have been associated with an increased risk of neonatal necrotizing enterocolitis.[18,19] Additional recent evidence suggests that naproxen, aspirin, and ibuprofen, when taken during pregnancy, can be associated with a significantly increased risk for PPHN.[20,21] Based on this findings it would appear prudent to restrict the use of NSAIDs to the short term relief of pain (i.e., less than 48 hours continuous use) during preterm gestation prior to 32 weeks when the risk of intrauterine ductal narrowing and subsequent compromise of the pulmonary circulation is minimized.[22]

Recommendations for the use of NSAIDs during pregnancy are as follows:

- Consider use of nonpharmacologic management or acetaminophen first.

- Continue aspirin or another NSAID if symptoms cannot be controlled nonpharmacolgically or with acetaminophen.
- Whenever possible, restrict NSAID use to the short term relief of pain (less than 48 hours of continuous use).
- Institute close fetal monitoring during the second trimester. If high doses of NSAID are required, periodic fetal ultrasound, including fetal echocardiography, should be employed to monitor amniotic fluid volume and patency of the ductus arteriosus.
- Discontinue the NSAID after week 32 to reduce the risks of peripartum bleeding, neonatal hemorrhage, and persistent fetal circulation.

In breast-feeding women, salicylate transport into breast milk is limited by its highly ionized state and high degree of protein binding. Caution should be used if more short-term use is contemplated during lactation because neonates have very slow elimination of salicylates.[23] Both ibuprofen and naproxen are also minimally transported into breast milk and are considered compatible with breast-feeding.[6] Little information is available on the safety of maternal ketorolac use during lactation; however, the American Academy of Pediatrics considers ketorolac to be compatible with breast-feeding.[6]

Acetaminophen provides similar analgesia without the anti-inflammatory effects seen in NSAIDs. Acetaminophen has no known teratogenic properties, does not inhibit prostaglandin synthesis or platelet function, and is hepatotoxic only in extreme overdose.[9,24] If persistent pain demands the use of a mild analgesic during pregnancy, acetaminophen appears to be a safe and effective first-choice agent. Acetaminophen does enter breast milk, although maximal neonatal ingestion would be less than 2% of a maternal dose.[25] Acetaminophen is considered compatible with breast-feeding.[6]

Opioid Analgesics

Much of the present knowledge about the effects of chronic opioid exposure during pregnancy comes from studies of opioid-abusing patients.[26–28] Opioids such as heroin are often adulterated with other substances that pose additional health risks. Bacterial and viral infections are often associated with intravenous (IV) drug abuse.

Most studies suggest that methadone maintenance is associated with longer gestation and increased birth weight when compared with outcomes in untreated opioid abusers. No increase in congenital defects has been observed in offspring of methadone-consuming patients. The Food and Drug Administration (FDA) has designated methadone a risk Category B unless the drug is used in high doses near term.

Fentanyl is one of the most common parenteral opioid analgesics administered during the perioperative period. As with all opioid analgesics, administration of fentanyl to the mother immediately before delivery may lead to respiratory depression in the newborn.[29] Maternal administration of fentanyl or other opioids may also cause loss of normal variability in fetal heart rate. Such loss can signal fetal hypoxemia; thus, administration of opioids during labor may deprive obstetrical caregivers of a useful tool for assessing fetal well-being.[30]

Although mixed agonist-antagonist opioid analgesic agents are widely used to provide analgesia during labor, they do not appear to offer any advantage when compared with pure opioid agonists.

Fentanyl, morphine, and hydromorphone are all safe and effective alternatives when a potent opioid is needed for parenteral administration:

1. For mild pain, acetaminophen either alone or in combination with hydrocodone is a good alternative.
2. For moderate pain, oxycodone alone or in combination with acetaminophen is effective.
3. Patients with more severe pain may require morphine or hydromorphone, which are both available for oral administration.

Narcotic analgesics can also be administered into the intrathecal or epidural compartment to provide postoperative analgesia. Such neuraxial administration of hydrophilic agents (e.g., morphine) greatly reduces total postoperative opioid requirements while providing excellent analgesia.[31]

Opioids are excreted into breast milk. Pharmacokinetic analysis has demonstrated that breast milk concentrations of codeine and morphine are equal to or somewhat greater than maternal plasma concentrations.[32] Meperidine use in breast-feeding mothers via patient-controlled analgesia (PCA) resulted in significantly greater neurobehavioral depression of the breast-feeding newborn than equianalgesic doses of morphine.[33] After absorption from the infant's gastrointestinal tract, opioids contained in ingested breast milk undergo glucuronidation to inactive metabolites.[32] Meperidine undergoes N-demethylation to the active metabolite normeperidine.[34] Normeperidine's half-life is markedly prolonged in the newborn,[35] so that regular breast-feeding leads to accumulation and the resultant risks of neurobehavioral depression and seizures. The American Academy of Pediatrics considers use of many opioid analgesics, including codeine, fentanyl, methadone, morphine, and propoxyphene, to be compatible with breast-feeding.[6]

Local Anesthetics

Few studies have focused on the potential teratogenicity of local anesthetic agents. Lidocaine and bupivacaine do not appear to pose significant developmental risk to the fetus. In the Collaborative Perinatal Project,[7] only mepivacaine had any suggestion of teratogenicity; however, the number of patient exposures was inadequate to draw conclusions.

Neither lidocaine nor bupivacaine appear in measurable quantities in the breast milk after epidural local anesthetic administration during labor.[36] IV infusion of high doses (2 to 4 mg/min) of lidocaine for suppression of cardiac arrhythmias led to minimal levels in breast milk.[37] Based on these observations, continuous epidural infusion of dilute local anesthetic solutions for postoperative analgesia should result in only small quantities of drug actually reaching the fetus. The American Academy of Pediatrics considers local anesthetics to be safe for use in the nursing mother.[6]

Mexiletine is a newer, orally active, antiarrhythmic agent with structural and pharmacologic properties similar to those of lidocaine. This agent has shown promise in the treatment of neuropathic pain. Mexiletine is lipid soluble and freely crosses the placenta. Mexiletine appears to be concentrated in breast milk; however, based on expected breast milk concentrations and average daily intake of breast milk, the infant would receive only a small fraction of the usual pediatric maintenance does of mexiletine.[38] Mexiletine is rated risk Category C by the FDA, and it should be used cautiously during pregnancy. The American Academy of Pediatrics considers mexiletine use to be compatible with breast-feeding.[6]

Steroids

Most corticosteroids cross the placenta, although prednisone and prednisolone are inactivated by the placenta.[2] The use of corticosteroids during a limited trial of epidural steroid therapy in the pregnant patient probably poses minimal fetal risk.

In the mother who is breast-feeding, less than 1% of a maternal prednisone dose appears in the nursing infant over the next 3 days.[39] This amount of steroid exposure is unlikely to impact infant endogenous cortisol secretion.[39]

Benzodiazepines

Benzodiazepines are among the most frequently prescribed of all drugs and are often used as anxiolytic agents, as sleep aids in patients with insomnia, and as skeletal muscle relaxants in patients with chronic pain.[40] First-trimester exposure to benzodiazepines may be associated with an increased risk of congenital malformations. Diazepam may be associated with cleft lip, cleft palate,[41] and congenital inguinal hernia.[42]

In the breast-feeding mother, diazepam and its metabolite desmethyldiazepam can be detected in infant serum for up to 10 days after a single maternal dose. This is due to the slower metabolism in neonates than in adults.[43] Clinically, infants who are nursing from mothers receiving diazepam may show sedation and poor feeding.[43] It appears most prudent to avoid any use of benzodiazepines during organogenesis, near the time of delivery, and during lactation.

Antidepressants

Antidepressants are often employed in the management of migraine headaches and for analgesic and antidepressant purposes in chronic pain states. Amitriptyline, nortriptyline, and imipramine are all rated risk Category D by the FDA. The selective serotonin reuptake inhibitors (SSRIs) fluoxetine and paroxetine are rated FDA risk Category B. Desipramine and all other conventional antidepressant medications are Category C.[44]

The American Academy of Pediatrics considers antidepressants to have unknown risk during lactation.[6]

Anticonvulsants

Most data regarding the fetal risk of major malformation in women taking anticonvulsants are derived from the women receiving phenytoin, carbamazepine, or valproic acid; the risk of a congenital defect was approximately 5%[45] or twice that of the general population. Neural tube defects and, to a lesser extent, cardiac abnormalities predominate in the offspring of women taking carbamazepine and valproic acid[46] and can be detected during routine prenatal screening (elevated α-fetoprotein level).

The *fetal hydantoin syndrome* has been associated with phenytoin, carbamazepine, and valproate use during pregnancy; the syndrome consists of variable dysmorphic features, including microcephaly, mental deficiency, and craniofacial abnormalities.[46] The appearance of this syndrome may be predicted either by fetal genetic screening[47] or by measuring amniocyte levels of the enzyme responsible for phenytoin metabolism.[48] Although anticonvulsants have teratogenic risk, epilepsy may be partially responsible for fetal malformations.[46] Perhaps pregnant women taking anticonvulsants for chronic pain have a lower risk of fetal malformations than patients taking the same medications for seizure control.

For patients contemplating childbearing who are receiving anticonvulsants, their pharmacologic therapy should be critically evaluated. Women who are taking anticonvulsants for neuropathic pain should strongly consider discontinuation during pregnancy, particularly during the first trimester. Consultation with a perinatologist is recommended if continued use of anticonvulsants during pregnancy is considered. Frequent monitoring of serum anticonvulsant levels and folate supplementation should be initiated, and maternal α-fetoprotein screening may be considered to detect fetal neural tube defects.

The use of anticonvulsants during lactation does not seem to be harmful to infants. Phenytoin, carbamazepine, and valproic acid appear in small amounts in breast milk, but no adverse effects have been noted.[9]

Ergot Alkaloids

Ergotamine can have significant therapeutic efficacy in the episodic treatment of migraine headaches. However, even low doses of ergotamine are associated with significant teratogenic risk, and higher doses have caused uterine contractions and abortions.[44] During lactation, ergot alkaloids are associated with neonatal convulsions and severe gastrointestinal disturbances.[9] Occasionally, methergonovine is systemically administered to treat uterine atony and maternal hemorrhage immediately after delivery. This brief exposure does not contraindicate breast-feeding.[49]

Caffeine

Caffeine is often used in combination analgesics for the management of vascular headaches. It has been found that there are no added risks with moderate caffeine ingestion, although ingestion of more than 300 mg/day was associated with decreased birth weight.[50] Caffeine ingestion combined with tobacco use increases the risk for delivery of a low-birth-weight infant.[51]

Ingestion of modest doses of caffeine (100 mg/m^2, a dose similar to that found in 2 cups of brewed coffee) in caffeine-naïve subjects produces modest cardiovascular changes in both mother and fetus, including increased maternal heart rate and mean arterial pressure, increased peak aortic flow velocities, and decreased fetal heart rate.[52] Caffeine ingestion is also associated with an increased incidence of tachyarrhythmias in the newborn. Many over-the-counter analgesic formulations contain caffeine (from 30 to 65 mg per dose), and one must consider the use of these preparations when determining total caffeine exposure.

Moderate ingestion of caffeine during lactation does not appear to affect the infant. However, excessive use may cause increased wakefulness and irritability in the infant.[53]

Sumatriptan

Sumatriptan is a selective serotonin agonist that has achieved widespread use because of its efficacy in the abortive therapy of migraine headaches. The limited data available in humans have not demonstrated any strong teratogenic effects.[44,54] Glaxo-Wellcome established a registry to prospectively evaluate the risk of sumatriptan use during pregnancy in 1996.[55] At the time of this writing, 124 pregnant women had early exposure to sumatriptan, with a 4% birth defect rate. This is close to the expected rate in the general population, and no particular clustering of defects has been noted. Sumatriptan is labeled risk Category C by the FDA.

Beta Blockers

Propranolol and other beta blockers are used in chronic prophylaxis against migraine and nonmigraine vascular headaches. There is no evidence that propranolol is teratogenic. Fetal effects that are noted with maternal consumption of propranolol include decreased weight, potentially because of a modest decrease in maternal cardiac output with consequent diminished placental perfusion.[56]

In the lactating mother, propranolol doses of up to 240 mg/day appear to have minimal neonatal effects.

EVALUATION AND TREATMENT OF PAIN DURING PREGNANCY

Often, severe pain arises from an extreme form of one of the more common musculoskeletal pain syndromes of pregnancy. Thus, a working knowledge of the painful musculoskeletal conditions that occur during pregnancy is essential. Evaluation of back pain and migraine headaches is also needed, because these are among the most common problems encountered in practice.

Musculoskeletal Consideration

Abdominal Wall and Ligamentous Pain

Pain in the abdomen brings pregnant woman to the obstetrician early. In most cases, the problem is not serious and diagnosis is based on the physical examination alone. One of the most common causes of abdominal pain early in pregnancy

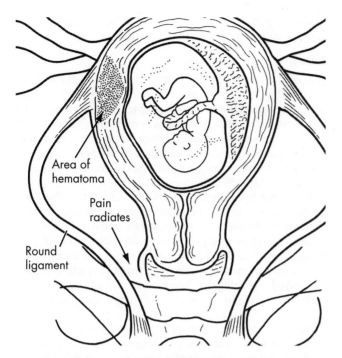

FIG. 8–1 Abdominal pain arising from stretch and hematoma formation in the round ligament typically presents between 16 and 20 weeks' gestation with pain and tenderness over the round ligament, which radiates to the pubic symphysis.

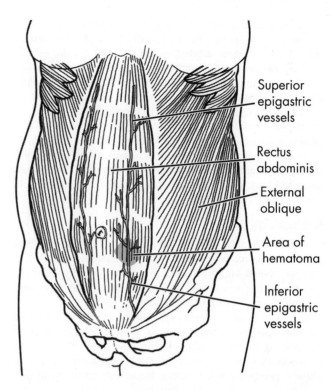

FIG. 8–2 Stretch of the abdominal wall in pregnancy can lead to tearing of the rectus abdominis muscle or inferior epigastric veins and formation of a painful hematoma within the rectus sheath. Pain is well localized and can be severe, often started after a bout of coughing or sneezing.

is miscarriage, which appears as abdominal pain and bleeding. Unruptured ectopic pregnancy and ovarian torsion may be seen with vague hypogastric pain and suprapubic tenderness. Once these conditions that require the immediate attention of the obstetrician are ruled out, myofascial causes of abdominal pain should be considered.

The round ligaments stretch as the uterus rises in the abdomen. If the pull is too rapid, small hematomas may develop in the ligaments (Fig. 8–1). Treatment consists of bed rest and local warmth along with oral analgesics in more severe cases.

Less common is abdominal pain arising from hematoma formation within the sheath of the rectus abdominis muscle (Fig. 8–2). As the uterus expands, the muscles of the abdominal wall become greatly overstretched. Rarely, the rectus abdominis may dehisce, or the inferior epigastric veins may rupture behind the muscles. Conservative management with bed rest, local heat, and mild analgesics is often all that is needed.

Hip Pain

Two relatively rare conditions—osteonecrosis and transient osteoporosis of the hip—both occur with somewhat greater frequency during pregnancy.[57] High levels of estrogen and progesterone in the maternal circulation and increased interosseous pressure may contribute to the development of osteonecrosis.[58] Transient osteoporosis of the hip is a rare disorder characterized by pain and limitation of motion of the hip and osteopenia of the femoral head.[59]

Both conditions are managed symptomatically during pregnancy. Limited weight bearing is essential in transient osteoporosis of the hip to avoid fracture of the femoral neck.[59]

Posterior Pelvic Pain and Back Pain
Etiology and Clinical Presentation

The hormonal changes that occur during pregnancy lead to widening and increasing mobility of the sacroiliac synchondroses and the symphysis pubis as early as the 10th to 12th weeks of pregnancy. This type of pain is often described by pregnant women and is located in the posterior part of the pelvis distal and lateral to the lumbosacral junction.[60] The pain radiates to the posterior part of the thigh and may extend below the knee, often resulting in misinterpretation as sciatica. The pain is less specific than sciatica in distribution and does not extend to the ankle or foot. Differentiating back problems from posterior pelvic problems is a challenge, but typical signs and symptoms of posterior pelvic pain are[60]:

- A history of time-related and weight-bearing-related pain in the posterior pelvis, deep to the gluteal area
- A positive "posterior pelvic pain provocation test"
- A pain drawing with well-defined markings of stabbing in the buttocks distal and lateral to the L5-S1 area, with or without radiation to the posterior thigh or knee but not into the foot
- Free movements in the hips and spine and no nerve root symptoms
- Pain when the patient is turning in bed[60]

Back pain occurs at some time in about 50% of pregnant women[61-63] and is also so common that it is often seen as a normal part of pregnancy. The lumbar lordosis becomes markedly accentuated during pregnancy and may contribute to the development of low back pain.[64] Endocrine changes during pregnancy may also play a role in the development of back pain. Relaxin, a polypeptide secreted by the corpus luteum, softens the ligaments around the pelvic joints and cervix, allowing accommodation of the developing fetus and facilitating vaginal delivery. This laxity may cause pain by producing an exaggerated range of motion.[65]

Ostgaard and co-workers[63] prospectively followed 855 pregnant women from the 12th week of gestation until childbirth. Back pain occurred in 49% of women at some point during the average 28 weeks of the observation. The authors classified back pain into three groups: sacroiliac, high back, and low back (Fig. 8–3).

Evaluation

Evaluation begins with a thorough history that often points the clinician to other causes.[65] Physical examination should include complete back and neurologic evaluations. Particular attention should be directed toward the pelvis and sacroiliac joint during the examination.

Electrophysiologic tests including electromyography and peripheral nerve conduction velocity studies provide good screening tests of the patient with new onset of low back pain accompanied by sensory or motor symptoms. When the clinical presentation is unclear, these tests can help to differentiate peripheral nerve lesions, polyneuropathies, and plexopathies from single radiculopathies.

Prevention and Treatment

Few of the commonly used strategies to prevent low back pain during pregnancy are universally effective. Patients who were instructed in basic lifting techniques experienced significantly less backache than a control group who did not receive similar instruction.[61] Aerobic exercise can be prescribed safely throughout pregnancy,[66] but maintenance of good physical shape may not alter the incidence of back pain during pregnancy.[67]

Treatment begins with counseling the patient about the common causes of back pain during pregnancy. Reassurance and simple changes in the patient's activity level often suffice to reduce symptoms to a tolerable level. If pain remains poorly controlled, referral to a physical therapist for evaluation and instruction on body mechanics and low back pain may be beneficial.[68] Aquatic exercise programs can be particularly helpful, as well as massage and the surface application of heat or ice.[69]

Although rigorous clinical trials are lacking, transcutaneous electrical nerve stimulation (TENS) appears to produce clinically meaningful pain relief in a variety of painful disorders in which pain has a limited distribution.[70,71]

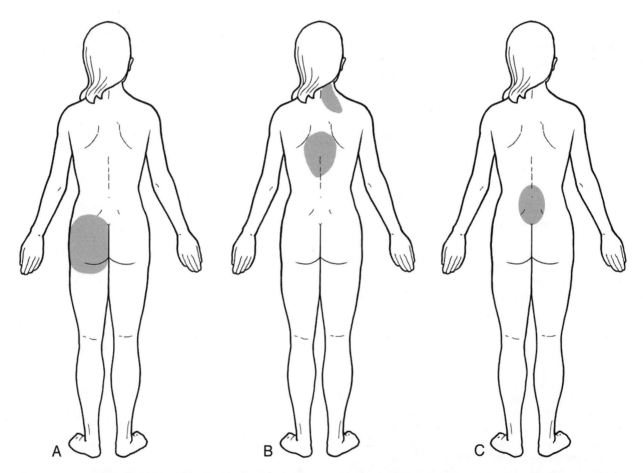

FIG. 8–3 Three types of pain were reported by a group of 855 women studied between 12 menstrual weeks of pregnancy and delivery. Forty-nine percent of the women reported back pain at some point during pregnancy: *A,* Sacroiliac pain by 50%; *B,* High back pain by 10%; *C,* Low back pain by 40%. *(Redrawn from Ostgaard HC, Andersson GBJ, Karlsson K: Prevalence of back pain in pregnancy. Spine 16:549, 1991).*

For posterior pelvic pain of sacroiliac origin, Daly and associates[72] described the successful treatment of 91% of women using rotational manipulation of the sacroiliac joint. Some pain relief was reported by most women with posterior pelvic pain who used a nonelastic trochanteric belt (Fig. 8–4).[60]

Although the incidence of herniated nucleus pulposus during pregnancy is low, radicular symptoms are common and often accompany sacroiliac subluxation and myofascial pain syndromes. The strongest evidence for efficacy of epidural steroids appears to be in patients with symptoms attributable to disk pathology.[73] Although the risk to the fetus after a single dose of epidural corticosteroid appears to be low, it is our opinion that epidural steroids should be reserved for the parturient with the new onset of signs and symptoms consistent with lumbar nerve root compression.

Acetaminophen is the first analgesic to consider for management of minor back pain. The use of NSAIDs during pregnancy remains controversial. Short-term use of ibuprofen and naproxen appears to be safe during the first and second trimesters.[9] Severe back pain may require treatment with narcotics and necessitate hospital admission for parenteral administration of opioid analgesics.

Migraine Headache

Etiology and Clinical Presentation

Nearly 25% of women suffer from migraine headaches,[74] with the peak period incidence during childbearing years. Migraines occur more often during menstruation, which has been attributed to a sudden decline in estrogen levels.[75]

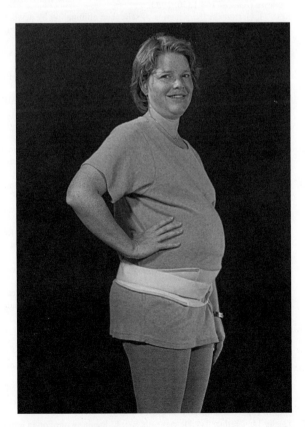

FIG. 8–4 Proper placement of a trochanteric belt to stabilize painful pelvic joints and decrease back pain.

During pregnancy, a sustained 50- to 100-fold increase in estradiol occurs. Indeed, 70% of woman report improvement or remission during pregnancy.[44]

Migraine headaches rarely begin during pregnancy. Many clinicians believe that initial presentation of headaches during pregnancy should signal the need for a thorough search for potentially serious causes.[44,76]

Evaluation

Patients who have their first severe headache during pregnancy should receive a complete neurologic examination and should be strongly considered for magnetic resonance imaging (MRI), toxicology screen, and serum coagulation profiles. In the patient who has sudden onset of the "worst headache of my life," a subarachnoid hemorrhage should be ruled out.[44] Progressively worsening headaches in the setting of sudden weight gain should suggest preeclampsia or pseudotumor cerebri.

Treatment and Prevention

For pregnant women with a history of migraines before pregnancy and normal neurologic findings, the therapeutic challenge is to achieve control of the headaches while minimizing risk to the fetus. Nonpharmacologic techniques, including relaxation, biofeedback, and elimination of certain foods, often suffice for treatment.

If pharmacologic therapy appears warranted, acetaminophen with or without caffeine is safe and effective.[77] Ibuprofen and naproxen appear to be safe for use during the first two trimesters.[9] The short-term use of mild opioid analgesics, such as hydrocodone alone or in combination with acetaminophen, also appears to carry little risk. When oral analgesics prove ineffective, hospital admission and administration of parenteral opioids may be required.

A history of three to four incapacitating headaches per month warrants consideration of prophylactic therapy.[77] Daily oral propranolol or atenolol is a reasonable choice, although patients should understand that its use is associated with small-for-gestational-age infants.

Sickle Cell Disease

Etiology and Clinical Presentation

Sickle cell disease is an inherited multisystem disorder. The presence of abnormal hemoglobin within red blood cells leads to the cardinal features of the disease—chronic hemolytic anemia and recurrent painful episodes. Vaso-occlusive crises are the most common maternal complication noted in parturients with sickle cell hemoglobinopathy.[78] Vaso-occlusive crises follow a characteristic pattern of recurrent sudden attacks of pain, usually involving the abdomen, vertebrae, and extremities.

Most crises during pregnancy are vaso-occlusive and are often precipitated by urinary tract infection, preeclampsia or eclampsia, thrombophlebitis, or pneumonia. Clinically, the individual describes the pain in the bones or joints but may also perceive pain in the soft tissue. Visceral pain is also common and may be related to events in the liver or spleen.

Evaluation

Because laboratory evaluation is nonspecific, diagnosis of vaso-occlusive crisis begins with excluding other causes for the painful episode, particularly occult infections.[78]

Complete assessment of the acute management of sickle cell crisis in pregnancy has been reviewed by Martin and colleagues.[79]

Treatment

Management of vaso-occlusive crisis during pregnancy is primarily supportive and symptomatic. General management begins with aggressive hydration to increase intravascular volume and decrease blood viscosity.[79] Supplemental oxygen is essential in those patients with hypoxemia. Partial exchange transfusions to reduce polymerized hemoglobin S remain an integral part of the management of sickle cell disease[80]; prophylactic transfusion may reduce the incidence of severe sickling complications during pregnancy.[81]

Educating the patient on how pregnancy interacts with sickle cell disease can help to reduce depression or anxiety, which often decreases the pain that the patient is experiencing. Biofeedback has been shown to reduce pain of sickle cell crisis and the number of days that analgesics were needed.[82] Physical therapy techniques can also be helpful.[83] TENS may be helpful when pain is isolated to a limited region.[84]

The severity of pain dictates the pharmacologic approach to managing sickle cell pain. Although nonopioid analgesics may suffice, oral or parenteral opioids are often required. Acetaminophen remains the nonopioid analgesic of choice during pregnancy.

For the hospitalized patient with severe sickle cell pain, potent opioid analgesics administered intravenously may be necessary to adequately control pain. Morphine sulfate is well tolerated and effective for the control of severe sickle cell pain.[85]

SUMMARY

Many physicians are apprehensive about treating pain in pregnant patients. Evaluation and treatment are limited by the relative contraindication of radiography in the evaluation and the risks associated with pharmacologic therapy during pregnancy. Nonetheless, familiarity with common pain problems and the maternal and fetal risks of pain medications can allow the pain practitioner to help women achieve a more comfortable pregnancy. A single health care provider should be designated to coordinate specialist evaluations and integrate their suggestions into an individual, integrated plan of care.

References

1. Rice SA: Anesthesia in pregnancy and the fetus: toxicology aspects. In Reynolds F, editor: *Effects on the baby of maternal analgesia and anaesthesia.* London, WB Saunders, 1993.
2. Niebyl JR: Nonanesthetic drugs during pregnancy and lactation. In Chestnut DH, editor: *Obstetric anesthesia: Principles and practice.* St. Louis, Mosby, 1994.
3. American Academy of Pediatrics Committee on Drugs: The transfer of drugs and other chemicals into human milk. *Pediatrics* 84:924, 1989.
4. Berlin CM: Pharmacological considerations of drug use in the lactating mother. *Obstet Gynecol* 58:175, 1981.
5. Verger H: Drug excretion in breast milk. *Post Grad Med J* 56:97, 1974.
6. American Academy of Pediatrics Committee on Drugs: The transfer of drugs and other chemicals into human milk. *Pediatrics* 93:137, 1994.
7. Slone D, Siskind V, Heinonen OP et al: Aspirin and congenital malformations. *Lancet* 1(7974):1373, 1976.
8. Stuart MJ, Gross SJ, Elrad H et al: Effects of acetylsalicylic acid injection on maternal and neonatal hemostasis. *N Engl J Med* 307:909, 1982.
9. Briggs GG, Freeman RK, Yaffe SJ: *Drugs in pregnancy and lactation.* Baltimore, Williams & Wilkins, 1994.
10. Niebyl JR, Blake DA, White RD et al: The inhibition of premature labor with indomethacin. *Am J Obstet Gynecol* 136:1024, 1980.
11. Moise KJ Jr, Huhta JC, Sharif DS et al: Indomethacin in the treatment of premature labor: Effects on the fetal ductus arteriosus. *N Engl J Med* 319:327, 1988.
12. Leal SD, Cavalle-Garrido T, Ryan G et al: Isolated ductal closure in utero diagnosed by fetal echocardiography. *Am J Perinatol* 14:205, 1997.
13. Hennessey MD, Livingston ED: The incidence of ductal constriction and oligohydramnios during tocolytic therapy with ibuprofen (abstract). *Am J Obstet Gynecol* 166:324, 1992.
14. Syntex Laboratories, Palo Alto, Calif, 1997.
15. Dordoni PL, Della Ventura M, Stefanelli A et al: Effect of ketorolac, ketoprofen, and nefopam on platelet function. *Anaesthesia* 49:1046, 1994.
16. van der Heijden B, Carlus C, Narcy F et al: Persistent anuria, neonatal death, and renal microcystic lesions after prenatal exposure to indomethacin. *Am J Obstet Gynecol* 171:617, 1994.
17. Besinger RE, Niebyl JR, Keyes WG, Johnson TRB: Randomized comparative trial of indomethacin and ritodrine for the long-term treatment of preterm labor. *Am J Obstet Gynecol* 164:981, 1991.
18. Major CA, Lewis DF, Harding JA et al: Tocolysis with indomethacin increases the incidence of necrotizing enterocolitis in the low-birth-weight neonate. *Am J Obstet Gynecol* 170:102, 1994.
19. Norton ME, Merrill J, Cooper BA et al: Neonatal complications after the administration of indomethacin for preterm labor. *N Engl J Med* 329:1602, 1993.
20. Van Marter LJ, Leviton A, Allred EN et al: Persistent pulmonary hypertension of the newborn and smoking and aspirin and nonsteroidal anti-inflammatory drug consumption during pregnancy. *Pediatrics* 97:658, 1996.
21. Alano MA, Ngougmna E, Ostrea EM Jr, Konduri GG. Analysis of nonsteroidal antiinflammatory drugs in meconium and its relation to persistent pulmonary hypertension of the newborn. *Pediatrics* 107:519, 2001.
22. Moise KJ. Effect of advancing gestational age on the frequency of fetal ductal constriction in association with maternal indomethacin use. *Am J Obstet Gynecol* 168:1350, 1993.
23. Levy G, Garrettson JK: Kinetics of salicylate elimination by newborn infants of mothers who ingested aspirin before delivery. *Pediatrics* 62:201, 1974.
24. IARC: Paracetamol (acetaminophen). *IARC Monogr Eval Carcinog Risks Hum* 50:307, 1990.
25. Notorianni LJ, Oldham HG: Passage of paracetamol into human milk. *Br J Clin Pharmacol* 24:63, 1987.
26. MacGregor SN: Drug addiction and pregnancy. In Dilts PV, Sciarra JJ, editors: *Gynecology and Obstetrics.* Philadelphia, JB Lippincott, 1976.
27. Zelson M, Lee SJ, Casalino M: Neonatal narcotic addition. *N Engl J Med* 289:1216, 1973.
28. Strauss ME, Andresko M, Stryker JC et al: Methadone maintenance during pregnancy: Pregnancy, birth and neonate characteristics. *Am J Obstet Gynecol* 120:895, 1974.
29. Carrie LES, O'Sullivan CM, Seegobin R: Epidural fentanyl in labour. *Anaesthesia* 36:965, 1981.
30. Rayburn W, Rathke A, Leuschen MP et al: Fentanyl citrate analgesia during labor. *Am J Obstet Gynecol* 161:202, 1989.
31. Eisenach JC, Grice SC, Dewan DW: Patient controlled analgesia following cesarean delivery: A comparison with epidural and intramuscular narcotics. *Anesthesiology* 68:444, 1988.
32. Finlay JW, DeAngelis RL, Kearney MF et al: Analgesic drugs in breast milk and plasma. *Clin Pharmacol Ther* 29:625, 1981.
33. Wittels B, Scott DT, Sinatra RS: Exogenous opioids in human breast milk and acute neonatal neurobehavior: A preliminary study. *Anesthesiology* 73:864, 1990.
34. O'Donoghue SEF: Distribution of pethidine and chlorpromazine in maternal, fetal and neonatal biologic fluids. *Nature* 229:124, 1971.
35. Kuhnert BR, Kuhnert PA, Philipson EH, Syracuse CD: Disposition of meperidine and normeperidine following multiple doses in labor. *Am J Obstet Gynecol* 151:410, 1985.
36. Dailland P: Analgesia and anesthesia and breast feeding. In Reynolds F, editor: *Effects on the baby of maternal analgesia and anaesthesia.* London, WB Saunders, 1993.
37. Zeisler JA, Gardner TD, DeMesquita SA: Lidocaine excretion in breast milk. *Drug Intell Clin Pharm* 20:691, 1986.

38. Lewis AM, Patel L, Johnston A et al: Mexiletine in human blood and breast milk. *Postgrad Med J* 57:546, 1981.
39. Katz FH, Duncan BR: Entry of prednisone into human milk. *N Engl J Med* 293:1154, 1975.
40. Dellemijn PLI, Fields H: Do benzodiazepines have a role in chronic pain management? *Pain* 57:137, 1994.
41. Safra MJ, Oakley GP Jr: Association between cleft lip with and without cleft palate and prenatal exposure to diazepam. *Lancet* 2(7933):47, 1975.
42. Laegreid L et al: Abnormalities in children exposed to benzodiazepines in utero. *Lancet* 1(8524):108, 1987.
43. Erkkola R, Kanto J: Diazepam and breast feeding. *Lancet* 1(7762):1235, 1972.
44. Hainline B: Neurologic complications of pregnancy: Headache. *Neurol Clin* 12:443, 1994.
45. Speidel BD, Meadow SR: Maternal epilepsy and abnormalities of the fetus and newborn. *Lancet* 2(7782):839, 1972.
46. Yerby MS: Pregnancy, teratogenesis, and epilepsy. *Neurol Clin* 12:749, 1994.
47. Strickler SM, Dansky LV, Miller MA et al: Genetic predisposition to phenytoin-induced birth defects. *Lancet* 2(8458):746, 1985.
48. Buehler BA, Delimont D, Van Waes M, Finnell RH: Prenatal prediction of the risk of the fetal hydantoin syndrome. *N Engl J Med* 322:1567, 1990.
49. Del Pozo E, Brun Del Re R, Hindselmann M: Lack of effects of methergonavine on postpartum breast lactation. *Am J Obstet Gynecol* 123:845, 1975.
50. Martin TR, Bracken MB: The association between low birth weight and caffeine consumption during pregnancy. *Am J Epidemiol* 126:813, 1987.
51. Beaulac-Baillargeon L, Desrosiers C: Caffeine-cigarette interaction on fetal growth. *Am J Obstet Gynecol* 157:1236, 1987.
52. Miller RC, Watson WJ, Hackney AC, Seeds JW: Acute maternal and fetal cardiovascular effects of caffeine ingestion. *Am J Perinatol* 11:132, 1994.
53. Findlay JWA, Deangelis RL, Kearney MF et al: Analgesic drugs in breast milk and plasma. *Clin Pharmacol Ther* 29:625, 1981.
54. Humphrey PPA, Feniuk W, Marriott AS et al: Pre-clinical studies on the anti-migraine drug, sumatriptan. *Eur Neurol* 31:282, 1991.
55. Eldridge R, Senior Pregnancy Registry Monitor. Personal communication, 1997.
56. Pruyn SC, Phelan JP, Buchanan GC: Long term propranolol therapy in pregnancy: Maternal and fetal outcome. *Am J Obstet Gynecol* 135:485, 1979.
57. Heckma JD, Sassard R: Musculoskeletal considerations in pregnancy. *BMJ* 302:1390, 1991.
58. Hungerford DS, Lennox DW: The importance of increased interosseous pressure in the development of osteonecrosis of the femoral head: Implications for treatment. *Orthop Clin North Am* 16:635, 1985.
59. Bruinsma BJ, LaBan MM: The ghost joint: Transient osteoporosis of the hip. *Arch Phys Med Rehabil* 71:295, 1990.
60. Ostgaard HC, Zetherstrom G, Roos-Hansson E et al: Reduction of back and posterior pelvic pain in pregnancy. *Spine* 19:894, 1994.
61. Mantle MJ, Holmes J, Currey HLF: Backache in pregnancy: II. Prophylactic influence of back care classes. *Rheum Rehabil* 20:227, 1981.
62. Fast A, Shapiro D, Ducommun EJ et al: Low back pain in pregnancy. *Spine* 12:368, 1987.
63. Ostgaard HC, Andersson GBJ, Karlsson K: Prevalence of back pain in pregnancy. *Spine* 16:549, 1991.
64. MacEvilly M, Buggy D: back pain and pregnancy: A review. *Pain* 64:405, 1996.
65. Rungee JL: Low back pain during pregnancy. *Orthopedics* 16:1339, 1993.
66. Wolfe LA, Hall P, Webb KA et al: Prescription of aerobic exercise during pregnancy. *Sports Med* 8:273, 1989.
67. Berg G, Hammar M, Moller-Nielsen J. et al: Low back pain during pregnancy. *Obstet Gynecol* 71:71, 1988.
68. Gleeson PB, Pauls JA: Obstetrical physical therapy. *Phys Ther* 68:1699, 1988.
69. Pauls JA: *Therapeutic approaches to women's health: a program exercise and education.* Gaithersburg, Md, Aspen, 1995.
70. Robinson AJ: Transcutaneous electrical nerve stimulation for control of pain in musculoskeletal disorders. *J Orthop Sports Phys Ther* 24:208, 1996.
71. Reeve J, Menon D, Corabian P: Transcutaneous electrical nerve stimulation (TENS): A technology assessment. *J Technol Assess Health Care* 12:299, 1996.
72. Daly JM, Frame PS, Rapoza PA: Sacroiliac subluxation: A common, treatable cause of low-back pain in pregnancy. *Fam Pract Res J* 11:149, 1991.
73. Benzon HT: Epidural steroid injections for low back pain and lumbosacral radiculopathy. *Pain* 24:277, 1986.
74. Rasmussen BK, Rigmor J, Schroll M: Epidemiology of headache in a general population: A prevalence study. *J Clin Epidemiol* 44:1147, 1991.
75. Sommerville BW: The role of estradiol withdrawal in the etiology of menstrual migraine. *Neurology* 22:355, 1972.
76. Chanceller MD, Wroe SJ: Migraine occurring for the first time during pregnancy. *Headache* 30:224, 1990.
77. Silerstein SD: Headaches and women: Treatment of the pregnant and lactating migraineur. *Headache* 33:533, 1993.
78. Powars DR, Sandhu M, Niland-Weiss J et al: Pregnancy in sickle cell disease. *Obstet Gynecol* 67:217, 1986.
79. Martin JN, Martin RW, Morrison JC: Acute management of sickle cell crisis in pregnancy. *Clin Perinatol* 13:853, 1986.
80. Wayne AS, Kevy SV, Nathan DG: Transfusion management of sickle cell disease. *Blood* 81:1109, 1993.
81. Howard RJ, Tuck SM, Pearson TC: Pregnancy in sickle cell disease in the UK: Results of a multicentre survey of the effect of prophylactic blood transfusion on maternal and fetal outcome. *Br J Obstet Gynaecol* 102:947, 1995.
82. Cozzi L, Tyron WW, Sedlaceck K: The effectiveness of biofeedback assisted relaxation in modifying sickle cell crisis. *Biofeedback Self Regul* 12:51, 1987.
83. Alcorn R, Bowser B, Henley EJ et al: Fluidotherapy and exercise in the management of sickle cell anemia. *Phys Ther* 64:1520, 1984.
84. Wang WC, George SL, Wilimas JA: Transcutaneous nerve stimulation treatment of sickle cell pain. *Acta Haematol* 80:99, 1988.
85. Chamberlain G: Medical problems in pregnancy: II. *BMJ* 302:1327, 1991.

1. Codeine, fentanyl, and methadone are considered to be in which of the following categories of maternal medication use during pregnancy

   A. Category 1—These medication should not be consumed
   B. Category 2—The pharmacologic effects in human infants are unknown
   C. Category 3—These medications are compatible with breast-feeding
   D. Category 4—These medications are incompatible with breast-feeding

2. Studies show that methadone maintenance in the mother is associated with

   A. Shorter gestation and increased birth weight
   B. Longer gestation and increased birth weight
   C. Shorter gestation and decreased birth weight
   D. Longer gestation and decreased birth weight

3. Use of which of the following opioids by breast-feeding mothers via PCA depresses the behavior of the infant more than the equianalgesic dose of morphine

   A. Fentanyl
   B. Meperidine
   C. Nubain
   D. Buprenorphine

4. The use of epidural steroid during a limited trial during pregnancy probably poses

   A. Severe fetal risk
   B. Moderate fetal risk
   C. Minimal fetal risk
   D. No fetal risk

5. The hormonal changes that occur during pregnancy lead to widening of the sacroiliac joints and symphysis pubis. After 10 to 12 weeks of pregnancy, posterior pelvic and back pain can occur from this widening. The characteristics of these are all of the following except

   A. Pain radiating to the posterior part of the thigh, often extending below the knee
   B. Pain radiating to the upper thoracic back and shoulders
   C. Pain confined to the perineum
   D. Headache

ANSWERS

1. C

2. B

3. B

4. C

5. A

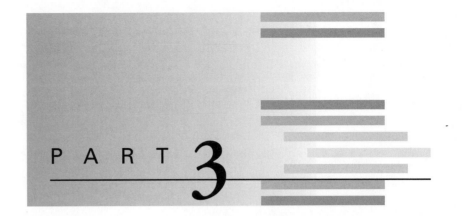

PART 3

Chronic Pain Syndromes

CHAPTER 9

Nociceptive Pain

NICOLAS E. WALSH, SOMAYAJI RAMAMURTY,
TERRENCE M. CALDER, JOHN C. ROWLINGSON,
AND ROBERT J. BURTON, JR

Nociceptive pain originates in tissues other than peripheral and central nervous system (CNS). Common sites are skin, muscles, bones, ligaments, and visceral structures. In this chapter differential diagnosis of neck and shoulder and lower back pain is described, with comments on management rationale.

NECK AND SHOULDER PAIN

The patient complaining of neck, shoulder, and arm pain should be examined for anatomic location of the pain, derangement of mechanical structures, and underlying pathologic conditions. A careful history and examination are required to reach a diagnosis. Laboratory tests and x-ray films may be necessary but may have limited diagnostic value.

The neck and upper extremity are composed of numerous pain-sensitive tissues including nerves, vessels, muscles, ligaments, and joints. Pain may result from irritation, injury, inflammation, or infection of any of these tissues. Conditions causing pain in this region are those of neurogenic, musculoskeletal, soft tissue, referred, and autonomic origin (Box 9–1).

Pain of Neurogenic Origin

Neurogenic pain in the neck and upper extremities may commonly be caused by spinal cord and nerve root compression, myelopathy, postherpetic neuralgia, neuritis, peripheral nerve compression, and peripheral neuropathy.

Pain Caused by Spinal Cord and Nerve Root Compression

Compression at the cervical level characteristically produces spinal and radicular signs in the upper limbs and long tract signs in the lower extremities. Also, the muscles of the shoulder girdle and arms lose power and bulk.

When cord or nerve root compression produces only pain, localization by clinical examination alone is difficult. Myelography, electromyography, computed tomography (CT) scan, magnetic resonance imaging (MRI), or surgical exploration are often more accurate. Pain alone in the neck, shoulder, upper arm, scapula, or interscapular area is nonlocalizing. Most of the lesions in this area involve C5, C6, C7, and C8 nerve roots (Table 9–1).

Objective weakness is much more specific for localizing root level lesions. A C5 nerve root lesion is best located by

---

BOX 9–1 Common Origins of Neck and Upper Extremity Pain

NEUROGENIC PAIN
Cervical spinal cord compression
Nerve root compression
Neuritis
Peripheral nerve compression
Peripheral neuropathy
Torticollis
Herpetic neuralgia
Cervical myelopathy
Neoplasm
Meningitis
Neuroma

SOFT-TISSUE PAIN
Acute cervical strain
Myofascial pain
Fibromyalgia

REFERRED PAIN
Cardiac
Neoplasm
Myofascial pain
Viscera

MUSCULOSKELETAL PAIN
Degenerative joint disease
Tendinitis and bursitis
Cervical spondylosis
Degenerative disk disease
Rheumatoid arthritis
Fracture
Neoplasm
Osteomyelitis

SYMPATHETIC PAIN
Reflex sympathetic dystrophy
Causalgia

---

weakness in the deltoid, supraspinatus, and infraspinatus muscles. This may be tested by abduction and external arm rotation. Weakness of the brachialis and biceps muscle is a result of a C6 nerve root lesion. A C7 nerve root lesion is localized by eliciting weakness primarily in the triceps and to a lesser degree in the flexor carpi ulnaris and radialis, pronator teres, and extensor pollicis longus (see Figs. 9–1 through 9–6).

TABLE 9–1 Sign and Symptoms of Nerve Root Compression of the Cervical Region

Location of Lesion	Referred Pain	Motor Dysfunction	Sensory Dysfunction	Reflex Changes
C5	Shoulder and upper arm	Shoulder muscles (deltoid-supraspinatus infraspinatus) abduction and external rotation	Upper and lateral aspect of the shoulder	Biceps reflex
C6	Radial aspect of forearm	Biceps and brachialis muscles flexion of the elbow and supination wrist extensors	Radial aspect of forearm and thumb	Thumb reflex and brachioradialis reflex
C7	Dorsal aspect of forearm	Triceps muscle extension of the elbow	Index and middle digits	Triceps reflex
C8	Ulnar aspect of forearm	Intrinsics of the hand adduction and abduction	Ring and little digits	No change

Objective hypoesthesia and hypoalgesia in the appropriate dermatomal patterns are useful in localizing nerve root lesions. The deep tendon reflexes mainly depend on the integrity of the reflex arcs; however, testing deep tendon reflexes must be done properly.

Differential Diagnosis

The most common causes of cervical nerve compression are cervical spondylosis, disk degeneration, and acute disk herniation; however, there are numerous other causes. Radicular pain is a shooting, radiating type of pain that is accompanied by objective neurologic signs such as loss of sensation and changes in the reflex and muscle strength. Radiculopathy may be caused by other etiologic factors such as primary or secondary malignancy of the bone, involvement of the nerve root by carcinoma of the lung, and the degenerative changes of the cervical spine. Compression of the spinal cord from a herniated disk may produce symptoms very similar to those of nerve root compression.

Compression of the spinal cord in the neck may result in cervical myelopathy, which produces radicular symptoms in the upper extremities and long tract signs in the lower extremities.

Pain associated with degenerative disk disease may be local and limit neck movement. Pain referred to the upper back, shoulders, and upper extremity suggests that the pathology lies in the intervertebral foramina and the adjacent tissues. Myofascial pain may also produce pain in the neck and arms, but the character of the pain is different.

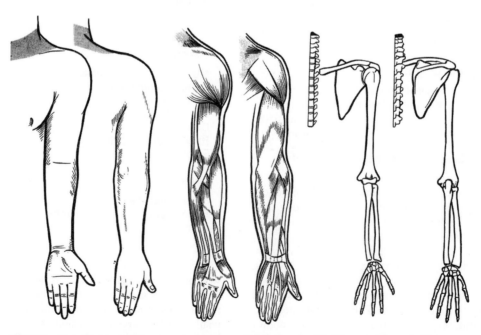

FIG. 9–1 Dermatome, myotome, and sclerotome distribution for C3. Dermatome: neck. Myotome: paraspinals, trapezius, diaphragm. Sclerotome: bones—vertebra and periosteum; joints—facet; ligaments—longitudinal, ligamentum flavum, interspinous. *(From Walsh NE, Ramamurthy S: Neck and upper extremity pain. In Raj PP, editor:* Practical management of pain, *ed 2. St. Louis, Mosby, 1992).*

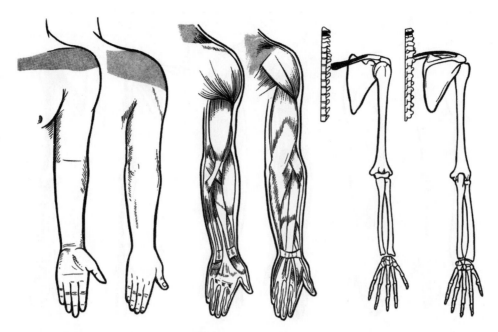

FIG. 9–2 Dermatome, myotome, and sclerotome distribution for C4. Dermatome: shoulder. Myotome: paraspinals, trapezius, diaphragm, scapular abductors. Sclerotome: bones—vertebra and periosteum, clavicle; joints—facet; ligaments—longitudinal, ligamentum flavum, interspinous. *(From Walsh NE, Ramamurthy S: Neck and upper extremity pain. In Raj PP, editor: Practical management of pain, ed 2. St. Louis, Mosby, 1992).*

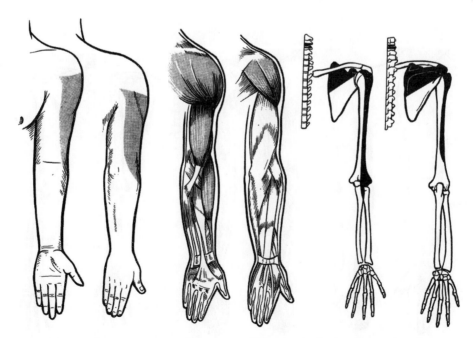

FIG. 9–3 Dermatome, myotome, and sclerotome distribution for C5. Dermatome: lateral arm. Myotome: paraspinals, scapular abductors, scapular elevators, shoulder extensors, shoulder rotators, level flexors. Sclerotome: bones—vertebra and periosteum, scapula, humerus; joints—facet; ligaments—rotator cuff, longitudinal, ligamentum flavum, interspinous. *(From Walsh NE, Ramamurthy S: Neck and upper extremity pain. In Raj PP, editor: Practical management of pain, ed 2. St. Louis, Mosby, 1992).*

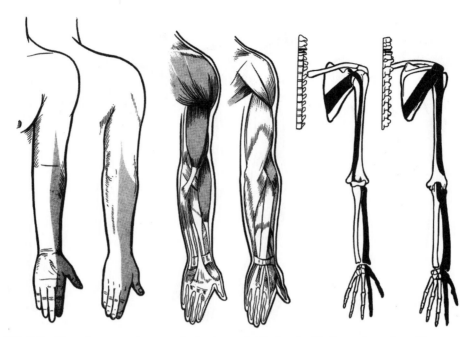

FIG. 9–4 Dermatome, myotome, and sclerotome distribution for C6. Dermatome: lateral forearm, lateral hand. Myotome: paraspinals, level flexors, wrist flexors, pronators, supinators. Sclerotome: bones—scapula, humerus, radius, lateral fingers; joints—facet, shoulder, elbow; ligaments—longitudinal, ligamentum flavum, interspinous. *(From Walsh NE, Ramamurthy S: Neck and upper extremity pain. In Raj PP, editor:* Practical management of pain, *ed 2. St. Louis, Mosby, 1992).*

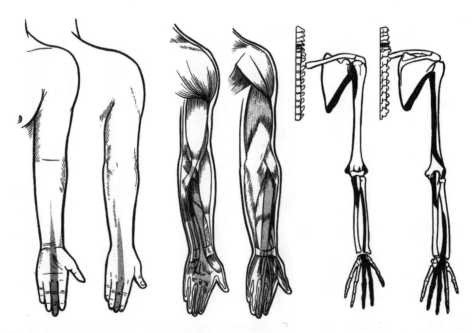

FIG. 9–5 Dermatome, myotome, and sclerotome distribution for C7. Dermatome: midhand, middle finger. Myotome: paraspinals, pronators, elbow, extensor, wrist extensor. Sclerotome: bones—scapula, humerus, radius, ulna, middle fingers; joints—facet, wrist; ligaments—longitudinal, ligamentum flavum, interspinous. *(From Walsh NE, Ramamurthy S: Neck and upper extremity pain. In Raj PP, editor:* Practical management of pain, *ed 2. St. Louis, Mosby, 1992).*

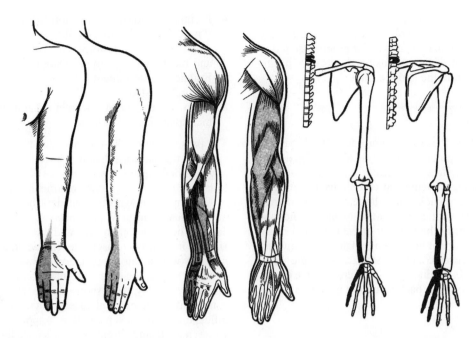

FIG. 9–6 Dermatome, myotome, and sclerotome distribution for C8. Dermatome: medial hand. Myotome: paraspinals, elbow extensors, wrist flexors, grip, finger abduction, finger flexion, finger adduction, finger opposition, finger extension. Sclerotome: bones—vertebra and periosteum, ulna, medial fingers; joints—facet, wrist; ligaments—longitudinal, ligamentum flavum, interspinous. *(From Walsh NE, Ramamurthy S: Neck and upper extremity pain. In Raj PP, editor:* Practical management of pain, *ed 2. St. Louis, Mosby, 1992).*

Investigation

Diagnostic tests may be helpful in differentiating the causes of neck and arm pain, but a thorough neurologic examination is one of the most important ways of making a diagnosis. To localize and establish the nature of lesions causing intraspinal compression, several diagnostic tests may be used. Roentgenographic investigations are the most useful, but electrophysiologic techniques, radioisotope scanning, and cerebrospinal fluid examination may also be helpful.

Management of Suspected Nerve Root and Spinal Cord Compression

A careful history and physical examination are essential for effective physiologic treatment of pain. The examination should ascertain the extent of the pathology and the mechanism of pain. The specific management of intraspinal compression of nerve roots of the cord depends on the suspected diagnosis, the severity of the symptoms, and the extent of the neurologic signs.

Conservative Management

Patients who should be treated conservatively are those with acute localized pain in the spinal or paraspinal region with or without peripheral radicular radiation. These patients do not have neurologic deficits indicative of spinal cord or severe nerve root compression. The most likely diagnosis is an acute intervertebral disk protrusion, and with time complete recovery can usually be anticipated.

If symptoms persist despite conservative treatment, an epidural steroid injection should be considered. If neurologic deficits and pain continue or worsen despite the con-

servative treatment, surgical treatment is indicated. The most commonly performed surgery is anterior cervical diskectomy.

Signs of moderate sensory or motor deficit in a root distribution may accompany acute pain. Some loss of strength, paresthesia, and mild sensory impairment or loss of muscle stretch reflexes represents such signs. If these signs worsen or do not subside after a trial of conservative treatment, the patient should be admitted to the hospital to ensure immobilization and rest and to allow further investigation.

Even if the patient's symptoms completely subside with any of the modalities, the patient should be given appropriate exercise to stretch and strengthen the muscles.

Management Aimed at Possible Surgical Decompression

Surgical decompression is indicated for patients showing signs of spinal cord compression. This is also advisable for patients with nerve root compression if there is intractable or severe progressive recurrent pain or if there are signs of severe neurologic deficit, particularly marked weakness and muscle atrophy with long tract signs attributable to cervical pathology.

Patients in whom spinal cord compression rapidly develops require prompt investigation and surgical decompression. Such investigations usually include plain x-ray films of the spine and an emergency myelogram.

Physical Therapy Program

The physical therapy depends on past medical intervention, the extent of the lesion, and the stage of recovery. During the acute stage the patient may be treated with bed rest and immobilization. When the condition reaches the subacute stage, the patient should begin an exercise program suited to the level and direction of the protrusion. Aggressive physical therapy may begin in the chronic stage.

LOW BACK PAIN

Most adults have had at least one episode of back pain in their lifetime. Its vast potential for physical, emotional, and economic impact requires that health care professionals have an understanding of acute and chronic back pain. The differential diagnosis of back pain is large, physical findings can vary markedly from one examination to another, no laboratory test can quantify the severity of the pain, and many causes of back pain cannot be proven by laboratory studies. Furthermore, the musculoskeletal structures of the back rarely operate alone in producing pain. Therefore, the evaluation of the patient with low back pain must be thorough and systematic.

Prevalence

Low back pain is second only to the common cold as a cause for absence from work in people younger than age 55, and second only to headache as a cause of chronic pain. In one survey, 56% of Americans reported back pain in the preceding year.[1] The incidence of low back pain decreased with advancing age, but the percentage of those with more than 100 days of backache was higher in those older than 50 years. The 7.5% of patients with low back pain who did not improve with therapy accounted for 75% of the money spent on back pain, according to the Quebec Task Force on Spinal Disorders.[2] That study group also showed that, despite its high prevalence, most low back pain resolves in less than 2 months.[3,4] The problem seems to be worsening, with costs of long-term disability in the United States increasing 163% for 1970 to 1981.[5] Back pain is the leading cause of disability in people younger than 45 years.[6] The overall incidence of claims for low back pain covered by industrial health insurance is 1% to 2%, and those claims are disproportionately expensive compared with other claims.[7,8]

Etiology

Low back pain usually involves changes in the musculoskeletal structures of the lumbosacral area. Less frequent causes must be excluded in the workup.[9] Sullivan's[10] functional approach to diagnosis is presented in Box 9–2. Although there are many causes, several have the same mechanism for pain.

Evaluation of the Patient with Back Pain

Given the number of possible causes for low back pain, the evaluation protocol must be thorough and comprehensive, including:

1. Pertinent record review
2. Questionnaire to elicit pain and drug, medical, and psychologic history
3. Pain scaling: draw-your-pain, visual analog scale (VAS), verbal rating

4. Formal psychologic evaluation for selected patients
5. Physical examination: walk; bend; lift; stand; sit; lie down; and the more formal neurologic, musculoskeletal, and functional capacity evaluations
6. Ergonomic assessment
7. Laboratory studies
8. Team conference to document diagnosis and for treatment planning

The pain specialist should scrutinize the relevant records to validate the patient's history, become familiar with past physical findings, review the results of diagnostic laboratory tests, and acknowledge past treatments and outcomes.

A complete diagnosis considers both the physical and nonphysical aspects of pain because appropriate treatment cannot be comprehensive without this understanding. History includes the onset, site, character, and quality of the pain, as well as an appreciation for what makes the pain better or worse, the degree of interference with desired and necessary activity, the response to past treatment, coexisting complaints, and medical disease that may be causing or influencing the back pain. It is important to differentiate between acute and chronic pain, because the management is different, and to consider the psychosocial aspects (nonphysical factors).

Physical examination includes evaluation of the nervous, musculoskeletal, and vascular systems and a search for bone disorders. In chronic pain patients, the examination may not

---

BOX 9–2 Etiology of Low Back Pain

VERTEBRAL AND PARAVERTEBRAL CAUSES OF BACK PAIN (± RADICULOPATHY)
Herniated nucleus pulposus: cervical, thoracic, and most commonly lumbar
Degenerative joint disease: disk space narrowing, spinal stenosis, facet abnormality
Arachnoiditis: postsurgical, postradiographic contrast-material study
Musculoskeletal disorder: strain, sprain, spasm
Neoplastic: metastatic, multiple myeloma, other primary spinal tumors
Infectious: epidural abscess, vertebral osteomyelitis, Pott's disease, herpes zoster
Rheumatic conditions: ankylosing spondylitis, Reiter's syndrome, fibromyalgia

REFERRED CAUSE OF BACK PAIN (USUALLY WITHOUT RADICULOPATHY)
Vascular origin: abdominal aortic aneurysm, arterial occlusive disease
Biliary origin: obstructed bile duct, distended gallbladder
Gastrointestinal: perforated viscus
Pancreatic origin: pancreatic carcinoma, endometrial carcinoma
Renal origin: renal carcinoma, kidney stones, ureteral stones, pyelonephritis, bladder carcinoma

From Cailliet R: Low back pain. In Cailliet R, editor: *Soft tissue pain and disability.* Philadelphia, FA Davis, 1977.

substantiate earlier assessments because of progression or regression of disease with and without treatment. Findings and physical changes may vary over time. Furthermore, serial examinations help determine if treatment is resulting in improvement.

There is no diagnostic laboratory test that reveals every cause of low back pain.[9,11] The main sites of origin of low back pain are the posterior longitudinal ligament, the interspinous ligaments, the nerve roots and dural coverings, the facet joints, and the deep muscles.[12] Because only two of these are really evaluated by routine laboratory studies, it is easy to explain the many false negatives. Up to 85% of patients with low back pain cannot be given definitive diagnosis because of the poor association among symptoms, pathologic findings, and imaging results.[13] Thirty percent to 40% of CT scans, myelograms, and discograms can show abnormalities in asymptomatic individuals.

Plain posteroanterior and lateral x-ray films of the lumbosacral spine can reveal anatomic changes, bony tumors, compression fractures, scoliosis, and disk space narrowing.[14-16] Oblique views can show spondylosis, which is a defect in the lamina that may separate the anterior body from the posterior elements, and spondylolisthesis, the sliding of one vertebral body anteriorly relative to the one inferior. Myelography, most appropriate preoperatively, will show disk herniation, nerve root compression, and space-occupying lesions. CT and MRI scans can reveal much of the same information noninvasively while assessing the relationship of the lumbosacral structures to neural elements.[17]

In persistent or chronic pain, nonphysical and psychosocial aspects should be evaluated. It must be determined whether psychologic conflicts are being expressed through physical complaints.

Chronic pain can affect the quality of life for the entire family, both socially and economically. Ergonomic evaluation considers human factors in the interactions with equipment and the total work environment.

Anatomic Considerations

In normal posture the anterior vertebral column carries most of the weight in the low back, and the disks absorb shocks and allow flexion yet limit motion. The disks comprise one third of the height of the vertebral column in the lumbar region and one fifth of the height in other regions.[18] With age the disks become less resilient and lose the ability to distribute mechanical forces evenly.[19] The posterior longitudinal ligament narrows from L2 to L5 and is, thus, less of a barrier to posterolateral disk protrusion. It is not surprising that 85% of herniated disks occur at L4-L5 or L5-S1. Whereas the cervical nerves exit the foramina above the corresponding vertebrae, the thoracic, lumbar, and sacral nerves exit below the corresponding vertebrae. The nerve roots run from the spinal cord caudally along the posterior portion of the body and disk of the vertebrae before exiting through the intervertebral foramina. Therefore, when the L4-L5 disk herniates, it impinges in the L5 and S1. Only 1% to 2% of patients with low back pain have a herniated disk.

The posterior elements of the spine include the lamina, pedicles, and facet joints, which together encircle and protect the spinal cord and emerging nerve roots (Fig. 9–7). The purpose of the posterior elements is to restrict range of motion and anchor muscles, ligaments, and tendons. If the

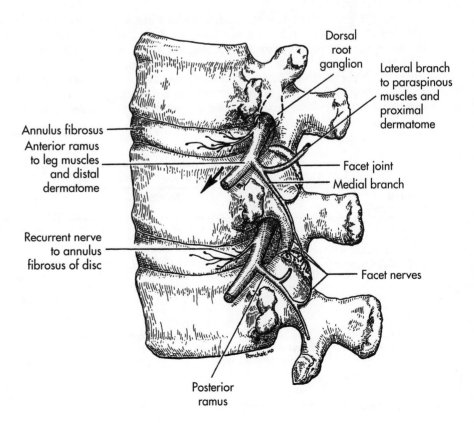

FIG. 9–7 Anatomic features of a typical lumbar nerve root. Branches to the spinal facet joints, disk annulus, and back muscles are present and may be sources of pain referred to as sciatica. *(Adapted from illustration by Stephen Ponchak MD).*

spine is not in optimal position because of disruption in coordination of the musculoskeletal system, lifting, bending, or twisting can result in injury.

Common Low Back Pain Syndromes

The most common cause of low back pain is postural change associated with primary or secondary injury to supporting muscles and ligaments. Of all low back pain, 80% to 90% is postural. Cailliet[12] proposes that the lumbar lordotic curve increases secondary to pain-initiated reflex muscle spasm. Then weight bearing is transferred from the anterior structures of the spine to the posterior structures, the facet joint is maximally loaded, sheer forces on the disks increase (especially in the posterior axis), and the intervertebral foramina may be compressed, causing nerve root impingement.

Eventually, *postural pain* may lead to herniated disks, facet joint pain, and myofascial pain. Diffuse lumbosacral pain is described by the patient as dull and aching with no radiation except perhaps into the buttocks or hips. Pain at rest suggests causes other than mechanical low back pain.[9] Patients with *degenerative joint disease* may have similar symptoms, but their diagnosis suggests some baseline disorder of the facet joints in addition to the postural changes.

Facet syndrome (zygapophyseal joint)[20] is related to physical stress on the facet joint or an anatomic derangement of the facet joint and is associated with pain that is most often referred to the gluteal region or thigh but can be felt anywhere in the leg. Facet syndrome[21,22] may accompany degenerative joint disease and spinal stenosis, presenting with unilateral back pain that radiates from a site off the (lumbar) midline down the back of the thigh to the knee. Pain is aggravated by hyperextension or lateral flexion. Lateral bending with the extension of the spine often causes the most intense pain.

Acute disk syndromes often are associated with a history of a specific initiating event such as lifting in a bent and twisted stance. The pain is sharp and stabbing and shoots in a dermatomal fashion into the lower extremity but decreases when the patient lies down. Increasing intra-abdominal pressure, as with straining during bowel movement or coughing, may exacerbate pain because the pressure increase is transmitted to the spine and the already bulging disk. Typical changes in neurologic examination include decreased deep tendon reflex, decreased sensation, paresthesias, positive straight leg raise when supine and/or seated, and the indication that sitting causes radicular symptoms (Table 9–2).

Disk injury can result in the release of even small amounts of phospholipase-A$_2$, causing marked nerve root inflammation without obvious structural changes. Phospholipase-A$_2$ is an enzyme that releases arachidonic acid from cell membranes. Its action is blocked by steroids and *not* antiprostaglandin agents such as nonsteroidal anti-inflammatory drugs.

After lumbar laminectomy (with or without fusion) some patients continue to have pain. Presumably this is due to scar tissue in and around the spinal nerves. Their complaints are diffuse, ill-defined, low back pain that is dull and aching in nature, with occasional shaper pain. Pain commonly involves hips, buttocks, and upper posterior thighs. Pain may begin early in the day because of progressive muscle fatigue, which imposes greater physical stress on the already compromised musculoskeletal system.

Both *primary* and *metastatic cancer* can cause back pain.[23] Night pain, fever, a palpable and often tender spinal mass, or a combination of these findings are the usual presenting symptoms. These can be related to bony involvement, pressure on neurologic or vascular elements, or inherent properties of the lesion. Tumor and infection must be considered in any patient who has weight loss, fever, chills, significant neurologic involvement, or atypical blood and urine tests. A specific diagnosis is made using radiologic studies with consideration to patient age, location, density, type of deformity, and host reaction.

Treatment Issues

With an acute bout of low back pain, patients expect an evaluation that readily identifies the cause for the pain and then treatment that at least reduces, but hopefully eliminates, the pain. Pain becomes chronic when it lasts more than 6 to 7 weeks. Treatment goals for chronic pain are necessarily different than for acute pain.

Realistic goals for chronic pain management are to decrease the frequency and intensity of the patient's pain

---

TABLE 9–2 Differentiation of Level of Disk Herniation by Physical Examination and History

Level of Herniation	Pain	Numbness	Weakness	Atrophy	Reflexes
L3-L4 disk (fourth lumbar nerve root)	Lower back, hip, posterolateral thigh, anterior leg	Anteromedial thigh and knee	Quadriceps	Quadriceps	Knee jerk diminished
L4-L5 disk (L5 nerve root)	Over sacroiliac joint, hip, lateral thigh, and leg	Lateral leg, first three toes	Dorsiflexion of great toe and foot; difficulty walking on heels, foot drop possible	Minor	Uncommon in knee and ankle (internal hamstring diminished or absent)
L5-S1 disk (first sacral nerve root)	Sacroiliac joint, hip, and posterior and lateral thigh and leg to heel	Back of calf, lateral heel, foot, and toe	Plantar flexion of foot and great toe may be affected; difficulty walking on toes	Gastrocnemius and soleus	Ankle jerk diminished or absent

(using medications, surgery, nerve blocks, and stimulation techniques), help the patient cope with the residual pain (using psychologic strategies), and restore function (using physical therapy). The usual plan is to decrease the pain enough to allow physical therapy to strengthen muscles, improve posture, and increase activity. Psychotherapy to provide the patient with insight into the intense interaction of physical and nonphysical components may be indicated.

Nachemson[24] found that 70% of patients with discogenic low back pain and sciatica had relief with conservative treatment in 3 weeks; 90% had relief in 2 months. Conservative treatment included decreased activity, time off work, or less strenuous physical activity. Also, the inclination for rest was reinforced by potent analgesics nd indirect-acting muscle relaxants, which are mild to moderate sedatives. Physical therapy was used in many cases. As pain subsided, normal activity was resumed. Pain that does not resolve may need evaluation by a pain specialist.

Treatment Options

Medications

Proper compliance on the patient's part is needed to assume an adequate trial with any drugs. Medications need to be used purposefully; if pain is from inflammatory process within the musculoskeletal system, then aspirin or another nonsteroidal anti-inflammatory drug should be used. If nonsteroidal anti-inflammatory drugs are contraindicated, then acetaminophen is an alternative; however, it does not have potent anti-inflammatory actions, so it may offer less pain relief.

Indirect muscle relaxants can relieve reflex muscle spasm and allow increased range of motion and activity, but many have sedative side effects.

Narcotics should be used for moderate to severe acute pain and in patients with acute flare-ups above and beyond their usual chronic pain.

Adjuncts to narcotics and nonnarcotic medications include hydroxyzine, promethazine, doxepin, amitriptyline, and trazodone. Sedative hypnotics such as the benzodiazepines are not recommended because of the potential for physical dependence and an analgesic effect assumed to be related to the CNS serotonin depletion.

As pain becomes chronic, a simple pharmacologic answer is less likely. If a long trial of drugs has been ineffective, the patient will benefit from gradual detoxification and reevaluation for alternative management strategies.

Surgery

Success is about 80% for the first surgery, but it is invasive, involves an interruption of normal activities, necessitates a variable period of hospitalization, and requires some recovery time. A specific diagnosis that can be corrected surgically is desirable. Surgery is usually done for those who fail conservative therapy, have foraminal encroachment on the nerve root, or have progressive neurologic deficit.

Nonphysical aspects that influence pain need to be considered preoperatively. As pain becomes more chronic and factors other than soft-tissue damage contribute to pain, surgery may be inadequate or even inadvisable. After a long exposure to pain, the nervous system may compensate for pain transmission interruption by the mechanisms of plas-

ticity and neuron recruitment. This neural repair and recovery process may ultimately cause more pain after surgery.[25]

Nerve Blocks

Nerve blocks can be used for diagnosis or therapy. The effectiveness of nerve blocks is diluted if they are used indiscriminately, as in patients with an incomplete database or when used with faulty technique. However, when done appropriately and within the framework of a treatment program that provides pain relief and encourages physical and emotional rehabilitation in patients with lifestyle distribution caused by the pain, they can be effective.

Epidural steroid injections are effective in about 66% of selected patients.[26] Box 9–3 reviews the advantages and disadvantages of epidural steroid injections, which must be weighed for each patient. Box 9–4 suggests the types of patients who might benefit from epidural steroid injections. All patients who have received epidural steroid injections must be reassessed.

An additional mechanism for low back pain that is proposed and that may also be more frequent after surgery is as follows: Persistent low back pain with subsequent injury to peripheral nerves or nerve roots can trigger changes in the nervous system, which affect the central modulation of afferent and efferent neuronal activity or encourage neuroma formation.[23] Corticosteroids can inhibit a neuroma's abnormal, spontaneous discharge.[27]

BOX 9–3 Advantages and Disadvantages of Epidural Steroid Injections

ADVANTAGES
- The technique is known to many practitioners and is widely available.
- The procedure can be done on an outpatient basis.
- The procedure is normally of low risk and can be done at all clinically necessary spinal levels.
- When the patient is given local anesthetics and steroids, this is two active treatments at once.
- The positive results change the patient's attitude about medication use, the need for surgery, and participation in rehabilitation.
- Money can be saved if surgery, long convalescence, and work interruption are avoided.

DISADVANTAGES
- There is the potential for reaction to the local anesthetic drug or the corticosteroid drug injected.
- There is a risk of tissue with the occurrence of bleeding, infection, ligamentous pain, or postdural puncture headache.
- The treatment may not help the patient, thereby increasing discouragement.
- There are not many studies that clearly define which patients are the most appropriate for this treatment.

BOX 9–4 Patients to Consider for Epidural Steroid Injections

- Patients with radicular pain and a corresponding sensory change
- Patients with symptoms caused by a herniated disk who have not improved with 4 weeks of conservative therapy
- Patients with cancer in whom tumor infiltration of the nerve roots may be causing the radicular pain
- Active patients with chronic back pain who suffer an acute flare-up, manifest symptoms that have radicular-like features, and do not respond to conservative therapy
- Motivated patients with postdural back pain that has radicular-like features and a poor response to conservative therapy
- Selected patients with chronic back pain for whom epidural steroid injection is but one component of a comprehensive treatment program

---

Other useful blocks may include paravertebral and transsacral blocks when pain is away from the midline or when a midline approach is precluded by past surgery or traumatic change. Facet joint nerve blocks have been proposed as useful at least in the diagnosis of the source of low back pain.[28,29]

Trigger points are discrete areas in muscles or connective tissue that are exquisitely painful to palpation and can initiate some of the patient's pain. They are areas of focal ischemia that result when pain causes reflex muscle and vascular spasm. They may be the primary complaint but more often are secondary to prolonged imbalance in posture from chronic low back pain. Pain in the sacroiliac joint and that at the sciatic notch associated with the piriformis muscle can be considered as trigger points.[12,30] Trigger points are found during physical examination.

Stimulation Techniques

Based on Melzack and Wall's[31] gate control theory, small pain-fiber (C- or A-delta) input can be modified by faster A-alpha or beta neural input. Dorsal column stimulators or epidural stimulators can be used as a clinical application of this theory.[32] They have been found helpful in some patients who have failed conservative treatment and are poor candidates for surgery.[33]

Transcutaneous electrical nerve stimulation (TENS) is a noninvasive stimulation technique that is simple enough for home use, does not require a formal therapist for continued treatment, is used basically without age restriction, does not interfere with other therapy, has no systemic side effects, and is patient controlled. Use of TENS may not affect the primary cause of the pain but could relieve reflex muscle spasm, which may allow physical therapy that improves muscle tone, strength, and overall function.

Physical Rehabilitation

Physical rehabilitation is fundamental to patient's overall improvement. Enforced inactivity and disruption of routine may provoke anxiety, despair, anger, agitation, frustration, and depression and lead to loss of muscle tone and strength, decreased range of motion, inflexible posture, and weight gain. Attention must be directed to reversing the detrimental effects of inactivity. Formal physical therapy assessment is highly recommended in patients with chronic low back pain because the training ensures that the patient has been shown the proper procedure for exercises.

Psychologic Rehabilitation

Emotional response is a part of pain, and lack of positive identification of pathology does not mean that a psychiatric cause is predominant. In acute low back pain with its associated anxiety component, anxiolytics may be temporarily indicated. Benzodiazepines help with bed rest and reduce reflex muscle spasm.

Psychotherapeutic techniques for selected patients with chronic low back pain include biofeedback, self-regulation skills, and hypnosis; they help control muscle tension, anxiety, and spasm. There is less utility with these techniques in acute pain, because such episodes have resolved before they can be introduced, practiced, and learned.

Vocational Rehabilitation

Mayer and colleagues[34] found that return to work was based on improved physical motivation to become productive. More attention may need to be paid to matching an employee with a specific job that is based on the physical demands, his or her functional capacity, and the psychology of the work environment.

SUMMARY

Most acute episodes of back pain resolve on their own in a limited amount of time. Not all pain can be documented by testing, and positive results do not necessarily explain the patient's complaints. Sound medical practice dictates that tests should not be duplicated needlessly. Rather, only those that would change the course of referral or treatment should be ordered. When the pain persists, the cause can be complicated by reactive physical and psychosocial mechanisms that compound the signs and symptoms. Adding compensation, possible secondary gain, and pain behavior can further confuse the evaluation of the patient with chronic back pain. Following the Quebec Task Force on Spinal Disorders' recommendation to apply conservative measures for up to 6 weeks and then to obtain evaluation and treatment if needed at a multidisciplinary pain center seems prudent. The onus of improvement lies with the patient, because measures to alleviate the pain are usually aimed at allowing the patient to perform exercises to strengthen his or her back musculature. The role of back schools and work hardening is unproved in large studies but appears to support the idea of helping the patient take the lead in his or her own care. Finally, an understanding of the psychologic dynamics is needed in the proper evaluation and treatment of these patients.

MUSCULOSKELETAL PAIN

The musculoskeletal system consists of the bones and articulations of the skeleton and the ligaments, muscles, and tendons that connect and manipulate them. These are diverse tissues with radically different characteristics. Injuries or disorders may directly affect any of these component tissues and may indirectly affect the overlying integument, musculature, or neural elements associated with or contained within the skeletal framework. All of these tissues are represented in the spinal column, and all are richly innervated.

Myofascial and skeletal pain are common pain syndromes. Although many forms of skeletal pain have an identifiable cause, myofascial pain often lacks a pathologic definition. It is typically grouped under the umbrella of myofascial pain syndrome and is also referred to as myositis, fibromyalgic pain syndrome, fibrositis, fibromyalgia, myalgia, idiopathic myalgia, myelosis, and myofascitis.[35] Skeletal pain is considered any pain emanating from the bony or supporting connective tissue, including synovium, ligaments, or cartilage.

Pathophysiology of Pain in Paraspinous Muscles and Tendons

Muscular pain may be the result of a direct injury such as a blow or puncture, which disrupts or damages the muscle tissue and its intrafascicular nerve fibers, or a result of the distention and pressure produced by the ensuing hematoma and edema. Pain also results from indirect injuries such as athletic injuries, in which the muscle is torn or ruptured as it strains against an excessive resistance force. Inflammation and edema play a role in the mediation of pain symptoms. In major musculoskeletal injuries, persistent spasm may result in severe muscle pain and further trauma to the muscle and other tissues of the soft-tissue envelope.

The primary nociceptive endings in muscle are unencapsulated free nerve endings similar to those seen in periarticular tissues, which transmit their impulses centrally by way of type III and IV afferent fibers. Intramuscular mechanoreceptors may also produce pain impulses when exposed to noxious stimuli. In all, muscular pain receptors may be either chemonociceptive or mechanonociceptive and may respond to stimuli as either or polymodal receptors. Chemonociceptive endings may respond to metabolites that accumulate during anaerobic metabolism; to the products of cell injury produced by injury or ischemia; or to chemical irritants such as bradykinin, serotonin, or potassium. Mechanonociceptive units may respond to stretch, pressure, or disruption. Some receptors may also respond to thermal stimuli.[36,37]

A more ominous type of muscle pain occurs when excessive pressure in or around the muscle results in ischemia. Compartment syndromes occur in patients with bleeding disorders, vascular injuries, musculoskeletal trauma, systemic infections, and constrictive dressings or casts and, although rare, have been reported in the paraspinous muscular compartments.[38] Pain in compartment syndrome is severe and unremitting and out of proportion to any injury the patient may have sustained.

Pathophysiology of Intervertebral Disk Pain

A considerable controversy exists concerning if and how the intervertebral disk might produce back pain. The confusion arises, at least in part, from difficulties in separating out disk tissues from peridiscal tissues in some studies and frank differences of opinion as to the innervation of the disk. Some authors have failed to find any nerve fibers in the annulus fibrosis, contending that endings reported by others were actually residing in adherent portions of the posterior longitudinal ligament.[39–41] Other authors have reported finding nerve endings within the layers of the outer annulus but only in limited areas.[42] More recent studies, however, have consistently demonstrated fine nerve endings in the outer one third of the annulus.[43,44]

Pathophysiology of Bone and Periosteal Pain

Bone is a dynamic composite tissue involved in a variety of physiologic processes and capable of a number of biologic responses to injury or stress. Bone is a tissue capable of responding to both internal and external pressure changes, physical distortion, inflammation, and periosteal injury by transmitting pain signals proximally. Bone pain may be produced by microfracture and subsidence in osteoarthritis, by periosteal elevation and distortion in infection or tumor, by vascular congestion and infarction in sickle-cell crisis, and by mechanical disruption in traumatic conditions.

The tough periosteal sheath that adheres to the outer cortex of the vertebral body is highly vascular and copiously supplied with both free and encapsulated nerve endings; the complex free nerve endings are thought to generate painful discharges, and the encapsulated endings are thought to be sensitive to pressure.[45,46] The nerves found in periosteal tissues are immunoreactive to a wide variety of pain-related and vasoactive neuropeptides.[47]

Facet Joints

Facet joints are specialized to meet specific demands of function: Articular cartilage absorbs and distributes loads, subchondral bone resists deformation and supports and nourishes the cartilage, ligaments maintain alignment and constrain joint excursion, and musculotendinous units flex, extend, and stabilize the joint. Derangement of the joint may result in destruction of the articular cartilage, fracture of the subchondral bone, attenuation or disruption of the ligaments, and excessive strains and inflammation of the muscles.

Synovial joints enjoy a dual pattern of innervation: *Primary articular nerves* are independent branches from larger peripheral nerves, which specifically supply the joint capsule and ligaments; accessory articular nerves reach the joint after passing through muscular or cutaneous tissues, to which they provide primary innervation.[48,49] Both primary and accessory articular nerves are mixed afferents, containing both proprioceptive and nociceptive nerve fibers.

It was previously thought that the synovium was a relatively insensitive tissue[50] and that the pain of synovitis was produced by distortion of the capsule and the elaboration of inflammatory factors. Using antisera against specific neuronal markers, investigators reexamining synovial tissue found vastly greater numbers of small-diameter nerve fibers than were previously reported using standard histologic methods.[51,52]

Myofascial Pain

In the muscular system the muscle fibers are classified as skeletal, cardiac, and smooth. These fibers are long multinucleated cells having a characteristic cross-striated appearance under a microscope. Muscles are supplied by adjacent vessels, and each is supplied by one or more nerves containing motor and sensory fibers that are usually derived from several spinal groups. Histologically, muscle nociceptors are presumably free nerve endings that are connected to the spinal cord by fine afferent fibers.

More recent data suggest that free nerve endings are not free in the strict sense because they are almost completely ensheathed by Schwann cells. Only small areas of the axonal membrane remain uncovered by Schwann cell processes and are directly exposed to the interstitial fluid.[53] The exposed membrane areas are supplied with mitochondria and vesicles and show other structural specializations characteristic of receptive areas. They are assumed to be the site where external stimuli act.[54]

Causes of Myofascial Pain

Myofascial pain can be primary or secondary. Primary myofascial pain is considered to be caused by traumatic disease of the muscle, whereas secondary myofascial pain exhibits painful foci in the skeletal muscle, but the disorder arises outside the skeletal muscle. The hallmark of identification of both syndromes is the trigger point.[35] These trigger points are characterized by a discrete circumscribed painful area in the skeletal muscle. Although histologic evidence is debatable, trigger point areas appear to have structural changes observable by electron microscopy.[35] These areas show morphologic alterations that include myofibrillar degeneration, hyalin formation in the muscle fibers, and deposition of nonspecific inflammatory residue in the interstices of the skeletal muscle.[54]

It is believed that an initial muscle injury or overload results in rupture of sarcoplasmic reticulum and release of ionized calcium, which results in sustained vigorous contraction of a small band of muscles in the region involved.[55] This sustained sarcomere contractile state results in depletion of adenosine triphosphate (ATP) to a critical level, leading to local contraction and electrical silence, as observed in McArdle's disease or rigor mortis. Local ischemia and hypoxia are produced in these areas, along with the release of algogenic substances such as histamine, kinin, serotonin, and prostaglandin, which sensitize nociceptors.[56] Nociceptive impulses are carried to the CNS, resulting in increased muscle tension, sympathetic activity, and local ischemia. A vicious cycle is produced and the event becomes self-sustaining, eventually resulting in localized fibrosis.[35]

Diagnosis

The diagnosis of primary or secondary myofascial pain syndrome is established by demonstrating painful trigger points.[35,57,58]

Although myofascial pain has no distinct laboratory findings, many perpetuating factors may be identified by abnormal laboratory values.[35] Trigger points can be demonstrated with the help of an algometer or by electrical stimulation. Thermography, a noninvasive technique, uses the infrared radiation from the body for diagnostic purposes. It is useful for revealing dysfunction in microcirculation from autonomic response to disease and trauma. Trigger points may cause dysfunction of microcirculation with overlying skin showing an increase in temperature, but it alone is not sufficient to make the diagnosis of myofascial trigger points.[59]

Clinical Management

The goals of therapy in patients with myofascial pain are similar whether the syndrome is primary or secondary. They are structured to alleviate the patient's pain and enhance the patient's functional capabilities. Management of myofascial pain is empirical and should include education and psychologic intervention, which help the patient to understand and decrease the exacerbating factors that increase muscle tone, such as emotional stress, sudden overloading, or repetitive use.

Modalities for Management of Myofascial Pain

The physical modalities often used are heat and cryotherapy, with more recent acceptance of TENS, acupuncture, cold laser, iontophoresis, and H-wave as valuable adjuncts to the management of the syndrome.[60,61]

Cryotherapy

Cryotherapy is useful in myofascial pain syndromes because it alleviates pain by direct and indirect mechanisms. The direct effect is a decrease in temperature of the painful area, whereas reduced pain sensation is felt to result through an indirect effect on the fibers and sensory organs. It is speculated that activation of A-delta fibers helps to close the spinal cord gate and reduces C-fiber activity.[60]

Heat

Heat application is commonly used to treat myofascial pain. Its beneficial effect is secondary to increased collagen extensibility, blood flow, metabolic rate, and inflammation resolution. The pain threshold is believed to be raised by the direct and indirect actions of heat.

Stimulation Techniques

TENS, H-wave, and vibratory stimulation modalities are felt to suppress pain by similar mechanisms. This is believed to be via activation of large-diameter afferent nerve fibers, thereby inhibiting transmission of small-diameter pain fibers at the dorsal horn on the spinal cord. It has been postulated that through peripheral and central mechanisms these increase circulating intrinsic opioids and modulating autonomic responses.[62]

Iontophoresis

Iontophoresis is a modality treatment that involves transfer of ionized substances through intact skin by the passage of direct-current (DC) electrical current between two electrodes. This method can concentrate an anesthetic solution in a localized area, which avoids the trauma that may be associated with a hypodermic needle.

Physical Therapy

Physical therapy plays an important role in the treatment of primary, secondary, acute, and chronic myofascial pain. In physical therapy, patients are educated regarding their functional goals with exercise programs, postural corrections, and training in body mechanics. Patients following and maintaining a sensible regime can attain lasting results.

Fibromyalgia

Fibromyalgia is a syndrome of chronic, diffuse musculoskeletal pain with associated widespread discrete tender points. It occurs predominately in women (10:1) between the ages of 20 and 60 years. Approximately 75% of patients have associated fatigue, nonrestorative sleep, and widespread stiffness. Other common features in approximately 25% of patients include irritable bowel syndrome, subjective swelling, paresthesias, symptoms of anxiety or depression, and functional disability.[63]

The physical examination of a patient with fibromyalgia is notable only for the presence of specific areas of focal tenderness. These diagnostic tender points occur at characteristic muscle-tendon junctions, with digital palpation of a tender point resulting in local pain only.

The sensitivity of the criteria suggests that it may be useful for diagnosis and classification.[64] However, on an individual basis it may be useful to exclude other conditions such as polymyalgia rheumatica and endocrine myopathies, which can also present with widespread musculoskeletal pain and stiffness. Accordingly, a complete blood count, erythrocyte sedimentation rate, and thyroid function tests should be performed.

The etiology of fibromyalgia is unknown. It was originally termed *fibrositis* because of a presumed inflammatory cause of the diffuse muscle pain; however, analysis of muscle biopsy specimens showed only nonspecific or normal findings.[65]

Study regarding psychopathology in fibromyalgia has been complicated by the use of psychologic tests such as the Minnesota Multiphasic Personality Inventory (MMPI), which do not control for symptoms related to chronic pain and associated medical conditions.[66] Although there appears to be a greater prevalence of symptoms reflecting depression, anxiety, and somatoform disorders, most patients with fibromyalgia do not have an active psychiatric disorder.[67,68]

A potential neuroendocrinologic factor for pain-medicated pathways in fibromyalgia is under investigation by many centers, with attention focused on the serotonin pathway, substance P, and the hypothalamic-pituitary-adrenal axis.[69,70] An autoimmune disturbance has not been supported.[71]

In the few controlled therapeutic trials in fibromyalgia, beneficial results were reported with low-dose amitriptyline, cyclobenzaprine, and cardiovascular fitness training.[72-75] It is interesting to speculate that their benefit relates to the sleep disturbance and aerobically unfit muscles previously reported in fibromyalgia.[76,77]

Although nonsteroidal anti-inflammatory agents are the most commonly used medication in these patients, there is little evidence for efficacy.[75]

This common chronic pain syndrome will obviously be a continuing source of medical and economic problems until the pathophysiology is better delineated and subsequent improved treatment methods are formulated. Furthermore, understanding the neuropathophysiologic basis of fibromyalgia may have broader applicability towards an understanding of chronic pain per se.[78]

Skeletal Pain

The skeleton consists of bones and cartilage. Bones provide a framework of levers, protect organs from damage, and their marrow forms certain cells that substance provides for storage and exchange of calcium and phosphate ions. Cartilage is a tough, resilient connective tissue composed of cells and fibers embedded in a firm, gel-like intercellular matrix. Cartilage is an integral part of many bones, and some skeletal elements are entirely cartilaginous. Joints vary widely in structure and arrangement and are often specialized for particular functions. They are typically classified on the basis of their most characteristic structural features into three main types: fibrous, cartilaginous, and synovial.[79]

Bones are richly supplied with blood vessels (Fig. 9–8). This supply typically consists of a nutrient artery that pierces the compact bone of the shaft and divides into branches that supply the marrow and compact bone as far as the metaphysis. Many nerve fibers accompany these blood vessels. Pain felt in a bone may be felt locally at the site of stimulation; however, it often spreads or is referred. Epiphysial vessels are the major blood supply, and the principal distribution of nerves are the same trunks of nerve whose branches supply the groups of muscles moving the joint. They also furnish a distribution of nerves to the skin over the insertions of the same muscle. They are known as articular nerves and contain sensory autonomic fibers.[79]

Conditions Causing Skeletal Pain

Patients with skeletal pain usually complain of pain coming from the joints, surrounding soft tissue, or bone. Most pain presenting as skeletal pain emanates from the joints, because it is the area most richly endowed with nerve fibers. In evaluating joint pain, the clinician should determine whether the cause of the pain is a result of intrinsic or extrinsic disorder. Intrinsic disorders involve the structure (intra-articular surface, periarticular soft tissue, and adjacent bone), whereas extrinsic disorders involve pain arising outside of the structure.

The three intrinsic locations where pain arises occasionally have some overlap between anatomic regions, but a distinct location can usually be made by physical examination. Intra-articular diseases cause joint effusion and synovial or joint-line tenderness. Although periarticular conditions may also cause tenderness around the joint, they usually lack joint effusions. Intra-articular causes of skeletal pain may be divided into three broad categories: inflammatory joint diseases, intra-articular derangement, and osteoarthritis.

Inflammatory Causes

The major immunologic disorders causing intra-articular pain are rheumatoid arthritis, psoriatic arthritis, and systemic lupus erythematosus. Rheumatoid arthritis is by far the most common, afflicting an estimated 5 million Americans. Immunologic conditions are usually polyarticular and in the case of rheumatoid arthritis pursue a relentless

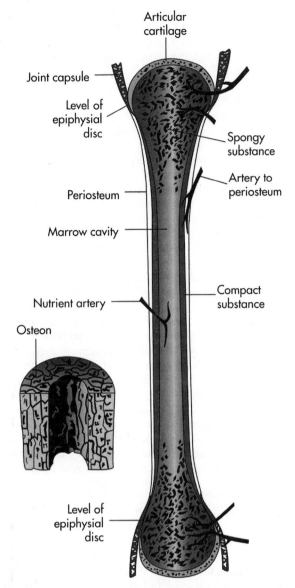

Articular
cartilage

Joint capsule

Level of
epiphysial
disc

Spongy
substance

Artery to
periosteum

Periosteum

Marrow cavity

Compact
substance

Nutrient artery

Osteon

Level of
epiphysial
disc

FIG. 9–8 Schematic diagram of a long bone and its blood supply. Inset shows lamellae of compacta arranged into osteons. *(From Gardner E: Skeleton. In Gardner E, editor: Anatomy: A Regional Study of Human Structure, ed 3. Philadelphia, WB Saunders, 1993).*

course with multiple remissions and reoccurrence until the articular cartilage is destroyed.

Inflammatory joint pain is caused by deposits of crystalline substances, including gout and pseudogout. Uric acid and calcium pyrophosphate crystals that precipitate into joint space can cause an inflammatory response. The symptoms are usually monarticular severe joint pain and swelling.

Joint infections causing inflammation and pain occur either through direct contact or hematogenously. The clinical course of the disease depends on the infectious agent. Symptoms can be indolent or fulminant, with a swollen, painful joint and systemic signs of fever.

Intra-articular Causes

Intra-articular derangement is mechanical blocking of the joint by a foreign body or abnormal joint structure. A history of episodic locking, giving way, and associated effusion is usually given; this is an indication of arthroscopy.[80] Loose bodies, torn menisci, and, in rare cases, tumors can be causative factors. Osteoarthritis, also known as degenerative joint disease, is the most common form of arthritis. It is characterized by progressive loss of articular cartilage, subchondral bony sclerosis, and cartilage, as well as proliferation at the joint margin and eventual osteophyte formation.

Periarticular Causes

Joint pain from periarticular soft-tissue disorders are caused by acute inflammatory conditions or mechanical instability. Overuse, unusual excessive activity, or trauma are the primary precipitating causes. Therapy for inflammatory conditions requires rest and anti-inflammatory medications, and, if symptoms persist, water-soluble glucocorticoid medication is sufficient.[81]

References

1. Taylor H, Curran NM: *The Nuprin pain report.* New York, Louis Harris & Associates, 1985.
2. Quebec Task Force on Spinal Disorders: Scientific approach to the assessment and management of activity-related spinal disorders. *Spine* 12(7S):S16, 1987.
3. National Institute on Disability and Rehabilitation Research: Report on workshop on low back pain. Charlottesville, VA, Rehabilitation Research and Training Center of the University of Virginia, Department of Orthopedics, 1989.
4. Roland M, Morris R: A study of the natural history of back pain. *Spine* 2:145, 1983.
5. Wood PHN, Badley EM: Epidemiology of back pain. In Jayson MJV, editor: *The lumbar spine and back pain.* London, Pitman Medical, 1980.
6. Waddell G: A new clinical model for the treatment of low back pain. *Spine* 12:632, 1987.
7. Klein BP, Jensen RC, Sanderson LM: Assessment of workers' compensation claims for back strains/sprains. *J Occup Med* 26:443, 1984.
8. Spengler DM: Back injuries in industry: A retrospective study. *Spine* 11:241, 1986.
9. McCulloch JA: Differential diagnosis of low back pain. In Tollison CD, editor: *Handbook of chronic pain management.* Baltimore, Williams & Wilkins, 1989.
10. Sullivan JGB: The anesthesiologist's approach to back pain. In Rothman RH, Simeone FA, editors: *The spine,* ed 3. Philadelphia, WB Saunders, 1992.
11. Frymoyer JW: Back pain and sciatica. *N Engl J Med* 318:291, 1988.
12. Cailliet R: Low back pain. In Cailliet R, editor: *Soft tissue pain and disability.* Philadelphia, FA Davis, 1977.
13. Deyo RA: Fads in the treatment of low back pain. *N Engl J Med* 325:1039, 1991.
14. Keim HA, Kirkaldy-Willis WH: Low back pain. *CIBA Clin Symp* 32(6):6, 1980.
15. Frymoyer JW et al: Spine radiographs in patients with low-back pain. *J Bone Joint Surg* 66A:1048, 1984.
16. Lowry PA: Radiology in the diagnosis and management of pain. In Raj PP, editor: *Practical management of pain,* ed 2. St. Louis, Mosby, 1992.
17. Thornbury JR, Fryback DG, Turski PA et al: Disk-caused nerve compression in patients with acute low-back pain: Diagnosis with MR, CT myelography, and plain CT. *Radiology* 186:731, 1993.
18. Finneson BE: *Low back pain,* ed 2. Philadelphia, JB Lippincott, 1981.
19. Moore KL: *Clinically oriented anatomy.* Baltimore, Williams & Wilkins, 1985.
20. Bogduk N: Back pain: Zygapophyseal blocks and epidural steroids. In Cousins MJ, Bridenbaugh PO, editors: *Neural blockade in clinical anesthesia and management of pain,* ed 2. Philadelphia, JB Lippincott, 1988.
21. Yank KH, King AI: Mechanism of facet load transmission as a hypothesis for low-back pain. *Spine* 9:557, 1984.
22. Namey TC: Differential diagnosis and treatment of sciatica: The nondiscgenic causes. *Adv Clin Updates* 1:33, 1985.

23. Loeser JD, Bigos SJ, Fordyce WE et al: Low back pain. In Bonica JJ, editor: *The management of pain,* ed 2. Philadelphia, Lea & Febiger, 1989.

24. Nachemson AL: The lumbar spine. An orthopedic challenge. *Spine* 1:59, 1976.

25. Loeser JD: Pain due to nerve injury. *Spine* 10:232, 1985.

26. Benzon HT: Epidural steroid injections for low back pain and lumbosacral radiculopathy. *Pain* 24:277, 1986.

27. Devor M, Govrin-Lippman R, Raber P: Corticosteriods suppress ectopic neural discharge originating in experimental neuromas. *Pain* 22:127, 1985.

28. Sauser DD, Neumann M: Facet block. In Raj PP, editor: *The practical management of pain,* ed 2. St. Louis, Mosby, 1992.

29. Sandrock NJG, Warfield CA: Epidural steroids and facet injections. In Warfield CA, editor: *Principles and practice of pain management.* New York, McGraw-Hill, 1993.

30. Wyant GM: Chronic pain syndromes and their treatment, III: The piriformis syndrome. *Can Anaesth Soc J* 26:305, 1979.

31. Melzack R, Wall PD: Pain mechanisms: A new theory. *Science* 150:971, 1965.

32. North RB: Neural stimulation techniques. In Tollison CD, editor: *Handbook of chronic pain management.* Baltimore, Williams & Wilkins, 1989.

33. North RB, Ewend MG, Lawton MT et al: Spinal cord stimulation for chronic, intractable pain: Superiority of "multi-channel" devices. *Pain* 44:119, 1991.

34. Mayer TG, Gatchel RJ, Mayer H et al: A prospective two-year study of functional restoration in industrial low back injury. An objective assessment procedure. *JAMA* 258:1763, 1987.

35. Sola AE, Bonica JJ: Myofascial pain syndromes. In Bonica JJ, editor: *The management of pain,* ed 2. Philadelphia, Lea & Febiger, 1990.

36. Kumazawa T, Mizumura K: Thin fiber receptors responding to mechanical, chemical, and thermal stimulation in the skeletal muscle of the dog. *J Physiol (Lond)* 273:179, 1977.

37. Mense S, Schmidt RF: Muscle pain: Which receptors are responsible for the transmission of noxious stimuli? In Rose CF, editor: *Physiological aspects of clinical neurology.* Oxford, Blackwell Scientific Publications, 1977.

38. Carr D, Gilbertson L, Frymoyer J: Lumbar paraspinal compartment syndrome: A case report with physiologic and anatomic studies. *Spine* 10:816, 1985.

39. Pedersen HE, Blunk CFJ, Gardner E: The anatomy of the lumbosacral posterior rami and meningeal branches of the spinal nerves (sinuvertebral nerves). *J Bone Joint Surg* 38A:377, 1956.

40. Stillwell DL: The nerve supply of the vertebral column and its associated structures in the monkey. *Anat Rec* 125:139, 1956.

41. Parke WW: The innervation of connective tissues of the spinal motion segment. Paper presented at the International Symposium on Percutaneous Lumbar Discectomy. Philadelphia, Pa, 1987.

42. Hirsch C: Studies on the mechanism of the low back pain. *Acta Orthop Scand* 20:261, 1951.

43. Bogduk N, Tynan W, Wilson AS: The innervation of the human lumbar intervertebral discs. *J Anat* 132:39, 1981.

44. Yoshizawa H, O'Brien JP, Smith WT: Neuropathology on the intervertebral disc removed for low back pain. *J Pathol* 132:95, 1980.

45. Cooper RR: Nerves in cortical bone. *Science* 160:327, 1968.

46. Ralston HJ, Miller MR, Kasahara M: Nerve endings in human fasciae, tendons, ligaments, periosteum, and joint synovial membrane. *Anat Rec* 136:137, 1960.

47. Wyke B: Articular neurology—A review. *Physiotherapy* 58:94, 1972.

48. Gardner E: The distribution and termination of nerves in the knee joint of the cat. *J Comp Neurol* 80:11, 1944.

49. Gardner E: The innervation of the knee joint. *Anat Rec* 101:109, 1948.

50. Kellgren JH, Samuel EP: Sensitivity and innervation of the articular cartilage. *J Bone Joint Surg* 32B:84, 1950.

51. Gronblad M et al: Neuropeptides in synovium of patients with rheumatoid arthritis and osteoarthritis. *J Rheumatol* 15:1807, 1988.

52. Kidd BL et al: Neurogenic influences in arthritis. *Ann Rheum Dis* 49:649, 1990.

53. Andres KH, von During M, Schmidt RF: Sensory innervation of the Achilles tendon by group III and IV afferent fibers. *Anat Embryol (Berl)* 172:145, 1854.

54. Zohn DA, Mennell J: *Musculoskeletal pain: Diagnosis and physical treatment.* Boston, Little, Brown & Co, 1976.

55. Simons DG: Electrogenic nature of palpable bands and "jump sign" associated with myofascial trigger points. In Bonica JJ, Albe Fessard D, editors: *Advances in pain research and therapy.* New York, Raven Press, 1976.

56. Mense S: Peripheral mechanisms of muscle nociception and local muscle pain. *J Musculoskeletal Pain* 1:1, 1993.

57. Travell JG, Simons DG: Myofascial pain and dysfunction. In *The trigger point manual.* Baltimore, Williams & Wilkins, 1983.

58. Simons DG: Myofascial pain syndromes due to trigger points. In Goodgold J: *Rehabilitation Medicine.* St. Louis, Mosby, 1987.

59. Edeiken J, Shaber G: Thermography: a reevaluation. *Skeletal Radiol* 15:545, 1986.

60. Lehmann JF, deLateur RJ: *Therapeutic heat and cold,* ed 3. Baltimore, Williams & Wilkins, 1982.

61. Lorenz KY: A neuromodulation technique for pain control. In Aronoff GM, editor: *Evaluation and treatment in chronic pain.* Baltimore, Urban & Schwarzenburg, 1985.

62. Phero JC, Raj TP, McDonald JS: Transcutaneous electrical nerve stimulation and myoneural injection therapy for the management of chronic myofascial pain. *Dent Clin North Am* 31:703, 1987.

63. Wolfe F: Fibromyalgia: the clinical syndrome. *Rheum Dis Clin North Am* 15:1, 1989.

64. Wolfe F, Smythe HA, Yunus MB et al: The American College of Rheumatology 1990 criteria for the classification of fibromyalgia. *Arthritis Rheum* 33:160, 1990.

65. Kalyan-Raman UP, Kalyan-Raman K, Yunus MB et al: Muscle pathology in primary fibromyalgia syndrome: A little microscopic, histochemical and ultrastructural study. *J Rheumatol* 11:808, 1984.

66. Smythe HA: Problems with the MMPI. *J Rheumatol* 11:417, 1985.

67. Ahles TA, Yunus MB, Riley SD et al: Psychological factors associated with primary fibromyalgia syndrome. *Arthritis Rheum* 27:1101, 1984.

68. Goldenberg DL: Psychological symptoms and psychiatric diagnosis in patients with fibromyalgia. *J Rheumatol Suppl* 19:127, 1989.

69. Russell IJ: Neurohormonal aspects of fibromyalgia syndrome. *Rheum Dis Clin North Am* 15:73, 1989.

70. Ferraccioli G, Cavalieri F, Salaffi F et al: Neuroendocrinologic findings in primary fibromyalgia (soft tissue chronic syndrome) and in other chronic rheumatic conditions (rheumatoid arthritis, low back pain). *J Rheumatol* 17:869, 1990.

71. Bengtsson A, Ernerudh J, Vrethem M et al: Absence of autoantibodies in primary fibromyalgia. *J Rheumatol* 17:1682, 1990.

72. Carette S, McCain GA, Bell DA et al: Evaluation of amitriptyline in primary fibrositis: A double blind, placebo-controlled study. *Arthritis Rheum* 29:655, 1986.

73. Goldenberg DL, Felson DT, Dinerman H: A randomized controlled trial of amitriptyline and naproxen in the treatment of patients with fibromyalgia. *Arthritis Rheum* 29:1371, 1986.

74. Bennett RM, Gatter RA, Campbell SM et al: A comparison of cyclobenzaprine and placebo in the management of fibrositis: A double-blind controlled study. *Arthritis Rheum* 31:1535, 1988.

75. McCain GA, Bell DA, Mai FM et al: A controlled study of the effect of a supervised cardiovascular fitness training program on the manifestations of primary fibromyalgia. *Arthritis Rheum* 31:1135, 1988.

76. Bennett RM, Clark SR, Goldberg L et al: Aerobic fitness in patients with fibrositis: A controlled study of respiratory gas exchange and xenon clearance from exercising muscle. *Arthritis Rheum* 32:454, 1989.

77. Moldofsky H, Scarisbrick P, England R et al: Musculoskeletal symptoms and non-REM sleep disturbance in patients with "fibrositis syndrome" and healthy subjects. *Psychosom Med* 37:341, 1975.

78. Reilly PA, Littlejohn GO: Fibrositis/fibromyalgia syndrome: the key to the puzzle of chronic pain. *Med J Aust* 152:226, 1990.

79. Gardner E: Skeleton. In Gardner, editor: *Anatomy: A regional study of human structure,* ed 3. Philadelphia, WB Saunders, 1993.

80. Zuckerman JD, Mirabello SC, Newman D et al: The painful shoulder: Part II. Intrinsic disorders and impingement syndrome. *Am Fam Physician* 43:497, 1991.

81. Gerhart T, Dohlman LE: Joint pain. In Warfield CA, editor: *Principles and practice of pain management.* New York, McGraw-Hill, 1993.

Questions • Nociceptive Pain

1. Pain caused by spinal cord and nerve root compressions, postherpetic neuralgia, and peripheral neuropathy is generally categorized as

   A. Nociceptive pain
   B. Visceral pain
   C. Neuropathic pain
   D. Myofascial pain

2. Radicular symptoms in the upper extremities with long tract signs in the lower extremities are generally caused by

   A. Cervical spinal cord compression
   B. Cervical facet syndrome
   C. Complex Regional Pain Syndrome (CRPS) of the upper extremity
   D. Stroke

3. Conservative management is appropriate for patients with paraspinal pain without radicular symptoms because these patients do not have

   A. Normal spinal canal
   B. Disc prolapse causing radiculopathy
   C. Aortic aneurysm
   D. Spinal cord or nerve root compression

4. In patients younger than age 55, low back pain is second to which of the following as a cause for absence from work

   A. Postherpetic neuralgia
   B. CRPS
   C. Common cold
   D. Cancer

5. Paraspinal pain that is associated with a radiating zone of pain to the gluteal region and thigh is usually due to

   A. Ilioinguinal neuralgia
   B. Genitofemoral neuralgia
   C. Facet syndrome
   D. Lumbar nerve root compression

ANSWERS

1. C
2. A
3. D
4. C
5. C

CHAPTER 10

Neuropathic Pain

DONALD C. MANNING, CHRISTOPHER M. LOAR, P. PRITHVI RAJ, AND ALLEN H. HORD

CENTRAL NERVOUS SYSTEM PAIN

Central pain is produced by lesions on the central nervous system (CNS); however, not all CNS lesions produce a central pain syndrome. Lesions can occur in the spinal cord, brainstem, and brain. Most cases of central pain are associated with spinal cord lesions.[1] Central pain syndromes often occur with complete or partial lesions of the somatosensory pathways, especially the spinothalamic tract, which carries pain and temperature sense. When central pain occurs with a lesion in the spinothalamic tract, it may be associated with all or part of the affected sensory deficit. Central pain states, however, have been observed in patients without clinically detectable somatosensory impairment.[2]

The clinical features of central pain are similar whether the lesion is located in the spinal cord, brainstem, or brain. There are generally two types of central pain: spontaneous pain and hyperesthesia.

Spontaneous pain is constant but may vary in intensity over time. The pain is often described as the sensation of tingling, burning, numbness, twisting, or pressing.

Hyperesthesia occurs when sensory stimuli in an area of partial sensory deficit produce discomfort. The sensation is often poorly localized and unpleasant. There are two types of hyperesthesia: hyperpathia and allodynia. Hyperpathia is intense discomfort produced by mild or moderately painful stimuli, whereas allodynia is an unpleasant sensation produced by a normally nonpainful stimulus. Hyperesthetic sensations may occur in volleys or paroxysms that can be excruciating. Often the stimulations appear sometime after the eliciting stimulus, and they may last much longer than the original stimulus.[1,2]

Spinal Cord Lesions

Spinal cord lesions are responsible for most central pain states. Lesions at any level and of varying pathologic origin can produce a central pain state. Pain is usually produced in an area of sensory impairment resulting from interruption of the spinothalamic tract.

There are numerous types of pathologic conditions that may produce a spinal cord lesion and cause central pain. Traumatic lesions are the most frequent cause; however, disk disease and vascular disease, including infarction and arteriovenous malformation (AVMs), have been reported to cause central pain of spinal cord origin.[2]

In evaluating central pain, the clinician should obtain a magnetic resonance imaging study of the affected level of the spinal cord to exclude post-traumatic syringomyelia.

The treatment of central pain of spinal cord origin is often frustrating and difficult. There is, unfortunately, no totally effective treatment. At best, treatment focuses on lessening the discomfort.

Brain and Brainstem Lesions

Brain and brainstem lesions may produce central pain states. They may be produced by many different pathologic conditions and at any level of the brain or brainstem. Central pain states may occur with lesions that produce alteration in sensory function, especially in those areas where there has been spinothalamic sensory loss.

Characteristics of central pain from brain and brainstem lesions are the same as pain from spinal cord lesions. There is both a spontaneous pain and hyperpathic pain that may affect all or part of the distribution of sensory loss.

Brainstem Lesions

Most brainstem lesions that produce pain are vascular in origin. The most common vascular cause of pain is Wallenberg's syndrome, also called the *lateral medullary syndrome*.[3,4] The neurologic presentation in this syndrome may be variable, but the syndrome characteristically presents with crossed sensory findings. There is ipsilateral facial sensory loss and contralateral body impairment of pain and temperature loss.

Other lesions besides Wallenberg's syndrome may cause brainstem origin central pain, including syringobulbia or hematobulbia, neoplasms in the brainstem, and tuberculomas in the pontine region.

Brain Lesions

One of the first central pain syndromes recognized was the thalamic pain syndrome, also referred to as Dejerine-Roussy syndrome.[5] There are many lesions in the thalamus that may produce central pain. Among these, infarctions are the most common. Other lesions include AVMs, neoplasms, abscesses, multiple sclerosis plaques, traumatic injury, nonspecific degenerations, and certain surgical lesions. The thalamic pain syndrome may also be mimicked by cortical lesions, which are caused by infarct, neoplasm, or head trauma.

Medical Treatment of Central Pain

Central pain is partially relieved by barbiturates but not by opiates. Anticonvulsants such as diphenylhydantoin, carbamazepine, and clonazepam may be effective. Amitriptyline in combination with anticonvulsants may also have some effect.

Surgical Treatment of Central Pain

There are two types of surgical therapy: those directed at interrupting the pain pathways and those directed at modulating sensory input.

Surgical procedures that interrupt pain pathways include rhizotomy, cordotomy, cordectomy, and dorsal root entry zone (DREZ) procedures. Unfortunately, these procedures rarely produce a long-lasting, pain-free state.

Neuromodulation techniques are more hopeful than surgical procedures that interrupt pain pathways. The technique involves chronic electrical stimulation of the dorsal columns or the medical lemniscal pathway, both of which carry light touch, joint position sense, and vibration sensation. The exact mechanism by which chronic electrical stimulation suppresses central pain and induces paresthesias in the painful body part is unknown.

PERIPHERAL NERVOUS SYSTEM PAIN

Peripheral nervous system pain results from peripheral nerve lesions. The peripheral nervous system is composed of the cranial nerves and spinal nerves that originate from the cervical, thoracic, lumbar, and sacral nerves. The peripheral nervous system is outside the CNS.

Spinal and Peripheral Nerve Pain

Peripheral nerve pain may occur because of reflex sympathetic dystrophy (RSD) or causalgia, herpes zoster, polyneuropathy, radiculopathy, plexopathy, and multiple entrapment neuropathies.

Polyneuropathy

Polyneuropathy, or peripheral neuropathy, is a common clinical syndrome and cause of peripheral nerve pain. It is clinically characterized by ascending and symmetric paresthesia and impairment of sensation distally more than proximally. It results in a common presentation of sensory and motor abnormalities termed *stocking/glove dysesthesia*. Polyneuropathies may present with primary sensory and primary motor abnormalities. Distally, at the level of hands and feet, sensation may be impaired but may be normal proximally.

The pathophysiology of peripheral neuropathy relates to the two major components of the peripheral nerve: the axon and the myelin sheath. In diseases in which the axon is primarily affected, there is axonal degeneration but perhaps intact myelin sheaths in the nerve. The myelin sheath may also be the primary site of the pathologic condition, and there may be a demyelination of the nerve axon. Demyelinating lesions can occur at multiple sites along the individual nerve in a pattern that is termed *segmental demyelination*. Most peripheral neuropathies can be classified into demyelinating, axonal, or a mixed pattern of both axonal and demyelinating abnormalities.[6,7]

The individual with polyneuropathy or peripheral neuropathy may have a wide variety of underlying causes. History, physical examination, and workup may be important in determining the underlying causes.

In situations in which the cause of the peripheral neuropathy can be determined, treatment of the underlying condition supersedes the treatment of the discomfort. In those situations in which the cause of the peripheral neuropathy cannot be determined, treatment of the painful state is primarily symptomatic.

Diabetic Peripheral Neuropathy

Diabetes mellitus may cause multiple peripheral nerve disorders. There may be mononeuropathies of the cranial nerves and a proximal amyotrophy affecting the femoral and lumbar roots, with pain and symmetric weakness of the proximal lower limb. Peripheral neuropathy or polyneuropathy is the most common peripheral nerve disease with long-standing diabetes mellitus.

Diabetic peripheral neuropathy is symmetric and involves both the sensory and motor nerves. Diabetic peripheral neuropathy can be disabling. The symptoms are usually gradually progressive and may begin with mild numbness, tingling, or a burning sensation in the feet. The discomfort progresses in a proximal direction over months or years, and pain may occur later in the course of the disease.

The pain of diabetic neuropathy has been treated with various medications including carbamazepine and phenytoin,[8] as well as antidepressants such as amitriptyline and desipramine.[9]

Alcoholic Neuropathy

Alcoholic neuropathy is probably the second most common type of peripheral neuropathy in North America. It is estimated that about 20% of chronic alcoholics have peripheral neuropathy. Clinical manifestations consist of mixed sensory and motor disorder that involves primarily the distal segments of the lower extremities. In mild cases there may be sensory symptoms only with complicates of burning feet or painful paresthesia. With more advanced cases, motor weakness is present. In this condition the legs are always more affected than the arms. In advanced cases the arms may also become involved.

Treatment of these individuals consists primarily of abstinence from alcohol and nutritional supplements containing thiamine and vitamin B complex.

Uremic Neuropathy

Uremic neuropathy is a complication of chronic renal failure that may be present in 20% to 50% of patients with uremia. The disease may be becoming less frequent because of more effective treatment for chronic renal failure, including chronic hemodialysis and renal transplant.

Like other peripheral neuropathies, it presents clinicians with a slowly progressive, predominantly sensory neuropathy. Cramps and unpleasant dysesthesias and paresthesia often occur primarily at rest; they appear to be relieved by moving around and walking. Muscle weakness may involve the distal foot muscles, toe extensors, or flexors.

The neuropathy usually stabilizes or improves with dialysis.

Cranial Nerve Pain

There are several disorders of the cranial nerves that can cause pain. These disorders may be caused by vascular compression, infection, or trauma, usually at one specific spot on the nerve. They are usually cause by metabolic disorders.

Trigeminal Neuralgia

Trigeminal neuralgia has been traditionally described as having five fundamental features.[10] These criteria, although they have been modified, are still useful today:

1. There are paroxysmal pains with pain-free intervals; pain is described as "sharp," "stabbing," or "electric shock-like" and lasts for only seconds. A burst of multiple shocks may even last up to 1 minute. In between flashes the patient is pain free.
2. There are no objective clinical or neurologic findings. This traditionally held view used to divide trigeminal neuralgia into structural (with neurologic abnormalities) or idiopathic (without neurologic abnormalities).
3. There are no pathologic findings postmortem.
4. Trigger zones are present. Studies of large groups of patients report that trigger zones are present in 91% of cases. Trigger zones may even be present in more than one division of the trigeminal nerve.
5. Pain is restricted to the area of the trigeminal nerve. Rarely, radiation outside the trigeminal distribution has been reported with trigeminal neuralgia.

Medical Treatment

Baclofen is currently considered the drug of choice for trigeminal neuralgia because of its favorable side effect profile and therapeutic efficacy. The most common side effects of baclofen are drowsiness, dizziness, and gastrointestinal distress. Side effects can be minimized by starting at a low dose.

Carbamazepine is currently the drug of second choice for trigeminal neuralgia. The effectiveness of this agent was proven in several double-blinded and controlled trials. Side effects are most commonly drowsiness, dizziness, unsteadiness, nausea, and anorexia; they occur more commonly if the drug is started at higher doses.

Phenytoin is now less commonly used for medical treatment of trigeminal neuralgia. It is estimated that only 25% of patients obtain sustained relief with this medication. For this reason it is only used in patients who cannot tolerate baclofen or carbamazepine. Symptoms of toxicity may occur above 20 µg/ml and may include dizziness, nausea, vomiting, nystagmus, diplopia, and ataxia.[10–12]

Surgical and Regional Anesthetic Treatment

Blocks of the trigeminal nerve branches of the trigeminal ganglion (gasserian ganglion) are often necessary in patients who are refractory to oral medication. There are several reasons for using this form of treatment:

1. It may allow the patient to experience the kind of numbness obtained after a destructive procedure on the nerve ganglion.
2. The rare debilitated patient may be allowed a period of oral intake and, thus, become a better surgical risk through a period of better nutrition.
3. It may have diagnostic significance by differentiating some forms of atypical facial pain that have a ticlike presentation.
4. It may help to relieve severe debilitating acute pain until medication can be started and become effective.
5. Some patients obtain prolonged or permanent relief. The procedures may be repeated when necessary.[10,11,13]

The second and third branches of the trigeminal nerve are the most often affected, and the blocking procedure must, therefore, be modified to selectively block those affected branches. Maxillary nerve block is usually performed in the pterygopalatine fossa. The mandibular branch may also be blocked through the pterygopalatine fossa. Glycerol gangliolysis is a common and useful technique for sustained relief of trigeminal neuralgia. This procedure is generally performed under fluoroscopic or computed tomography (CT) guidance.

Posterior fossa microvascular decompression of the trigeminal nerve is a procedure that is performed with the assumption that trigeminal neuralgia is caused by vascular compression of the nerve-root entry zone. This procedure carries the morbidity and mortality associated with an open procedure, but because it is not a neurodestructive procedure, there are no complications of facial anesthesia or anesthesia dolorosa.

Glossopharyngeal Neuralgia

Glossopharyngeal neuralgia is a disease of adults, more common in patients 50 years and older. Glossopharyngeal neuralgia is similar to trigeminal neuralgia but is much less common, occurring at ratios of 1:70 to 1:100 that of trigeminal neuralgia.[10,14] The pain of glossopharyngeal neuralgia is also shocklike in nature with spontaneous remissions. Areas that are affected include the ear, tonsils, larynx, and tongue.

Medical evaluation is similar to that for trigeminal neuralgia in that magnetic resonance imaging and CT are performed to evaluate for structural causes of the disorder. Carbamazepine and phenytoin have been reported to be effective in controlling the pain initially.

Herpes Zoster

Herpes zoster may produce two painful conditions: acute herpes zoster, also known as shingles, and postherpetic neuralgia.

Acute Herpes Zoster

Acute herpes zoster most commonly occurs in adults who have previously been infected with the chicken pox virus. An outbreak of the rash may be due to an infection or a malignancy, especially lymphoma, or the immunosuppressed state. Most cases occur without known cause. It is believed that the virus remains dormant in the dorsal root ganglion and then later becomes reactivated. It multiples in the dorsal root ganglion and then is transported down the sensory nerve to the nerve endings, where the zoster lesions erupt on the skin, producing the vesicular rash.

The management of acute herpes zoster today consists primarily of the use of acyclovir. Acyclovir is effective in reducing the length of time of the acute outbreak of lesions and in decreasing the pain and promoting healing.[15,16] The discomfort may also be treated with analgesic medications and anti-inflammatory medications. The use of corticosteroids is unclear but may help to reduce the risk of subsequent postherpetic neuralgia.

Nerve blocks may also be effective, and local infiltration of areas of eruption using triamcinolone 0.2% solution in normal saline have been used with excellent relief of discomfort. Epidural blocks may also be effective in the treatment of acute herpes zoster of the trunk and extremities.

Postherpetic Neuralgia

The pain of postherpetic neuralgia follows an acute outbreak of herpes zoster. Postherpetic neuralgia is said to occur when the discomfort of herpes zoster persists 1 month after the rash has healed. There are three primary components to the discomfort:

1. A constant burning or gnawing pain
2. Paroxysmal shooting or shocking pain
3. Sharp, radiating pain that is elicited by very light stimulation

There may also be scarring in the area of the healed rash, with altered touch or pinprick sensation.[12]

The treatment of postherpetic neuralgia is difficult. Corticosteroids may decrease the risk of developing postherpetic neuralgia. Capsaicin may also be of benefit in the treatment of postherpetic neuralgia. This topical agent is applied four to five times per day for several weeks.

Atypical Facial Pain

Atypical facial pain is a vague, ill-defined disorder. It is characterized by a steady, diffuse, aching discomfort that may last hours or days. The pain does not occur in paroxysms or in short lancinating bursts. There are no associated trigger zones or known precipitating factors of this discomfort. In addition, the pain is not limited to the distribution of the fifth cranial nerve. It may spread over a wide area of the face and also areas supplied by the upper cervical roots.[11,12] The discomfort of atypical facial pain is not improved by surgical section of cranial nerves V or IX.

Atypical facial pain may clinically resemble a form of migraine headache. Clinical symptoms with a throbbing pain are typical. Treatment is similar to that of migraine, including antidepressants or nonsteroidal anti-inflammatory drugs. Mild analgesics or sedatives can be used. Also, nerve blocks, electrical stimulation, or biofeedback can be helpful. Occasionally, treatment of atypical facial pain appears to resemble a trial-and-error approach.[11,12]

Post-traumatic Facial Neuralgia

Chronic facial pain may follow trauma to the head and face. More characteristic than the discomfort is the presence of anesthesia, paresthesias, dysesthesias, or a burning discomfort. The cause of the abnormal sensation is nerve injury to the branches of the fifth cranial nerve or to the ganglion.

Treatment of this form of facial pain is often unsatisfying because this discomfort typically does not respond to opiates or other analgesics. Tricyclic antidepressants (TCAs) and electrical nerve stimulation may be helpful.[11]

PHANTOM PAIN

Phantom sensation may occur in any appendage but is most often described in the extremities. Phantom sensation of the tongue, penis, breast, and nose have also been noted.[17–19]

Phantom limb sensation is the perception of the continued presence of the amputated limb. By definition, this sensation is nonpainful. Phantom limb pain describes painful sensations that are perceived to originate in the amputated portion of the extremity. In addition, patients may have localized pain following amputation, which originates in the stump.

Phantom Limb Sensation
Epidemiology

Phantom limb sensation is an almost universal occurrence at some time during the first month following surgery. Patients may have the perception of the amputation was not carried out as planned. The limb is described in terms of definite volume and length. Patients may try to reach out with, or stand on, the phantom limb.[20] Phantom limb sensation is strongest in above-elbow amputations and weakest in below-knee amputations[21] and is more frequent in the dominant limb of double amputees.[22]

Spinal or epidural anesthesia may be associated with phantom sensation in the anesthetized limbs. Prevoznik and Eckenhoff[23] reported a 24% incidence of phantom limb sensation that corresponded to the onset of proprioceptive blockade during spinal anesthesia. The phantom lower limbs were perceived to be raised (lithotomy position) even when the patient was supine.

Symptoms and Signs

Patients generally describe the sensations in their phantom limb either as normal in character or as pleasant warmth or tingling. The strongest sensations come from body parts with the highest brain cortical representation, such as the fingers and toes.[19,24] The phantom limb may undergo the phenomenon known as telescoping, in which the patient loses sensations from the midportion of the limb with subsequent shortening of the phantom.[25]

Treatment

Phantom limb sensations are a natural result of amputation and should not require treatment. However, before amputation, a patient should be prepared to expect these sensations so that the psychologic impact of their presence is minimized.

Phantom Limb Pain
Epidemiology

Recent studies have shown the incidence of phantom limb pain to be 60% to 85%.[25–28] The incidence of phantom limb pain increases with more proximal amputations. In the first month after amputation, 85% to 97% of patients experience phantom limb pain.[26,29,30] At 1 year after amputation, approximately 60% of patients continue to have phantom limb pain.[26,31] Pain may begin months to years after an amputation, but pain beginning 1 year after amputation occurs in less than 10% of patients.

Symptoms and Signs

Phantom limb pain is usually described as burning, aching, or cramping.[30,32] It is sometimes described as crushing, twisting, grinding, tingling, drawing, or like being stabbed with needles.[30] Up to one third of patients may report sharp, shocklike pains in the phantom limb, which are excruciating but brief.

Exacerbations of pain may be produced by trivial physical or emotional stimuli.[33] Fifty percent of patients have phantom limb pain that is provoked by emotional distress, urination, cough, defecation, or sexual activity.[25,31,33,34]

Sunderland[35] has suggested that patients can be divided into four groups based on the frequency and severity of pain and the degree to which it interferes with the patient's lifestyle.

- Group I—Mild, intermittent paresthesias that do not interfere with normal activity
- Group II—Paresthesias that are uncomfortable and annoying but do not interfere with activity
- Group III—Pain that is of sufficient intensity, frequency, or duration to cause stress but bearable and intermittently interferes with activities
- Group IV—Nearly constant severe pain that interferes with normal activities

When symptoms of phantom limb pain increase in severity or begin later than 1 month after amputation, the reasons should be investigated. Any patient who has undergone amputation because of cancer should have an evaluation for metastatic disease if phantom limb pain significantly increases.

Physical examination is generally unrevealing, although the stump should be examined for the presence of trigger areas that reproduce the phantom limb pain. Thermography may be a useful diagnostic tool if symptoms consistent with RSD are present.

Cause

Theories involving peripheral, central, and psychologic mechanisms have all been proposed. None of these theories, however, fully explains the clinical characteristics of this condition.

Peripheral Theories

Early investigators theorized that phantom pains originate from the cut end of nerves that previously innervated the extremity.[33] Studies support this neuroma theory.

The role of the sympathetic nervous system in phantom limb pain is unknown. An increase in the rate of spontaneous discharges originating in the neuroma occurs with stimulation of the sympathetic trunk or with intravenous (IV) injection of epinephrine.[36] Therefore, decreasing sympathetic activity may decrease pain originating from a neuroma.

However, peripheral theories do not fully explain phantom limb pain because complete sensory blockade does not provide pain relief in most patients. Neuromas have been found in only 20% of patients with phantom limb pain.[30]

Central Theories

The gate control theory of pain is commonly used to explain phantom limb pain. Following significant destruction of sensory axons by amputation, wide dynamic range neurons are freed from inhibitory control.[37] Self-sustaining neuronal activity may then occur in the spinal cord neurons.[37,38] If the spontaneous spinal cord neuronal activity exceeds a critical level, then pain may occur in the phantom limb. This loss of inhibitory control may lead to spontaneous discharges at any level in the CNS and explains the lack of analgesia in paraplegics with phantom body pain following complete cordectomy.[39]

Psychologic Theories

No consistent personality defect has been shown in patients with phantom limb pain, and there does not appear to be an increased incidence of neurosis or other psychologic disorders in amputees with phantom limb pain.[36,40–42] It is possible that phantom limb pain exists only as a psychopathic interpretation of phantom limb sensation.[43]

Treatment

Physical Therapy

Because phantom limb pain occurs more often in patients who are unable to use a prosthesis within 6 months after amputation,[27,44] attention must be paid to the conditioning of the stump and preparation for prosthesis use.

Transcutaneous Electrical Nerve Stimulation

Investigators have reported excellent results with the use of transcutaneous electrical nerve stimulation (TENS).

Acupuncture

Acupuncture has been used for treatment of phantom limb, but there are few reports in the English literature. Relief from phantom limb pain of the arm has been reported with electroacupuncture,[45] and relief was also obtained with the application of TENS over the same acupuncture points.

Psychologic Therapies

Kolb[40] has retrospectively reported good results with psychotherapy in some patients, and relaxation training has also been reported to benefit patients with phantom limb pain. Relaxation can be assisted by the use of electromyogram biofeedback recorded from either muscles in the stump or the forehead.[46,47]

Medications

Various medications have been used for the treatment of phantom limb pain, generally on the basis of anecdotal reports of success. The most commonly used classes of medications are antidepressants and anticonvulsants.[48] Of the anticonvulsants, carbamazepine is most commonly used. Narcotic analgesics are generally ineffective in producing long-term pain relief[28] and are, therefore, not currently recommended for phantom limb pain treatment because of the risk of addiction.[30]

Nerve Blocks

Nerve blocks are commonly used in treatment of phantom limb pain, and the physicians performing these blocks report a high success rate.[48] Trigger point or direct stump injections and sympathetic, peripheral nerve, and major conduction blocks have all been used in the treatment of pain.

Surgical Treatment

Phantom limb pain does not respond to surgical treatment. Sherman and colleagues[28,48] found that neither surgeons nor patients reported good success rates with currently recommended surgical procedures.

Stump Pain

Epidemiology

Stump pain is a significant clinical problem, because it occurs in up to 50% of amputees and results in disuse of the limb prosthesis in more than half of the patients who experience it.[49,50]

Symptoms and Signs

Pain in the stump may be spontaneous or may result from pressure by the prosthesis. It is varying in nature, character, and frequency. It may be described as sharp, stabbing, or burning.

The stump should be inspected for signs of trauma from the prosthesis or the presence of a neuroma or stitch abscess. Signs of increased sympathetic activity may be present.

Stump pain is often due to a poorly fitting prosthesis, which may cause ulceration or blistering of the skin and may lead to infection. Pain may be due to the development of bone spurs, osteomyelitis, or myofascial trigger points.

Treatment

Local injuries or infection should be appropriately treated and the prosthesis fit should be carefully examined and adjusted as needed. Desensitization of the stump with application of repetitive cutaneous stimulation may decrease pain. Surgical treatment may be necessary if vascular insufficiency is present or if a bone spur or neuroma is repeatedly traumatized by weight bearing.

COMPLEX REGIONAL PAIN SYNDROMES

Complex regional pain syndrome (CRPS) I applies to a variety of seemingly unrelated disorders having similar clinical features and manifesting the same fundamental disturbed physiology; CRPS II applies to similar unrelated disorders, in which there is a partial nerve injury to an identifiable nerve.

Regardless of the cause, CRPS I or CRPS II can be defined[51] as a syndrome of diffuse limb pain often burning in nature and usually consequent to injury or noxious stimulus with variable sensory, motor, autonomic, and trophic changes.[52] The syndrome may spread independently of the source or site of the precipitating event and often presents in a pattern inconsistent with dermatomal or peripheral nerve distributions. Clinical findings usually include autonomic dysregulation (e.g., alterations in blood flow, hyperhidrosis, edema), sensory abnormalities (e.g., hypoesthesia, hyperesthesia, allodynia to cold and mechanical stimulation), motor dysfunction (e.g., weakness, tremor, joint stiffness), reactive psychologic disturbances (e.g., anxiety, hopelessness, depression), and trophic changes (e.g., muscle atrophy, osteopenia arthropathy, glossy skin, brittle nails, altered hair growth).

Mechanism

CRPS may be thought of as prolonging the normal sympathetic response to injury.[53] A sympathetic reflex arc is the normal response to any traumatic injury. A sympathetic reflex is activated by efferent sympathetic impulses sent out of the spinal cord through the ventral roots to a ramus communications albus and then into the sympathetic chain to synapse in a sympathetic ganglion. If this sympathetic reflex arc does not shut down but continues to function and accelerate, a sympathetic hyperdynamic state ensues. This results in increased vasoconstriction and tissue ischemia, causing more pain and, thus, increasing the barrage of afferent pain impulses traveling to the spinal cord and reactivating the sympathetic reflex.

Peripheral Tissue Abnormalities

Vasoconstriction and Vasodilatation

Changes at the peripheral tissue level have been implicated by several authors as the cause of this persistent painful state. Both vasodilated and vasoconstricted states have been suggested.[52,54–56]

Leriche[57] believed that vasoconstriction at the site of injury led to tissue ischemia and pain. Abnormal vasomotor reflexes were stated to be the cause of the vasospasm. Lewis and Gatewood[56] postulated that causalgia was a state of painful vasodilatation caused by the liberation of pain-producing vasodilator substances in response to antidromic impulses arising from the area of nerve injury.

Peripheral Nerve Abnormalities

Role of Sympathetic Afferents

There is anatomic and physiologic evidence from animal studies that some afferent fibers from the affected limb travel through the sympathetic chain before entering the dorsal horn of the spinal cord.[58–61] Several clinical observations suggest that some types of pain may be mediated by afferent fibers in the sympathetic chain.

Artificial Synapse

Doupe and colleagues[62] ascribed the "peculiar" qualities of causalgic pain to stimulation of sensory fibers by efferent impulses in the sympathetic fibers. This theory states that an artificial synapse or ephapse is created at the damaged segment of the nerve by a breakdown in the normal insulation between adjacent fibers. Efferent sympathetic impulses that are tonically active can cross over to sensory fibers in the area of injury. This artificial synapse may produce several types of nerve impulses, which may account for many of the features of the disease. Impulses that cross over to the afferent pain fibers may be directed orthodromically (toward the CNS) and would be interpreted as pain. Impulses crossing to afferent pain fibers directed antidromically (toward the periphery) can also cause pain by sensitizing the peripheral nociceptor, possibly through the release of a vasodilating substance, neurokinin.[63]

Gate Theory

In 1965, Melzack and Wall[64] introduced the gate theory of pain, which is a refinement of the fiber dissociation theory. This theory proposed a balance of input by large A-beta and small A-delta and C-fibers to the CNS. This balance may be upset by any number of pathologic processes, including soft tissue or peripheral nerve injury as in the CRPSs. According to this theory, large fiber input inhibits, whereas small fiber input facilitates, the spinal cord transmission of afferent impulses. Causalgia is felt to be a result of selective damage of these large myelinated fibers, allowing the balance to favor small fiber activity, thus, opening the gate and increasing the central transmission of the painful afferent impulses. Large fiber stimulation, which may form the basis for the use of TENS, would close the gate and afford pain relief.

Neuroma Formation and Sprout Growth

The observation that properties of nerves change markedly after various types of nerve injury has spawned several theories based on neuroma formation and sprout outgrowth.[54,65–67]

The sensory fibers have their cell bodies in the dorsal root ganglia, just outside the spinal cord. When a nerve fiber is transected, the distal portion degenerates completely, for it is now separated from its cell body. The endoneural tube and Schwann cells surrounding the fiber remain intact, except at the point of injury. As the distal fiber degenerates, it is absorbed by neighboring cells. At the same time, the proximal portion of the fiber begins its regeneration of about 3 mm of growth daily until the fibers reach their original destination. If, however, the architecture is such that the sprouts do not find intact tubes nearby, they are surrounded by an area of tissue injury and inflammatory response. Multiple sprouts are sent out by each axon in an unsuccessful attempt to find the familiar endoneural structures. The end result of failed regeneration is called a neuroma and includes fibrous tissue and fine nerve sprouts trapped therein.[66]

Central Nervous System Abnormalities

Present Status

It is known that injured tissue results in spontaneous pain, hyperalgesia, and allodynia. More recently, it has become evident that tissue injury is followed by increased responsiveness of nociceptive neurons of the spinal cord. Under some pathologic conditions, especially after nerve injury, A-beta input gains access to, and triggers, the N-Methyl-d-aspartate (NMDA) receptor that is normally activated by C-afferent stimulation. Mechanical allodynia and slow temporal summation of allodynia may well be integrally related to the patient's ongoing spontaneous pain.[68]

Clinical Presentation

Trauma secondary to accidental injury is probably the most common cause of CRPS. In recent years it has become obvious that many visceral, neurologic, vascular, and musculoskeletal disorders may also produce CRPS, presumably by producing injury to nerves that initiates a physiopathologic mechanism similar if not identical to that produced by external trauma. Perhaps the most notable disease process that produces CRPS is myocardial infarction, although other thoracic disorders such as pneumonitis, carcinoma, and embolism may be followed several months later by CRPS of the upper extremity.

Signs and Symptoms

CRPS is manifested by pain; hyperesthesia; vasomotor and sudomotor disturbances; and increased muscular tone, followed by weakness, atrophy, and trophic changes involving the skin, and its appendages, muscles, bones and joints.

Pain is certainly the most prominent and characteristic feature. Although it usually has a burning quality, not infrequently the patient describes it as an aching pain. It may vary in severity from mild discomfort to excruciating and intolerable pain, such as occurs with classical causalgia. The pain is usually constant but with recurrent paroxysmal aggravations. Initially the pain is localized to the site of injury, but typically with time it spreads to involve the entire extremity; in certain cases, the pain even spreads beyond the affected extremity to the contralateral limb and sometimes even to the ipsilateral extremity or the entire side of the body.

The severity of the signs and symptoms varies among patients and in the same patient in different phases of the disease. However, common to all cases of sympathetic dystrophy is the fact that the pain and physical signs do not conform to known patterns of nerve distribution, either segmental or peripheral. Moreover, they have a tendency to spread proximally to involve the contralateral and ipsilateral extremity. Once CRPS has become established, the entire syndrome continues even after the causal mechanism has healed or disappeared. An important characteristic common to all of the sympathetic dystrophies is the fact that the symptoms can be abolished by sympathetic block at an appropriate level; if carried out before the point at which the syndrome becomes irreversible, repetitive interruption of the involved sympathetic pathways can result in resolution of the entire syndrome.

Diagnosis

A diagnosis of CRPS may be obvious if (1) there is a history of recent or remote trauma, infection, or disease; (2) there is persistent, spontaneous pain that is burning, aching, or throbbing in character; (3) there are vasomotor or submotor disturbances; and (4) there are obvious trophic changes. However, although the typical case of CRPS can be diagnosed without difficulty, many cases do not present with classic signs and symptoms but with vague and confusing symptomatology that not infrequently simulates other diseases.

Differential Diagnosis

Several postoperative or post-traumatic conditions have symptoms in common with CRPS I and II. Peripheral nerve injuries may produce burning dysesthetic pain without a sympathetic nervous system component. Hyperpathia is often encountered within the distribution of transected or entrapped nerves. Pain is limited to the distribution of the involved nerve, and a positive Tinel's sign is often elicited over the site of nerve injury.

Inflammatory lesions such as tenosynovitis or bursitis may produce post-traumatic pain, which may be burning in quality and may persist for months. Myofascial pain often develops after injury or surgery. It is nondermatomal in distribution, may be burning in nature, and is characterized by sensitive trigger points in affected muscles.[69] Although the truncal musculature is most often affected, such problems may also involve the extremities.

Raynaud's disease produces vasospasm of the extremities associated with cold skin, pallor, and often cyanosis. The condition is bilateral, involving the hands and sometimes all four extremities. The vasospasm may be relieved by sympathetic blocks, but most patients are not helped by such treatment. Patients who experience transient vasodilatation with sympathetic blocks may benefit from sympathectomy or systemic α-adrenergic blocking agents.

Raynaud's phenomenon, a similar vasospastic disorder, is associated with an underlying pathologic process, often one of the connective tissues diseases such as scleroderma, and is often unilateral. As in Raynaud's disease, sympathetic blocks are helpful in a minority of patients.

Establishing an absolute diagnosis for a chronic pain problem is usually difficult, because multiple pain mechanisms often exist. It is possible, however, to assess the importance of sympathetic mechanisms by comparing the degree and duration of pain relief achieved by sympathetic blocks with those produced by somatic blocks and placebo injections.

The response to a placebo injection is often helpful diagnostically. A true placebo response, which is elicited in about one third of chronic pain patients, is usually brief (10 to 30 minutes). Pain relief persisting for days or weeks probably signifies a psychogenic pain mechanism. A very transitory response to the placebo and prolonged analgesic effect from a sympathetic block provides some assurance that sympathetic pathways are involved in the pathogenesis of the pain. If no analgesia occurs after sympathetic block and pain is relieved by blocking the appropriate somatic nerves, then a somatic pain mechanism, such as neuralgia, myofascial syndrome, or radiculopathy, is likely. Failure of both sympathetic and somatic blocks to produce analgesia points to a central pain mechanism, which may be psychogenic or may result from neuronal activity within the CNS that is independent of peripheral input.

For lower extremity pain, a differential spinal block may be used to distinguish among sympathetic, somatic, and central pain mechanisms. Following introduction of a needle into the subarachnoid space and with the patient positioned laterally, 10 ml of normal saline is injected. Relief of pain is interpreted as a placebo response. If no analgesia occurs, 10 ml of 0.25% procaine is injected, which results in preganglionic sympathetic blockade. A sympathetic pain mechanism is likely if pain relief ensues. If no analgesia occurs, 10 ml of 0.5% procaine is injected, and pain is reassessed after the onset of somatic blockade. Analgesia is interpreted as evidence of a somatic mechanism. Lack of pain relief points to a central or psychogenic mechanism.

Clinical Investigations

Several clinical measurements and laboratory investigations, which are listed later, are helpful in a diagnosis and treatment of patients with CRPS:

- Temperature measurement
- Thermography
- Fine-detail radiography
- Triple phase scintigraphy
- Interpretation of bone scans
- Bone density measurement
- Electromyogram
- Tests of sudomotor function
- Psychologic evaluation

These studies can aid in confirmation of diagnosis and determination of phase and severity of the disease and provide objective baseline information that can then be used to monitor the patient's response to therapy.

Current Treatment

Because the pathophysiology of CRPS is predominantly a hyperactivity of the regional sympathetic nervous system, pain management in such patients should focus on interrupting the activity of the sympathetic nervous system. This interruption can be produced by different modalities classified as pharmacologic, nerve blocks, surgical or chemical sympathectomy, physical therapy, and psychologic. In addition, a serious effort has to be made toward maintaining function and alleviating the stresses produced by the syndrome on the CNS.

Pharmacologic Treatment

A wide variety of unrelated agents, such as those listed in Box 10–1, have been used in treating CRPS because a patient suffering from this syndrome can go through phases of severe pain, limited function, and depression and eventually develop a full-blown chronic pain syndrome.

Nerve Blocks

Although the causal mechanisms of CRPS are not limited purely to sympathetic hyperactivity, sympathetic blockade and physical therapy are the mainstays of current therapeutic management. Most patients respond in an impressive manner to sympathetic blockade, and permanent resolution is possible if therapy is instituted before irreversible changes have occurred.

A series of sympathetic blocks should be performed and continued until minimal discomfort persists. If repeat injections in this manner are not possible, the admission to the hospital for continuous infusion of local anesthetic at the

---

BOX 10–1 Drugs Used in the Treatment of Reflex Sympathetic Dystrophy (RSD)

Antidepressants
Sedative-hypnotics
Anxiolytics
Anticonvulsants
Muscle relaxants
Narcotic analgesics
Non-narcotic analgesics
Nonsteroidal anti-inflammatory agents
Corticosteroids
Local anesthetics
Sympathetic blocking agents
Vasodilators
Neurolytics

appropriate site is an alternative. For upper extremity CRPS, the site of block is either at the stellate ganglion or on the brachial plexus. Continuous stellate ganglion blockade has been reported with the use of an indwelling catheter.

There are numerous approaches available for blockade of the brachial plexus. For repetitive blocks, the axillary approach is the most convenient. The infraclavicular approach is excellent for continuous infusion techniques. The thoracic sympathetic chain is not a convenient site for repeated injections, is technically difficult, and requires the use of radiographic guidance. For lower extremity disease, the epidural space or the lumbar sympathetic chain is the preferred site for sympathetic blockade. Either of these sites can be used with repetitive injection and continuous infusion techniques.

Treatment methods gaining popularity include the IV regional block technique (Bier block) employing reserpine, guanethidine, and bretylium, as well as nifedipine, a calcium channel blocker, as a vasodilator.[70–76]

Intravenous Regional Block

IV or intra-arterial infusion of ganglionic blocking agents into the affected extremity have recently gained prominence in the treatment of CRPS.[70,72,74] There are two reasons why IV administration of ganglionic blockers is superior to intra-arterial injection for treatment of CRPS. First, the likelihood of systemic side effects from an injection of these vasodilating agents is significantly greater if administered intra-arterially than if administered in an IV regional block technique. Second, it has been proposed that when these drugs are administered by an IV regional anesthetic, they are permitted to have more protracted contact with the affected extremity, allowing them to fix to the tissue and hopefully produce more significant and prolonged improvement in symptomatology. Experience with IV regional reserpine techniques is controversial. Abrams[52] and Brown[72] have found the results of this technique to be sporadic, and side effects including postural hypotension, facial flushing, and burning or injection are relatively common.

In an attempt to improve results and lessen side effects during treatment of patients with CRPS, guanethidine has been substituted for reserpine in the IV regional block format. Results with the IV regional guanethidine technique from Europe and selected North American centers appear to be more consistent and more reliable than those with IV regional reserpine.[75,77,78] For upper extremity blocks, 20 mg guanethidine is diluted in 40 ml 0.25% lidocaine or 50 cc 0.25% lidocaine for lower extremity blocks. The solution is injected into an exsanguinated extremity with drug contact permitted for 30 to 45 minutes by tourniquet inflation.

IV regional bretylium has been used because of its ability to accumulate in adrenergic nerves and block norepinephrine release. In a report of four patients with CRPS, McLeskey and colleagues[79] noted good to excellent pain relief in all patients for up to 7 months after treatment. In addition, bretylium produced objective signs of prolonged sympatholytic activity and improved function in all four patients, and side effects were minimal. Thus, bretylium appears to be an attractive alternative to guanethidine or reserpine as an adrenergic blocking agent.[79]

Surgical Sympathectomy

Surgical sympathectomy has been advocated for patients who do not experience permanent relief from blocks or other conservative measures.

Before electing sympathectomy, the following criteria should be met:

1. The patient should experience pain relief from sympathetic blocks on several occasions.
2. Pain relief should last at least as long as the vascular effects of the block.
3. Placebo injection should produce no pain relief, or the relief should be less pronounced and of shorter duration than that achieved with local anesthetic sympathetic blocks.
4. Possible secondary gain motives and significant psychopathology should be ruled out as possible causes of pain complaints.

Chemical Sympathectomy

Neurolytic lumbar sympathetic block may be chosen as an alternative to surgical sympathectomy for lower extremity dystrophy.

Sympathectomy is not without potential problems. Patients are occasionally bothered by dermatologic problems associated with skin dryness. A painful condition, sometimes termed *sympathalgia,* may begin in the second or third postoperative week.[80] Patients experience muscle fatigue, heaviness, deep pain, and tenderness in the limb that may continue for weeks. When sympathectomy includes ablation of the stellate ganglion, the resultant ptosis, conjunctival injection, and nasal congestion may be distressing but can usually be controlled with the use of 10% phenylephrine eye drops. Recent trend has been to perform radiofrequency lesioning of T2-T3 sympathetic ganglia for upper extremity or of lumbar L1 to L4 sympathetic ganglion for lower extremity.

Physical Therapy

Physical therapy is an important adjunct to sympathetic blocks and may be effective alone for the treatment of mild cases of CRPS.[81] For longstanding cases, extensive physical rehabilitation may be necessary. Active and active assisted range-of-motion exercises, muscle strengthening and conditioning, massage, and heat are particularly useful.

Vigorous passive range-of-motion exercises and the use of heavy weights may retrigger symptoms. Exercises are best performed during analgesic periods following sympathetic blocks. Often pain is severe enough to interfere with the patient's ability to do meaningful physical therapy. These patients may require hospital admission and aggressive analgesia by way of the epidural, IV, or oral routes to participate in an effective physical therapy program.

Transcutaneous Electrical Nerve Stimulation

TENS has been effective as the sole treatment[82] and as an adjunctive therapy for sympathetic dystrophy. Pain control may be achieved with the regular use of TENS in some patients with longstanding sympathetic dystrophy who have not responded to sympathetic blocks. Increased skin temperature has been documented during TENS therapy.[83]

Spinal cord stimulation or peripheral nerve stimulation are now considered superior to surgical sympathectomy in persistent CRPS. Intrathecal analgesic programmable pumps have also been found to be helpful in difficult CRPS patients.

Psychology

Psychologic intervention in CRPS patients should have the following three purposes:

1. Help patients deal with the psychologic distress that results from the prolonged pain experience.
2. Address psychosocial factors that may adversely affect the patient's response to treatment.
3. Teach effective coping strategies.

The various interventions include psychotherapy, family therapy, stress management training, biofeedback, and relaxation training. Psychotherapy and family therapy are aimed at helping patients deal with the adverse effects of pain on functioning as well as with the factors that may have a negative impact on response to treatment. Stress management training, which includes biofeedback and relaxation training, helps the patient learn effective methods of dealing with the pain or with factors that cause the pain symptomatology to exacerbate.[84–86]

Even though a small number of patients with CRPS get better spontaneously or with minimal medical procedures, most suffer for 1 to 1½ years before they begin to approach a normal and productive state. Patients in the second and third phase of the syndrome require a multidisciplinary approach to manage pain, depression, functional disability, and possible drug abuse.

OUTCOME STUDIES ON NEUROPATHIC PAIN

Despite the wide range of therapies available for the treatment of pain-related nerve injury, most reports are anecdotal in nature. Although these data are important early in the development of a technique, they do not help when a clinician must select a treatment for a patient in the clinic. This task is greatly complicated by the lack of data comparing long-term follow-up after treatment. The least helpful piece of evidence is the single case report, next is the case series or review of the literature, followed by uncontrolled clinical trials. The usual "gold standard" for therapeutic assessment is the controlled clinical trial. These are usually performed on a carefully selected group of patients with well-defined pain characteristics and clear causes of pain. Three of the most commonly studied neuropathic pain types are postherpetic neuralgia, diabetic neuropathy, and trigeminal neuralgia.

Controlled trials can suffer from several shortcomings. The study procedures, although appropriate for the control of variables in the trial, may not represent the average practice in the clinician's office. Also, many trials may have small numbers of patients precluding statistical power or clear conclusions.

To address these concerns, several studies are grouped in a meta-analysis to improve power and yield clearer conclusions. The term *meta-analysis* refers to a study in which several original studies are combined statistically to produce a single estimate of an intervention's effect. For an adequate meta-analysis, the component studies need adequate numbers, clearly stated inclusion and exclusion criteria, case definition, and a clearly defined outcome of interest. In the pain field, several outcomes are appropriate in addition to pain, including function, psychosocial well-being, and adverse events as a result of the procedure or treatment. Meta-analytic techniques, however, depend on the quality of the data in the original papers.

Few studies carefully state the case definition used in the study. This deficit makes it difficult to interpret the results of a study and more difficult to apply the results to an individual practitioner's patient population. It is also difficult to evaluate the usefulness of an intervention when few agree as to what constitutes the diagnosis of the condition to be treated. Most of our efforts in treating patients with neuropathic pain are directed toward improving quality of life. Unfortunately, most studies of neuropathic pain medications use pain and pain relief as the primary outcome variables (when one is identified).

Side effects can be problematic in the performance and interpretation of clinical trials involving neuropathic pain. Few studies of pharmacologic agents for neuropathic pain have assessed the effect of patient blinding. The presence of side effects in almost all drug therapies, as well as interventional techniques, makes the interpretation of the results difficult.

It is often more difficult to prove that therapies are ineffective. It is much easier to show a beneficial effect and to determine its statistical significance. A negative trial is believable only if the study has been powered sufficiently to determine whether an effect was truly present. It is very easy to study a small number of patients and show no effect of a treatment because of truly no effect, a small effect, or variability in the data obscuring significance. A large placebo effect can also create a negative outcome, because the greater the placebo effect, the more difficult it is to determine drug effect.

The lack of well-designed studies of sufficient power to confidently direct therapy for neuropathic pain has led to a disorganized trial-and-error approach whereby the patient is indeed the experimental subject. A good description of the clinical trial design issues related to neuropathic pain therapies has been presented by Max.[87]

In discussions of treatment complications, the consequences of not treating the patient or treating with an ineffective agent or technique are seldom mentioned. In neuropathic pain, the dysfunction is often very prominent, and to do nothing would often be sentencing the patient to an ever-declining functional status. The decision to use a particular technique, which may have a chance of significant adverse effects, should be balanced with the consequences of not treating the patient adequately.

One must distinguish between side effects and complications. Confusion between those terms can lead to unnecessary anxiety and concern by both patient and care provider. For instance, dry mouth is an expected side effect of TCA therapy, but cardiac arrhythmia or anaphylactic reaction is a complication.

PHARMACOTHERAPY: OUTCOMES AND COMPLICATIONS

Methods of Evaluation

Clinical outcome studies mean little for the patient if the practitioner does not carry out adequate drug trials. Because pain relief can occur at a wide range of doses, the drug should be selected carefully and the patient educated as to the side-effect profile and the intended benefit, mainly because the side effects often appear before beneficial effects. It is inappropriate to refer to a treatment as a failure when the patient has not received an adequate trial in either time or dose. Dose-escalation regimens must take into account the particular kinetics of the drug and the rate at which side effects fade. Escalating the dose too rapidly can accentuate side effects without changing the onset of analgesia.

The practitioner and patient should also set realistic goals. The ability to increase function also relates to side effects. A successful outcome is *not* one in which pain is completely relieved but patients are so sedated or nauseated that they cannot function as desired.

Translation of clinical research results into clinical practice requires the synthesis of large amounts of data of variable quality. Several methods express the effectiveness of a treatment:

1. The probability that pain is reduced (or a component of pain) by a drug compared with the probability of reduced pain by a placebo or another active drug.
2. The result is qualified for significance and confidence.
3. Relative risk is defined as the probability of an event in the active treatment group divided by the probability of an event in the control group. If relative risk is subtracted by 1, the answer is relative risk reduction.
4. Odds ratios. The odds of an event in the active treatment group, divided by the odds of an event in the control group, has statistical but minimal clinical utility.
5. The number needed to treat (NNT) approach. This method is more clinician friendly because it expresses the number of patients a clinician must treat with a particular therapy to expect to prevent one adverse event (pain). Not all reviews use this method, but it is becoming popular because of its ease of use in the clinic and on the wards.

For neuropathic pain, both TCAs and antiepileptic drugs (AEDs) have been subjected to this analysis. This approach also allows drug classes to be compared with each other and can be used to express the relative adverse event rated.

Antidepressant Drugs

Tricyclics

McQuay and colleagues[88] reviewed the literature related to antidepressants and neuropathic pain and systematically selected reports based on design quality.

The common perception that TCAs are most effective against burning pain, whereas AEDs are more effective against lancinating episodic pain is not supported by controlled clinical trials.[3] When analgesia occurred, it was independent of pain character.

The tricyclic structure present in TCAs, carbamazepine, chlorpromazine, and related antipsychotic agents was derived from a chemical synthesis program to develop a treatment for surgical shock. In an attempt to suppress autonomic nervous system hyperactivity, thought to be responsible for surgical shock, an active antihistamine compound was modified to exert anticholinergic and antiadrenergic properties. Although this chemical led to the persistence of this structure in classical neuroleptic and antidepressant agents. The chemical design process provides a complex pharmacology consistent with the wide range of side effects observed.

Common side effects related to anticholinergic actions are dry mouth, constipation, urinary retention, tachycardia, blurred vision, and cognitive difficulties. Contraindications to TCAs include closed-angle glaucoma, benign prostatic hypertrophy, and acute myocardial infarction.

When patients are not responding to TCA therapy or when adverse effects occur at very low initial doses, the drug regimen of the patient with chronic pain should be carefully examined to rule out drug interactions.

Other Antidepressants

The introduction of the atypical antidepressants or non-TCAs was a great benefit to patients because the side-effect profiles were greatly improved. The pain management community also embraced these agents as an alternative to the TCAs for the treatment of neuropathic pain. Unfortunately, selective serotonin reuptake inhibitors (SSRIs) have been judged to be less effective for pain than TCAs in virtually all studies.[2] The rate of major adverse events, however, was half that seen with TCAs.

Antiepileptic Drugs

AEDs have been used for many years to treat neuropathic pain, especially when it is lancinating, episodic, or burning. The only Food and Drug Administration (FDA)-approved drug for relief of neuropathic pain is carbamazepine for trigeminal neuralgia. Other AEDs are used to treat neuropathic pain, but for many of them evidence is minimal, limited mostly to case reports and series. Because no study has compared one AED with another to treat neuropathic pain, relative recommendations are difficult to make. The many new AEDs have greatly expanded the treatment options for neuropathic pain patients. So far, few of these agents have been studied for analgesic efficacy.

Carbamazepine and phenytoin are the AEDs most commonly studied for neuropathic pain.[90] Trigeminal neuralgia is the most commonly studied neuropathic pain state.

There is a close association between analgesic effects and adverse events. What these data do not address is the effectiveness of the drug therapy when it is combined with other treatment modalities or when treatment is initiated at various stages in the course of a patient's pain state. Combination therapy, such as an AED and an antidepressant, may lead to greater efficacy but may also narrow the dose range between effectiveness and toxicity resulting from drug interactions and synergies.

Second-generation AEDs are now being examined for their antineuropathic pain properties. Lamotrigine, a once-a-day AED, is reported to be effective for trigeminal neuralgia.[91]

AEDs can produce a range of adverse effects from mild, "just bothersome" in some patients to serious adverse events, which range from 25% to 50% of patients in the studies. The most common side effects were drowsiness, dizziness, and gait disturbance.

Other adverse effects include mental clouding, vertigo, and dizziness. Ataxia can be seen with most AEDs as the dose is increased or when one or more are combined. These effects on the CNS are dose dependent and can usually be minimized by a careful dose reduction. The most troublesome effects of AEDs are hepatic toxicity and dermatologic effects ranging from rashes to life-threatening erythema, desquamation, and mucositis similar to Stevens-Johnson syndrome. Any report of maculopapular rash in a patient should be taken seriously; the drug should be stopped and the patient seen quickly.

Hepatic dysfunction has been rarely reported with carbamazepine, and baseline liver and renal function tests should be obtained at the start of therapy.

Opioids

Opioids have been traditionally avoided in neuropathic pain states because they were assumed to be ineffective. More recent trials and reports have led practitioners to reconsider this position. Open trials with opioid infusion and sustained-release opioids have demonstrated pain relief in postherpetic neuralgia. Responsiveness must be viewed in the context of adverse events, in that patients with intolerable adverse events cannot titrate the opioid dose to an effective level. In summary, the responsiveness to opioids cannot be predicted purely by the type of pain. The adverse effects of opioids are well known.

Capsaicin

Many pain-predominant neuropathies involving small afferent fibers are resistant to the antihyperalgesic agents already listed. Capsaicin, the vanniloid compound most commonly associated with hot peppers, can deplete the transmitter contents of small afferent fibers and, ultimately, can cause a degeneration of the small-caliber terminal.

Several claims have been made for capsaicin-induced analgesia in cutaneous hyperalgesia states mostly from uncontrolled studies. Topical 0.025% capsaicin has been reported to improve the pain associated with postherpetic neuralgia.[92,93]

In general, it is difficult to recommend capsaicin cream in the forms available for the treatment of painful neuropathies. The choice to use a therapy must take into account the adverse event profile versus potential benefit. For capsaicin, degranulation of primary afferent fibers can cause a variety of adverse events; when applied topically, it causes a burning sensation that can worsen the existing cutaneous hyperalgesia.

Although most of capsaicin's effect in these studies can be appropriately assigned to a large placebo effect, there appears to be some small beneficial effect of the available preparations. The efficacy of capsaicin can be improved by increasing the concentration and injecting it into the affected skin to deliver more agent to the afferent fiber.

Lidocaine

IV lidocaine infusion can reduce spontaneous abnormal activity in injured axons and neuromas,[94–96] and these findings have led to the use of IV lidocaine in patients with neuropathic pain. Many claims of success have been made, but few controlled clinical trials have been reported. Although the relief is typically short lived with IV lidocaine, some reports claim pain relief lasting days to weeks in 10% of subjects.

Risks of IV lidocaine include precipitation of seizures and cardiac arrhythmias at high plasma concentrations. Side effects commonly seen at moderate doses are paresthesias in the fingers, abnormal taste, tinnitus, blurred vision, drowsiness, and dysarthria.

Mexiletine

Mexiletine, an oral antiarrhythmic agent, has relieved neuropathic pain in diabetic neuropathy[97] and postherpetic neuralgia[98] in well-controlled studies. As with many other antineuropathic pain agents, there is no correlation between plasma level and degree of pain relief.

Because mexiletine is prone to many drug interactions, especially those resulting from the cytochrome P-450 2D6 system, it should be used with caution in patients already receiving TCAs and SSRIs. The most common side effects are related to the gastrointestinal tract and include heartburn and nausea. Also common are dizziness, tremor, nervousness, and headache, although these effects may fade with chronic dosing. The adverse effect of most concern is the ability of mexiletine to worsen preexisting cardiac arrhythmias, and it should not be used in patients with second-degree or third-degree heart block.

Given the multiple adverse reactions and drug interactions displayed by the common antineuropathic pain agents, the use of a topical agent would be welcome.

Clonidine

Clonidine, an α-adrenergic agonist, has analgesic activity when administered intrathecally. Topical clonidine relieved diabetic neuropathy pain in two well-controlled studies.[99,100] Transdermal clonidine appears to be effective for only a subpopulation of neuropathic pain patients, and prolonged use is associated with dermatitis-like reactions. The pain relief appears localized to the areas just beneath the patch. Adverse reactions include orthostatic hypotension, sedation, weakness, dizziness, and dry mouth.

Baclofen

Baclofen, a γ-aminobutyric acid-B (GABA-B) agonist, can facilitate inhibitory mechanisms in the spinal cord and decrease the hyperexcitation in neuropathic pain. The most convincing evidence for its antineuropathic pain activity is in trigeminal neuralgia.

The most common side effects are drowsiness, dizziness, and gastrointestinal upset.

Calcitonin

A few controlled studies of intranasal calcitonin have supported its use in patients with CRPS and patients with phantom limb pain.[101,102]

α-Adrenergic Blockers

Few data support the use of systemic α-adrenergic blockers in CRPS. Terazosin, prazosin, and phenoxybenzamine have all been effective in anecdotal reports, but the data are unconvincing. These drugs all tend to produce significant cardiovascular side effects and to worsen disability.

Preventive Therapy

Given the difficulty of treating postherpetic neuralgia, it may be more effective to prevent acute herpes zoster pain from becoming chronic.

Neural Blockade

The role of neural blockade in the management of neuropathic pain depends on the presumed origin of the pain. A central pain syndrome is not likely to respond over the long term to the blockade of peripheral nerves. A transient reduction in pain can be achieved by reduced total neural input to the CNS. An increase in peripheral afferent activity can be addressed via neural blockage, whereas a defect in central suppression systems probably can be handled by pharmacologic or neural augmentation techniques.

Neural blockade has become a staple in the collection of treatments for neuropathic pain, and reports have addressed its role in diagnosis. Often spinal root blockade is used to predict the response from surgery on that root or spinal level.

Epidural Steroid Injections for Radiculopathy

Epidural steroid injection is probably the most common nerve block performed for neuropathic or radicular pain. Accordingly, many studies have been published, although definitive outcome studies are lacking;[103–112] thus, the debate continues as to the efficacy of this treatment, although its safety has been well documented.[104]

Complications

Little is known about the true efficacy of neural blockade in neuropathic pain, but much is known regarding the potential complications of neural blockade. Great skill in both placement of the injection and approach to the patient is needed in neural blockade for pain management. If the intention is diagnosis of the problem, poorly performed or evaluated nerve block can lead to inappropriate treatment and delay pain relief. Inadequately performed sympathetic ganglia blocks can result in inappropriate repeated blocks or surgery for sympathectomy. Poorly performed nerve blocks can further traumatize patients and lead to further despair.

The physician must first be keenly aware of the objective of the proposed conduction block, and the patient must then be educated as well.

Everyone performing neural blockade therapy must have the skills, knowledge, and equipment available for resuscitation. Although compilations can occur with neural blockade, they are typically transient and not life threatening if the practitioner is vigilant and the appropriate treatment is initiated.

Many complications can be avoided by the proper selection of patient through a complete history and physical evaluation. There is no substitute for getting to know the patient and clarifying the clinician's plans and the patient's expectations.

Many patients are emotionally distraught because of their painful state. Any complications or even side effects are poorly tolerated and, if unexpected, can take on greater significance in the patient's mind.

Specific complications related to nerve injury can occur after direct injury to the nerve by the needle, from toxicity resulting from the injected material, and from ischemia because of the pressure exerted on the nerve after an intrafascicular injection.

Local anesthetics in general have reversible actions on neural function; with increasing concentrations, however, they become toxic to nerves and muscles. Local anesthetics can cause degeneration of muscle fibers after a single injection.[113] Regeneration usually occurs over 2 weeks with little or no consequence. Repeated injections over short intervals, however, may cause extensive and irreversible damage.

Intrafascicular injection of local anesthetic can lead to devastating consequences from cytotoxicity and edema. This effect grows with increasing local anesthetic concentration.[114,115] Additives can augment the neurotoxicity of the intrafascicular local anesthetics.

Nerve injuries can occur with direct insertion of the needle point into the nerve. The rent caused by the needle trauma can expose the nerve to edema and the toxic effects of the injected material. The endoneural contents can also extrude through the defect.

To avoid nerve injury,[116] the practitioner should:

1. Use a blunt needle ("B" bevel) when possible, and avoid paresthesias. If paresthesias are obtained, the clinician should not advance the needle and should consider withdrawing the needle slightly.
2. Stop the injection and move the needle more superficially, if paresthesias intensify during injection. Multiple injections during the same visit invite injury, as the nerve may be blocked enough to mask any warning paresthesias.
3. Avoid heavy sedation because it may not allow the patient to provide the feedback needed to prevent nerve injury.
4. Move the needle only along the axis of the shaft, not laterally. If the needle is to be redirected, the tip should be brought to the skin surface and then reinserted.

Complications can also occur because of pulmonary or vascular compromise. Inadvertent injection of even small volumes of local anesthetic into the cerebral circulation can lead to life-threatening consequences if the appropriate actions are not taken.

Hematomas can occur with neural blockade but usually do not present any significance unless they are located in the epidural space. Epidural hematomas can occur after spinal or epidural injection and, if unrecognized, can lead to permanent neurologic injury.

Respiratory complications can occur after blockade of the motor fibers to the intercostal muscles, as in epidural or spinal local anesthetic block, or as a result of phrenic nerve blockade, which impairs the diaphragm activity. Injection or spread of local anesthetic into the epidural space or cerebrospinal fluid can occur from paravertebral nerve block techniques, including deep cervical plexus block, intercostal nerve block, interscalene block, stellate ganglion block, and thoracic and lumbar nerve root and sympathetic ganglion in the neck region, including interscalene brachial plexus block and cervical nerve root blocks.

Allergic reactions to local anesthetics are rare. Injuries to nerve or soft tissue can occur if an extensive region is blocked. The loss of sensation, although allowing pain relief, may also result in the patient's self-injury.

Intravenous Regional Infusion

Indications and Efficacy

IV regional blockade is directly related to the Bier block employed intraoperatively for surgery on the distal extremities. Several variations of this technique exist, but most employ a means of exsanguinating an extremity and then isolating the regional blood flow by means of a single or double tourniquet. The now nearly empty vascular space is filled with the therapeutic agent of choice and then maintained in this space for a variable length of time, usually up to 2 hours.

IV regional infusions continue to be advocated by pain practitioners, and care reports and case series are offered as proof. The relative ease of performance and relative lack of complications continue to fuel this trend.

Complications

Complications can include infection from IV placement, compression, and subsequent ischemia of peripheral nerves resulting from tourniquet use. Toxicity of the infusion material results if the blood pressure cuff fails to isolate the region. The last problem should be minimized by the use of a double tourniquet. A relatively high concentration of agent in a small volume can be used in the restricted region of the isolated circulation. Potential complications can occur with high-concentration local anesthetic or α-adrenergic antagonists when the blood pressure cuff fails shortly after infusion, before the tissues have absorbed the material.

Neurostimulation

No surveys or controlled studies have been done of dorsal column stimulation in neuropathic pain caused by polyneuropathy. Neurostimulatory techniques include acupuncture, percutaneous electrical nerve stimulation, dorsal column stimulation, and deep brain stimulation.

Transcutaneous Electrical Nerve Stimulation

Conventional TENS has shown the best results in patients with postherpetic neuralgia. In a summary of long-term follow studies, Sjolund[117] found the most useful applications of TENS to be (1) when the pain was due to deafferentation, (2) when the pain was precisely localized, (3) when the treatment may be applied closely to the nervous structure supplying the painful area, and (4) when enough lemniscal fibers were preserved to transmit the stimulation.

Peripheral Nerve Stimulation

Peripheral nerve stimulation (PNS) has had limited use because of the requirement for surgical manipulation of the nerve, which may increase scarring. PNS is usually recommended for patients with pain associated with a single nerve without a correctable lesion, resulting from nerve trauma, postherpetic neuralgia, or CRPS.[118]

Spinal Cord Stimulation

Success with spinal cord stimulation requires the ability to superimpose paresthesias on the effected region, usually by a trial stimulation before the stimulator is implanted. North[119] listed several indications for spinal cord stimulation in order of reported success rates. Lumbar arachnoid fibrosis or failed back surgery syndrome with radiculopathy[120] were the most successful, followed by peripheral vascular disease with ischemic pain, peripheral nerve injury, neuralgia or causalgia, phantom limb or stump pain,[121] and spinal cord lesions.[122,123] The use of spinal cord stimulation for peripheral neuropathic pain was suggested by the findings of Tesfaye and colleagues.[124] Neurostimulation of the spinal cord in amputees has given mixed, if not poor, results.[125]

Complications

Complications associated with implantable stimulation devices occur at a high rate compared with other procedures. These complications often lead to secondary invasive procedures but are usually minor. Complications can include bleeding, infection, epidural abscess, meningitis, cerebrospinal fluid leak, postdural puncture headache, malposition of the subcutaneous pocket, accidental subcutaneous administration of the drug in the attempt to refill the reservoir, drug-related side effects, and battery or equipment failure in spinal cord stimulators.

Nerve Destruction Procedures

Neurolytic Blocks and Surgery

Indications and Efficacy

Frustration with nonsustainable analgesia from local anesthetic injections can tempt clinicians to employ neurolytic procedures. These attempts are ill advised and often lead to patient dissatisfaction and little defense for the clinician when adverse events occur. Peripheral neurolysis is not often performed in nonterminal patients because of the temporary nature of the block and the high risk of neuritis of deafferentation pain, as well as the risk of motor deficit. With proper patient selection, however, neurolysis may have a role in pain management. Based on clinical experience, the role of neurolytic blockade can be limited to patients with pain that is well characterized, well localized, somatic, or visceral in origin and that is not a component of a pain syndrome characterized by multifocal aches and pains.

Life expectancy has also been a criterion for neurolytic block. Neurolytic procedures have been estimated to last for 3 to 6 months. Long life expectancies have been incompatible with neurolytic blockade because of pain recurrence and the potential for worsening pain or neuritis. Neurolytic blockade is also limited to nerves without significant motor function.

In general, the use of invasive neurodestructive techniques has decreased with the advent of more effective pharmacologic agents for neuropathic pain. However, as the cost of these techniques and therapies increases, the use of neurolysis may undergo a resurgence.

Complications

Complications from local anesthetic administration are usually short lived, and most complications can be managed with vigilance and proper resuscitation skills, Neurolytic agents usually produce long-term, if not permanent, effects.

The general complications can be divided into effects on (1) adjacent peripheral nerves, (2) CNS, (3) non-neural tissues around the injection, and (4) the system generally.

Postsympathectomy Neuralgia

Postsympathectomy neuralgia is a common complication of sympathectomy whether open surgical procedures or percutaneous chemical or thermal methods are used. The estimated incidence varies from 30% to 50%. Pain typically starts abruptly 10 to 14 days after sympathectomy; lasts 1 to 5 weeks; is worse at night; and is described as deep, dull, and boring. Because the pain is self-limiting, supportive analgesic therapy is the mainstay of treatment.

Surgical exploration may play a role in nerve entrapments and neuromas in restricted regions such as the amputation stump. Most patients with deafferentation amputation pain experience a recurrence of pain after surgical interruption of a pain pathway.[126] The major exception is use of the DREZ lesion in certain plexus avulsion injuries.

Neurolytic Procedures for Trigeminal Neuralgia

Trigeminal neuralgia is now treated predominantly by pharmacologic agents. However, some refractory cases must be treated surgically. Techniques include (1) radiofrequency thermocoagulation, (2) cryoanalgesia, (3) microvascular decompression, (4) retrogasserian glycerol injection, and (5) balloon rhizolysis. Many of these techniques have been furthered by the use of CT or fluoroscopic or ultrasound guidance.

Radiofrequency Thermocoagulation

Radiofrequency thermocoagulation is considered the leading neurolytic technique for cases refractory to pharmacologic therapy, especially with carbamazepine. Its advantages include no need for a craniotomy, a high initial success rate, and low rate of recurrence.[127] Disadvantages include the requirement for a cooperative and, therefore, an awake patient and a low but finite incidence of corneal anesthesia and anesthesia dolorosa.

Microvascular Decompression

Microvascular decompression attempts to address the cause of the pain in trigeminal neuralgia by inserting a sponge between the nerve and the overlying vessels via a suboccipital craniotomy. The need for a craniotomy prevents its use in medically ill or older patients. Mortality and serious adverse events occur in 0.5% to 15% of operated patients.[127]

Advantages of this technique are a high rate of sustained pain relief up to 90% in some reports.[128]

References

1. White JC, Sweet WH: *Pain and the neurosurgeon. A forty-year experience.* Springfield, Ill, Charles C Thomas, 1969.
2. Tasker RR: Pain resulting from central nervous system pathology (Central pain). In Bonica JJ, editor: *Pain.* New York, Raven Press, 1980.
3. Pagni CA: Central pain due to spinal cord and brainstem damage. In Wall PD, Melzack R, editors: *Textbook of pain.* Edinburgh, Churchill Livingstone, 1984.
4. Cassinari V, Pagni CA: *Central pain: A neurosurgical survey.* Cambridge, Mass, Harvard University Press, 1969.
5. Lhermitte J, Levy G, Nicholas M: Les sensations de dechanges electriques, symptome precoce de la scleroser en plaque. Clinique et pathogenie. *Presse Med* 39:610, 1927.
6. Bosch EP, Mitsumoto H: Disorders of peripheral nerves, plexuses and nerve roots. In Bradley WG et al, editor: *Neurology in clinical practice.* Boston, Butterworth-Heinemann, 1991.
7. Oh SJ: *Clinical electromyography: Nerve conduction studies.* Baltimore, University Park Press, 1984.
8. Brown MJ, Asbury AK: Diabetic neuropathy. *Ann Neurol* 15:2, 1984.
9. Max MB, Lynch SA, Muir J et al: Effects of desipramine, amitriptyline and fluoxetine on pain in diabetic neuropathy. *N Engl J Med* 326:1250, 1992.
10. Fromm GH: *Medical and surgical management of trigeminal neuralgia.* Mount Kisco, NY, Futura Publishing, 1987.
11. Fromm GH: Neuralgias of the face and oral cavity. *Pain Dig* 1:67, 1991.
12. Dalessio DJ: Diagnostic and treatment of cranial neuralgias. *Med Clin North Am* 75:605, 1991.
13. Raj PP, Johnson KS, Murphy TM et al: Nerve blocks. In Raj PP, editor: *Practical management of pain.* St. Louis, Mosby, 1986.
14. Rushton JG, Stevens JC, Miller RH: Glossopharyngeal neuralgia. *Arch Neurol* 38:201, 1981.
15. Peterslund NA, Seyer-Hansen K, Ipsen J et al: Acyclovir in herpes zoster. *Lancet* 2(8251):8127, 1981.
16. McKendrick MW, McGill JL, White JE et al: Oral acyclovir in acute herpes zoster. *BMJ Neurology* 39(Suppl 1):327, 1989.
17. Hanowell ST, Kennedy SF: Phantom tongue pain and causalgia: Case presentation and treatment. *Anesth Analg* 58:436, 1979.
18. Jamison K, Wellisch DK, Katz RL et al: Phantom breast syndrome. *Arch Surg* 114:93, 1979.
19. Riddoch G: Phantom limbs and body shape. *Brain* 64:197, 1941.
20. Simmel ML: Phantoms in patients with leprosy and in elderly digital amputees. *Am J Psychol* 69:529, 1956.
21. Weiss SA, Fishman S: Extended and telescoped phantom limb in unilateral amputees. *J Abnorm Soc Psychol* 66:489, 1963.
22. Almagor M, Jaffe Y, Lomranz J: The relation between limb dominance, acceptance of disability, and the phantom limb phenomenon. *J Abnorm Psychol* 87:377, 1978.
23. Prevoznik SJ, Eckenhoff JE: Phantom sensations during spinal anesthesia. *Anesthesiology* 25:767, 1964.
24. Miles JE: Phantom limb syndrome occurring during spinal anesthesia: relationship to etiology. *J Nerv Ment Dis* 123:365, 1956.
25. Jensen TS, Krebs B, Nielsen J et al: Phantom limb, phantom pain and stump pain in amputees during the first 6 months following limb amputation. *Pain* 17:243, 1983.
26. Parker CM: Factors determining the persistence of phantom pain in the amputee. *J Psychosom Res* 17:97, 1973.
27. Sherman RA, Sherman CJ: Prevalence and characteristics of chronic phantom limb pain among American veterans. Results of a trial survey. *Am J Phys Med* 62:227, 1983.
28. Sherman RA, Sherman CJ, Parker L: Chronic phantom and stump pain among American veterans: Results of a survey. *Pain* 18:83, 1984.
29. Roth YF, Sugarbaker PH: Pains and sensations after amputations: Character and clinical significance. *Arch Phys Med Rehabil* 61:490, 1980.
30. Bailey AA, Moersch EP: Phantom limb. *Can Med Assoc J* 45:37, 1941.
31. Jensen TS et al: Immediate and long-term phantom limb pain in amputees: Incidence, clinical characteristics and relationship to preamputation limb pain. *Pain* 21:267, 1985.
32. Saris SC, Iacono RP, Nashold BS Jr: Dorsal root entry zone lesions for post-amputation pain. *J Neurosurg* 62:72, 1985.
33. Frazier SH: Psychiatric aspects of causalgia, the phantom limb, and phantom pain. *Dis Nerv Syst* 27:441, 1966.
34. Wall R, Novotny-Joseph P, MacNamara TE: Does preamputation pain influence phantom limb pain in cancer patients? *South Med J* 78:34, 1985.
35. Sunderland S, editor: *Nerves and nerve injuries.* New York, Churchill Livingstone, 1978.
36. Matzner O, Devor M: Contrasting thermal sensitivity of spontaneously active A- and C-fibers in experimental nerve-end neuromas. *Pain* 30:373, 1987.
37. Omer GE Jr: Nerve, neuroma, and pain problems related to upper limb amputations. *Orthop Clin North Am* 12:751, 1981.
38. Livingston WK: *Pain mechanism: A physiologic interpretation of causalgia and its related states.* New York, MacMillan, 1944.
39. Melzack R, Loeser JD: Phantom body pain in paraplegics: Evidence for a central "pattern generating mechanism" for pain. *Pain* 4:195, 1978.
40. Kolb LC: *The painful phantom.* Springfield, Ill, Charles C Thomas, 1954.
41. University of California: *Progress report of the advisory committee on artificial limbs,* ed 2. Berkley, Calif, University of California Press, 1952.

42. Ewalt JR, Randall GC, Morris H: The phantom limb. *Psychosom Med* 9:118, 1947.

43. Frazier SH, Kolb LC: Psychiatric aspects of pain and the phantom limb. *Orthop Clin North Am* 1:481, 1970.

44. Steinbach TV, Nadvorna H, Arazi D: A five year follow-up study of phantom limb pain in posttraumatic amputees. *Scand J Rehabil Med* 14:203, 1982.

45. Monga TN, Jaksic T: Acupuncture in phantom limb pain. *Arch Phys Med Rehabil* 62:229, 1981.

46. Dougherty J: Relief of phantom limb pain after EMG biofeedback-assisted relaxation: a case report. *Behav Res Ther* 18:355, 1980.

47. Sherman RA, Gall N, Gormley J: Treatment of phantom limb pain with muscular relaxation training to disrupt the pain-anxiety-tension cycle. *Pain* 6:47, 1979.

48. Sherman RA, Sherman CA, Call NG: A survey of current phantom limb pain treatment in the Untied States. *Pain* 8:85, 1980.

49. Sherman RA, Sherman CJ: A comparison of phantom sensations among amputees whose amputations were of civilian and military origins. *Pain* 21:91, 1985.

50. Helm P, Engel T, Holm A et al: Function after lower limb amputation. *Acta Orthop Scand* 57:154, 1986.

51. International Symposium on Reflex Sympathetic Dystrophy. *Reflex sympathetic dystrophy.* Mainz, Germany, June 1988.

52. Abrams SE: Intravenous reserpine. *Anesth Analg* 59:889, 1980.

53. Bonica JJ: Causalgia and other reflex sympathetic dystrophies. *Postgrad Med* 53:143, 1973.

54. Bonica JJ: Causalgia and other reflex sympathetic dystrophies. In Bonica J, editor: *Advances in pain research and therapy,* vol 3. New York, Raven Press, 1979.

55. De Takats G: Causalgia states in peace and war. *JAMA* 128:699, 1945.

56. Lewis D, Gatewood W: Treatment of causalgia: Results of intraneural injections of 60% alcohol. *JAMA* 74:1, 1920.

57. Leriche R: Causalgia envisage comme une neurite du sympathetique et son traitement par la denudation et l'excision de plexus nervuex periarterials. *Presse Med* 23:184, 1916.

58. Kuntz A, Farnsworth D: Distribution of afferent fibers via the sympathetic trunk and gray communication rami to the brachial and lumbosacral plexuses. *Comp Neurol* 53:389, 1973.

59. Kuntz A: Afferent innervation of peripheral blood vessels through sympathetic trunks. *J South Med Assoc* 44:673, 1951.

60. Kuntz A, Saccomanno G: Afferent conduction from extremities through dorsal root fibers via sympathetic trunks. *Arch Surg* 14:606, 1942.

61. Threadgill FD, Solnitzky O: Anatomical studies of afferency within the lumbosacral sympathetic ganglia. *Anat Rec* 103:96, 1949.

62. Doupe J, Cullen CR, Chance GQ: Post-traumatic pain and the causalgia syndromes. *J Neurol Neurosurg Psychiatry* 7:33, 1944.

63. Chapman LF, Dingman HF, Ginzberg SP et al: Neurohumoral features of afferent fibers in man. *Arch Neurol* 49:82, 1961.

64. Melzack R and Wall: Clinical aspects of pain. In *The puzzle of pain.* New York, Basic Books, 1973.

65. Devor M: Nerve pathophysiology and mechanisms of pain in causalgia. *J Auton Nerv Sys* 7:371, 1983.

66. Melzack R, Wall PD: Pain after injuries of the nervous system. In *The challenge of pain.* New York, Basic Books, 1983.

67. Wall PD, Gutnick M: Ongoing activity in peripheral nerves: The physiology and pharmacology of impulses originating from a neuroma by stimulation of the sympathetic supply in the rat. *Neurosci Lett* 24:43, 1981.

68. Price DD, Mao J, Mayer DJ: Neural mechanisms of normal and abnormal pain states. In Raj PP, editor: *Current review of pain.* Philadelphia, Current Medicine, 1994.

69. McCain G, Scudds R: The concept of primary fibromyalgia. *Pain* 33:273, 1988.

70. Benzon HT, Chomka CM, Brenner EA: Treatment of reflex sympathetic dystrophy with regional intravenous reserpine. *Anesth Analg* 59:500, 1980.

71. Bonelli S, Conoscente F, Movilia PG et al: Regional intravenous guanethidine vs. stellate ganglion block in reflex sympathetic dystrophies: a randomized trial. *Pain* 16:297, 1983.

72. Brown BR: Intra-arterial reserpine. *Anesth Analg* 59:889, 1980.

73. Davies JAH, Beswick T, Dickson G: Ketanserin and guanethidine in the treatment of causalgia. *Anesth Analg* 66:575, 1987.

74. Kepes ER: Regional intravenous guanethidine for sympathetic blockade. Report of 10 cases. *Reg Anaesth* 7:52, 1982.

75. Sonnoeveld GJ, Vander Nuelen JC, Smith AR: Quantitative oxygen measurements before and after intravascular guanethidine blocks. *J Hand Surg* 8:435, 1983.

76. Thomsen MB, Bengtsson M, Lassvik C et al: Changes in human forearm blood flow after intravenous regional sympathetic blockade with guanethidine. *Acta Chir (Scand)* 48:657, 1982.

77. Kozin F, Ryan LM, Carerra GF et al: The reflex sympathetic dystrophy syndrome (RSDS). III. Scintigraphic studies, further evidence for the therapeutic efficacy of systemic corticosteroids, and proposed diagnostic criteria. *Am J Med* 70:23, 1981.

78. Hannington-Kiff JG: Intravenous regional sympathetic block with guanethidine. *Lancet* 1:1019, 1974.

79. McLeskey CH: Use of cold-stress test and IV regional reserpine block to diagnose and treat reflex sympathetic dystrophy. *Anesthesiology* 59:199, 1983.

80. Hermann LG, Reineke HG, Caldwell JA: Post-traumatic painful osteoporosis: A clinical and roentgenological entity. *Am J Radiol* 47:353, 1942.

81. Pak TJ, Martin GM, Magness JL et al: Reflex sympathetic dystrophy: Review of 140 cases. *Minn Med* 53:507, 1970.

82. Stilz RJ, Carron H, Sanders DB: Reflex sympathetic dystrophy in a 6-year-old. Successful treatment by transcutaneous nerve stimulation. *Anesth Analg* 56:438, 1977.

83. Abrams SE, Asiddao CB, Reynolds AC: Increased skin temperature during transcutaneous electrical simulation. *Anesth Analg* 59:22, 1980.

84. Raj PP, Cannella J, Kelly J et al: Multidisciplinary management of reflex sympathetic dystrophy. In Stanton-Hicks M, editor: *Reflex sympathetic dystrophy.* Boston, Kluwer Academic, 1990.

85. Barowsky E, Zweig J, Moskowitz J: Thermal biofeedback in the treatment of symptoms associated with reflex sympathetic dystrophy. *J Child Neurol* 2:229, 1987.

86. Sherry D, Weisman R: Psychologic aspects of childhood reflex neurovascular dystrophy. *Pediatrics* 88:572, 1988.

87. Max MB: Neuropathic pain syndromes. In Max M, Portenoy R, Laska E, editors: *Advances in pain research and therapy,* vol 18. New York, Raven Press, 1991.

88. McQuay HJ, Tramer M, Nye BA et al: A systematic review of antidepressants in neuropathic pain. *Pain* 68:217, 1996.

89. Max MB, Lynch SA, Muir J et al: Effects of desipramine, amitriptyline and fluoxetine on pain in diabetic neuropathy. *N Engl J Med* 326:3, 1992.

90. McQuay H, Carroll D, Jadad AR et al: Anticonvulsant drugs for management of pain: A systematic review. *BMJ* 311:1047, 1995.

91. Zakrzewska JM, Chaudhry Z, Nurmikko TJ et al: Lamotrigine (Lamictal) in refractory trigeminal neuralgia: Results from a double-blind placebo controlled crossover trial. *Pain* 73:223, 1997.

92. Bernstein JE, Bickers DR, Dahl MV et al: Treatment of chronic postherpetic neuralgia with tropical capsaicin. *J Am Acad Dermatol* 17:93, 1987.

93. Watson CPN, Evans RJ, Watt VR: Postherpetic pain and topical capsaicin. *Pain* 33:333, 1988.

94. Sotgiu ML, Lacerenza M, Marchettini P: Effect of systemic lidocaine on dorsal horn neuron hyperactivity following chronic peripheral nerve injury in rats. *Somatosensory Motor Res* 9:227, 1992.

95. Chabal C, Russell L, Burchiel K: The effect of intravenous lidocaine, tocainide and mexiletine on spontaneously active fibers originating in rat sciatic neuromas. *Pain* 38:333, 1989.

96. Tanelian D, MacIver M: Analgesic concentrations of lidocaine suppress tonic A-delta and C fiber discharges produced by acute injury. *Anesthesiology* 74:934, 1991.

97. Dejgard A, Petersen P, Kastrup J: Mexiletine for treatment of chronic diabetic neuropathy. *Lancet* 1(8575-6):9, 1988.

98. Chabal C, Jacobson L, Mariano A et al: The use of oral mexiletine for the treatment of pain after peripheral nerve injury. *Anesthesiology* 76:513, 1992.

99. Zeigler D, Lynch SA, Muir J et al: Transdermal clonidine versus placebo in painful diabetic neuropathy. *Pain* 48:403, 1992.

100. Byas-Smith MG, Max MB, Muir J et al: Transdermal clonidine compared to placebo in painful diabetic neuropathy using a "two-stage" enriched enrollment design. *Pain* 60:267, 1995.

101. Gobelet C, Waldburger M, Meier GAL: The effect of adding calcitonin to physical treatment of reflex sympathetic dystrophy. *Pain* 48:171, 1992.

102. Jaeger H, Maier C: Calcitonin in phantom limb pain: a double blind study. *Pain* 48:21, 1992.

103. Beliveau P: A comparison between epidural anesthesia with and without corticosteroid in the treatment of sciatica. *Rheum Phys Med* 11:40, 1971.

104. Benzon HT: Epidural steroid injections for low back pain and lumbosacral radiculopathy. *Pain* 24:277, 1986.

105. Breivik H: Treatment of chronic low back pain and sciatica: Comparison of caudal epidural injections of bupivacaine and methylprednisolone with bupivacaine followed by saline. In Bonica JJ, Albe-Fessard D, editors: *Advances in pain research and therapy.* New York, Raven Press, 1976.

106. Coomes EN: A comparison between epidural anaesthesia and bedrest in sciatica. *Br Med J* 1:20, 1961.

107. Dilke TFW, Burry HC, Grahame R: Extradural corticosteroid injection in management of lumbar nerve root compression. *Br Med J* 2:635, 1973.

108. Goebert HW: Painful radiculopathy treated with epidural injections of procaine and hydrocortisone acetate: Results in 113 patients. *Anesth Analg* 40:130, 1961.

109. Snoek W, Weber H, Jorgensen B: Double blind evaluation of extradural methyl prednisolone for herniated lumbar discs. *Acta Orthop Scand* 48:635, 1977.

110. Swerdlow M, Sayle-Creer W: A study of extradural medication in the relief of the lumbosciatic syndrome. *Anesthesia* 25:341, 1970.

111. Winnie AP, Hartman JT, Meyers HL Jr et al: Pain clinic II: Intradural and extradural corticosteroids for sciatica. *Anesth Analg* 51:990, 1972.

112. Yates DW: A comparison of the types of epidural injection commonly used in treatment of low back pain and sciatica. *Rheum Rehab* 17:181, 1978.

113. Benoit PW, Belt WD: Destruction and regeneration of skeletal muscle after treatment with a local anesthetic, bupivacaine (Marcaine). *J Anat* 107:547, 1970.

114. Selander D, Brattsand R, Lundborg G et al: Local anesthetics: Importance of mode of application, concentration and adrenaline for the appearance of nerve lesions. *Acta Anesth Scand* 23:127, 1979.

115. Gentili F, Hudson AR, Hunter D et al: Nerve injection injury with local anesthetic agents: A light and electron microscopic, fluorescent microscopic, and horseradish peroxidase study. *Neurosurgery* 6:263, 1980.

116. Abram SE, Hoan QH: Complications of nerve blocks. In Benumof JL, Saidman LJ, editors: *Anesthesia and perioperative complications.* St. Louis, Mosby, 1992.

117. Sjolund BH: Transcutaneous electrical stimulation (TENS) in neuropathic pain. *Pain Dig* 3:23, 1993.

118. Heavner FE, Racz G, Diede JM: Peripheral nerve stimulation: Current concepts. In Waldman SD, Winnie AP, editors: *Interventional pain management.* Philadelphia, WB Saunders, 1996.

119. North RB: The role of spinal cord stimulation in contemporary pain management. *APS J* 2:91, 1993.

120. Law JD: Targeting a spinal stimulator to treat the 'failed back surgery syndrome.' *Appl Neurophysiol* 50:437, 1987.

121. Krainick JU, Thoden U, Riechert T: Pain reduction in amputees by long-term spinal cord stimulation: Long-term follow-up study over 5 years. *J Neurosurg* 52:346, 1980.

122. North RB, Ewend MG, Lawton MT et al: Spinal cord stimulation for chronic, intractable pain: Superiority of 'multichannel' devices. *Pain* 44:119, 1991.

123. North RB, Kidd DH, Zahurak M et al: Spinal cord stimulation for chronic, intractable pain: Experience over two decades. *Neurosurgery* 32:384, 1993.

124. Tesfaye S, Watt J, Benbow SJ et al: Electrical spinal cord stimulation for painful diabetic peripheral neuropathy. *Lancet* 348:1698, 1996.

125. Krainick JU, Thorden U, Reichert T: Pain reduction in amputees by long-term spinal cord stimulation. *J Neurosurg* 52:346, 1980.

126. Tasker RR, Dostrovsky JO: Deafferentation and central pain. In Wall PD, Melzack R, editors: *Textbook of pain,* ed 2. Edinburgh, Churchill Livingstone, 1989.

127. Mauskop A: Trigeminal neuralgia (tic douloureux). *J Pain Symptom Manage,* 8:148, 1993.

128. Loeser JD: Tic douloureux and atypical facial pain. In Wall PD, Melzack R, editors: *Textbook of pain,* ed 3. Edinburgh, Churchill Livingstone, 1994.

1. A study in which several general original studies are combined statistically to produce a single estimate of an intervention's effects is termed

   A. Placebo controlled study
   B. Epidemiologic study
   C. Meta-analysis
   D. Double-blind study

2. What kind of event does the numbers needed to treat (NNT) approach express, with a particular therapy?

   A. An expected event
   B. An adverse event
   C. An improvement in the patient's condition
   D. An improvement in longevity

3. One of the common side effects resulting from cholinergic action of antidepressant agents is

   A. Dry mouth
   B. Diarrhea
   C. Frequency of micturition
   D. Bradycardia

4. When injected intrathecally, clonidine, an α-adrenergic agonist, is a

   A. Neurolytic
   B. Analgesic
   C. Spasmogenic
   D. Muscle relaxant

5. Dorsal column stimulation is indicated in which of the following pain states

   A. Peripheral swelling with hyperemia
   B. Lumbar arachnoid fibrosis with radiculopathy
   C. Diabetic gangrene
   D. Acute femoral fracture

ANSWERS

1. C

2. B

3. A

4. B

5. B

CHAPTER 11

Visceral Pain

P. PRITHVI RAJ AND RICHARD B. PATT

Visceral pain originates from organ tissues of the thorax, abdomen, or pelvis. It is a deep, vague, difficult-to-locate pain that radiates away from the affected organ. It is usually accompanied by an increase in sympathetic outflow and spasm of adjacent musculature. The nonspecific features are probably due to a wide divergence and small number of visceral afferents activating a large area with extensive ramifications. The main factors capable of inducing pain in visceral structures are[1]:

- Abnormal distention and contraction of hollow visceral walls
- Rapid stretching of the capsule of solid visceral organs
- Ischemia of visceral musculature
- Formation and accumulation of algogenic substances
- Direct action of chemical stimuli on compromised mucosa
- Traction or compression of ligaments, vessels, or mesentery

Significantly cutting or burning normal viscera does not induce pain. Slow distention of hollow viscera associated with a pathologic condition is not painful, and visceral pleura, peritoneum, and parenchyma are insensitive to handling. Characteristics of visceral and somatic (superficial and deep) pain are given in Table 11–1.

True visceral pain is usually perceived during the initial episodes of a painful visceral disease.[2] Whatever the viscus in question, this pain is usually felt in the same site. Whether the pain originates from the heart, esophagus, stomach, duodenum, gallbladder, or pancreas, it is always at this site (Fig. 11–1). It is generally perceived as a deep, dull, vague, and poorly defined sensation; in most cases, it cannot even be clearly described. It is a sense of discomfort, malaise, or oppression rather than real pain. It can vary from slight to maximal intensity and is characteristically associated with marked autonomic phenomena. Strong emotional reactions are often present and consist of anxiety, anguish, and sometimes even a sense of impending death.

Over time, the symptom can be continuous, undulating, or occasional. Its duration is always limited, varying from a few minutes to a few hours, after which it either ceases or radiates to superficial or parietal somatic areas.

INITIATION OF VISCERAL PAINFUL STIMULI

Stimuli that are known to induce pain in viscera differ from those that evoke the symptom in somatic structures, and there is often no relationship between internal injury and visceral pain.[3–6] Crushing, cutting, and burning—all of

TABLE 11–1 Clinical Features of Pain of Viscera and Radiating Sites

Characteristic	Visceral Pain*	Superficial Somatic Pain	Deep Somatic Pain
Site	Thoracoabdominal, generally along the central axis and mainly in the low sternal and epigastric regions	Limited skin area	Structure involved, sometimes with a scleromeric or myomeric pattern with extension to the dermatome
Spatial discrimination	Poorly discriminated, diffused	Perfectly discriminated, circumscribed	Fairly well discriminated, of medium diffusion
Quality	Dull, heavy, oppressing, tensive	Pricking, burning, depending on the stimulus	Piercing, cramplike, constrictive, lacerating, burning, heavy
Intensity	Slight to intolerable	Slight to intolerable	Slight to intolerable
Evolution in time	Continuous, subcontinuous, undulating, occasional (colic)	Immediate, continuous, subcontinuous, undulating	Continuous, subcontinuous, occasional
Duration	A few minutes to a few hours, after which pain stops or becomes referred (parietalized)	Variable in relation to the noxa	Variable in relation to the noxa
Emotional reaction	Severe anxiety, anguish, sense of impending death	Absent	Absent
Accompanying neurovegetative signs	Pallor, sweating, nausea, vomiting, bradycardia or tachycardia, pollakiuria, alveus disturbances	Generally absent	Pallor; sweating, nausea
Additional stimuli	Do not increase pain	Increases pain	Increases pain

*Clinical features of true visceral pain in contrast to those of superficial (i.e., skin) and deep somatic (i.e., muscle, ligament, joint) pain. Adapted from Giamberardino MS, Vecchiet L: Pathophysiology of visceral pain. *Curr Rev Pain* 1:23, 1996.

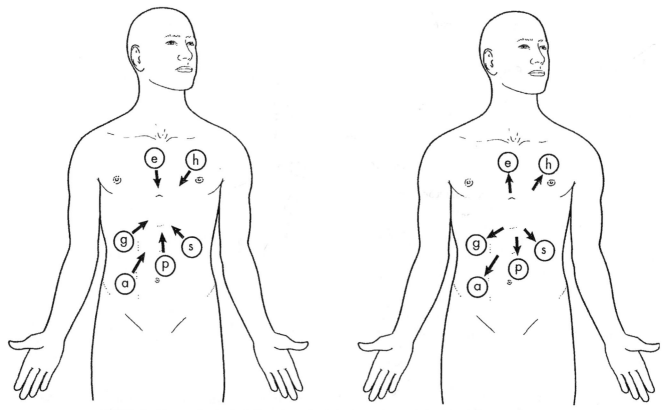

FIG. 11–1 Phases of pain. *Left,* True visceral pain is always perceived in the same site whether it originates from the esophagus (e), heart (h), gallbladder (g), spleen (s), pancreas (p), or appendix (a). *Right,* Referred pain from viscera is perceived in different areas according to the viscus of origin (*arrows*). *(Adapted from Giamberardino MA, Vecchiet L: Pathophysiology of visceral pain. Curr Rev Pain 1:23, 1996).*

which are clearly damaging and painful stimuli for somatic tissues—generally have no algogenic effect in the viscera.

Adequate visceral stimuli include mechanical stimulation, ischemia, and chemical stimulation, which may act individually or in various combinations in the different domains. Contraction of a hollow viscus under isometric conditions produces pain of much greater severity than that produced by contraction under isotonic conditions.

Inflammatory states, which cause visceral pain directly as well as indirectly by sensitizing visceral tissues to nonpainful stimuli, play and important role.

Not all viscera have the same sensitivity to pain. Solid visceral organs are the least sensitive followed by the wall of hollow organs. The serosal membranes are the most sensitive of all.

The visceral pain pathway is initiated by tissue damage activating visceral nociceptors, which can be of high or low (silent) threshold.[2]

Visceral Nociceptors

Some researchers claim that painful stimuli in viscera are encoded in the activity of specific nociceptors that are similar to those described in the skin, muscles, and joints. This is known as the *specificity theory.* Others claim that noxious events in the visceral domain are encoded in the discharge intensity of the same population of visceral receptors

that is responsive to innocuous events; this is known as the *intensity theory.*

The controversy over intensity versus specificity in the visceral domain has subsided because it has now become apparent that the two mechanisms of receptor activation are not mutually exclusive. Their relative importance may vary according to the individual viscus that is involved.[7]

A special class of nociceptors is *silent* or *sleeping* nociceptors. These receptors either are unresponsive or have a very high threshold for activation under normal conditions, but they can be "awakened" by prolonged noxious stimulation, leading to inflammation or frank damage in tissues. Activation of silent nociceptors could be an important mechanism beyond the sensitizing effect of inflammation in viscera.

Visceral Afferent Fibers

Sensory fibers in the viscera are constituents of the spinal and cranial nerves, having their cell bodies in the posterior root ganglia of spinal nerves or the ganglia of cranial nerves. Their distal processes course along with mostly sympathetic but also parasympathetic nerves, reaching the viscera, and their central processes pass via the dorsal roots.[8]

The density of innervation of the viscera by spinal afferents is small compared with the density of afferent innervation in the skin and probably also in many deep somatic tissues. A few visceral afferent fibers can activate many neurons in the spinal cord through extensive functional divergence.[9]

Nociceptive Convergence

Viscerosomatic Convergence

The second-order neurons that receive inputs are mostly located in laminae I and V of the dorsal horn, as well as in the ventral horn of the spinal cord.[10] Viscerosomatic convergence is normal, and visceral sensations can be mediated only through the convergent signals via somatosensory pathways.

Cervero[10] classified viscerosomatic neurons as:

1. A minority of neurons located mainly in the superficial dorsal horn, having a limited, ipsilateral visceral input and a cutaneous input (with restricted receptive fields activated only by noxious stimuli) and subject to descending inhibitory control. They project to the brain via spinothalamic pathways.
2. Most neurons located in the deep dorsal and ventral horn, having a diffuse and bilateral visceral input and a somatic input, often from deep tissues (with large and multireceptive fields), and subject to descending excitatory and inhibitory control. The excitatory control probably originates from the rostral medullary centers. A number of these neurons project to the reticular formation of the brainstem.

Viscerovisceral Convergence

Along with viscerosomatic convergence, there exists viscerovisceral convergence onto the same second-order neurons. Both viscerosomatic convergence and viscerovisceral convergence are maintained at the supraspinal level.[2,11,12]

REFERRAL OF TRUE VISCERAL PAIN

Referral is one of the fundamental features of visceral pain.[3] When a visceral algogenic process either recurs or becomes particularly intense and prolonged, the sensation is no longer felt in a common site, irrespective of the viscus of origin. Instead, it tends to be perceived in superficial somatic structures. Referral sites differ according to the viscera and are often remote from the primary source of the algogenic impulses. The painful sensation becomes sharper, qualitatively more similar to pain of somatic origin, and better defined and localized. It is no longer accompanied by marked autonomic phenomena. Two types of referred pain from viscera have been characterized: (1) without hyperalgesia and (2) with hyperalgesia.[2]

Referred pain without hyperalgesia is also called *irradiated segmental pain*. It is felt in wide areas of the parietal metameres that are related to the viscus in question. It may also extend to adjoining metameres (Fig. 11–2).

Referred pain with hyperalgesia, or true parietal pain, is more complex than simple referred pain, and the convergence-projection mechanism alone is inadequate to account for hyperalgesia. Two theories have been proposed:

1. **Convergence-facilitation:** Abnormal visceral input produces an "irritable focus" in the related spinal cord

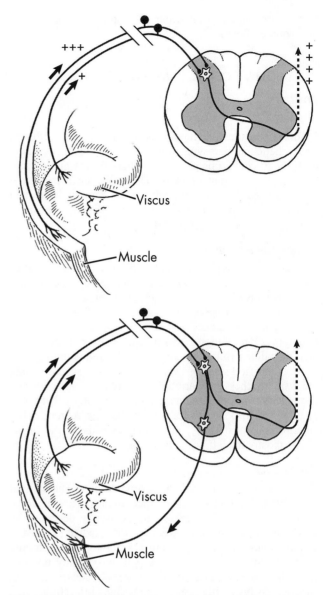

FIG. 11–2 Theories of referred pain with hyperalgesia from viscera. Skeletal muscle is used here as the site of referred pain or hyperalgesia in parietal tissues. *Top,* Convergence-facilitation theory. *Bottom,* Reflex arc theory.

segment, thus facilitating messages from somatic structures.[10] The central effect of the normal somatic input from the area of referral is amplified. According to this theory, referred pain with hyperalgesia is caused mainly by central mechanisms.

2. **Reflex arc:** Algogenic conditions develop in the periphery with subsequent excitation of pain receptors because of several viscerocutaneous and visceromuscular reflexes that are triggered by the afferent visceral barrage.[3]

Hyperalgesia and related phenomena at the skin level are induced by sympathetic efferents because a local anesthetic block of the sympathetic ganglia leads to disappearance or marked decrease of referred pain and hyperalgesia. In contrast, hyperalgesia in muscle is caused by somatic efferents. These efferents are responsible for a sustained contraction that in turn sensitizes muscular nociceptors and becomes a new source of pain.[3,13]

COMMON VISCERAL PAIN SYNDROMES

Thorax

Cardiac Pain

Cardiac structures are innervated by afferent and efferent sympathetic and parasympathetic fibers. Sympathetic fibers to the heart contain preganglionic fibers for the intermediolateral cell column at T1 to T4. These fibers exit the spinal cord via ventral roots to the white rami communicates and paravertebral sympathetic chain to the inferior, middle, or superior cervical ganglia (Fig. 11–3).

Myocardial Infarction

One of the most typical examples of visceral pain is that of myocardial infarction.[14] During the first phase, true visceral pain is perceived in the lowest sternal or epigastric areas and sometimes also in the interscapular region. The symptom is only vaguely localized; has an oppressive or constrictive quality; is often of high intensity; and is generally accompanied by pallor, profuse sweating, nausea, and vomiting.

After a period varying from 10 minutes to several hours, the pain reaches the parietal structures and assumes the characteristics of deep somatic pain. It becomes sharper in quality; tends to be located in the thoracic region, either anteriorly or posteriorly; and often extends to the upper limbs, mostly the left one (Fig. 11–4).

Pericarditis

The visceral pericardium is insensitive to pain. The parietal pericardium has no pain fibers expect in the portion adjacent to the diaphragm. Pericardial pain is usually described as sharp, burning, and precordial. It may radiate from the diaphragmatic parietal pericardium through the phrenic nerves to the left shoulder. The pain is typically relieved when the patient sits and leans forward. Causes of pericarditis include infection, myocardial infarction, cardiotomy, trauma, collagen vascular disease, irradiation, uremia, and metastatic cancer.

Aortic Dissection

Patients with dissecting aortic aneurysms often have chest pain. Anterior chest pain with radiation to the interscapular area is the typical pattern of presentation. Ascending aortic dissection is frequently associated with anterior chest pain; dissection of the descending thoracic aorta usually causes posterior chest pain. Patients with a history of hypertension, Marfan's syndrome, cystic medial necrosis, and blunt chest trauma are at risk for aortic dissection.

Lung

Lung innervation arises from T2 to T6 and the vagus via the pulmonary plexus. The lung has two types of pain receptors: J receptors (lining the interstitial space) and lung irritant receptors (found in the epithelial lining.) Mechanical or chemical damage is mediated through these receptors and the vagus nerve. Lung parenchyma is not nociceptive (Fig. 11–5).

Chest pain may be present in various pleuropulmonary diseases. Most parenchymal lung disorders cause pain by involving the pleura and mediastinum. Obstructive lung diseases can cause chest pressure by overworking the accessory muscles of respiration. Pain of pleural origin is usually exacerbated by respiration, as is pericardial and chest wall pain.

Pleurisy

Inflammation of the pleura is a common cause of chest pain. The visceral pleura has no sensory innervation; pain arises from the parietal pleura. Intercostal nerves innervate the costal part of the parietal pleura and the lateral portion of the diaphragmatic pleura, and phrenic nerves innervate the central part of the diaphragm. Therefore, radiation to the ipsilateral shoulder may occur in pain caused by diaphragmatic pleurisy.

Pulmonary Embolism

Massive pulmonary embolism can cause acute pulmonary hypertension with substernal chest pain similar to that of angina. The mechanism of chest pain is unclear. It may result from the acute distention of the pulmonary artery or from right ventricular ischemia secondary to the acute rise in afterload. A smaller embolism usually causes pleuritic pain, probably as a result of pulmonary infarction and subsequent pleural inflammation. Dyspnea and tachycardia are usually present with pulmonary emboli.

Mediastinal Disease

Mediastinitis and mediastinal tumors can result in dull poorly localized chest pain. Alcohol ingestion often causes acute chest pain in patients with mediastinal Hodgkin's lymphoma. Chest radiographs help to confirm the presence of mediastinal disease.

Pneumomediastinum can be caused by pneumothorax, acute airway obstruction, or a Valsalva's maneuver during labor. The resultant pain is substernal or precordial and can radiate to the jaw, neck, and arm. Dyspnea usually occurs.

Esophagus

Substernal chest pain is often esophageal in origin and is caused by reflux, motility disorders, infection, cancer, or connective tissue diseases and esophageal dysmotility.[15]

Heartburn is the result of esophageal reflux of gastric acid. It is a burning retrosternal pain that can be severe especially after meals and when the patient is recumbent. Heavy chest pressure with meals or physical exertion can also be caused by esophageal spasm. It can mimic angina so closely that nitroglycerin or calcium channel blockers relieve the pain.

Abdomen

Abdominal pain is usually caused by pathologic conditions in the viscera in the abdominal cavity. Thoracic referral complicates the differential diagnosis because the abdomen and the thorax have a common somatic and visceral nerve supply. Pathologic conditions in these adjacent structures can refer pain to a similar location.

The sympathetic supply of abdominal viscera is via thoracic and lumbar splanchnic nerves with synapses in subsidiary plexuses. The parasympathetic supply is via efferent

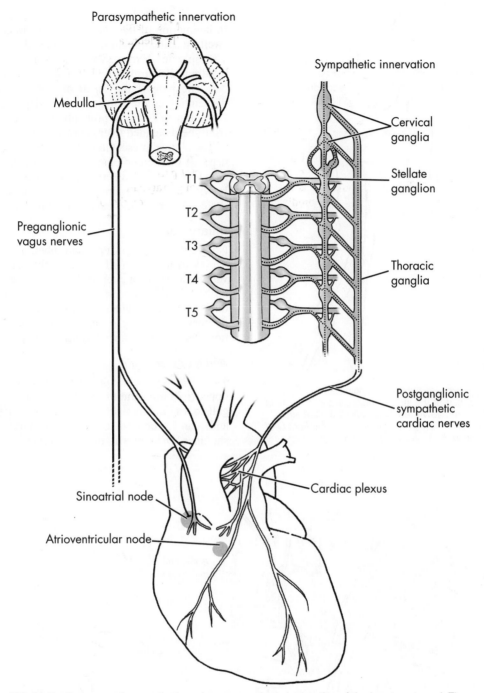

Parasympathetic innervation

Sympathetic innervation

Medulla

Cervical ganglia

Stellate ganglion

Preganglionic vagus nerves

T1
T2
T3
T4
T5

Thoracic ganglia

Postganglionic sympathetic cardiac nerves

Cardiac plexus

Sinoatrial node

Atrioventricular node

FIG. 11–3 Pathways of sympathetic and parasympathetic innervation of the heart are traced. The heart's afferent sensory fibers pass through the sympathetic chain and enter the spinal cord in the upper thoracic posterior roots (T1 to T5). *(Redrawn from Lin A, Warfield CA: Differentiating causes of chest pain.* Hosp Pract *24:44, 1989).*

and afferent innervation conducted by the vagus nerve and nervi erigentes. Pain travels with sympathetic and parasympathetic nerve fibers.

Abdominal visceral pain is present in the midline, and parietal pain is secondary to inflammation of the involved viscus, with pain referred to the lateral regions. Inspection of respiratory movements can help to differentiate between thoracic and abdominal causes.

Stomach and Duodenum

Little is known about gastrointestinal tract pain receptors. Nociception is probably via sympathetic fibers to the celiac plexus and spinal cord through splanchnic nerves T5 to T9. Nociception from the distal duodenum occurs via T8 to T11 splanchnic nerves. Common disorders affecting the stomach and duodenum are gastritis, peptic ulcer disease, and neoplasm.

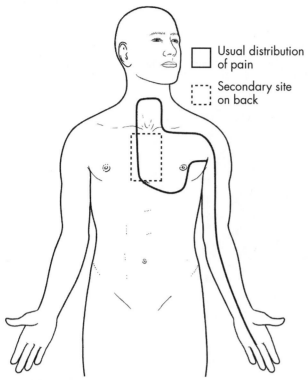

FIG. 11–4 Myocardial ischemia produces anginal pain, which is commonly felt in all or part of the sternal region, in the left side of the chest, in the neck, and down the ulnar side of the left arm. Other sites are sometimes involved, as shown. (Redrawn from Lin A, Warfield CA: Differentiating causes of chest pain. Hosp Pract 24:48, 1989).

Liver or Spleen

Inflammation of the liver or spleen can cause subcapsular swelling and pain that radiates to the diaphragmatic pleura. The splenic flexure syndrome is marked by left upper quadrant discomfort, which may radiate to the left shoulder. The pain is the result of gaseous distention of the descending colon with secondary diaphragmatic irritation. Pain transmission is probably via afferent sympathetics from the distended liver capsule.

The clinical presentation of hepatic pathologic conditions depends on the etiologic agent. In viral hepatitis, diagnosis is made by elevated serum transaminase values. Treatment for viral hepatitis is supportive, involving nutrition and analgesics. Abscess requires incision and drainage.

Biliary Pain

Nociception is via sympathetic fibers and right splanchnic nerves to the T6 to T10 level at the spinal cord. Because vagotomy does not alter pain transmission, vagal fibers play no role in pain transmission. Inflammatory disease of the biliary system stimulates afferent nerve fibers of the parietal peritoneum, causing somatic pain in the T6 to T9 distribution that is well localized to the right upper quadrant.

Acute Cholecystitis

The clinical presentation reveals pain well localized to the upper right quadrant of the abdomen and is associated with gallstones. Inflammation reaches the parietal peritoneum, and pain is referred to the intrascapular region and right shoulder. Diagnosis is made by ultrasonography, although

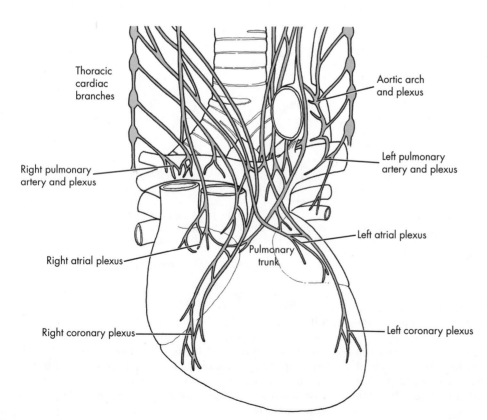

Thoracic cardiac branches

Aortic arch and plexus

Right pulmonary artery and plexus

Left pulmonary artery and plexus

Left atrial plexus

Right atrial plexus

Pulmonary trunk

Right coronary plexus

Left coronary plexus

FIG. 11–5 The cardiac plexus and its subsidiary plexuses.

cholangiography is useful preoperatively and intraoperatively. Treatment is by cholecystectomy, which relieves visceral pain in almost all patients.

Postcholecystectomy Pain

Postcholecystectomy pain is found in 5% or more of patients after cholecystectomy. It can be caused by retained stones, postoperative biliary stricture, or common bile duct obstruction. A functional disorder of biliary emptying may cause biliary dyskinesia. The clinical presentation usually involves pain in the right upper quadrant of the abdomen after a brief hiatus or postcholecystectomy pain relief. Diagnosis is made by biliary manometry, which records pressures in the common bile duct. Treatment is medical and surgical.

Pancreas

Sympathetic afferents carry nociception from the pancreas to thoracic splanchnic nerves T5 to T9 via the celiac plexus and ganglion and then to the spinal cord. Vagal afferents do not appear to mediate pancreatic pain.

Acute Pancreatitis

Chronic alcohol abuse remains the most common cause of acute pancreatitis. Gallstones are the most common cause in nonalcoholic patients. Diagnosis is made by clinical presentation and investigations. Treatment should be aggressive because acute pancreatitis is a medical emergency. The patient should be resuscitated by restoring intravascular volume, and respiration should be supported.

Chronic Pancreatitis

Chronic pancreatitis in most patients is caused by chronic alcoholism. Biliary calculus is a rare cause. The clinical presentation is one of a constant, epigastric gnawing pain that radiates to the back and is aggravated by food and alcohol. Diagnosis is made by clinical presentation; serum enzymes are of little value. Treatment includes abstinence from alcohol, support of endocrine and exocrine insufficiency, and palliation of pain.

Cancer

Pancreatic cancer is a lethal disease, with less than 2% survival over 5 years. The clinical presentation is that of an epigastric, gnawing, dull ache that radiates to the back in 25% of patients. Diagnosis is made by computed tomography (CT) scanning, endoscopic retrograde cholangiopancreatography, or percutaneous biopsy. Treatment is rarely effective.

Small and Large Intestine

Pain fibers arising from the jejunum to the ileum travel with sympathetic afferents via splanchnic nerves through the superior mesenteric plexus to the spinal cord at T8 to T12. Large-bowel nociceptive impulses are conducted through sympathetic afferents via the superior and inferior mesenteric plexus to the spinal cord at T10 to L2 and via parasympathetic afferents to the pelvic plexus and spinal cord at S2 to S4. Examples of visceral pathologic processes involving the large and small intestines include Crohn's disease and ulcerative colitis.

Genitourinary Pain

Innervation of the kidney involves sympathetic, parasympathetic, pathetic, and sensory contributions. Preganglionic sympathetic fibers from T10 to L1 convey afferent information via the white rami and paravertebral ganglia and synapse in celiac and aorticorenal ganglia. Postganglionic fibers pass to the renal plexus. Parasympathetic fibers from the vagus nerve traverse the celiac plexus and synapse in the renal plexus.

Ureter

The upper half of the ureter receives the same nerve supply as the kidney. The lower half is innervated by fibers traveling with lumbar splanchnic nerves via the aortic and then the superior hypogastric plexus. Sympathetic fibers from the sacral trunk also contribute to innervation of the ureter. Parasympathetic fibers from S2 to S4 travel with pelvic splanchnic nerves via the inferior hypogastric plexus to the ureter. Sensory fibers travel with sympathetic fibers to T12 and L1 and sometimes L2 of the spinal cord. Midureteral pain is referred to the inguinal region, and distal ureter pain is referred to the suprapubic region.

Renal and Ureteric Calculi

Patients with calculus have an acute onset of severe, colicky flank pain caused by passing of the calculus. Pain referral is dependent on the position of the stone, and the pain is not relieved by position changes. It is associated with ipsilateral costovertebral angle tenderness, nausea, vomiting, urgency, extreme restlessness, and mild shock. Diagnosis is made by clinical presentation, presence of hematuria, and radiography showing renal calculi. Treatment depends on the size of the stone, the presence of sepsis, and pain control.

Renal Tumor

Renal cell carcinoma has an unknown cause and is seen predominately in older men. Metastases can be widespread to the lung, liver, bone, and lymph nodes. Clinical presentation of flank pain, palpable mass, and hematuria are good warning signs. Diagnosis is confirmed by CT scanning and angiography. Treatment involves nephrectomy if the tumor is confined to the kidney.

Pelvis

The cyclic course of many types of pelvic pain is the reason for much misdiagnosis and mistreatment. When the diagnosis is uncertain, the patient is most commonly thought to have pelvic inflammatory disease and treated with antibiotics. In reality, many of these patients have endometriosis, a functional ovarian cyst, *Mittelschmerz,* or pelvic pain of nongynecologic origin. The pain associated with many of these noninfectious entities resolves spontaneously without treatment. The assumption that antibiotics have alleviated the pain only confirms the misdiagnosis and delays proper evaluation.

Most patients with pelvic pain who are seen in pain clinics suffer from chronic or recurrent episodes of pelvic pain and have not responded to most of the conventional forms of therapy.

Acute pelvic pain is usually organic in nature. It is easily treatable by common surgical or medical intervention if an accurate diagnosis can be established in the primary care setting. Causes of acute pelvic pain include appendicitis, torsion testis, prostatitis, salpingo-oophoritis, ectopic pregnancy, fibroid degeneration, occult pelvic fractures, dislocations, muscle sprains, and renal colic.

Diagnostic Procedures

Diagnostic procedures should be governed by a review of the patient's workup and the likely diagnosis after a meticulous history and physical examination. Complete blood count, erythrocyte sedimentation rate, cervical swabs, Papanicolaou smear, urinalysis, pregnancy test, and other inexpensive tests are used for a large number of differential diagnoses and are commonly performed very early. Other tests such as pelvic ultrasonography, magnetic resonance imaging, abdominal-pelvic CT, and determinations of CA 125 and alpha-fetoprotein levels are generally ordered in consultation with a gynecologist or an oncologist.

Pain Syndromes

Adnexal Disorders

Recurrent, painful, functional ovarian cyst occurs in young women with dull, cyclic, lower abdominal pain. Adnexal torsion leads to severe unilateral pain, which subsequently spreads.

Pelvic Muscle Spasm

Levator spasm causes pain deep in the lower abdomen, pelvis, vagina, and perineum that is triggered by intercourse or pelvic examination.

Gynecologic Cancer

Early cancer of the pelvic viscera rarely produces pain. Regular screening is of the utmost importance to identify early cancer. Abnormal bleeding, foul discharge, dyspareunia, cervical induration, and an abnormal Papanicolaou smear are often early presentations of pelvic cancer. Early spread to lumbosacral plexus, blood vessels, and bones leads to intense pain.

Endometriosis

Endometriosis can occur anywhere in the pelvic cavity but most commonly occurs in the pouch of Douglas, the uterosacral ligaments, and the peritoneal cavity. Pain is commonly cyclic and is relieved at menopause. Dysmenorrhea, dyspareunia, rectal pain, and a deep postcoital pelvic ache are common presenting symptoms.

Pelvic Congestion

Many patients with chronic pelvic pain who have no identifiable pathologic condition may be suffering from excessive pelvic congestion.[16] Characteristically, this kind of pain is dull, achy, and suprapubic with accompanying psychosomatic features such as headaches, backaches, urinary symptoms, and menstrual disorders. Pelvic congestion is probably secondary to estrogen influence and tends to disappear in postmenopausal women.

Ovarian Remnant Syndrome

Patients with ovarian remnant syndrome have adnexal tenderness and chronic cyclical pelvic pain and a history of difficult hysterectomy and bilateral salpingo-oophorectomy 2 to 3 years before the onset of pain.

Gastrointestinal Causes of Chronic Pelvic Pain

The lower gastrointestinal tract shares sensory innervation with the pelvic viscera. Gastrointestinal cases account for a large number of causes of pelvic pain. Irritable bowel syndrome, a common cause of lower abdominal pain, is often seen in gynecologic clinics and may account for 7% to 60% of all referrals.[17] Pain is generally cramping in nature and diffuse in distribution, accompanied by bowel disturbances and associated psychosomatic pathologic findings.

Urologic Causes of Chronic Pelvic Pain

Infections such as cystitis, ureteritis, prostatitis, and epididymitis may be associated with acute, recurrent, or chronic pain, usually accompanied by frequency dysuria and pyuria and positive urine cultures. Failure of treatment is accounted for by the development of drug resistance, use of inappropriate antibiotics, and inadequate treatment. Urethral syndrome is similar but more recalcitrant. A urologist should be consulted to manage all suspected urologic causes of pelvic pain.

Rationale for Patients with Pelvic Pain

To minimize further frustration, a meticulous search for causes and cost-effective management of this complex syndrome require a well thought out approach. A careful and complete evaluation of the presenting problem should be done at the outset.

A detailed history should be elicited including a full description of the pain complaint, associated disease, past interventions, psychosexual problems, and sexual history. A detailed interview with a specialist psychologist should be obtained.

Physical examination should focus largely on the area of interest while keeping in perspective the broad-based differential diagnosis and signs of associated causes of pelvic pain. Examination of the lower part of the abdomen should be performed last.

Treatment

Treatment of chronic pelvic pain syndromes of uncertain cause requires a multidisciplinary approach for best results. A psychologist, a physiatrist, and appropriate consultants are used in an exhaustive search for the cause. A pain management specialist is recruited to control pain when all else either has failed or is not considered an option. A more conservative approach at the outset involving oral nonsteroidal agents and coanalgesics is followed by narcotics, nerve blocks, and other interventional pain techniques (see Fig. 11–1). Some of these techniques include:

- Laparoscopy
- Hysterectomy
- Presacral neurectomy
- Percutaneous superior hypogastric plexus block (Fig. 11–6)
- Ganglion impar block (Fig. 11–7)
- Lumbar sympathetic block
- Somatic nerve block

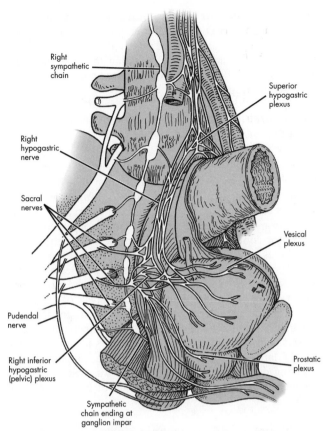

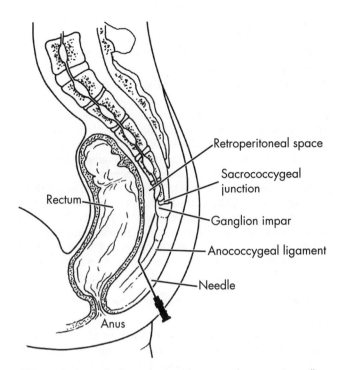

FIG. 11–7 Lateral schematic view demonstrating correct needle placement for blockade of ganglion impar and anatomic relations.

FIG. 11–6 Simplified anatomy of the pelvis. *(Modified from Bonica JJ, editor: The management of pain, ed 2. Philadelphia, Lea & Febiger, 1990).*

- Subarachnoid and epidural neurolytic block
- Spinal cord stimulation and sacral stimulation
- Neuraxial opioids and clonidine

SYMPATHETIC AXIS: AN ENTICING TARGET FOR NEUROABLATION

Several observations have led to the acceptance of sympathetic nerve block in the management of pain, especially pain from incurable cancer. First is the widespread recognition that the sympathetic nervous system plays a critical role in the transmission of visceral pain.[18] The second equally fundamental observation is a recognition that, in the absence of technical errors or rare unexpected mishaps, interruption of the pertinent components of the sympathetic axis (even when taken to the extreme of chemical, thermal, or surgical destruction) is typically accompanied by pain relief with no accompanying tactile insensibility (numbness) or motor weakness and with only a modest risk of postablative dysesthesias. Given the presence of discrete neural targets that are accessible and can be transgressed with minimal risk of neurologic morbidity, it is not surprising that these ablative therapies have been met with considerable enthusiasm both historically and in contemporary practice.

Methodologic Difficulties

Unfortunately, because of features peculiar to the target symptom of pain and the nature of intervention,[19] the methods employed to determine outcome often do not provide certainty to the discriminating clinician's decision making.[20–22] However, the more critical and scientific approach adopted by some investigations,[23–28] combined with the overall volume of reports in the literature,[29–31] is sufficient to serve as a reasonable guide to clinicians seeking to integrate these techniques into their practice.

The contemporary clinician must be conversant with all the literature, including its deficiencies and possible interpretations, while ideally undertaking the broader obligation of serving as clinician-investigator or at least supporting the scientific initiatives of appropriate funding agencies and professional societies.

Historical Aspects

Since Kappis[32] introduced the percutaneous splanchnic nerve block in 1914, pain emanating from the abdominal viscera has been managed by blocking sympathetic nervous system components. Because reliably safe general anesthetic agents were not yet introduced, this technique and early modifications were limited to providing intraoperative and, later, postoperative analgesia. In the late 1940s, local anesthetic blockade of the splanchnic nerves and celiac plexus was first advocated to relieve nonsurgical abdominal pain[31]; in 1957, alcohol neurolysis was first reported by Jones.[33]

The literature of the 1980s increasingly reported the use of modified techniques (transcrural,[34,35] transaortic,[36] anterior percutaneous,[37] transcatheter neurolysis[38]) that, despite an increased emphasis on anatomic detail and diagnostic imaging support, still generally lacked scientific controls. Reports published in the 1990s were generally better designed and provided greater clinical detail.[23–28]

Alternative Approaches

"Classic" Techniques of Kappis (Retroaortic Splanchnic Nerve Block)

As recounted by Labat,[39] the classic Kappis technique was actually conducted with patients in a lateral decubitus position, thus requiring that they be repositioned on their opposite side between injections. Introduced just below the 12th rib and 7 cm lateral to the spine, needles were advanced toward the anterolateral margin of the thoracolumbar vertebral column at an angle of about 30 degrees. Depending on patient gender and habitus, a total of 50 to 70 ml of procaine was deposited at three distinct sites per side, which reached through three separate paravertebral skin weals. In a later modification of his own technique, Kappis reverted to a single skin weal, recognizing that he could reach all three sites by withdrawing the needle into the subcutaneous tissue and adjusting it cephalocaudad.

First Anterior Percutaneous Approach

Wendling[40] suggested the first anterior percutaneous approach to the splanchnic nerves. It involved a single needle introduced through the intact abdominal wall, 0.5 cm to the left of the midline and 1 cm below the xiphoid process. Inserted perpendicular to the skin, the needle was advanced through the left lobe of the liver and the lesser omentum until the anterior surface of the 12th vertebral body was encountered at a depth of about 6 cm, where 50 to 80 ml of solution was injected. Criticized by contemporary authorities, this technique was quickly abandoned until a similar, CT-guided approach, reintroduced by Matamala and coworkers,[37] was received enthusiastically 60 years later.

Injection during Laparotomy and Other Surgical Approaches

Braun[41] and later Pauchet first advocated a so-called anterior approach to splanchnic anesthesia, undertaken at the time of laparotomy.[41,42] Whether this approach is best regarded as truly anterior is debatable; although undertaken from an anterior vantage point, the injectate is ultimately deposited in about the same location as more traditional posterior approaches. Isolated reports of paraplegia with this approach highlight the importance of this distinction on the basis of theoretical concerns that needle trajectory may influence the risk of neurologic morbidity.

When this technique was pioneered, laparotomy was initially facilitated by local infiltration anesthesia, then retraction of the left lobe of the liver and lesser curvature of the stomach exposed the anterior surface of the first lumbar vertebrae.

Although reports are few,[43–45] thoracoscopic splanchnicectomy performed with contemporary endoscopic technique shows considerable promise.

Early Modifications to Kappis' Posterior Technique

While acknowledging Kappis' contributions, Finsterer[42] strongly decried the lateral position, opting instead for the performance of splanchnic anesthesia with the patient seated, for reasons of safety. Attributing numerous reported fatalities with splanchnic anesthesia to unrecognized intravascular and intrathecal injections, he surmised that the effects of gravity and pressure in the seated patient would facilitate the recognition of aberrant placement. Expressing a similar concern regarding the potential for local anesthetic toxicity, he also advocated eliminating the satellite injections above and below the principal site of drug deposition proposed by Kappis and later by Labat.

Transcrural (Precural) Celiac Block Versus Retrocrural (Deep Splanchnic) Block

In 1978, Boas[35] emphasized the importance of *retrocrural* and *transcrural (precrural)* needle placement, a distinction further refined by Singler's[34] introduction of a CT-guided transcrural approach in 1982. Using CT, Singler noted that Moore's classic posterior technique resulted in a retrocrural disposition of the needle tips. He further observed a tendency for contrast to accumulate in the retroaortic space, sometimes tracking backward toward the lumbar plexus, and noted poor spread anterior to the aorta. Singler advanced needles through the diaphragmatic crura and positioned their tips on each side of the anterior aspect of the aorta, using CT guidance to calculate insertion points and trajectories that ensured avoidance of renal parenchyma and major vessels. Attributing the success of Moore's technique to the use of large volumes of injectable to accommodate for injecting distant to the plexus, Singler was able to achieve excellent results with just 10 to 20 ml of 50% alcohol on each side.

Traditional (High) Splanchnic Block and Its Modifications

The so-called classic (modified Kappis) approach to celiac plexus block is best regarded as a deep splanchnic block[46] and must be distinguished from the traditional paravertebral approach to splanchnic block. The greater, lesser, and least splanchnic nerves run together along the anterolateral aspect of the T11 and T12 vertebral bodies before piercing the diaphragm and synapsing in the celiac plexus. Although the technique for high splanchnic block has been known since the time of Kappis, until recently it has not enjoyed much popularity relative to celiac (and deep splanchnic) block. The splanchnic nerve block technique is similar to that of the classic retrocrural approach to the celiac plexus.

Transaortic Approach

In 1983, Ischia and colleagues[36] introduced the concept of deliberately transgressing the abdominal aorta with a single, posteriorly placed needle to ensure preaortic spread of injected solutions. One strength of the technique is reliance on the predictable juxtaposition of the targeted nerve and an easily identified vessel. Probable safety was suggested by documented experience with both transarterial axillary blocks and translumbar aortograms.

Although the potential for aortic tears, dissection, and abrupt or occult retroperitoneal hemorrhage was recognized, early experience with the transaortic approach, including one study that measured serial hematocrits and another that introduced postprocedural CT scanning, implied safety.[36,47,48] Potential advantages of the transaortic method include reliance on a single needle, elimination of the need for costly CT scanning, and assurance that drug is deposited both near where the plexus is concentrated and distant from the spinal axis.

Contemporary Anterior Percutaneous Techniques

A percutaneous anterior approach to the plexus was advocated early in the 20th century, only to be abandoned later.[40] The advent of fine needles, improvements in radiologic techniques, and advances in interventional radiology have since revitalized this option for blocking the celiac plexus. Consensus that anterior percutaneous approaches may be associated with less risk of paraplegia supports an increase in this technique's popularity in coming years.

Anterior Approach with CT Guidance

Anterior techniques involve the use of CT scout films to target either the L1 vertebral body[49] or, more commonly, the root of the celiac artery[37] and then to plot coordinates to determine the optimal point of insertion, needle trajectory, and depth. For neurolytic block, a preliminary injection of local anesthetic is recommended to further verify placement.

Anterior Approach with Ultrasound Guidance

Although slow to be adopted in the United States, ultrasonographically guided celiac neurolysis, performed generally via a percutaneous anterior approach, has been described in a number of reports.[50–52]

Complications Associated with Celiac and Splanchnic Block

The consideration of complications is especially pertinent when informed consent is being obtained. Operationally, complications can be regarded as minor, moderate, or severe; fortunately, those that are relatively common are of minor significance and are readily reversible. Complications of a moderate nature occur infrequently and, although generally reversible, entail more demanding management, including possible hospitalization and additional procedures. Finally, the most severe complications are extraordinarily infrequent but, regrettably, are rarely associated with recovery.

Minor Complications

Hypotension[53] and *diarrhea,* the most common complications of celiac block, are usually transient and, when anticipated, innocuous. Because they are sufficiently common, a combination of prophylaxis, patient education, monitoring, and a well-conceived management plan are warranted. The clinician should be aware that despite their usual benign outcomes, hypotension and diarrhea are occasionally prolonged, severe, and, without intervention, potentially even life threatening. Other minor complications can include self-limited *pain* (manifesting as dull backache or pleuritic pain) or *metabolic* and *chemical complications.*

Moderate Complications

Complications of moderate severity generally involve accidental mechanical or chemical injury to structures within the path of needle insertion or adjacent to the targeted nerves. Given the location of the plexus at the body's epicenter, the proximity of many major vulnerable structures, and the anatomic changes wrought by advanced cancer, it is

surprising that such events do not occur with greater frequency. Nevertheless, complications stemming from injury to nearby structures are so infrequent that they are described almost exclusively in case reports, and few studies describe more than one (if any) complication of a particular type. A busy pain specialist might conceivably complete an entire career without encountering a single example of complication. Such complications, should they be encountered, generally can be described as *either visceral injury* or *minor neurologic complications.*

Major Complications

Although extremely infrequent outcomes of celiac neurolysis, major complications are important not only because of their serious and usually lasting nature but also because their occurrence appears to be largely idiosyncratic, so that even impeccable technique is not necessarily protective. Although discussion of these consequences may add to anxiety on the part of the clinician, patient, and family, it is an important part of the informed consent. Major complications include *paraplegia* and *vascular problems.*

Efficacy of Celiac and Splanchnic Nerve Blocks

Despite general agreement that celiac plexus block is indeed efficacious, significant controversy persists regarding (1) its efficacy relative to opioid therapy, (2) the relative efficacy among different approaches and techniques, and (3) whether even a remote risk of paraplegia warrants a commitment to neurolysis, especially when treatment with analgesics usually provides adequate relief. Regrettably, despite the legacy of a richly descriptive literature, these questions remain largely unresolved because of persisting scientific inadequacies.

Unfortunately, most early reports were anecdotal in nature, suffered from poor study design, and lacked careful longitudinal follow-up until, spurred by the outcomes movement of the 1990s, more elegantly designed trials began to appear in the literature.

Outcome Data

The trend toward a more critical appraisal of outcome is suggested by the decline in favorable results from 98% to 80% reported from the same center for treatment rendered between 1948 and 1964 and between 1978 and 1985, respectively. Thus, a careful analysis of available clinical data is warranted to make even limited conclusions regarding efficacy.

A survey of the literature reviewed data from 23 studies on celiac neurolysis performed on 1126 patients, 64% of whom had pancreatic cancer pain and 36% of whom had pain caused by other intra-abdominal malignancies.[29] Good to excellent pain relief was achieved in 90% of evaluable patients during the first 2 weeks after treatment, only 6% of whom required a repeated procedure for inadequate analgesia. Partial or complete pain relief was observed in 95% of patients alive at the time of last follow-up and 87% of patients at time of death.

Pancreatic Cancer Versus Other Painful Disorders

Classically, viscerally medicated abdominal pain is vague and poorly localized. It is described as a deep, dull, aching, dragging, boring, squeezing, or pressure-like sensation. Pain from pancreatic cancer[54,55] and other retroperitoneal pathologic conditions[56] is classically characterized as relentless midepigastric pain radiating through or around to the back. Additional abdominal symptoms consistent with obstruction, infection, or other pathologic conditions suggests the need for further diagnostic studies and alternative therapies such as surgery or antibiotics.

Other Intra-abdominal Neoplasms

Although, based on its contribution to the innervation of all intra-abdominal viscera derived from the embryonic foregut (gastrointestinal tract from the distal esophagus through the proximal transverse colon, pancreas, adrenals, spleen, liver, and biliary tree), celiac neurolysis has potential utility for treating pain emanating from diverse conditions, its most important indication remains pain resulting from pancreatic cancer. Despite its identification with pancreatic cancer pain, however, it appears to be a reasonable alternative for extrapancreatic abdominal pain of malignant origin, especially hepatic, as long as pain is visceral in origin and is not associated with diffuse disease, as in the case of peritoneal seeding and malignant ascites.

An association between neoplastic invasion of the retroperitoneum and referred back pain is supported by findings of a 21% incidence of back pain in a series of patients with testicular germ cell tumors and periaortic nodal metastases.[54] The appropriateness of celiac plexus block for abdominal pain resulting from malignancies other than pancreatic cancer includes evidence for perineural and plexus invasion in 10 of 16 patients with cancer originating in the common bile duct.[57]

Acquired Immunodeficiency Syndrome

Although experience is limited, case reports suggest that celiac plexus neurolysis should be considered for refractory pain in acquired immunodeficiency syndrome (AIDS) patients. A report of three patients with intractable abdominal pain secondary to sclerosing cholangitis revealed complete eradication of pain at follow-up checks ranging from 2 to 11 months. Interestingly, the onset of pain relief was delayed for 3 days in one patient.[58]

Pancreatitis

Based on anecdotal experience and a few small trials, most authorities discourage the consideration of celiac neurolysis for pain resulting from chronic pancreatitis except when special circumstances arise in carefully selected patients.[59,60]

Early Intervention

The most common reason for considering an anesthetic intervention for pain relief in any setting is the presence of a side effect that interferes with the process of upward titration to effect.[61,62] A number of factors, generally applicable to medically ill populations and specific to patients with abdominal pain, however, reduce the likelihood of attaining adequate pain control with systemic analgesics alone.

Although a high proportion of patients with intra-abdominal malignancies are not candidates for curative therapy, their life-extending palliative treatments may render pharmacologic-based pain control more difficult to achieve because concomitant asthenia and cachexia increase the

likelihood of side effects from opioids titrated to therapeutic effect.

Celiac block ideally should be applied early, both to maximize potential benefits and to minimize difficulties caused by disease-related and patient-related factors. Failure of celiac plexus block appears to be more common when treatment is withheld until late in the disease course, presumably as a result of poor spread of the neurolytic drug because of tumor spread. Early implementation may result in better pain control and may improve overall ease of management by increasing performance status. Reduced sympathetic tone (and unopposed parasympathetic activity) may enhance gastrointestinal motility, often with improvement of ileus, constipation, and anorexia, effects that are in stark contrast to the obstipating effects of opioids.

Choice of Technique

Authorities recommend different approaches to celiac block (e.g., retrocrural, transcrural, transaortic, transdiskal, splanchnic, anterior, intraoperative), various techniques (e.g., one to four needles positioned based on anatomic landmarks alone, plain radiography, fluoroscopy, sonography, CT), and the use of various volumes and agents (e.g., 15 to 50 ml of 50% to 100% alcohol or 6% to 10% phenol). Because studies comparing the efficacy of these alternatives are unavailable, poorly controlled, or inconclusive, the choice of technique should be individualized based on available resources, the patient's physical status, the pattern of tumor spread, the clinician's experience, and a careful assessment of the apparent relative merits of each approach.

Making Clinical Decisions Despite Inadequate Data

Recognizing the paucity of outcome data regarding celiac block does not excuse the skilled clinician from providing treatment but should serve to stimulate better research while mandating careful scrutiny of all available data to ensure the best clinical decision making possible. Although the literature comparing the various available approaches to neural blockade is flawed, overall efficacy and safety appear to be established. Celiac block has a therapeutic role, ideally early in the course of disease, because of its global record and because pain from pancreatic cancer and other abdominal malignancies is a common and vexing problem, often responding inadequately to standard pharmacotherapies.

Radiologic Guidance

Although radiographic guidance does not prevent complications, some form of radiographic guidance is indicated whenever a neurolytic block is undertaken because of the serious and potentially lasting nature of potential complications.

Although inexpensive and usually accessible, plain radiography is least preferred because it is time consuming and provides no real-time information. The obvious advantage of CT scanning relates to its capacity to directly demonstrate tumor spread and details of visceral and vascular anatomy, thus minimizing the likelihood of anatomic injury. These advantages are to some extent offset by the limited availability of CT, its cost, the requirement for cooperation from a knowledgeable radiologist, time required, and limited acceptance in claustrophobic patients.

Fluoroscopy is an adequate alternative, especially when anatomy is grossly normal and when special techniques are not undertaken.

Anatomic Approach

Some anatomic approaches include:

- Retrocrural (deep splanchnic) approach
- Transcrural approach
- Transaortic approach
- High splanchnic block
- Blockade at the time of laparotomy

Percutaneous Anterior Approaches: The Technique of Choice?

Potential advantages of both CT and sonographically guided anterior techniques include enhancing the likelihood of preferential spread anterior to the celiac trunk where fibers may be concentrated, less pain because of the avoidance of bony structures, and rapidity of performance. These features, combined with the absence of a need for the prone position, make treatment much less demanding for the patient who, as a consequence, is less likely to recall the procedure as distressing. The most important advantage, however, appears to relate to the risk of neurologic morbidity; a report of paraplegia after an anterior percutaneous approach (CT or ultrasonographically guided) has never been disclosed.

An obvious disadvantage to the anterior approach is the need for CT or ultrasound guidance that may be costly, inconvenient, or unavailable. Other potential disadvantages include risk of infection, abscess, hemorrhage, and fistula formation. Although preliminary findings indicate that the risks of these complications are low, further experience is needed to make a definitive conclusion.

Changing Trends in Practice

Preliminary Diagnostic Block

Early series advocating the routine performance of a local anesthetic and neurolytic block on separate occasions have given way to a trend toward performing both together, especially for radiographically guided procedures in patients with cancer pain. Subjected to careful analysis, the older tradition fails the test of logic. Performing a local anesthetic and neurolytic block on separate days is stressful to patients who are debilitated, uses costly resources unnecessarily, and indeed fails to predict outcome with any certainty. It should be recognized that when two separate blocks are performed, needles are always ultimately positioned in slightly different tissue planes, even with the same anatomic technique.

Finally, when blocks are performed with radiologic guidance and careful attention to technical details, including the use of test doses, the risk of serious complications is low, and, in well-selected patients, the likelihood of efficacy is high. The separate performance of diagnostic and therapeutic blocks is strongly indicated, however, when a diagnosis is uncertain and when treatment is undertaken for a chronic, non-neoplastic process.

Outpatient Celiac Neurolysis

The infrequency of serious or persistent side effects and complications of celiac neurolysis, combined with contemporary fiscal pressures that discourage inpatient hospitalization, has resulted in a trend toward outpatient treatment. Routine outpatient celiac neurolysis appears to be warranted for relatively fit patients as long as they are prehydrated, observed for several hours, and provided discharge instructions that include information on contacting a knowledgeable physician.

References

1. Procacci P, Maresca M, Cersosimo R: Visceral pain: Pathophysiology and clinical aspects. In Costa M, editor: *Sensory nerve and neuropeptides in gastroenterology.* New York, Plenum Press, 1991.
2. Vecchiet L, Giamberardino MA, Dragani L. et al: Pain from renal/ureteral calculosis: Evaluation of sensory thresholds in the lumbar area. *Pain* 36:289, 1989.
3. Bonica JJ: General considerations of acute pain. In Bonica JJ, editor: *The management of pain.* Philadelphia, Lea & Febiger, 1990.
4. Cervero F: Sensory innervation of the viscera: Peripheral basis of visceral pain. *Physiol Rev* 74:95, 1994.
5. Gebhart GF, Sengupta JN: On visceral nociceptors. In Besson JM, Guilbaud G, Ollat H, editors: *Peripheral neurons in nociception: Physiopharmacological aspects.* Paris, Eurotext, 1994.
6. Ness TJ, Gebhart GF: Visceral pain: A review of experimental studies. *Pain* 41:167, 1990.
7. Cervero F, Jänig W: Visceral nociceptors: A new world order? *Trends Neurosci* 15:374, 1992.
8. McMahon SB, Koltzenburg M: Silent afferents and visceral pain. In *Pharmacological approaches to the treatment of chronic pain: New concepts and critical issues. Progress in pain research and management,* vol 1. Seattle, IASP Press, 1994.
9. Jänig W, Morrison JFB: Functional properties of spinal visceral afferent supplying abdominal and pelvic organs with special emphasis on visceral nociception. In Cervero F, Morrison JFB, editors: *Visceral sensation: Progress in brain research,* vol 67. Amsterdam, Elsevier, 1986.
10. Cervero F: Pathophysiology of referred pain and hyperalgesia from viscera. In Vecchiet L, Albe-Fessard D, Lindblom U et al, editors: *New trends in referred pain and hyperalgesia, pain research and clinical management.* Amsterdam, Elsevier Science, 1993.
11. Giamberardino MA, Vecchiet L: Experimental studies on pelvic pain. *Pain Rev* 1:104, 1994.
12. Berkley KJ, Guilbaud G, Benoist JM et al: Responses of neurons in and near the thalamic ventrobasal complex of the rat to stimulation of uterus, cervix, vagina, colon, and skin. *J Neurophysiol* 69:557, 1993.
13. Procacci P, Zoppi M, Maresca M: Clinical approach to visceral sensation. In Cervero F, Morrison JFB, editors: *Visceral sensation: Progress in brain research,* vol 67. Amsterdam, Elsevier, 1986.
14. Hammermeister KE: Cardiac and aortic pain. In Bonica JJ, editor: *The management of pain.* Philadelphia, Lea & Febiger, 1990.
15. Fine PG, Karwande SV: Sternal wire-induced persistent chest pain: A possible hypersensitivity reaction. *Ann Thorac Surg* 49:135, 1991.
16. Taylor HC Jr: Pelvic pain based on a vascular and autonomic nervous system disorder. *Am J Obstet Gynecol* 67:1177, 1954.
17. Reiter RC, Gambone JC: Demographic and historic variables in women with idiopathic chronic pelvic pain. *Obstet Gynecol* 75:428, 1990.
18. Dargent M: Role of sympathetic nerve in cancerous pain. *Br Med J* 1:440, 1948.
19. Chapman CR, Donaldson GW: Issues in designing trials of nonpharmacologic treatments for pain. *Adv Pain Res Ther* 18:699, 1991.
20. Sharfman WH, Walsh TD: Has the efficacy of celiac plexus block been demonstrated in pancreatic cancer pain? *Pain* 41:267, 1990.
21. Chapman CR, Donaldson GW: Issues in designing trials of nonpharmacologic treatments for pain. *Adv Pain Res Ther* 18:699, 1991.
22. Patt RB, Jain S, Ketchedjain AG: The outcomes movement and neurolytic blockade for cancer pain management. *Pain Dig* 5:268, 1995.
23. Lillemoe KD, Cameron JL, Kaufman HS et al: Chemical splanchnicectomy in patients with unresectable pancreatic cancer: a prospective randomized trial. *Ann Surg* 217:447, 1993.
24. Kawamata M, Ishitani K, Ishikawa K et al: Comparison between celiac plexus block and morphine treatment on quality of life in patients with pancreatic cancer pain. *Pain* 64:597, 1996.

25. Mercadante S: Celiac plexus block versus analgesics in pancreatic cancer pain. *Pain* 52:187, 1993.
26. Ischia S, Ischia A, Polati E et al: Three posterior percutaneous celiac plexus block techniques: A prospective, randomized study in 61 patients with pancreatic cancer pain. *Anesthesiology* 76:534, 1992.
27. De Cicco M, Matovic M, Balestreri L et al: Single-needle celiac plexus block: Is needle tip position critical in patients with no regional anatomic distortions? *Anesthesiology* 87:1301, 1997.
28. Polati E, Finco G, Gottin L et al: Prospective randomized double-blind trial of neurolytic coeliac plexus block in patients with pancreatic cancer. *Br J Surg* 85:199, 1998.
29. Eisenberg E, Carr DB, Chalmers TC: Neurolytic celiac plexus block for treatment of cancer pain: A meta-analysis. *Anesth Analg* 80:290, 1995.
30. Mercadante S, Nicosia F: Celiac plexus block: A reappraisal. *Reg Anesth Pain Med* 23:37, 1998.
31. Patt RB, Cousins MJ: Techniques for neurolytic neural blockade. In Cousins MJ, Bridenbaugh PO, editors: *Neural blockade,* ed 3. Philadelphia, JB Lippincott, 1998.
32. Kappis M: Erfahrungen mit lokalanästhesie bei bauchoperationen. *Verhandl Deutsch Gesellsch Cir* 43:87, 1914.
33. Jones RR: A technique of injection of the splanchnic nerves with alcohol. *Anesth Analg* 36:75, 1957.
34. Singler RC: An improved technique for alcohol neurolysis of the celiac plexus. *Anesthesiology* 56:137, 1982.
35. Boas RA: Sympathetic blocks in clinical practice. *Int Anesthesiol Clin* 16:149, 1978.
36. Ischia S, Luzzani A, Ischia A et al: A new approach to the neurolytic block of the celiac plexus: The transaortic technique. *Pain* 16:333, 1983.
37. Matamala AM, Lopez FV, Martinez LI: Percutaneous approach to the celiac plexus using CT guidance. *Pain* 34:285, 1988.
38. Haaga JR, Kori SH, Eastwood DW et al: Improved technique for CT-guided celiac ganglia block. *Am J Radiol* 142:1201, 1984.
39. Labat G, editor: Operations on the abdomen. In *Regional anesthesia: Its technique and clinical application.* Philadelphia, WB Saunders, 1924.
40. Wendling H: Ausschaltung der nervi splanchnici durch leitungsanäs-thesie bei magenoperationen und anderen eingriffen in der oberen bauchhöhle. *Beitr z Klin Chur* 110:517, 1918.
41. Braun H: Ein Hilfsinstrument zur ausfuhrung der splanchnicusanäs-thesie. *Zentralbl Chir* 48:1544, 1921.
42. Finsterer H: *Local anesthesia methods and results in abdominal surgery.* New York, Rebman, 1923.
43. Olak J, Gore D: Thoracoscopic splanchnicectomy: Technique and case report. *Surg Laparosc Endosc* 6:228, 1996.
44. Rossi M, Zaninotto G, Finco C et al: Thoracoscopic bilateral splanch-nicotomy for pain control in unresectable pancreatic cancer. *Chir Ital* 47:55, 1995.
45. Takahashi T, Kakita A, Izumika H et al: Thoracoscopic splanchnicec-tomy for the relief of intractable abdominal pain. *Surg Endosc* 10:65, 1996.
46. Moore DC, Bush WH, Burnett LL: Celiac plexus block: A roentgeno-graphic, anatomic study of technique and spread of solution in patients and corpses. *Anesth Analg* 60:369, 1981.
47. Lieberman RP, Waldman SD: Celiac plexus neurolysis with modified transaortic approach. *Radiology* 175:274, 1990.
48. Feldstein GS, Waldman SD: Loss of resistance technique for transaor-tic celiac plexus block. *Anesth Analg* 65:1092, 1986.
49. McAfee JG: A survey of complications of abdominal aortography. *Radiology* 68:825, 1957.
50. Caratozzolo M, Lirici MM, Consalvo M et al: Ultrasound-guided alco-holization of celiac plexus for pain control in oncology. *Surg Endosc* 11:239, 1997.
51. Gimenez A, Martinez-Noguera A, Donoso L et al: Percutaneous neu-rolysis of the celiac plexus via the anterior approach with sonographic guidance. *AJR Am J Roentgenol* 161:1061, 1993.
52. Zenz M, Kurz-Muller K, Strumpf M et al: The anterior sonographic guided celiac plexus blockade: review and personal observations. *Anaesthesist* 42:246, 1993.
53. Myhre J, Hilsted J, Tronier B et al: Monitoring of celiac plexus block in chronic pancreatitis. *Pain* 38:269, 1989.
54. Foley KM: Pain syndromes and pharmacologic management of pan-creatic cancer pain. *J Pain Symptom Manage* 3:176, 1988.
55. Reber HA, Foley KM: Pancreatic cancer pain: Presentation, pathogen-esis and management. *J Pain Symptom Manage* 3:163, 1988.
56. Cantwell BM, Mannix KA, Harris AL: Back pain: A presentation of metastatic testicular germ cell tumors. *Lancet* 1(8527):262, 1987.
57. Fukuda T, Iwanaga S, Sakamoto I, et al: CT of neural plexus invasion in common bile duct carcinoma. *J Comput Assist Tomogr* 22:351, 1998.
58. Collazos J, Mayo J, Martinez E et al: Celiac plexus block as treatment for refractory pain related to sclerosing cholangitis in AIDS patients. *J Clin Gastroenterol* 23:47, 1996.
59. Malfertheiner P, Dominguez-Munoz JE, Buchler MW: Chronic pan-creatitis: Management of pain. *Digestion* 55(Suppl 1):29, 1994.
60. Leung JW, Bowen-Wright M, Aveling W et al: Celiac plexus block for cancer and chronic pancreatitis. *Br J Surg* 70:730, 1983.
61. Jacox A, Carr DB, Payne R et al: Management of cancer pain: Clinical practice guideline No. 9. AHCPR Publication No. 94-0592. Rockville, Md, 1994.
62. American Pain Society: *Principles of analgesic use in the treatment of acute pain and chronic cancer pain,* ed 3. Skokie, Ill, American Pain Society, 1992.

1. The visceral pain can be caused by

   A. Normal hollow visceral wall
   B. Vascularity of visceral musculature
   C. Rapid stretching of the capsule of solid visceral organ
   D. Relaxation of ligaments

2. A special class of nociceptors in the viscera is called

   A. Awake nociceptors
   B. Silent nociceptors
   C. Stretch nociceptors
   D. Pressure nociceptors

3. Sympathetic afferents carry nociception from pancreas to thoracic splanchnic nerves

   A. From T10 to T11
   B. From T5 to T9
   C. From T12
   D. In vagus

4. The nerve supply of which following organ travels with lumbar splanchnic nerves via the aorta and then the superior hypogastric plexus?

   A. Kidney
   B. Lower half of the ureter
   C. Pancreas
   D. Ascending colon

5. The classic Kappis technique of retroaortic splanchnic nerve block requires the patient to be positioned in the

   A. Sitting position
   B. Supine position
   C. Prone position
   D. Lateral decubitus position

ANSWERS

1. C

2. B

3. B

4. B

5. D

CHAPTER 12

Cancer Pain

MARK J. LEMA, MILES DAY,
DAVID P. MYERS, VICTOR A. FILADORA,
AND EDWARD T. PLATA

Advances in cancer treatment continue to lengthen survival among cancer patients. As patients live longer, the need for effective pain control has gained increased importance for improving the quality of life. Patients with advanced cancer often have pain as their chief complaint. The incidence of pain varies, depending on the type of neoplasm, stage, and the extent of spread. Because pain is a common symptom in cancer patients, next to incurability, it is the most feared complication.

With the current therapeutic modalities available to the clinician, about 80% to 90% of cancer pain can be controlled.[1,2] However, studies by Cleeland, using Eastern Cooperative Oncology Group (ECOG) physicians, showed that most cancer pain is undertreated, especially in regard to women, minorities, and older adults.[2,3] Major barriers to effective cancer pain control include:

1. Inadequate assessment by practitioners
2. Under-reporting by patients and families
3. Lack of knowledge regarding current treatment by practitioners
4. Lack of accountability for effectively treating pain
5. Fear of over-regulation by government officials
6. Inadequate reimbursement or excessive paperwork by payers for treatment of pain by health care providers

In an attempt to rectify the problems, the World Health Organization (WHO), the American Society of Anesthesiologists, and the Agency for Health Care Policy and Research (AHCPR) have developed guidelines for the treatment of cancer pain.[4,5]

PATHOPHYSIOLOGY

Etiology

There are essentially five different causes of pain in cancer patients (Table 12–1):

1. Acute cancer-related pain
2. Chronic cancer-related pain
3. Pain unrelated to cancer
4. Chronic nonmalignant pain in opioid-tolerant patients
5. End-of-life pain

Classification

Cancer pain is classified according to pain duration and pain quality. Pain duration denotes the degree of chronicity. The three temporal conditions are *acute* pain, *chronic* pain, and *incidental* pain. Pathophysiologic components are:

1. Somatic (nociceptive) pain
2. Visceral pain
3. Neuropathic pain
4. Central pain
5. Sympathetic pain

Breakthrough pain, which is experienced in up to 93% of cancer patients, is a clinical term describing the episodic exacerbations of pain above the established baseline.[5] Doses of morphine, oxycodone, or hydromorphone, for example, are given every 2 to 4 hours, as needed, to combat breakthrough pain while the patient continues taking a long-acting oral opioid agent. If a patient routinely uses breakthrough medications, the daily total amount should be converted to a sustained-release dose and added to the current maintenance dose.[6]

Cancer Pain Syndromes

Although clinicians classify pain according to its onset, duration, and nature, cancer pain is often experienced as several

TABLE 12–1 Types of Pain Experienced by Cancer Patients

Acute Cancer-Related Pain
Tumor spread
Chemotherapy, radiotherapy, or surgery
Debilitating effects of chronic illness

Chronic Cancer-Related Pain
Tumor destruction
Cancer therapies
Paraneoplastic pain

Pain Unrelated to Cancer
Acute injury pain
Disease-related pain
Chronic pain not resulting from malignancy

Pain in Opioid-Tolerant Cancer Patients
Current and previous drug addicts
Patients taking opioids daily for several months
Previous drug addict receiving methadone

End-of-Life Pain
Acute pain related to cachectic state
Chronic pain
Continuous acute pain associated with tumor progression

CANCER PAIN / 111

different types of pain. Combined somatic and neuropathic types are the most frequent.[7] During the course of the disease, the pain changes as a result of tumor progression or regression after treatment. These changes may occur rapidly and illustrate the dynamic nature of cancer pain.

Acute Pain

Pain is often the presenting symptom of a patient with cancer. If it occurs early in the disease, patients may endure high levels of pain in the expectation that adequate anticancer therapy will relieve their symptoms. If it occurs late in the course, pain often signifies disease recurrence, which is associated with anxiety, apprehension, and suffering.

Pain is also associated with diagnostic procedures such as lumbar puncture or bone marrow biopsy, for example. In addition, postoperative pain can persist after surgery for tumor recurrence and may be complicated in patients who are tolerant of opioids (Table 12–2).

Anticancer therapy is often associated with painful sequelae such as skin burns, mucositis, pharyngitis, and cystitis after radiation therapy. Similarly, while receiving drug chemotherapy, some patients experience myalgias, gastroin-

testinal distention, or local irritation, for example. Acute pain caused by the treatment occasionally progresses to chronic pain. Usually, acute pain is self-limiting and is most effectively treated with opioid analgesics and nonsteroidal anti-inflammatory drugs (NSAIDs).

Chronic Pain Related to Cancer

Chronic pain related to cancer can be considered according to the following categories (Table 12–3):

1. Tumor-induced pain
2. Chemotherapy-induced pain
3. Radiation therapy-induced pain

TABLE 12–2 Acute Cancer Pain Syndromes

Diagnostic and therapeutic interventions
    Lumbar puncture headache
    Arterial or venous blood sampling
    Bone marrow biopsy
    Lumbar puncture
Postoperative
Therapeutic interventions
    Pleurodesis
    Tumor embolization
Analgesic techniques
    Injection pain
    Spinal opioid hyperalgesia syndrome
    Epidural injection pain
Anticancer therapies
Chemotherapy infusion techniques
    Intravenous infusion pain
        Venous spasm
        Chemical phlebitis
        Vesicant extravasation
        Anthracycline-associated flare reaction
    Hepatic artery infusion pain
    Intraperitoneal chemotherapy abdominal pain
Chemotherapy toxicity
    Mucositis
    Corticosteroid-induced perineal discomfort
    Painful peripheral neuropathy
    Diffuse bone pain from *trans*-retinoic acid or colony-
        stimulating factors
Hormonal therapy
    Luteinizing hormone-releasing factor tumor flare in prostate
        cancer
    Hormone-induced acute pain flare in breast cancer
Radiation therapy
    Incidental pains
    Oropharyngeal mucositis
    Acute radiation enteritis and proctocolitis
Infection
    Acute herpetic neuralgia

Adapted from Cherny NI, Portenoy RK: The management of cancer pain. *CA Cancer J Clin* 44:262, 1994.

TABLE 12–3. Chronic Cancer Pain Syndromes

Tumor-Related Pain Syndromes	Cancer Therapy-Related Pain Syndromes

Bone Pain
Multifocal or generalized
  bone pain
    Multiple bony metastases
    Marrow expansion
Vertebral syndromes
    Atlantoaxial destruction
      and odontoid fractures
    C7 to T11 syndrome
    T12 to L1 syndrome
    Sacral syndrome
Back pain and epidural
  compression
Pain syndromes of the body
  pelvis and hip
	Postchemotherapy Pain Syndromes
	Chronic painful peripheral
	  neuropathy
	Avascular necrosis of femoral or
	  humeral head
	Plexopathy associated with
	  intra-arterial infusion
	
	Chronic Pain Associated with Hormonal Therapy
	Gynecomastia with hormonal
	  therapy for prostate cancer

Headache and Facial Pain Intracerebral tumor Leptomeningeal metastases Base of skull metastases Painful cranial neuralgias	**Chronic Postsurgical Pain Syndromes** Postmastectomy pain syndrome Post-radical neck dissection pain Post-thoracotomy pain Postoperative frozen shoulder Phantom pain syndromes Stump pain Postsurgical pelvic floor myalgia

Tumor Involvement of the Peripheral Nervous System
Tumor-related radiculopathy
    Postherpetic neuralgia
Cervical plexopathy
Brachial plexopathy
Malignant lumbosacral
  plexopathy
Tumor-related mononeuropathy
Paraneoplastic painful peripheral
  neuropathy
	Chronic Postradiation Pain Syndromes
	Plexopathies
	Chronic radiation myelopathy
	Chronic radiation enteritis and
	  proctitis
	Burning perineum syndrome
	Osteoradionecrosis

Pain Syndromes of the Viscera and Miscellaneous Tumor-Related Syndromes Hepatic distention syndrome Midline retroperitoneal syndrome Chronic intestinal obstruction Peritoneal carcinomatosis Malignant perineal pain Ureteric obstruction	
Paraneoplastic Nociceptive Pain Syndrome Tumor-related gynecomastia	

Adapted from Cherny NI, Portenoy RK: The management of cancer pain. *CA Cancer J Clin* 44:262, 1994.

POSTSURGICAL PAIN SYNDROMES

Pain After Thoracotomy

After thoracotomy, pain develops in the distribution of the intercostal nerves in a small number or patients as a result of partial or complete injury from retractors, sutures, wires, or transection.[8] Pain usually develops 1 to 2 months after the operation and is described as constant in the area of sensory loss, with occasional lancinating pain.

Pain After Mastectomy

Patients who have has a radical mastectomy may experience pain in the posterior part of the arm, axilla, and anterior chest wall as a result of damage to the intercostobrachial nerve.[8] Pain typically develops 1 to 2 months after the operation and is tight, constricting, and burning in nature. Patients tend to keep the arm in a flexed position close to the chest wall, because movement exacerbates the pain. As a result, a frozen shoulder may develop from reduced joint motion. Reports of phantom breast pain occasionally appear in the literature.[9]

Pain After Radical Neck Dissection

Pain can arise as a result of surgical intervention, including radical neck dissection. This pain is characterized as being constant, with dysesthesia and shock-like sensation as a result of interruption of the cervical plexus nerves and peripheral nerves serving those areas.[10]

Phantom Limb Pain

Phantom limb pain occurs in a large number of patients after amputation and usually produces a burning and cramping sensation in the area of the original limb. It can easily be differentiated from stump pain, which occurs at the site of the amputation and is elicited by palpation or percussion of the stump area.[11]

PAIN UNRELATED TO CANCER

Approximately 3% of the pain syndromes that occur in cancer patients have no relation to the underlying cancer or cancer treatment.[12] Most commonly, pain is caused by degenerative disk disease, arthritis, fibromyalgia, or migraine and has often predated the diagnosis of cancer. In these patients, pain does not necessarily signify recurrent disease; however, a chronic illness behavior has already developed in many patients. Careful assessment and early psychologic intervention are required.

CANCER PAIN AND OPIOID-TOLERANT PATIENTS

Opioid-tolerant pain patients are a challenging group. These patients may have used opioids illicitly in the past but are no longer using them. Many are reluctant to take opioids for their cancer pain, fearing an addiction potential. These patients require support and understanding of the necessity to treat the pain. The liberal use of adjuvant therapies allowing for decreased opioid doses is also beneficial.

Cancer pain that develops in patients who have been taking opioids for other medical conditions requires higher doses of opioids.[12] In these cases, the use of adjuvants and early intervention with block techniques or the use of more potent opioid receptor agonists may avoid dose escalation without good pain control.[13] Patients who use more than 50 mg of oral morphine for longer than 3 months often require three times more drug for a three times longer duration than opioid-naïve patients after surgery.[12]

ASSESSMENT OF CANCER PAIN

Assessment of cancer pain begins with a thorough understanding of the complex nature of pain. The International Association for the Study of Pain defined pain in 1979 as "an unpleasant sensory and emotional experience associated with actual or potential tissue damage or described in terms of such damage." This definition stresses the importance of the emotional and suffering aspects of pain.

Clinical Assessment

Treatment failure can often be directly attributed to an inadequate assessment by the physician of the patient with cancer pain. Initial treatment should be based on the cause and type of pain. Before beginning treatment, the clinician should perform a detailed history and physical examination. Based on the findings of the examination, diagnostic studies should be ordered; a preliminary diagnosis, treatment goals, and a treatment plan are then established. Following the initial evaluation, on subsequent visits, the patient's status should be reassessed, because tumor growth is a dynamic and evolving process (Table 12–4).

TABLE 12–4   Clinical Assessment for Effective Cancer Pain Management

I. Pain-related information
   A. Pain history
      1. Palliative/provocative factors
      2. Quality of pain
      3. Radiation of pain
      4. Severity
      5. Temporal aspects
   B. Significant medical history, including tumor locations
   C. Laboratory and radiologic reports
   D. Pertinent physical examination
II. Working diagnosis
   A. Provisional pain diagnoses
   B. Progressive and survival estimates
   C. Total pain management concerns
III. Continued diagnostic evaluation
   A. Causes of various pains
   B. Psychologic impact of pain and disease
IV. Problem list development
   A. Extent and course of disease
   B. Palliative issues
   C. Contingency plans
V. Patient feedback
   A. Initial therapy results
   B. Recognition of unmasked pain sites
   C. Psychologic assessment
   D. Side effect assessment

History and Physical Examination

To determine what further testing a patient may require, the location, quality, and duration of the patient's pain should be elicited. A complete review of the past medical history and what, if any, therapeutic measures have been previously tried to relieve pain may provide valuable information for developing a treatment plan. Physical examination should include a complete neurologic examination. Neurologic deficits from direct tumor invasion or compression are common and are often painful.

In addition to pain, most patients with cancer have numerous other symptoms.[14,15] They often suffer from insomnia, depression, fatigue, and the side effects from therapeutic intervention such as headache and nausea, for example. One should take into account all the symptoms and develop a therapeutic plan that will improve quality of life for the patient.

Pain Intensity

One of the most difficult aspects of pain control is the accurate assessment of pain intensity.[16] Although intensity is difficult to gauge, it is important because it provides a basis for developing a treatment plan and evaluating the effectiveness of therapeutic interventions. Also, if a patient's pain level increases during treatment, it may indicate disease progression. The best methods for determining pain intensity are the Verbal Scale or the Visual Analogue Pain Scale (VAPS) and the McGill Pain Questionnaire.

Diagnostic Testing

The patient's prior results should be reviewed, especially modalities such as computed tomography (CT) scans, magnetic resonance imaging (MRI), bone scans, endoscopies, and staging procedures. Additional tests may be necessary and should be ordered only if their results could potentially alter therapy.

Treatment Strategies

Following a thorough review of the patient's medical condition, a preliminary treatment plan should be established. Functional status and quality-of-life issues are also critically important to assess. Provisions for supportive care should be discussed, and the emotional stress on family members as well as the psychologic well-being of the patient should be considered.

Goals

After a treatment plan has been established, the patient's expectations in terms of pain control should be discussed (Table 12–5). Often patient's have unrealistic goals and may not understand the extent of the disease. If necessary, the help of the primary care physician can be obtained to communicate with the patient.

TREATMENT OPTIONS

Oral and Parenteral Analgesia

Pharmacotherapy is the most widely used method of pain control. Three categories of analgesic medications are commonly available: NSAIDs, opioid analgesics, and adjuvant agents.

TABLE 12–5 Cancer Pain Management Treatment Strategy

I. Clinical assessment
II. Therapeutic interventions
    A. Antitumor therapy
    B. Systemic analgesic therapy
       1. Non-opioid analgesics
       2. Opioid analgesics
       3. Adjuvant agents
       4. Side effects management
    B. Psychosocial therapy
    C. Invasive therapy
       1. Peripheral nerve blocks
       2. Plexus blocks
       3. Neuraxial therapy
       4. Neuroablative techniques
    D. Nonpharmacologic therapy
       1. Heat or cold application
       2. Exercise
       3. Counterstimulation (transcutaneous electrical nerve stimulation)
       4. Relaxation/imagery
       5. Distraction/reframing
       6. Hypnosis
       7. Peer group support
       8. Pastoral counseling
       9. Occupational therapy aids
     10. Physical therapy appliances

Nonsteroidal Anti-inflammatory Drugs

The peripheral effects of NSAIDs inhibit the enzyme cyclooxygenase, decreasing tissue levels of prostaglandins, which are the inflammatory mediators that sensitize peripheral nociceptors in the skin.[17] NSAIDs have an anti-inflammatory action and an inhibitory effect on bone tumor growth by the inhibition of prostaglandin E_2 release. They may also have a centrally medicated analgesic effect.[18]

Acetaminophen has an analgesic effect by inhibiting nitric oxide synthetase, an action that is centrally and spinally mediated[19] and similar in efficacy to that of aspirin. Also, NSAIDs possess a therapeutic ceiling dose, above which further dose increments provide little relief. Toxicity, however, increases and includes nausea, gastritis, and platelet dysfunction.

Opioid Analgesics

Opioid analgesics are the mainstay of therapy for cancer pain. The objective is to control pain while minimizing distressing side effects. The success of this therapy depends on the expertise of the prescriber, who must know the nuances of pharmacologic features among various opioids and must be experienced in their use to make an appropriate selection for each patient.

Agonist-antagonist agents are not effective in the treatment of cancer pain because of their ceiling effect of analgesia, potential to precipitate withdrawal, and associated psychotropic side effects with increasing dose. The *pure opioid agonists* should be used exclusively for patients with moderate pain from agonist-antignonist opioids on the second step of the analgesic ladder (Fig. 12–1). These drugs include codeine, oxycodone, and hydrocodone, and they are usually available in combination with acetaminophen compounds to

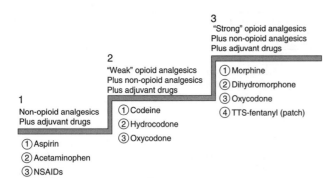

FIG. 12–1 World Health Organization (WHO) three-step ladder oral analgesic program for managing cancer pain. NSAIDs, nonsteroidal anti-inflammatory drugs; TTS, transdermal therapeutic system. *(Adapted from WHO: Cancer pain relief, ed. 2. Geneva, World Health Organization, 1996).*

prevent renal or hepatic dysfunction (Table 12–6). Ibuprofen-containing compounds are generally restricted to 3200 mg daily.

Patients who do not respond to second-step opioids are switched to opioids on the third step of the ladder, most often morphine, hydromorphone, oxycodone, or fentanyl. Morphine has been used extensively worldwide and has been endorsed by the WHO.[4] It is also available in several formulations and lends itself to administration by different routes.

When a physician selects a route for administration, factors such as gastrointestinal upset or obstruction, outpatient versus inpatient setting, and patient compliance should be addressed. Oral administration is the preferred and most economical route, although some medications may be given rectally when doses by both routes are considered equivalent.

A widely accepted principle of effective management of cancer pain with opioids is dose administration at fixed intervals on an around-the-clock basis. This approach provides sustained analgesia and avoids the peak and trough effects of medication given as needed. When sustained-release agents are used, additional opioids should also be available for breakthrough pain at all times during the course of treatment. Doses must be titrated to the patient's need, thereby avoiding side effects from overdosing or persistent pain from inadequate analgesia.

Adjuvant Therapy

Adjuvant medications are used in conjunction with oral or parenteral analgesics. They may have inherent analgesic action; improve mood or sleep; or alleviate nausea, anxiety, and somnolence:

- The tricyclic antidepressants are known to have analgesic action. They alleviate depression, improve sleep, and benefit patients with neuropathic pain.
- The tertiary amines are often the first line of therapy because of their greater analgesic effect. If they cause excessive sedation, a secondary amine can be used.
- Anticonvulsive drugs and the antispasmodic baclofen are helpful in patients with lancinating pain.
- Mexiletine has been used in neuropathic pain from cancer after its success in the treatment of painful diabetic neuropathy.
- Corticosteriods are useful adjuvants and have been shown to improve analgesia, mood, and appetite in the short term.[20]

A list of commonly used adjuvant drugs is provided in Table 12–7.

Transdermal Delivery

The transdermal therapeutic system with fentanyl (patch) has simplified the concept of continuous parenteral administration of opioid by using a noninvasive method. This method, which has high patient preference, has been beneficial in the treatment of cancer pain. Fentanyl is the sole opioid available by this method because of its high lipid solubility.[21,22]

After initial application of the patch, serum levels gradually increase to peak concentration in 12 to 24 hours, and effective analgesia occurs as early as 6 hours.[23] The patches are marketed in doses of 25, 50, 75, and 100 µg/hr and are applied for 72 hours. Because these doses are additive, a patient requiring 150 µg/hr of transdermal fentanyl may have two 75-µg/hr patches.

Patient-Controlled Analgesia

Patient-controlled analgesia (PCA) allows patients to treat their own pain by self-administering prescribed doses of opioids parenterally by means of a small, sophisticated programmable, computerized pump. The pump can be programmed to deliver a continuous infusion; in addition, the patient can administer bolus injections at a preset dose and time interval. There appears to be no difference in the effects on respiratory function compared with other therapies.[13]

Neurosurgical Procedures

With the development of the multidisciplinary approach to pain management and with an increasing range of available

TABLE 12–6 Opioid Agonist Analgesic Drugs* for Treating Cancer Pain

Drug	Equianalgesic Dose (mg)		Duration of Action (hr)	Comment
	IM	Oral		
Morphine	10	30	3–4	
Oxycodone	15	20	2–4	
Codeine	130	200	2–4	
Hydromorphone	1.5	7.5	2–4	
Oxymorphone	1	10 (rectal)	3–4	No oral form
Levorphanol	2	4	4–8	Delayed toxicity (accumulation)
Methadone	10	20	4–8	Delayed toxicity (accumulation)
Fentanyl	0.1	†	2–4	Transdermal delivery available

*Not recommended for cancer pain: propoxyphene, meperidine, partial opioid agonists, and opioid agonist-antagonists.
†No oral dose-equivalent established.
IM, intramuscular.

TABLE 12–7 Adjuvant Drugs for Treating Cancer Pain

Class and Generic Name	Dosage Range (mg/day)	Comment
Antidepressants		
Amitriptyline	10–300	Burning or lancinating neuropathic pain; helpful in treating insomnia and depression
Imipramine	10–30	
Doxepin	30–300	
Desipramine	75–300	Start with lowest dose and titrate to effect
Nortriptyline	25–100	
Maprotiline	75–300	
Paroxetine	20–60	
Venlafaxine	75–225	
Anticonvulsants		
Carbamazepine	300–1600	Lancinating neuropathic pain; considered the first line of therapy
Phenytoin	300–400	
Clonazepam	2–8	
Valproate	375–3000	
Gabapentin	100–3600	
Local Anesthetics		
Mexiletine	300–900	Lancinating neuropathic pain refractory to other agents
Tocainide	600–1200	Safest agents compared with others in this table
Corticosteroids		
Cortisone	100–300	Neuropathic pain from nerve compression or inflammation or bone pain
Methylprednisolone	10–30	
Dexamethasone	4–8	
Miscellaneous		
Baclofen	20–120	Antispasmodic, antineuropathic vasodilator for RDS pain; opioid potentiator, adrenergic agent, anxiolytic, major tranquilizer
Nifedipine	10–60	
Clonidine	0.1–0.3	
Benzodiazepines		
Phenothiazines		
Psychostimulants		Enhance alertness
Dextroamphetamine	10–80	
Methylphenidate	10–40	

RSD, reflex sympathetic dystrophy.

pharmacologic agents, fewer patients require surgical intervention. The aim of surgery is to interrupt the nociceptive pathways in the peripheral nerves or at certain sites in the neuraxis.

The most commonly performed surgical procedure for cancer pain relief is *anterolateral* cordotomy, which targets the spinothalamic tract. This can be done by open technique, which carries significant morbidity; complications include hemiparesis, urinary retention, and sexual impotence.

Percutaneous cordotomy has largely replaced the open method. It is usually performed with the patient under local anesthesia by advancement of a thermal coagulation probe with fluoroscopic guidance. It is ineffective for those with neuropathic pain caused by a central mechanism and has only limited use for visceral pain.

Intraspinal Therapies

Intraspinal administration of opioids is often used in the treatment of pain, especially pain that in not controlled with oral medications. Opioids can be delivered by the spinal or epidural route. Advantages include profound analgesia, often at a much lower opioid dose without the motor, sensory, or sympathetic block associated with intraspinal local anesthetic administration.[24]

The opioid dose is usually much lower; approximately 20% to 40% of the systemic dose is given epidurally, and only 10% of the epidural dose is used if given intrathecally, thereby lowering the risk of side effects.[25] Placement of an intrathecal pump initially is a much more complex and costly procedure in comparison to epidural catheter placement. However, the high cost of implantation may be negated by the sustained home maintenance costs of epidural infusion after 4 to 6 months.[26]

Three systems used for chronic intraspinal opioid administration include:

1. Percutaneous tunneled epidural catheters
2. Tunneled epidural or spinal catheters connected to subcutaneously implanted injection ports
3. Implanted spinal infusion pump systems

Regional Blocks

Patients suffering from cancer pain localized in a certain area of the body, which manifests as peripheral neuralgia or visceral pain, are excellent candidates for regional block with neurolytic agents. These techniques are also appropriate in patients who are extremely ill or debilitated.

Ganglion Blocks

Pain originating from most viscera is transmitted to the dorsal horn by unmyelinated afferent fibers in the sympathetic and parasympathetic nerves.[27] These fibers terminate in the dorsal horn and synapse with ascending neurons in the contralateral spinothalamic tract.

Regional nerve blocks are rarely used as the only means of pain relief in cancer patients. However, it is assumed that traditional pharmacotherapy and other conservative measures have failed to provide the patient with adequate analgesia when a regional block is employed.[28] As with any invasive procedure, a thorough risk-benefit analysis must be undertaken so as not to put the patient in danger of any unnecessary therapy or to prematurely employ invasive techniques before a reasonable trial of conservative therapy has been attempted.

The stellate (cervicothoracic) ganglion lies anterior to the lateral process of the C7 vertebra. Sympathetic nerve conduction to the ipsilateral head and upper extremity is interrupted by a block of this ganglion. Because of the proximity to other vital structures, many clinicians hesitate to perform blocks in this area. However, serial blocks with local anesthetic or neurolytic agents in dilute concentrations (3% to 6% phenol) after a diagnostic local anesthetic block have been recommended.[29] Potential complications include intravascular injection of the vertebral artery, phrenic and superior laryngeal nerve block, and, rarely, intrathecal injection.[30]

Celiac Plexus Block

The celiac plexus lies on the anterolateral surface of the aorta from the T12 to L2 vertebral level. A block of this plexus affects visceral pain in many abdominal organs and has gained widespread acceptance, especially for the treatment of pancreatic cancer pain. The incidence of pain relief[31] has been reported to be more than 84%, although occasionally repeat blocks are required. Possible complications include: hypotension; intrathecal, epidural, or interpsoas injection; intravascular injection of the aorta or vena cava; puncture of the kidney, intestine, or lung; paraplegia; and anterior spinal artery syndrome.

Hypogastric Plexus Block

Cancer patients with extensive tumor growth into the pelvis may experience pelvic pain that is unresponsive to traditional opioid therapy. Pelvic pain associated with cancer arises from visceral involvement, from tumor extension into the pelvic muscles, and from neuropathic involvement. Indirect evidence suggests that visceral pain may contribute a significant component to overall pain in advanced-stage pelvic cancer, thereby making neurolytic blocks a useful analgesic adjuvant.[32,33]

The hypogastric plexus lies anterior to the bodies of the L5 to S1 vertebrae and controls sympathetic activity to the pelvis and lower limbs. Injury to sacral nerves, bladder or bowel perforation, intravascular injection, and urinary or fecal incontinence are potential complications.

Ganglion Impar Block

Intractable perineal pain affects somatic, visceral, and autonomic nerves controlling excretory and sexual functions. A block of the ganglion impar, also known as the sacrococcygeal ganglion or ganglion of Walther, can provide relief without significant somatovisceral dysfunction in many patients with advanced cancer. The ganglion impar contributes to the innervation of the perineum, distal rectum and anus, distal urethra, vulva, and distal third of the vagina. Characteristically, pain in this region tends to be vague in nature, associated with tenesmus, a burning sensation, and poorly localized discomfort. The patient may also complain of a sense of bladder or bowel urgency. The ganglion impar is the only solitary ganglion and is a retroperitoneal structure. The ganglion impar lies anterior to the sacrococcygeal junction and can be blocked with 5 to 10 ml of solution.[34]

Interpleural Analgesia

Another technique employed in the treatment of cancer pain, interpleural analgesia, has been successfully used for surgical anesthesia and in the management of some chronic states such as pancreatic pain[35] and post-thoracotomy pain syndrome.[36,37] This block has also been used to alleviate acute exacerbations in various advanced cancer conditions. Possible complications associated with technique include

tension pneumothorax, pleural infection, and local anesthetic systemic toxicity from rapid tissue absorption.

SUMMARY

The management of patients with cancer pain can be a challenging task, even for physicians trained in cancer pain management. The use of a systemic approach in assessing such pain can simplify management. Without a thorough assessment, the possibility of misdiagnosis and undertreatment exists. Appropriate and frequent assessments form the basis for the development of an effective pain treatment plan. An understanding of the various etiologic mechanisms of cancer and the different types of pain that they can produce is essential to providing appropriate therapeutic interventions. Finally, a multidisciplinary approach addressing pain, anger, anxiety, depression, and associated symptoms is essential in providing the best quality of life during this life-threatening experience.

ACKNOWLEDGMENT

A portion of this chapter was adapted from Harrison P, Lema MJ: Cancer pain. In Brown DL, editor: *Regional anesthesia and analgesia.* Philadelphia, WB Saunders, 1996, pp 709–720, Copyright Mayo Clinic; and Lema MJ, Adlaka R: The assessment and etiology of pain in the cancer patient. In Ashburn MA, Rice LJ, editors: *The management of pain,* New York, Churchill Livingstone, 1998, pp 447–455.

References

1. Stjernsward J, Eeoh N: The scope of the cancer pain problem. In Foley KM, Bonica JJ, Ventafridda V, editors: *Advances in pain research and therapy,* vol 16. Second International Congress on Cancer Pain. Philadelphia, Lippincott-Raven, 1990.
2. Cleeland CS, Gonin R, Hatfield AK et al: Pain and its treatment in outpatients with metastatic cancer. *N Engl J Med* 330:592, 1994.
3. Bernabei R, Gambassi G, Lapane K et al, for the SAGE Study Group: Management of pain in elderly patients with cancer. *JAMA* 279:1877, 1998.
4. World Health Organization (WHO): *Cancer pain relief.* Geneva, WHO, 1986.
5. Clinical Practice Guideline No. 9: Management of cancer pain. Washington, DC, U.S. Department of Health and Human Services, 1994.
6. Bruera E, Fainsinger R, MacEachern T et al: The use of methylphenidate in patients with incident cancer receiving regular opiates: A preliminary report. Pain 50:75, 1992.
7. Zech DF, Grond S, Lynch J et al: Validation of World Health Organization Guidelines for cancer pain relief: A 10-year prospective study. *Pain* 63:65, 1995.
8. Kanner R: Postsurgical pain syndromes. In Foley KM, editor: Management of cancer pain. Syllabus of the Postgraduate Course of Memorial Sloan-Kettering Cancer Center, New York, 1985.
9. Weinstein S, Vetter RJ, Serson EA: Phantoms following breast amputation. *Neuropsychologia* 3:185, 1970.
10. Sist T, Lema MJ: Head and neck cancer pain. *Curr Rev Pain* 1:1, 1997.
11. Kao J, Wesolowski JA, Lema MJ: Phantom pain: Current insights into its neuropathophysiology and therapy. *Pain Diag* 7:333, 1997.
12. de Leon-Casasola OA, Myers DP, Donaparthi S et al: A comparison of postoperative epidural analgesia between patients with chronic cancer taking high doses of oral opioids versus opioid-naive patients. *Anesth Analg* 76:302, 1993.
13. Lema MJ: Cancer pain management: An overview of current therapeutic regimens. *Semin Anesth* 12:109, 1993.

14. Reuben DB, Mor V, Hiris J: Clinical symptoms and length of survival in patients with terminal cancer. *Arch Intern Med* 148:1586, 1998.

15. Coyle N, Adelhardt J, Foley KM et al: Character of terminal illness in the advanced cancer patient: Pain and other symptoms during the last four weeks of life. *J Pain Symptom Manage* 5:83, 1990.

16. Maguire P: The psychological and social sequelae of mastectomy. In Howell JG, editor: *Modern perspectives in the psychiatric aspects of surgery.* New York, Brunner/Mazel, 1976.

17. Vane JR: Inhibition of prostaglandin synthesis as a mechanism of action for aspirin-like drugs. *Nature New Biol* 231:232, 1971.

18. Willer JC, De Broucker T, Bussel B et al: Central analgesic effect of ketoprofen in humans: Electrophysiological evidence for a supraspinal mechanism in a double-blind and cross-over study. *Pain* 38:1, 1989.

19. Piletta P, Porchett HC, Dayer P: Central analgesic effect of acetaminophen but not of aspirin. *Clin Plarmacol Ther* 49:350, 1991.

20. Bruera E, Roca E, Cedaro L et al: Action of oral methylprednisolone in terminal cancer patients: A prospective randomized double-blind study. *Cancer Treat Rep* 69:751, 1985.

21. Miser AW, Narang PK, Dothage JA et al: Transdermal fentanyl for pain control in patients with cancer. *Pain* 37:15, 1989.

22. Maves TJ, Barcellos WA: Management of cancer pain with transdermal fentanyl: Phase IV trial. University of Iowa. *J Pain Symptom Manage* 7(Suppl 3):558, 1992.

23. Plezia PM, Kramer TH, Linford J et al: Transdermal fentanyl: Pharmacokinetics and preliminary clinical evaluation. *Pharmacotherapy* 9:2, 1989.

24. Plummer JL, Cherry DA, Cousins MJ et al: Long-term spinal administration of morphine in cancer and non-cancer pain: A retrospective study. *Pain* 44:215, 1991.

25. Lubenow T, Ivankovich A: Intraspinal narcotics for treatment of cancer pain. *Semin Surg Oncol* 6:173, 1990.

26. Bedder MD, Burchiel K, Larson A: Cost analysis of two implantable narcotic delivery systems. *J Pain Symptom Manage* 6:368, 1991.

27. Gebhart GF: Visceral pain mechanisms. In Chapman CR, Foley KM, editors: *Current and emerging issues in cancer pain: Research and practice.* New York, Raven Press, 1993.

28. Ventafridda V: Continuing care: A major issue in cancer pain management. *Pain* 36:137, 1989.

29. Lofstrom JB, Cousins MJ: Sympathetic neural blockade of upper and lower extremity. In Cousins MJ, Bridenbaugh PO, editors: *Neural blockade in clinical anesthesia and management of pain,* ed 2. Philadelphia, JB Lippincott, 1988.

30. Wells DG, Bjorksten AR: Monoamine oxidase inhibitors revisited. *Can J Anaesth* 36:67, 1989.

31. Brown DL, Bulley CK, Quiel EL: Neurolytic celiac plexus block for pancreatic cancer pain. *Anesth Analg* 66:869, 1987.

32. DeLeon-Casasola OA, Kent E, Lema MJ: Neurolytic superior hypogastric plexus block for chronic pelvic pain associated with cancer. *Pain* 54:145, 1993.

33. Plancarte R et al: Superior hypogastric plexus block for pelvic cancer pain. *Anesthesiology* 73:236, 1990.

34. de Leon-Casasola OA: Superior hypogastric plexus block and ganglion impar neurolysis for pain associated with cancer. *Tech Reg Anesth Pain Manage* 1:27, 1997.

35. Durani Z, Winnie AP, Ikuta P: Interpleural catheter analgesia for pancreatic pain. *Anesth Analg* 67:479, 1988.

36. Fineman SP: Long-term post-thoracotomy cancer pain management with interpleural bupivacaine. *Anesth Analg* 68:694, 1989.

37. Myers DP, Lema MJ, de Leon-Casasola OA et al: Interpleural analgesia for the treatment of severe cancer pain in terminally ill patients. *J Pain Symptom Manage* 8:505, 1993.

Questions • Cancer Pain

1. All of the following are causes of cancer pain except

   A. Acute cancer-related pain
   B. Chronic cancer-related pain
   C. Pain resulting from HIV
   D. End-of-life pain

2. Conservative treatment options for cancer pain includes all of the following except

   A. Oral and parenteral analgesics
   B. Nonsteroidal anti-inflammatory drugs
   C. Opioid analgesics
   D. Intrathecal narcotics

3. Systems used for chronic intraspinal opioid administration include all of the following except

   A. Percutaneous tunneled epidural catheter
   B. Tunneled epidural or spinal catheters connected to subcutaneously implanted injection ports
   C. Patient-controlled anesthesia
   D. Implanted spinal infusion pump systems

4. Cancer patients with extensive tumor growth into the pelvis may experience pelvic pain that may be responsive to

   A. Lumbar sympathetic block
   B. Hypogastric plexus block
   C. Myofascial injection of the low back
   D. Facet blocks

5. The ganglion impar innervates all of the following structures except

   A. Distal rectus and anus
   B. Distal urethra
   C. Distal third of vagina
   D. Lower half of ureter

ANSWERS

1. C

2. D

3. C

4. B

5. D

CHAPTER 13

Miscellaneous Pain Syndromes

P. PRITHVI RAJ

COCCYGODYNIA*

The term coccygodynia, first used by Simpson[1] in 1859 to describe a painful coccyx, is more properly identified as a symptom than a syndrome. Pelvic, anorectal, and spinal cord diseases are the leading sources for referred coccygeal pain.[2]

Although most coccygeal pain is related to benign underlying causes, some rare tumors of the sacrum and spinal cord can cause coccygodynia. Adjacent structures are associated with the symptom complex of coccygodynia. The levator syndrome[3]—a symptom complex consisting of pain and pressure in the rectum, sacrum, and coccyx—is often misdiagnosed as coccygodynia. This syndrome is related to muscular spasms of the levator ani muscles that insert on the anterior aspect of the coccyx. On physical examination, the tip of the coccyx is usually not tender. Treatment for this problem is directed toward massage therapy and muscle relaxants.

Anatomy

The coccyx consists of three to five segments that are attached inferiorly to the sacrum by the sacrococcygeal joint. The joint represents a synarthrosis, complete with intervertebral disk. A disk is also present between the first and second coccygeal segments. Lower segments usually undergo bony fusion with aging. The coccyx serves as the insertion site for the levator ani and coccygeus muscles on its ventral surface and for the gluteus maximus on the lateral aspect of the dorsal side. These muscles work together to flex the coccygeal extensors, which leads to an anterior angulation of the coccyx off the sacrum. The actual angle and morphology of the coccyx vary considerably within the normal population. There is some evidence, however, to suggest that more acutely angled coccyxes represent a risk factor for coccygeal injury.[4] The innervation of the coccyx is supplied by the coccygeal sacral nerves in conjunction with the coccygeal nerve. Occasionally, the third sacral nerve also makes a contribution.[5]

Acute Coccygodynia

Acute coccygodynia is usually related to a fall that exposes the coccyx to direct trauma. Less commonly, it may also occur during childbirth at the time of delivery. Acute coccy-

godynia is far more common in women than men, possibly because of the wider distance between female ischial tuberosities, thereby affording less protection to the coccygeal area.[6,7] The complaint is relentless aching and, occasionally, stabbing pain. This discomfort may be limited to the coccyx or may radiate to the buttock. Invariably, sustained sitting aggravates the pain, and many patients prefer to stand during the history-taking interview. Physical examination demonstrates impressive tenderness from the coccyx by either rectal or external palpation. X-ray examinations of the coccyx are of limited value when the history of coccygeal trauma is elicited. Often, x-ray films are entirely normal.[5]

Idiopathic Coccygodynia

Although the pain pattern and physical examination findings of idiopathic coccygodynia are identical to those of acute coccygodynia, the history of trauma is notably absent. It is currently believed that idiopathic coccygodynia may be related to a series of subacute coccygeal injuries or to a normal variation in coccygeal structure that lends itself more susceptible to injury.[4]

Treatment

Treatment for acute and chronic coccygodynia is directed toward minimizing pressure on the coccyx. The use of cushions or rubber donuts when sitting redistributes weight bearing away from the coccyx. Sitz baths and heating pads are often helpful in relaxing the traction of the pelvic musculature. Mild analgesics, anti-inflammatory drugs, and muscle relaxants may be required. In most cases, resolution of symptoms occurs within 3 months.

When coccygeal symptoms fail to resolve spontaneously, a more aggressive approach is warranted. Digital manipulation of the coccyx, using requiring an anesthetic, may prove helpful.[8] Injections of local anesthetics and steroids into and around the sacrococcygeal joint may offer significant relief when osteoarthritis is present.[8,9]

Coccygectomy is the definitive surgical procedure when conservative measures fail and the origin of the pain is believed to be confined to the coccyx. Bayne and colleagues[10] reviewed 48 cases of coccygectomy to assess the influence of different causes of pain on patient outcome. Those patients with a history of direct trauma or postpartum coccygodynia obtained good results in 22 of 29 (76%) cases. It is essential to rule out lumbar disk disease as a cause of coccygodynia before considering a coccygectomy.

---

*Excerpted from Gold MD: Coccygodynia. In Raj PP, editor: *Practical management of pain,* ed 2, St. Louis, Mosby, 1992.

OROFACIAL PAIN*

Pain of Dental Origin

Diagnosis of Tooth-Related Pain

Tooth-related pain has been described as one of the most extreme kinds of pain to endure. Often, the patient can precisely point to the affected tooth. The practitioner can then confirm the diagnosis by a positive painful or tender reaction to the tests of percussion or palpation adjacent to the tooth apex.

Typically, tooth-related pain is easy to identify. However, when the pain is diffuse and spread over a region of several teeth, diagnosis becomes a challenge. If the patient and practitioner are willing to delay diagnosis and treatment of this diffuse odontologic pain, the pain may localize and the offending tooth can be identified and treated.

In instances of persistent diffuse pain often progressing from one tooth to another and back again, the diagnosis of atypical odontalgia must be considered. Often these patients have a history of root-canal therapy or extraction without remission of pain.

One of the most difficult conditions to evaluate is the cracked tooth syndrome. The pain occurs when chewing, and clinically the split cannot be seen radiographically or through diagnostic testing of the teeth. The practitioner can become suspicious when the pain is reproduced when the patient bites on a hard object. A split tooth can refer pain to the head and neck and be a continual source of pain.

Temporomandibular Joint Disorders

A differential diagnosis is the first step in the workup of a patient with pain that might be of craniomandibular origin and is related to dental apparatus. Besides looking for obvious odontologic or periodontal disease, the practitioner evaluates the patient to see if a relationship exists among the functioning movements of the jaw, temporomandibular joint (TMJ), muscles, ligaments, and tooth occlusion. If the pain appears related to the TMJ, the examiner must ascertain whether the problem is extracapsular or intracapsular, because the treatment differs. Extracapsular problems of the masticatory apparatus are mainly muscular in origin. Intracapsular problems such as an arthritic condition, ankylosis, or displacement or dislocation of the TMJ disk, may result in inflammation or dysfunction of the jaw and result in pain.

Most disorders of the masticatory system manifest either as pain or as dysfunction with jaw movement. Most patients treated for TMJ disorders have several problems including malocclusions, psychologic stress, joint disease, pain, dysfunction, poor body mechanics, and myofascial pain.

Causes of Temporomandibular Joint Dysfunction

Extracapsular problems suggested as causes of TMJ dysfunction include possible trigger areas in masticatory muscles, psychophysiologic causes, and occlusal mechanisms.

Trigger Areas in Masticatory Muscles

Travell[11] observed areas in muscles called trigger zones, which are responsible for referred pain patterns. She suggests that these trigger areas "are a small zone of hypersensitivity located within the muscle in spasm or in fascia. Deep pressure on the trigger area, or touching it with a needle, reproduces a spontaneous pain at a distance, and infiltrating it locally with procaine eliminates the related reference of pain."

She classified these areas located within the masticatory muscles as follows:

1. Masseter muscle: Superficial layer refers pain to the jaws, molar teeth, and surrounding gingiva. From the anterior border of the masseter muscle and upper part of the muscle, pain is referred to the upper teeth; from the lower part, pain is referred to the lower molars. From trigger areas at the angle of the mandible, pain travels upward in and over the temporalis and around the outer portion of the eyebrow. Trigger areas in the deep layer of the masseter refer to the TMJ and deep in the ear.
2. Temporalis muscle: This muscle refers pain to the side of the head and to the maxillary teeth, depending on which area of the temporalis is injected. The anterior temporalis refers pain to the supraorbital ridge and maxillary incisors. The medial temporalis refers pain to the bicuspid area and the posterior temporalis to the upper molars and occiput.
3. External pterygoid muscle: This refers pain deep into the MJ and maxillary region.
4. Internal pterygoid muscle: This refers pain mainly to structures within the mouth, tongue, hard palate, and the TMJ and neck muscles.
5. Trapezius muscle: The suprascapular portion refers pain to the angle of the mandible, posterolateral neck, mastoid process, temporal area, and back of the orbit. Spasms of the trapezius muscle cause stiff neck, with limitation of motion on the contralateral side.
6. Sternocleidomastoid muscle: This muscle refers pain to the forehead, supraorbital ridge, inner angle of the eye, middle ear, posterior auricular region, the point of the chin, and the pharynx, with diffuse pain in the neck.

To confirm joint discomfort, pain in the TMJ may be elicited by palpating the external auditory meatus. Patients with psychologic stress may exhibit teeth clenching and/or bruxism, which may increase the intracapsular pressure in the TMJ, leading to improper joint movement.

THORACIC PAIN OF MUSCULOSKELETAL ORIGIN*

Thoracic musculoskeletal pain is a frequent complaint. It may be related to trauma, postsurgical changes, infectious processes, degenerative changes, overuse phenomenon, and inflammatory processes. The site of the pain may involve the vertebrae, the bony thorax, and the soft tissue or musculoligamentous structures.

---

*Excerpted from Phero JC McDonald JS, Green DB et al: Orofacial pain and other related syndromes. In Raj PP, editor: *Practical management of pain,* ed 2. St. Louis, Mosby, 1992.

*Excerpted from Neumann M: Trunk pain. In Raj PP, editor: *Practical management of pain,* ed 2, St. Louis, Mosby, 1992.

Costochondritis (Tietze's Syndrome)

Pain of the costochondral junctions along the anterior chest wall may follow blunt chest trauma, persistent coughing as with chronic obstructive pulmonary disease or acute respiratory infections, overuse of the upper extremity, or chest surgery. Tietze's syndrome is most often unilateral, involving the second and third costal cartilages.

Costochondritis presents as inflammation of multiple costosternal articulations. It may radiate widely and mimic intrathoracic and intra-abdominal disease. Because multiple articulations are usually involved, local tenderness is elicited with palpation, which may reproduce radiating pain symptoms. Costochondritis most often occurs in adults 40 years and older.

Vertebral Pain

Painful disorders of the vertebrae may include osteoporosis, compression fractures, thoracic facet syndrome, ankylosing spondylitis, postural abnormalities, and injuries involving forced or violent flexion or extension movement of the spine. Compression fractures of the thoracic vertebrae resulting from trauma, osteoporosis secondary to aging or corticosteroid use, and degenerative changes are often encountered. The patients complain of encircling pain along the intercostal nerves, aggravated by twisting motions, coughing, or postural changes. In the acute setting, fractured vertebrae and ribs produce severe, constricting pain of the thorax, which may inhibit respiration. The pain is generally accompanies by severe muscle spasm of the intercostal and paraspinous muscles, inhibiting the patient from obtaining adequate sleep or movement. Treatment consists of local heat or ice, transcutaneous electrical nerve stimulation (TENS), nonsteroidal anti-inflammatory medications, and nonopioid and opioid analgesics. Nerve-blocking techniques such as single-shot or continuous epidural blocks, single- or multiple-level intercostal blocks, paravertebral somatic nerve blocks, and intrapleural catheter techniques can also be used.

Myofascial Pain

Pain arising from paravertebral muscles and iliocostalis muscles is a frequent cause of thoracic pain. Pain can be reproduced by pressure on the trigger area and is often relieved by massage, vapocoolant spray, or by injection of a local anesthetic/steroid mixture.

Tender trigger points located in the pectoral and serratus anterior muscles and accompanied by spasm in those muscles are a frequent cause of anterior chest pain. Pain is reproduced by pressure on the trigger point and relieved by a local anesthetic injection or vapocoolant spray technique. The pain is not relieved by intercostal block, because the branches of the brachial plexus innervate the pectoral muscles. TENS and physical therapy involving stretching exercises, deep massage, and passive then active range-of-motion techniques are helpful in preventing recurrence.

Post-thoracotomy Pain

Chronic pain after thoracotomy can be due to various causes. Many of the common causes of post-thoracotomy pain are amenable to therapeutic interventions.

Entrapment of Nerve Fibers in the Scar Tissue

A light touch on the scar tissue produces intense radiating pain, sometimes accompanied by burning pain from associated reflex dystrophy. Injection of the scar tissue with a local anesthetic agent is diagnostic. Repeated injections of a local anesthetic mixed with a steroid are likely to provide long-term relief.

Neuroma

A palpable neuroma in the scar, loss of pinprick sensation over the skin, and elicitation of pain on palpation are diagnostic. Repeated injection of a local anesthetic/steroid mixture may relieve the pain. Persistent pain from a localized neuroma may respond well to neurolytic injection of phenol or to cryolysis.

Sympathetically Mediated Pain

Burning pain associated with hyperpathia, decreased skin temperature over the area, and increased sweating characterize this syndrome. Pain is relieved by blocking the sympathetic fibers with a paravertebral sympathetic block, nerve root block, or epidural block. This pain may also respond to calcium channel blocking drugs, antidepressants, anti-inflammatory medications, and neural stabilizing agents such as fluphenazine.

Myofascial Trigger Points

These points can also be the source of post-thoracotomy pain. They can be located by careful palpation of the paravertebral tissues. Local injections, TENS, and epidural blocks may be helpful, as well as local heat or ice, physical therapy, and anti-inflammatory agents.

Neurogenic Pain

When reviewing pain syndromes of the thorax, acute herpes zoster and chronic postherpetic neuralgia should be included. Additional pain syndromes in the thoracic region involving nerve tissue or damage to nerve tissue include causalgia and intercostal neuropathies after trauma, surgical intervention, or intraneural injection.

Cutaneous Pain

Scars

In the thoracoabdominal region, one can encounter noxious input from cutaneous receptors of a mild-to-severe degree secondary to scar tissue formation or nerve entrapment in the scar tissue. The pain is described as dull and aching, with frequent bouts of sharp, shooting pain associated with particular movement. Localized pain can be aggravated by direct pressure on the scar, and one might find referred pain to areas more closely associated with the scar tissue or more remote. The patients complain of exquisite tenderness over areas of the scar, hyperalgesia, and incapacitation. Infiltration of the scar with local anesthetic agents and steroid combinations often can be helpful.

References

1. Simpson JY: On coccygodynia, the diseases and deformities of the coccyx. *M Times and Gaz* 40:1, 1859.
2. Thiele GH: Coccygodynia: Cause and treatment. *Dis Colon Rectum* 6:422, 1963.

3. Grant SR, Salvati EP, Rubin RJ: Levator syndrome—An analysis of 316 cases. *Dis Colon Rectum* 18:161, 1975.
4. Postacchini F. Massobrio M: Idiopathic coccygodynia. Analysis of fifty-one cases and a radiographic study of the normal coccyx. *J Bone Joint Surg Am* 65:1116, 1983.
5. Traycott RB, Crayton H, Dodson R: Sacrococcygeal pain syndromes: diagnosis and treatment. *Orthopedics* 12:1373, 1980.
6. Frazier LM: Coccygodynia: a tail of woe. *N C Med J* 46:209, 1985.
7. Johnson PH: Coccygodynia. *J Ark Med Soc* 77:421, 1981.
8. Stern FH: Coccygodynia among the geriatric population. *J Am Geriatr Soc* 15:100, 1967.
9. Kersey PJ: Non-operative management of coccygodynia. *Lancet* 1:318, 1990.
10. Bayne O, Bateman JE, Cameron HU: The influence of etiology on the results of coccygectomy. *Clin Orthop* 190:266, 1984.
11. Travell JJ: Temporomandibular joint pain referred back from the head and neck. *Prosthet Dent* 10:745, 1960.

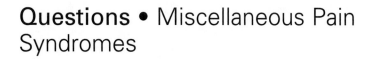

Questions • Miscellaneous Pain Syndromes

1. The symptoms of coccygodynia can consist of all of all of the following except

   A. Pains and pressure in the rectum
   B. Relentless aching and, rarely, stabbing pain
   C. Pain in the buttock
   D. Pain in the anterior aspect of the thigh

2. Intracapsular TMJ pain is mainly due to

   A. Arthritis
   B. Ankylosis
   C. Dislocation of disk
   D. Masticatory muscle

3. The pain of internal pterygoid muscle is mainly in the following structures except

   A. Eyeball
   B. Hard palate
   C. TMJ and neck muscles
   D. Tongue

4. In costochondritis the following signs and symptoms are present except

   A. Tenderness occurs at the costochondral junction
   B. Pain radiates widely
   C. Symptoms mimic intercostal neuralgia
   D. Symptoms occur in patient with musculoskeletal pain

5. Burning associated with hyperpathia, decreased skin temperature over the area, and increased sweating characterize which of the following syndromes

   A. Myofascial pain
   B. Sympathetically mediated pain
   C. Sympathetically independent pain
   D. Visceral pain

ANSWERS

1. D
2. D
3. A
4. C
5. B

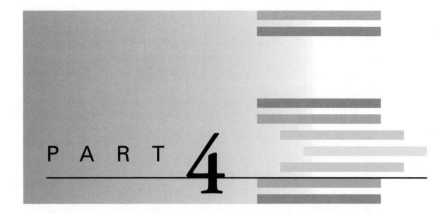

PART **4**

Evaluation and Investigation of Pain Patients

CHAPTER 14

History Taking of the Patient in Pain

BERNARD M. ABRAMS

Proper diagnosis should precede treatment. It forms the basis for management of the individual patient and for the acquisition of experience in evaluating the treatment of a group of patients sharing common symptoms or diagnoses. Of the diagnostic techniques available to the pain practitioner, the history still remains the most important despite the explosion of technology that is now available to help in diagnostic evaluations.

The patient history has several purposes:

1. Delineation of factors enabling diagnosis
2. Establishment of rapport with the patient
3. Assessment of previous treatments
4. Elimination of irrelevant data
5. Assessment of the patient's psychologic, legal, vocational, and disability status
6. Recognition of danger signals that may impede the diagnosis and management of the patient

There are two main issues in the acquisition of a history. They involve technique and a knowledge of the proper questions to ask a patient.

TECHNIQUE

First, a decision must be made whether to conduct a face-to-face interview or to use standardized forms. The forms may be of a generalized nature or modified for specific complaints. Although the ease of standardized forms may seem appealing, they do rob both the patient and physician of an opportunity to develop a rapport through conversation. In addition, the physician loses the opportunity to assess the style of the patient and to obtain a feeling for the patient's individual suffering and personal circumstances. This type of perception on the part of the physician is best obtained by unhurried listening.[1] Raj[2] has pointed out:

> The patient with a persisting pain who has already been to many physicians and clinics without relief must be considered a failure of the health care delivery system. A new approach is necessary and based on increased one-to-one patient-physician contact.

THE INTERVIEW

The interview should be conducted at an unhurried pace in a setting that ensures the patient's privacy and dignity. If the patient is competent to give a personal history, family members and other individuals should be excluded from the interview. Putting the patient at ease by having both the patient and examiner assume a comfortable posture helps build confidence and rapport, which certainly extends into the treatment phase and adds to the well-being of the patient.

Language and cross-cultural factors may play a significant role in the attempt to obtain an accurate history.

Some prediction of the difficulty and course of the interview may be made from the individual's circumstances. For example:

- In an *acute* pain setting, the patient is generally anxious from the pain, but the complaints are of short duration and brief in history. The site and cause are not obscure, and, although distressed, the patient is usually not discouraged with, or skeptical of, the pain physician.
- In a *chronic* pain setting, the history becomes more convoluted; the site of the pain production, mechanism, and cause are more obscure. Also, the patient is more disaffected with the physician.

In an independent medical examination, frank suspicion and hostility may appear. The physician must be prepared for a variety of responses, ranging from tears to verbally assaultive behavior. Generally, after a reasonable period, the situation is diffused and the interview proceeds on a more productive course.

The interview should be as nondirective as possible, but sometimes it is necessary to pace the interview so that there is an adequate amount of time spent on each portion of the interview.

ORDERING OF QUESTIONS

Experience dictates that questions be asked in a generally routine and orderly fashion. This includes the chief complaint, history of the presenting complaint, past medical history, systems review, family history, and occupational and social history (Table 14–1).[3] A list of 12 specific questions to ask the patient follows. Asking these questions in the order presented is important because they help to:

1. Differentiate acute from chronic pain
2. Differentiate painful conditions that threaten life or limb from chronic or recurrent conditions that warrant remediation, but that are not life threatening or limb threatening

TABLE 14–1 Sequence of Data Collection for Obtaining a Medical History of the Pain Patient

Chief Complaint

History of the Presenting Complaint
Condition at onset
Spatial distribution
Qualitative aspects
Temporal distribution
Provocative factors
Palliative factors
Current treatment
Quantitative aspects

Past Medical History
Similar symptoms
Similar region
Past treatment
Trauma or surgery
General past health

Systems Review
Pain in each system
General systems health
Tobacco, alcohol, drugs

Family History
Members with similar pain
Members with other pain
Members with disabling illness
Members with other illnesses
Deceased members and causes of death

Occupational and Social History
Marital status
Dependents
Education
Occupation
Current employment or disability status
Financial support
Rest and recreation
Attendance at external social functions
Social effects of pain

Modified from Longmire DR: Tutorial: The medical pain history. *Pain Dig* 1:29, 1992.

3. Identify the relative underlying tissue and mechanism involved in pain production (i.e., muscles, tendons, ligaments, nerves, nerve roots, plexuses, central nervous system, bony structures) and to elucidate the nature of the disease process[4]
4. Identify syndrome of pain or pain referral[5]

THE TWELVE QUESTIONS

Question 1: What Is the Matter?

This open-ended question allows patients to tell their story in their own fashion. This method quickly exposes whether or not the patient is talking about pain or another symptom and also allows a quick insight into the style of the patient. This method also eliminates any premature conclusion on the part of the physician. As much information should be derived under this general question as possible given the physician's time and the ability of the patient to stay on track. Recording the patient's complaints in quotations ensures a fair rendering of the complaints and allows for a retrospective analysis of what the patient really meant. Also,

the patient may offer a diagnosis rather than a history. Without offending the patient, the physician must progress beyond this point and resume the history.

Question 2: How Did This Complaint Develop?

Using this open-ended question may help to disclose bonus information such as an inciting injury, that is, a fall or other accident. However, assumptions should not be made, because sometimes patients relate the onset of pain to the occurrence of some meaningful event in their lives even though the pain is not related.

Gathering a summary of physicians who have previously treated the patient under these circumstances can be helpful. Securing records that appear to be pertinent in any way also help lead to a proper diagnosis.

Question 3: What Has Happened Since You First Experienced the Pain?

The temporal benchmark includes the differentiation between acute pain and chronic pain. It also helps to distinguish those conditions that are life threatening and those that are benign.

- Acute pain is pain of recent onset (according to Wall[6]) that usually ends within a period of days to weeks. Acute pain has a strong relationship with *nociception,* which is a term applied to activity induced in neural pathways by potentially tissue-damaging stimuli.
- Chronic pain persists or recurs frequently. Bonica[7] defined this pain as persisting for a month beyond the usual course of an acute illness or after a reasonable duration for an injury to disappear or pain that recurs at intervals for months or years.

Question 4: What Is the Pain Like? Describe It.

Although patients vary in how they describe pain and may even describe phenomena other than pain, such as vertigo or dizziness, the following terms are useful[8]:

- *Hyperpathia* is a particularly unpleasant dysesthesia or abnormal sensation characterized by an exaggerated pain response to either noxious or non-noxious stimulation.
- *Allodynia* refers to a situation in which a non-noxious stimulus is perceived as painful.
- *Hyperalgesia* is an increased pain response to a noxious stimulus.
- *Nociceptive* pains generally are familiar.[5] They may be sharp if musculoskeletal, gnawing or aching if muscular, and crampy if originating from an internal viscus.
- *Neuropathic* pains[5] are more difficult to describe and may be more diffuse; they may be burning, lancinating, sharp, or tearing.[9,10]

Sometimes unusual descriptions of pain may tempt the physician to try to speed up the interview by offering adjectives such as sharp, dull, or knife-like. This temptation must be resisted so that words are not put in the patient's mouth that could lead to an erroneous response.

Question 5: How Intense Is the Pain?

Individuals vary widely on their interpretation of pain intensity. It is, however, important to keep two factors in mind:

1. The description of pain intensity is often the patient's "red badge of courage" and indicates a style of suffering and veracity; to ignore it dismisses both the patient's style and an opportunity for empathy and rapport on the physician's part.
2. The description forms a basis for assessing treatment results.

Question 6: Where Is the Pain Located? Does It Radiate or Spread to Another Part of the Body?

Sometimes, at this point, a pain diagram is used to understand the location of the pain and any radiation of pain. Pain may be focal (experienced at one site), multifocal, or general. Often unexpected patterns of referred pain occur, and close inquiry may reveal that there is more than one type of pain.

Question 7: Do You Have Any Associated Medical Conditions?

Medical conditions that might affect the diagnosis should be discussed. Some examples of these conditions are a remote history of cancer, a present history of diabetes mellitus, or a history of arthritis.

Question 8: Which Treatments Have Been Attempted for This Pain Condition?

Although this question tends to be answered in a rather cursory fashion, it is important because it often sets the stage for assessing whether earlier diagnoses have been correct and which future treatments might be effective. The possible responses include:

1. "Red flag" drugs (narcotics, benzodiazepines, other sedatives, muscle relaxants),[1] which may conceivably interact with other drugs used by the patient
2. Drugs contraindicated for the patient's medical condition

A precise history should be obtained regarding neural blockade. Often neural blockade is perceived as ineffective, when in fact, it did not succeed in blocking the affected part of the body.

Question 9: Which Medications Are You Currently Taking and Have You Had Any Allergic Reactions?

All medications should be confirmed with regard to dose and duration of use.

Question 10: What Are the Factors That Make You Better or Worse?

Certain conditions are clearly associated with inciting factors. For example, lifting may produce abdominal hernia pain. Rest is generally a benefiting factor for most pains, but exceptional pain (i.e., that of bursitis) may be exacerbated at night. Sometimes the proper positioning of a patient while at rest is a key element in the relief of pain.

Question 11: What Has Been the Effect of This Pain on Your Life—Vocationally, Socially, and Interpersonally?

Much of this information may have already come to light, but new information may be disclosed at this point. The question should be delivered in a conversational tone that encourages patients to share their feelings about their suffering with the physician.[11]

Question 12: Is There Any History of Drug Addiction, Substance Abuse, or Psychiatric Disorder?

If a sympathetic approach with good patient rapport has been obtained, this is a routine, well-accepted question. If the question is not received well, the success of the history or the patient's motivation must be reconsidered. For patients in whom all treatments except narcotics seem to have been ineffective, a high level of suspicion should be maintained. In addition, a history of psychiatric illness or behavior does not preclude a legitimate current pain syndrome. A person with prior substance abuse who is in a addictive recovery program generally is wary of mind-altering substances and is deserving of respectful, trusting behavior on the part of the physician.

INFORMATION ACQUISITION

For each type of pain complaint, physicians must develop their own set of questions. However, certain factors in history taking, common to all pain complaints, have been covered earlier in the text. For each region of the body, a knowledge of disease entities causing pain, patterns of referred pain, and a scheme of questioning should be ascertained. For the physician with less experience, a good starting point is the diagnostic criteria for the particular entity.

SUMMARY

The patient history should attempt to:

1. Establish physician rapport with the patient
2. Establish a putative tissue and mechanism diagnosis for the patient's pain
3. Differentiate between acute and chronic pain as well as nociceptive and neuropathic pain
4. Assess prior treatment as a guideline to future treatments

References

1. Donohoe CD: Targeted history and physical examination. In Waldman S, Winnie A, editors: *Interventional pain management*. Philadelphia, WB Saunders, 1996.
2. Raj PP: History and physical examination of the pain patient. In Raj PP, editor: *Practical management of pain*, ed 2. St. Louis, Mosby, 1992.
3. Longmire DR: Tutorial: The medical pain history. *Pain Dig* 1:29, 1992.
4. Judge RD, Quidema GD, Fitzgerald FT, editors: *Clinical diagnosis: A physiologic approach*, ed 5. Boston, Little, Brown, 1989.
5. Portenoy RK, Kanner RM, editors: Definition and assessment of pain. In *Pain management: theory and practice*. Philadelphia, FA Davis, 1996.
6. Wall PD: On the relation of pain injury to pain. *Pain* 6:253, 1979.
7. Bonica JJ, editor: Definitions in taxonomy of pain. In *The management of pain*. Philadelphia, Lea & Febiger, 1990.
8. Mersky H, Bogduku P, editors: *Classification of chronic pain*, ed 2. Seattle, IASP Press, 1994.
9. Illis LS: Central pain: Much can be offered from a methodical approach. *Br Med J* 300:1284, 1993.
10. Fields HL, editor: *Pain syndromes in neurology*. London, Butterworth, 1990.
11. Cassel EJ: The nature of suffering and the goals of medicine. *N Engl J Med* 306:639, 1982.

Questions • History Taking of the Patient in Pain

1. Patient history taking has several purposes in a pain patient. All of the following are true except

   A. Delineation of factors enabling diagnosis
   B. Establishment of rapport with patient
   C. Discarding the previous treatment of patients
   D. Elimination of irrelevant data

2. Experience dictates that the questions should be asked in a routine and orderly fashion. These include a chief complaint, history of the chief complaint, past medical history, systems review, family history, and occupational and social history. Asking specific questions in the order presented is important because they will help all of the following except

   A. Differentiate acute from chronic pain
   B. Identify the relative underlying tissue and mechanism involved
   C. Identify the syndrome of pain
   D. Allow the patient to be referred to another physician

3. A particular unpleasant dysesthesia or abnormal sensation characterized by exaggerated pain response to either noxious or non-noxious stimulation is termed

   A. Allodynia
   B. Hyperpathia
   C. Nociceptive pain
   D. Hyperalgesia

4. Nociceptive pain is characterized by all of the following except

   A. Sharp pain
   B. Gnawing or aching pain
   C. Crampy pain
   D. Burning pain

5. Nociceptive pain of recent onset that does not last longer than 3 months is termed

   A. Cancer pain
   B. Sympathetically maintained pain
   C. Acute pain
   D. Neuropathic pain

ANSWERS

1. C
2. D
3. B
4. D
5. C

CHAPTER 15

Physical Examination

S T E V E N   S I M O N

The goal of the physical examination is to verify suspicions raised by the history and arrive at an accurate diagnosis. Physical medicine considers the relationship of pain to function and its effect on the whole patient, including vocational and avocational changes. The key to efficiency is performing the same examination in the same fashion for each patient.

VITAL SIGNS

Vital signs provide information about the general health status of the patients in pain. Blood pressure, pulse, respiratory rate, and temperature should be taken at each examination and rechecked after activity if cardiopulmonary debilitation is suspected.

GENERAL DESCRIPTION

The general description includes appropriateness of dress as well as the anxiety and comfort level of the patient. Effects of pain often show in the face and movement patterns and should correlate with complaints of distress. Body alterations such as amputation, contractures, deformities, or unusual size should be noted and considered regarding mechanical causes of pain syndromes. Postural assessment can lead to recognition of ergonomic reality of chronic muscle strain. Note should be made of weight bearing in either leg observed in stance or gait along with the symmetry of arm swing, hip rotation, knee excursion, and foot placement.

GAIT

Examination begins with gait analysis, which describes the walking mobilization efforts of the patient. Familiarization with normal patterns of heel strike, foot flat (midstance), and toe-off is necessary to recognize abnormal patterns.

Essential elements include reciprocating pattern, weight bearing, stance width, and use of braces and assistive devices (canes, crutches, walkers). Gross balance (general walking on a level surface) and higher level balance (tandem walking) should be tested (Fig. 15–1).

Five determinants of gait have been described that produce stability during changes in acceleration, deceleration, and direction:

1. Pelvic rotation occurs with advancement of one leg; the pelvic rotates 4 degrees in the opposite direction.

2. Pelvic tilt or pelvic drop on the ipsilateral side with swing phase is controlled by the gluteus medius and gluteus minimus of the contralateral stance leg.
3. Knee flexion occurs during midstance to shorten the leg and lower the center of gravity.
4. Knee and ankle motion of foot flat and toe-off allows a smooth pattern and shortened vertical displacement.
5. Center of gravity motion between the feet allows balance and efficiency in the horizontal plane.

Gait Examination

The walking cycle is described in two phases, stance and swing. About 60% of gait is spent in stance and 40% in swing. Stance includes the weight-bearing functions of heel strike, foot flat, and toe-off, and swing is divided into acceleration, midswing, and deceleration. Normal findings include a base width of 2 to 4 inches between the heels, center of gravity rising less than 2 inches, flexion of the knee until heel strike, pelvic shift of 1 inch from side to side, stride length of 15 inches, cadence of 90 to 120 steps per minute, and forward hip rotation of 40 degrees around the leg in stance (Fig. 15–2).

Common Abnormal Patterns of Painful Gait

Avoidance of weight bearing is the hallmark of *antalgic* gait. Because this is a stance function, the problem may be due to joint disease or various types of foot pathology including heel spurs, corns, and calluses.

In patients with a painful hip, the shoulder is dipped on the *affected* side to shift the center of gravity onto the joint. In lumbar disk disease, stenosis, or radiculopathy the opposite occurs in an effort to shift as much weight as possible away from the painful side. Weakness of the quadriceps group of muscles requires the patient to push the knee manually into extension in stance.

Abnormalities of the knee joint that result in varus or valgus deformities shorten leg length and produce a noticeable pelvic drop during stance. Ankle range deficits result in toe scrapes or steppage gait alterations. Foot pathology causes the patient to shift weight away from the painful area.

EXAMINATION ROOM

The examination that takes place on the table can yield extensive insights into the proper workings of the body. Attention should be paid to symmetry at the body sides of each tested area as a first indication of pathology, and all

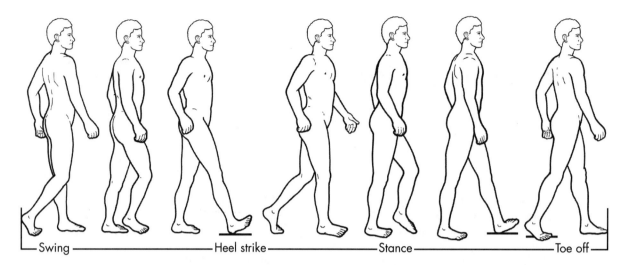

FIG. 15–1 Phases of gait from swing (non–weight bearing) through stance (full weight bearing) to swing. Heel strike begins weight-bearing phase, which ends with toe-off position.

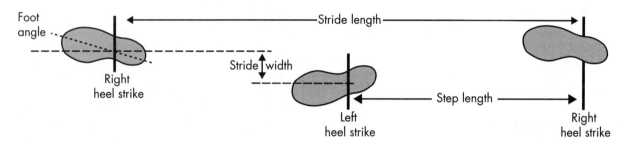

FIG. 15–2 Schematic representation of stride dimensions: step length (one half of stride) is about 80 cm and stride width is about 8 cm with a foot angle of about 7 degrees.

clinical findings collected should be recorded to support presumed diagnosis. Anatomic awareness of motor, reflex, and sensory distribution is essential for proper understanding of normal and pathologic states. Most sources use a five-point scale to measure motor power.

REFLEXES

Muscle stretch reflexes are measured on a four-point scale:

- (0/4)—Absent reflexes; cannot be elicited with typical reflex hammer testing
- (1/4)—Trace reflexes; palpable, but not visible and are weaker than physiologic reflexes
- (2/4)—Physiologic reflexes; muscle stretch that is both palpable and visible
- (3/4)—Brisk reflexes; visible, quick, and palpable responses, generally of a wider than physiologic arc
- (4/4)—Spastic reflexes; barely require tapping to elicit response and may include clonus or repetitive contractions

Typically measured reflexes include C5 (biceps), C6 (brachioradialis), C7 (triceps), C8 (finger flexors), L2 to L4 (quadriceps), and L5 to S2 (triceps surae). Special superficial segmental reflexes may also be examined for better localization of a pathologic process.

Pathologic reflexes for the feet include the Babinski, Chaddock, and Oppenheim 2 reflexes, which indicate upper motor neuron disease with fanning of toes and dorsiflexed great toe (Fig. 15–3).

SENSORY-DERMATOMAL EXAMINATION

Abnormalities in sensation result in an increased, decreased, or altered awareness of stimulation. Using the knowledge of anatomic pathways, the examiner can localize pathologic states and determine central versus peripheral etiology. Physiologic dermatomes[1,2] are described later in this chapter (Fig. 15–4).

Alterations of sensation can be felt as a phantom sensation, paresthesia, or dysesthesia. Words such as numbness, burning, pressure, swelling, tingling, itching, constricting, or heavy are used by patients and suggested to them to describe their sensory awareness. The following medical terms and definitions are used to describe sensation in peripheral and cortical awareness in the tested area:

1. Anesthesia or alganesthesia: loss of sensation
2. Topoanesthesia: loss of tactile localization (cortical sensation)
3. Hypoesthesia: decreased awareness of sensation
4. Dysesthesia: abnormal sensation

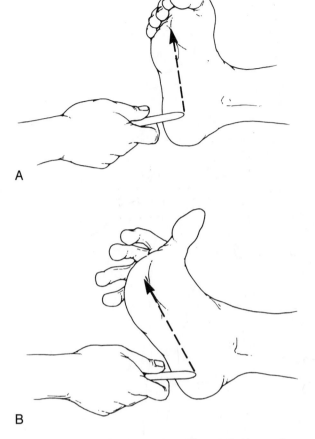

FIG. 15–3 Babinski test. *A*, Normal. *B*, Abnormal.

5. Hyperesthesia: increased awareness of sensation
6. Thigmesthesia: loss of light touch
7. Trichoanesthesia: loss of awareness of hair movement (cortical sensation)
8. Kinesthesia: sensation of muscle motion (cortical sensation)
9. Myesthesia: sensations coming from muscles (cortical sensation)
10. Bathyesthesia: deep sensation coming from muscle or joint (cortical sensation)
11. Arthresthesia: sensation of joint motion (cortical sensation)
12. Statagnosis: postural awareness
13. Pallesthesia: sensation of vibration over a bony prominence on use of an oscillating stimulus such as a tuning fork
14. Pallanesthesia: loss of sensation
15. Piesesthesia: awareness of differences in weight (cortical sensation)
16. Paresthesia: an abnormal spontaneous sensation
17. Baresthesia: awareness of pressure or weight (cortical sensation)
18. Baragnosis: ability to differentiate objects of different weights (cortical sensation)
19. Stereognosis: ability to identify objects by touch (astereognosis or loss of tactile identification is often present in right hemispheric stroke) (cortical sensation)

Exteroceptive Sensations

Exteroceptive sensations include pain, temperature, and touch.[3,4] They arise from superficial receptors in skin or mucous membrane and reach the spinal cord via corresponding peripheral nerves. A reasonable pattern of examination is to alternate stimulation between sharp and dull, move from less sensitive to more sensitive areas, and ask patients to note differences in intensity.

A tuning fork can be used to perform a "poor man's" nerve conduction study of the peripheral nervous system. Typically the (C) tuning fork is struck, the base is placed against the skin covering a nerve, and the patient asked to report when the vibration ceases.

Peripheral nerve sensations correspond to known patterns of distribution that are outlined in Figures 15–5 and 15–6. In testing situations, midline overlap blurs the true end point, but hysterical patients may lose sensation either before or at midline consistently.

Nerve root lesions cause changes in sensation that follow the segmental patterns of that nerve root, often producing radicular or girdle sensation changes. Dermatomes refer to skin innervated by nerve roots, spinal cord segments, or dorsal root ganglia (see Fig 15–4).

Proprioceptive Sensations

Proprioceptive sensations arise from muscles, ligaments, bones, tendons, or joints and produce the sense of motion and position. Normal awareness of movement requires only 1 to 2 degrees of displacement in the digits, and loss generally occurs distally to proximally, with position sense before movement sense.

Pressure sensations may be assessed by pinching tissue or applying direct touch.

Combined sensations (*cortical sensations*) use cognitive and sensory awareness resulting in discrimination perception, such as the recognition of hand-held objects, textures, and different weights.

Cranial Nerves

I. Olfactory nerve. Sense of smell, tested one nostril at a time using pungent aromas.
II. Optic nerve. Visual sense evaluation should include acuity, fields, depth perception, day and night vision, and color.
III. Oculomotor nerve. Coordinated motor control of the eye globe results from a balance of the visual axis and external muscles (including IV and VI).
IV. Trochlear nerve.
V. Trigeminal nerve. Facial and jaw motion sensation is conveyed by this motor and sensory nerve, which connects with cranial nerves III, IV, VI, VII, and IX.
VI. Abducens nerve.
VII. Facial nerve. Muscles of facial expression are innervated by the primarily motor seventh cranial nerve. Taste to the anterior two thirds of the tongue and mixed sensation to the tympanic membrane are the sensory component.
VIII. Acoustic or auditory nerve. Hearing and balance are provided by this mixed nerve, which carries fibers of the cochlear and vestibular nerves. Superficial

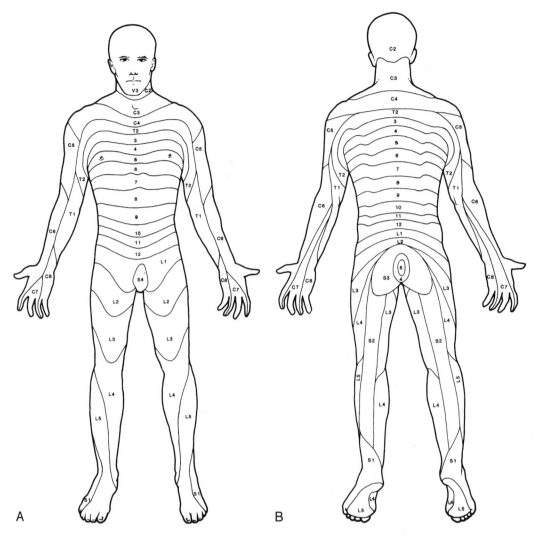

FIG. 15–4 Anterior (A) and posterior (B) dermatomes of the body. *(From Baker AB, Baker LH:* Clinical neurology, *vol 1. New York, Harper & Row, 1983.)*

auditory acuity testing may be performed by using a watch or rubbing fingers by the ear canal. Special equipment is indicated to differentiate soft versus loud and high-pitched versus low-pitched tomes. Otoscopic examination should be preformed to evaluate the tympanic membrane and ear canal.

IX. Glossopharyngeal nerve. Motor, sensory, and autonomic functions of the posterior pharynx.

X. Vagus nerve. Posterior pharynx motor and autonomic functions.

XI. Spinal accessory nerve. Pure motor function to the trapezius and sternocleidomastoid (SCM) muscles.

XII. Hypoglossal nerve. Pure motor supply to the tongue muscle.

TROPHIC EXAMINATION

Skin quality reflects muscle mass and blood flow, nutrition, and overall appearance and can yield clues to abnormality or asymmetry. The examiner should observe and document any signs of edema, discoloration, atrophy, hypertrophy, or temperature changes.

MUSCULOSKELETAL SYSTEM

The musculoskeletal system includes the coordinated use of muscle, nerve, and joint. Range of joint motion should be assessed for significant difference or limitation. Range and strength testing can be conducted simultaneously, which saves time and allows an assisted examination. Knowledge that pain can arise or refer from multiple structures such as skin, muscles, subcutaneous tissues, tendons, joints, ligaments, periosteum, nerve, or organs allows a complete assessment of the complaint.

Nociceptive pain results from lesions in the musculoskeletal system and is transmitted through an intact nervous system. Neuropathic pain results from nerve lesions and is transmitted through an abnormal nervous system.

Range of Motion

Cervical Spine

Cervical ranges of lateral bending, rotation, flexion, and extension are measured. Accurate goniometric studies can be preformed if needed, but side-to-side comparison and rule of thumb measures are usually adequate (Fig. 15–7; Box 15–1).

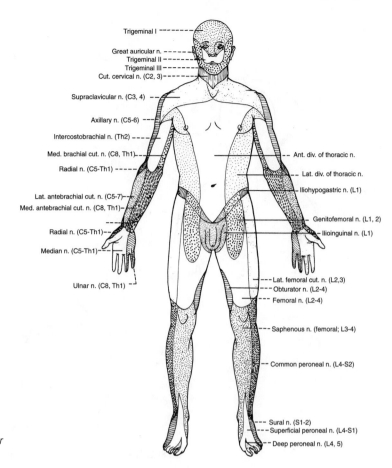

FIG. 15–5 Cutaneous distribution of the peripheral nerves on the anterior aspect of the body. *(From Baker AB, Baker LH: Clinical neurology, vol 1. New York, Harper & Row, 1983.)*

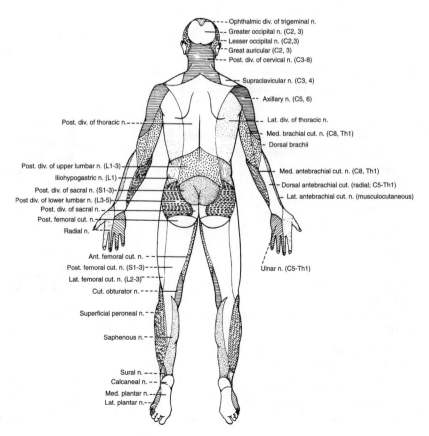

FIG. 15–6 Cutaneous distribution of the peripheral nerves on the posterior aspect of the body. *(From Baker AB, Baker LH: Clinical neurology, vol 1. New York, Harper & Row, 1983.)*

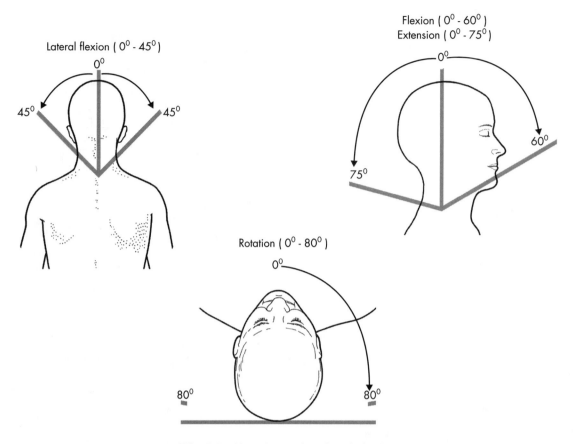

FIG. 15–7 Normal excursion of cervical spine.

BOX 15–1 Common Sources of Cervical Pain

Trauma
Hyperflexion-extension injury (whiplash)
Cervical vertebral fracture, subluxation

Infection
Cervical lymphangitis
Parotiditis
Meningitis
Salivary duct stone
Pleuritis

Referred
Angina
Myocardial infarction

Muscle
Myofascial overuse of trapezius, posterior cervicals
Torticollis

Cervical Degenerative Disease
Disk degeneration
Cervical spondylosis
Cervical foraminal stenosis
Rheumatoid atlantoaxial subluxation

Performing tests with the patient supine not only releases the muscles that oppose gravity but also gives the examiner a chance to test consistency in the patient's responses. A joint limitation remains fixed regardless of position, whereas muscles may release when positioned in a relaxed fashion.

Thoracolumbar Spine

Spinal range of motion can be tested efficiently after gait analysis with the patient standing. Asking the patient to touch the toes and then with hands on hips to look at the ceiling by bending backward from the waist tests flexion and extension. Lateral bending and rotation are often enhanced by the examiner assisting with range. Observations about asymmetry and range loss are then recorded (Fig. 15–8).

Extremities

Depending on the problem area, focused examination of any joints can be accomplished with manual range of motion and power testing. Shoulder examination can be performed by having the patient move hanging arms from the sides to an overhead clap, place hands on opposite shoulder tips, and place thumbs on opposite shoulder blades. Elbow range is assessed by placing the hand on the ipsilateral shoulder and stretching arms away from the body. Wrists are assessed by pressing the palms together and then the dorsa of the hands together, and ulnar and radial motion from a neutral wrist position is evaluated by movements in the appropriate direc-

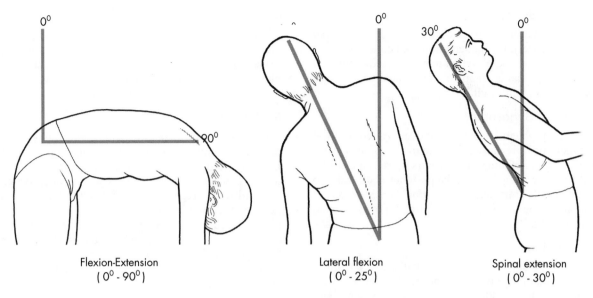

Flexion-Extension
(0° - 90°)

Lateral flexion
(0° - 25°)

Spinal extension
(0° - 30°)

FIG. 15–8 Normal excursion of lumbar spine.

tions. Finger motion can be assessed by having the patient form a tight fist and then open the hand fully. Touching the thumb to each digit pad tests adduction movements.

The significance of limitation of joint motion should be mentioned, as well as an indication of whether the shortening is in the muscle or the joint. Abnormal joint deformities such as swan neck, boutonnière, or mallet of the fingers or hammer toe or hallux valgus of the feet also must be listed.

Evaluation of Major Joints

There are several methods that should provide similar results, but use of a systematic routine rewards the examiner with increased efficacy and completeness. Knowledge of bone anatomy; muscle, nerve, and vascular supply; and pain referral patterns is assumed for the purpose of this chapter.

General technique should involve a visual inspection with focus on symmetry, range of motion or contractures, and manual strength testing. Abnormalities noted may dictate more specific testing such as radiography or electrical studies, which can then be performed as needed.

Evaluation of the Shoulder

Visual examination should indicate bilateral symmetry between the deltoid bulk and the level of the shoulder tips as well as general posture. Range of motion and power should be tested in the:

- Flexion and extension (0 to 180 degrees) sagittal plane
- Abduction and adduction (0 to 180 degrees) frontal plane
- External rotation (0 to 90 degrees) sagittal plane
- Internal rotation (0 to 40 degrees) sagittal plane
- Combination motions are also evaluated. External rotation and abduction: patient reaches over ipsilateral ear to touch tip of contralateral shoulder blade. Internal rotation and adduction: patient reaches behind

---

BOX 15–2 Common Sources of Shoulder Pain

Trauma
Humeral fracture
Anterior glenohumeral dislocation
Acromioclavicular separation
Clavicle fracture

Referred
Gallbladder disease
Myocardial infarction
Pericarditis
Pleuritis

Degenerative Disease
Calcific tendinitis
Subdeltoid bursitis
Rotator cuff tear, rupture
Biceps tendinitis

Muscle
Myofascial overuse of suprascapular muscles

---

the back to touch lower tip of contralateral shoulder blade

Common painful lesions are listed in Box 15–2, which suggests both symptoms and findings.

Special Tests

- Yergason test for biceps tendon stability: Should the long biceps tendon pop out of its groove while conducting this test, pain arises near the anterior lateral humeral head.
- Drop arm test for rotator cuff competence: A complete rotator cuff tear does not allow the arm to remain abducted, but partial tears can also be assessed by this test.

Impingement Syndrome

Impingement syndrome involves a mechanical entrapment of soft tissue between the humeral head and coracoacromial arch with abduction and elevation movements. Rotator cuff injuries such as partial or complete tears, tendinitis, and subacromial bursitis often result.[5,6]

Scapulocostal Syndrome

This common problem is also descriptively called postural fatigue syndrome. It is caused by inflammation of the levator scapulae and scapulothoracic bursa, and referred pain can be reported from the occiput down the posterior neck and into the deltoid muscle at its humeral insertion. Dysesthesias are common along the anterior chest wall and into the dorsal forearm and hand.[5,6]

Frozen Shoulder

This descriptive diagnosis includes any pathologic condition that limits normal range of motion at the glenohumeral and scapulothoracic joints. Physiologic range occurs at both areas with movement in a 2:1 ratio. Typical abduction occurs to 90 degrees at the glenohumeral joint before scapular movement is detected, but absent or very limited motion is found here in a patient with frozen shoulder.[5,6]

Subacromial Bursitis

Shoulder bursitis can be a result of impingement syndrome or strain. Pain referral is typically felt by the patient at the midhumerus and forearm.[5,6]

Evaluation of the Elbow

Visual examination should include bilateral symmetry of the humerus for radial-ulnar bulks. Epicondyles are easily visible and palpable on both medial and lateral surfaces. Range of motion and power should be tested. The radial head is also a source of elbow pain and should be manually examined if discomforted is noted.[5,7]

Lateral Epicondylitis Test (Tennis Elbow)

Common exterior insertional irritation at the lateral elbow epicondyle can be tested with resisted wrist extension.[5,7]

Evaluation of the Wrist

Visual examination should include bilateral symmetry of the forearm muscle bulk, tremors, or joint deviations.[5,7]

Special Tests

- Phalen's maneuver (carpal tunnel compression test). Compression of the median nerve can be exacerbated with forced wrist flexion.
- Reverse Phalen's maneuver (carpal tunnel compression test). Compression of the median nerve can also be exacerbated with forced wrist extension.

Evaluation of the Fingers

Visual examination should include bilateral symmetry of finger bulk, including thenar and hypothenar eminence, joint deviations, and contractures. The ability of the patient to close and open a tight fist provides a quick range test. The range of motion of metacarpophalangeal (MCP) joints in flexion and extension is 0 to 90 degrees in the sagittal plane.

Evaluation of the Thumb (First MCP Joint)

Visual examination should include bilateral symmetry of the thumb bulk, including the thenar eminence, and any joint deviation. Plane of motion is parallel to the palm. Range of motion is abduction and adduction is 0 to 50 degrees. Range of motion in opposition is 0 to 35 degrees.

Evaluation of the Hip

Visual examination should include bilateral symmetry of muscle bulk, surgery scars, and bruising. Hip pain can come from the fibrous capsule and its ligaments, muscle attachments, periosteum, and synovial joint lining. Typical pain reported in this region may be related to pathologic conditions of the lumbar spine, whereas a true hip pathologic process produces symptoms in the groin, anterior medial central or lateral thigh, or greater trochanteric region. Radiographic evaluation is helpful in identifying fractures, avascular necrosis, arthritic changes, tumors, and metastases[5,8] (Box 15–3).

Trochanteric Bursitis

Trochanteric bursitis is a commonly occurring problem because there are three bursae, the largest lying between the gluteus maximus and gluteus medius tendons. Smaller ones are located between the gluteus medius and gluteus minimus tendons and greater trochanter. Complaints are of a deep, dull or aching pain with radiation to the lateral hip region; the pain is worse at night.[8]

Iliotibial Band Syndrome (Snapping Hip Syndrome)

The patient describes an audible snapping sensation in the lower lateral hip with forward mobility that may not be painful. Hip flexion and internal thigh rotation reproduce this sign, which is found mostly in adolescents and young women.

BOX 15–3 Common Sources of Inguinal or Thigh Pain

Fracture of Femur
Traumatic
Pathologic
Stress

Muscle
Strain
Fever-related myalgias
Dermatomyositis
Polymyositis

Vascular Disease
Sickle cell crisis
Iliofemoral venous thrombosis
Avascular necrosis of femoral head

Referred
Inguinal or femoral hernia
Inguinal or femoral lymphadenitis
Degenerative arthritis of the hip (severe)

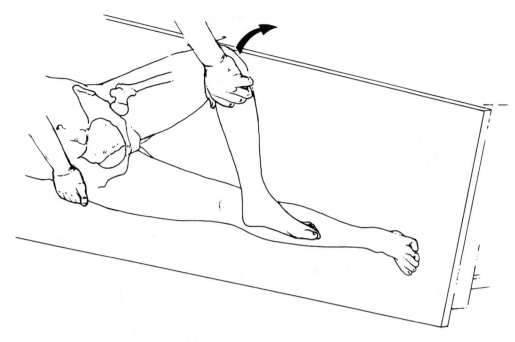

FIG. 15–9 The Patrick or Fabere test.

The cause is thickening of the posterior border of the iliotibial band, which slips over the greater trochanter in motion.[8]

Special Tests

- Fabere (flexion-abduction-external rotation [-extension]) test. This maneuver tests for sacroiliac or hip pathologic conditions (Fig. 15–9).
- Leg length discrepancy. A common source of back or hip pain that is often overlooked is uneven leg length, causing a mechanical repetitive strain on the lumbosacral muscles.
- Straight leg raising test: Lasègue's sign and Gower's sign. This maneuver can test for sciatic irritation (pain radiating to the ankle of the tested leg), but sciatic nerve irritation must be differentiated from hamstring tightness (pain descending to the posterior thigh only) (Figs. 15–10 and 15–11).
- Ober's test (contraction of iliotibial band). If a contracture of the fascia lata or iliotibial band exists, the leg remains abducted during the test. The leg may also remain abducted in cases of polio or meningomyelocele.
- Thomas test. The Thomas test evaluates flexion contracture of the hip.

Evaluation of the Knee

Visual examination should include bilateral symmetry of bone markings, patella positioning and movement, and surgery scars. Excess angulation should be noted on a unilateral or bilateral basis. Loss of the medial compartment produces a valgus knee, and loss of the lateral compartment results in a varus knee. Bilateral finding of genu varum (bowed legs), genu valgum (knock knee), or genu recurvatum (back knees) should also be listed. Pes anserinus and prepatellar bursae are often causes of pain in and around the knee and should be manually examined

with compression over these sites if discomfort is noted[9] (Box 15–4).

Special Tests

- McMurray test. This maneuver was developed to assess for posterior meniscal tears and provides an excellent clinical evaluation[8] (Fig. 15–12).
- Apley's compression or grinding test. A confirmatory test for meniscal tears can be accomplished by compressing the meniscus[8] (Fig. 15–13).
- Patellar femoral grinding test. Chondromalacia patellae is a common problem in degenerative knees, and there are common complaints of increasing pain on arising from a chair or climbing stairs. Exacerbation of symptoms can be elicited by compressing the patella into the femoral groove.[8]
- Drawer signs. These tests were designed to examine injury or disruption of the cruciate ligaments (Fig. 15–14).

Evaluation of the Ankle

Visual examination should include bilateral symmetry of bone markings and edema. Flexing the knee to 90 degrees with release of the gastrocnemius muscles allows the examiner to differentiate between footdrop caused by the soleus alone and that caused by the gastrocsoleus complex[10] (Fig. 15–15, Box 15–5).

Tarsal Tunnel Syndrome

Entrapment of the tibial nerve at the medial ankle by the laciniate ligament can cause a burning pain and dysesthesias along the medial border of the foot. Tarsal tunnel syndrome is somewhat analogous to carpal tunnel syndrome and can be identified by electromyography and nerve conduction studies (Fig. 15–16).

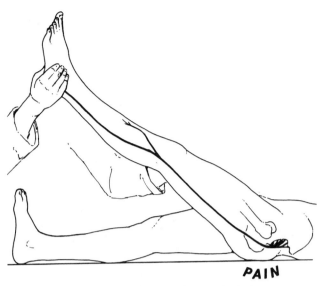

FIG. 15–10 Straight leg raising test (Lasègue's sign).

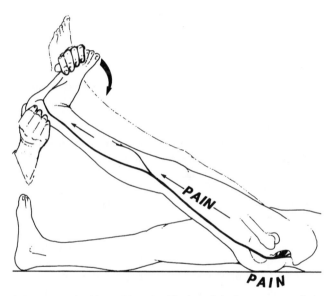

FIG. 15–11 In this position, dorsiflexion of the foot causes pain in the sciatic nerve distribution (Gowers' sign).

Evaluation of the Foot

Evaluation of the foot presents the examiner with a unique clinical opportunity to view, palpate, and mechanically test a body part completely (Fig. 15–17). Structural boundaries allow the plantar foot to be divided into three segments—anterior (5 metatarsal and 14 phalangeal bones), middle (navicular, cuboid, and three cuneiform bones), and posterior (talus and calcaneus)—and stepwise assessment can be performed. Sites of common painful foot problems are identified in Fig. 15–18.[10]

Morton's Neuroma

Morton's neuroma is the most common form of interdigital neuritis. It typically occurs between the third and fourth toes and rarely between the second and third toes. Pain can be produced between the metatarsal heads, which differentiates this condition from metatarsalgia.

Metatarsalgia

Pain along the plantar surface of the metatarsal heads causes weight-bearing discomfort with each step and can be replicated with manual compression. Pain is typically increased in combined pronation and eversion, and this gait pattern should be identified and can be used to make this diagnosis.

BOX 15–4   Common Sources of Knee Pain

Fractures
Traumatic

Monoarthritis
Pseudogout, gout, traumatic synovitis
Degenerative arthritis of knee joint (severe)

Polyarthritis
Reactive, crystal-induced, infectious

Trauma
Internal joint structures

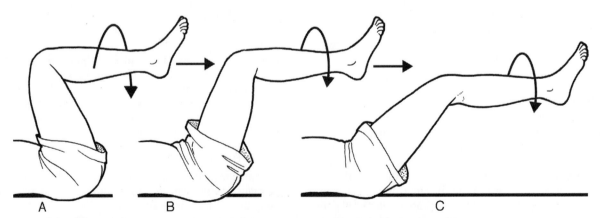

FIG. 15–12 Examination for meniscus injury. *A* to *C*, Stages of McMurray test. With the patient supine, the knee is fully flexed. The leg is internally rotated (lateral meniscus test) or externally rotated (medial meniscus test), and the knee is then fully extended.

Foot Strain

Foot strain reflects pain in the middle portion of the foot. It can occur acutely, as in weekend athletes who demand more of the structures than they readily deliver, or chronically, as the result of prolonged strain of normal structures and abnormal mechanics[11]:

- Plantar fasciitis. Commonly found in those who must stand on hard floors for long periods of time, is an inflammation of tendon and fascia and as they insert into the calcaneal periosteum.[11] Bone growth in the direction of the pull is often found as a calcaneal spur.
- Painful heel syndrome. This syndrome is often diagnosed in morbidly overweight people or those who stand or walk excessively.[12] Degeneration of the normal heel compression allows injury to weight-bearing surfaces of the calcaneus.

Coordination of Motion

Coordinated, fluid motion is considered physiologic. Jerky, stiff, or asymmetric patterns can suggest imbalances in nerve, muscle, joint, or central processing. Attention should be paid to reflex testing for spasticity, which can alter gait with crossed adduction, steppage patterns, or stiffness,

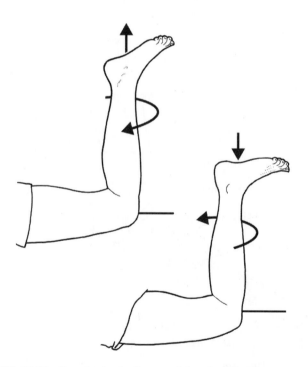

FIG. 15–13 Examination for ligament injury, including the meniscus (Apley test). The Apley test checks the integrity of the knee ligamentous structures and of the menisci. It is performed in two aspects. *Left,* with the patient prone and the knee flexed to a right angle, downward pressure is put on the lower leg. The leg is then rotated to test the menisci. This maneuver compresses the menisci between the femoral condyles and the tibial plateau, as in the McMurray test. With the lower leg internally rotated, the medial meniscus is tested. Grating, crepitation, limitation, and pain imply meniscal damage. From the same position, the leg is elevated (*right*), which places traction on the ligaments. Excessive motion, deduced by a comparison to the contralateral side, indicates laxity or injury to the knee ligaments and capsule.

and typical patterning of the arm in elbow flexion, pronation, and fisted palm, suggesting an upper motor neuron lesion.

Reproduction of Pain

One goal in the identification of pain is reproduction of the pain complaint. Generally, the patient can be helpful in initial localization, after which the examiner must maneuver the painful areas to test further for activation sites. The rule for myofascial examination is to press hard enough with the finger pad to blanch the fingernail. Information about whether the painful site is over a bone and the tone of the muscle (spasm) and trigger responses can be gained from this examination. Positioning can also be helpful in the examination by allowing gravity-dependent postures and gravity-eliminated ones to be compared.[13,14]

SPECIAL DIAGNOSTIC TESTS

The use of special tests can help to identify malingering or help isolate true causation of disease. The following are some of the more helpful tests that can be worked into a regular examination and not be detected as something out of the ordinary:

Cervical Compression Test (Axial Loading)

The cervical compression test is used for referral pain to arms and to examine for narrowing of the neural foramen by disk or facet disease.

Cervical Decompression Test (Distraction Test)

With the patient supine, distraction of the skull from the trunk stretches muscles and decreases pressure on facet joints. If the muscles are in spasm, this maneuver may be painful in the area from the neck to the midback.

Adson Test

The Adson test is used for subclavian artery compression. The examiner palpates a drop in pulse pressure or loss of pulse during the test, suggesting compression of the artery.

Valsalva Test

The Valsalva test is performed to increase intrathecal pressure. If a tumor, disk, or abscess is present in the cervical

---

BOX 15–5   Common Sources of Ankle Pain

Degenerative arthritis (severe)

Lateral Ankle
Traumatic fracture or sprains
Stress fracture of the tibia

Medial Ankle
Traumatic fracture or sprains
Stress fracture of the tibia

Posterior Ankle
Traumatic fracture
Achilles tendinitis, bursitis

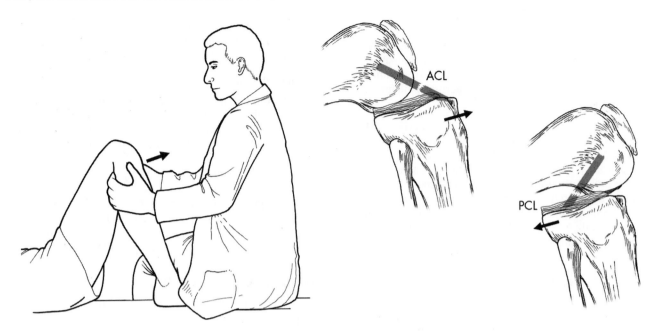

FIG. 15–14 Drawer sign test for cruciate ligaments. The standard drawer sign test for cruciate ligaments immobilizes the foot and stresses the lower leg on the femur. Pulling the leg forward tests the anterior cruciate ligament (ACL), and posterior pressure tests the posterior cruciate ligament (PCL).

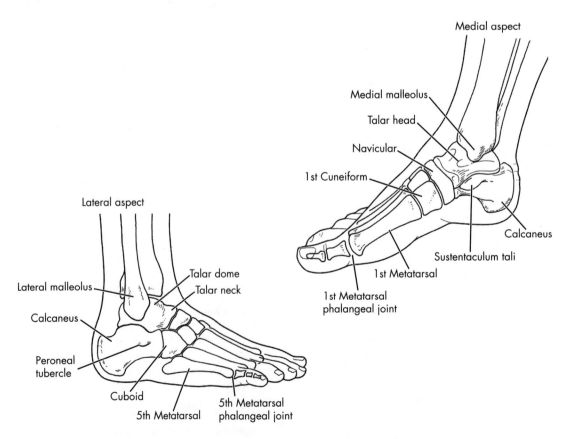

FIG. 15–15 Anatomic view of the bony foot, medial and lateral aspects.

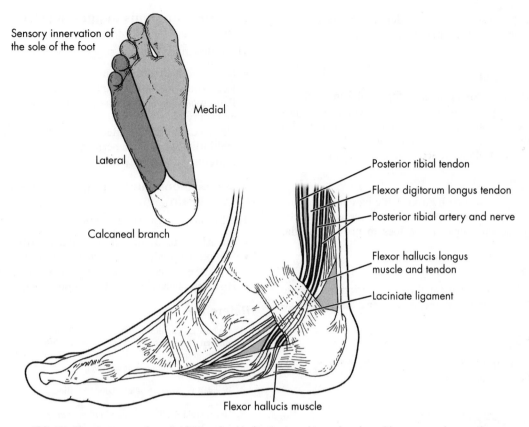

FIG. 15–16 Anatomy of medial foot and ankle for the tarsal tunnel and resulting sensory innervation.

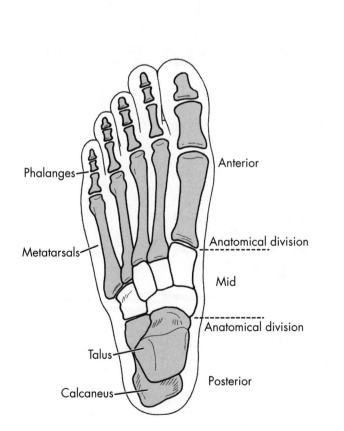

FIG. 15–17 Anatomy of the foot with functional segmentation.

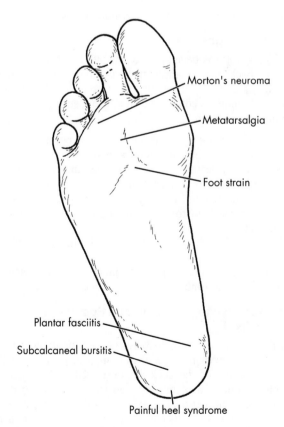

FIG. 15–18 Location of common painful conditions in the plantar foot.

spine canal, this test can help to identify its presence as well as its location if dermatomal referral patterns are reproduced.

Jaw Opening Test

The jaw opening test is performed for temporomandibular joint evaluation. Typical joint motion is vertical; as the jaw opens and closes, the examiner can watch the incisors for abnormal side-to-side motion, an indication of disk and joint abnormality and an often-missed source of facial pain.

Hopping Test

Calf strength can be tested by asking the patient to hop on the ball of the foot. Those who cannot balance well enough for this may use push-ups on the toes to provide similar results.

Kernig Test

Shooting pain in the spinal canal or legs during the Kernig test may indicate nerve root, meningeal, or dural inflammation (Fig. 15–19).

Milgram Test

This test can be used to help determine the presence of a mass lesion or herniated disk.

VALIDATION TESTS

Hoover Test

This test can be used to help determine malingering.

Waddell's Signs

Waddell's test was developed to evaluate functional overlay in low back pain complaints.[15] Each of the following findings is considered positive if present; a total of three positive findings is considered significant, strongly suggesting nonorganic pain:

1. Tenderness: poorly localized and does not follow dermatomal or documented referral patterns
2. Stimulation testing: should not be uncomfortable or cause discomfort in distant sites
3. Distraction testing: inconsistent findings with the same test performed in formal fashion and when attention is distracted
4. Regional disturbance: nonanatomic findings on sensory and motor testing
5. Over-reaction: inappropriate facial or verbal expressions, withdrawal of limbs from touch, or posture contortions

Tests for Psychogenic Pain and Positioning (Pillow Test)

The pillow test is performed to assess the patient's complaint of restricted cervical range of motion. The position of the head and angle of the neck are examined for stiffness in various positions to determine consistency with the complaint. The examiner may perform a similar test by distracting the patient with other activity or conversation and by then watching the patient's head positions.

Tests for Symptoms Suggesting Nonorganic Cervical Pain

The following symptoms suggest nonorganic cervical pain:

- Nonanatomic distribution
- Rest pain without change in various positions assessed
- Pain, dysesthesia, or weakness throughout the entire extremity
- Unsuccessful results after multiple treatments or inability of tests to be performed
- Extremity giving way to weakness

Tests for Signs Suggesting Nonorganic Cervical Pain

The following signs suggest nonorganic cervical pain:

- Superficial tenderness in nonanatomic distribution
- Symptoms produced by distribution tests
- Weakness or numbness throughout entire extremity
- Histrionic behaviors, including posturing and yelling

References

1. Foerster O: The dermatomes in man. *Brain* 56:1, 993.
2. Keegan JJ, Garrett FD: The segmental distribution of the cutaneous nerves in the limbs of man. *Anat Rec* 102:409, 1948.
3. Sinclair D: *Cutaneous sensation.* London, Oxford University Press, 1967.
4. Weddell G, Miller S: Cutaneous sensation. *Annu Rev Physiol* 24:199, 1962.
5. Hoppenfeld S: *Physical examination of the spine and extremities.* New York, Appleton-Century-Crofts, 1976.
6. Abrams B: Neck, arm and shoulder pain evaluation and treatment. *Pain Dig* 7:142, 1997.
7. Drachman DA: Bell's palsy: A neurological point of view. *Arch Otolaryngol* 89:173, 1969.
8. Abrams B: Tutorial 30: Painful conditions of the hip: Evaluation and treatment. *Pain Dig* 7:214, 1997.
9. Abrams BM, Glaser LF: Tutorial 31: Painful conditions of the knee: Evaluation and treatment. *Pain Dig* 7:282, 1997.

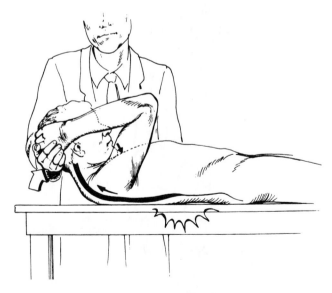

FIG. 15–19 The test for meningeal irritation. There is resistance to passive flexion and the chin cannot be placed on the chest. Pain is produced in the back.

10. Abrams B, Glaser L: Painful conditions of the foot and ankle: Evaluation and treatment. *Pain Dig* 7:351, 1997.

11. Edwards H: Neurological disease of the pharynx and larynx. *Practitioner* 211:729, 1973.

12. Head H: Six clinical lectures on diagnostic value of sensory changes in disease of the nervous system. *Clin J Neurol* 40:337, 1912; and 42:23, 1913.

13. Travell JG, Simons DG: *Myofascial pain and dysfunction: The trigger point manual.* Baltimore, Williams & Wilkins, 1983.

14. Calliet R: *Soft tissue pain and disability,* ed 2. Philadelphia, FA Davis, 1988.

15. Waddell G, Bircher M, Finlayson D et al: Symptoms and signs: Physical disease or illness behavior? *Br Med J* 289:739, 1984.

1. An abnormal spontaneous sensation is termed

   A. Kinesthesia
   B. Topoanesthesia
   C. Paresthesia
   D. Hyperesthesia

2. A syndrome that is caused by inflammation of the levator scapulae and the scapulothoracic bursa with referred pain from the occiput to the posterior neck into the deltoid muscles at its humeral insertion and dysesthesia along the anterior chest wall and into the dorsal forearm and hand is called

   A. Impingement syndrome
   B. Scapulocostal syndrome
   C. Frozen shoulder
   D. Subacromial bursitis

3. Compression of the median nerve that is exacerbated with forced wrist flexion is called

   A. Carpal compression test (Phalen's test)
   B. Carpal tunnel compression test (reversed Phalen's test)
   C. Tinel's sign
   D. Hoffman's sign

4. Fabere's test is used for sacroiliac or hip pathology. It consists of

   A. Test evaluating flexure and contracture of the hip
   B. Test evaluating contracture of the fascia lata or iliotibial band
   C. Test for evaluating sciatic irritation (pain radiating to the ankle of the tested leg)
   D. Test with flexion, abduction, and internal rotation of the hip

5. Lasegue's sign is a maneuver for testing

   A. Sciatic irritation
   B. Femoral neuralgia
   C. Saphenous neuralgia
   D. Genitofemoral neuralgia

ANSWERS

1. C

2. B

3. A

4. D

5. A

CHAPTER 16

Laboratory Investigation

L. DOUGLAS KENNEDY

There is no laboratory substitute for a careful history and physical examination on the initial consultation and on follow-up visits.[1] Laboratory tests, when applied in a logical, systematic method, can enhance the process. This not only improves patient care but also reduces cost. The step after the history and physical examination is development of a laboratory "database."[2]

History + Physical Examination + Database =
Initial Evaluation

After the initial evaluation, a problem list is made, and this results in a differential diagnosis. The differential diagnosis is confirmed or denied based on specific diagnostic tests. In this systematic approach, laboratory and other tests are not used in a random "shotgun" manner.

Medical laboratory investigations in the clinical pain practice serve three main purposes:

1. They aid in diagnosis of the disease that is responsible for producing the pain.
2. They aid in following the disease course. A progression or regression of the disease with a subsequent response to treatment may be determined. Serum carcinoembryonic antigen (CEA) can be used to follow the course of colonic cancer if a baseline CEA is drawn at the time of diagnosis. An increase in CEA may precede clinical advancement of colon cancer by 2 to 6 months.[3]
3. They help prevent iatrogenic complications. For example, by testing the periodic blood urea nitrogen and creatinine in a geriatric patient, the laboratory results can determine if nonsteroidal anti-inflammatory drugs (NSAIDs) are causing a decrease in renal function.

REVIEW OF PREVIOUS LABORATORY TESTS

By conservative estimate, many patients referred for consultation to the pain medicine physician have already been evaluated and treated by more than five other physicians. Previous reports must be evaluated to prevent unnecessary duplication of testing, which in turn reduces cost and risk to the patient. The trade-off is in increased time and cost to physicians and their staff to locate and record those test results. Therefore, the physician's staff should be in the habit of requesting patients to obtain their own previous records.

LABORATORY DATABASE

A laboratory database for the pain patient generally consists of the following:

1. Complete blood count (CBC)
2. Biochemical profile (renal function, liver function, electrolytes)
3. Urinalysis (U/A)
4. Sedimentation rate
5. Specific tests as indicated by the results of the history, physical examination, and database

These laboratory results not only help in the diagnosis of the underlying illness but also help estimate the patient's ability to distribute, metabolize, and eliminate a drug (i.e., the patient's pharmacokinetic drug profile).

Certain facts should be remembered when interpreting laboratory results. For any laboratory result, a "normal value" range is given based on the assumption that each test has been derived from a curve containing 95% of the sample or control population. Therefore, by definition 5% of the "normal" population will have "abnormal" laboratory values. The selection of these control populations must be assessed within this equation, and features such as age, sex, and ethnicity must be taken into account. False-positive results may occur in some instances in individual patients. If there is a question, the local clinical pathologist can provide helpful insight. Clinical reference manuals are published nationally for physicians and for allied health pofesionals.[3,4]

Complete Blood Count (Hemogram)

The CBC is performed from a peripheral blood sample. It is routinely automated but can be preformed manually and is commonly called a hemogram when a white blood cell (WBC) differential count is included. Components include, WBC, WBC differential (WBC diff), RBC count (RBC count), hematocrit (HCT), hemoglobin (HGB), RBC indices, and platelet count. RBC indices include the mean red cell volume (MCV), mean red cell hemoglobin concentration (MCHC), and mean red cell hemoglobin (MCH).

White Blood Cell Count

The adult normal range WBC or leukocyte count is 5000 to 10,000/μL. The WBCs are integrally involved with the body's immune response; change in absolute number and relative number of types of leukocytes provides important clinical information. An increase in the leukocyte absolute number (WBC count greater than 10,000/µL) is termed leukocytosis. A decrease in the leukocyte count (less than 5000/µL) is termed leukopenia. Usually one type of leukocyte is elevated or decreased. Thus, the differential leukocyte count is helpful in further limiting the differential diagnosis.

An increase or decrease in the relative type of leukocytes also provides important clinical information. The types of leukocytes and a partial differential of leukocytosis and leukopenia follows:

- Neutrophils (polymorphonuclear neutrophils [PMNs], segs, polys)—normally 50% to 60% of the total leukocyte count. They can be further differentiated into immature and mature neutrophils. PMNs are elevated with ongoing infection, particularly bacterial; this elevation is also known as a "left shift" (neutrophilia). A shift toward the mature neutrophils is known as a "right shift." This may be seen with allergies, tissue necrosis or injury, and hemolysis. A neutropenia of less than 500/µL is a medical emergency.
- Eosinophils—normally 1% to 4% of the total leukocyte count. Their number greater than 5% (eosinophilia) may indicate a pathologic condition.
- Monocytes—capable of phagocytosis and production of interferon. The normal monocyte range in the WBC differential is 2% to 6%.
- Lymphocytes—normally range from 20% to 40% of the leukocyte count. They are migratory cells and move toward sites of inflammation. Lymphocytes produce serum immunoglobulins and are important in cellular immunity. A lymphocytopenia of less than 500/µL is a medical emergency.

Hemoglobin and Hematocrit (H&H)

HCT determines the space occupied by RBCs in the blood, and HGB determines the content and concentration of the oxygen-carrying molecules within the RBC. Normal values for each are age- and sex-dependent. HCT range in the adult man is 40% to 54% and in the adult woman is 37% to 47% of the packed red cell volume. HGB range in the adult woman is 12 to 16 g/dl. H&H are important in determining the amount of oxygen-carrying material in the bloodstream, but they do not ensure the quality of that material. Increased HCT values may be seen in polycythemia and dehydration. Decreased HCT may be seen in leukemia, blood loss, collagen vascular disease, hyperthyroidism, and other conditions.

Red Blood Cell Indices

The RBC count indices define the size and HGB content of the RBC. They are helpful in differentiating the anemias. However, these indices are averaged values and are but one of the assays in the diagnosis of anemia. Examination of the peripheral blood smear and bone marrow aspiration and the examination are essential tools to be used in the differential diagnosis of anemia; if average values or indices alone are used, diagnoses may be missed.

Platelet Count

The platelet count is included with the hemogram. Platelets (thrombocytes) are formed in the bone marrow and are fragments of megakaryocytes. Platelet life span is approximately 8 days. This becomes important to the algologist when using NSAIDs. Acetylated salicylates (aspirin) inhibit platelet function in an irreversible fashion for the life of the platelet (8 days). Nonacetylated salicylates (most NSAIDs) inhibit platelet function in a reversible fashion. Their platelet inhibition relates to their elimination half-life, which is important when planning procedures with anticipated blood loss and for postoperative and post-traumatic analgesia. One commercially available salicylate, choline magnesium trisalicylate (Trilisate), does not appreciably inhibit platelet function, and it has been useful in treatment for thrombocytopenic cancer pain patients.

One third of the platelets available for immediate clotting are located in the reticuloendothelial system, mainly in the spleen. The rest (two thirds) are found in the circulating bloodstream. The normal adult platelet count is 150,000 to 350,000/µL. An increased platelet count (thrombocythemia) may occur with cancer, splenectomy, trauma, and infection. Decreased platelet count (thrombocytopenia) may occur with infection, chemotherapy, drug toxicity, allergic conditions, pulmonary embolism, disseminated intravascular coagulation (DIC), and idiopathic thrombocytopenia purpura.

Biochemical Profiles

Automated biochemical profiles have become the norm, resulting in a relatively less expensive, reliable, and rapid method of obtaining body chemistry results. A clinical pathologist, who determines what is included with each standard biochemical profile, directs each clinical laboratory. Some common acronyms are Chem 7, Astra 7, and SMA 7. Renal function is determined. This is particularly important with the use of NSAIDs in the geriatric population because nephrotoxicity can occur rapidly in this patient population.

Biochemical profiles can also indicate the homeostasis between the cardiovascular and renal systems. This is especially important to the algologist in determining how a patient will distribute and eliminate a particular drug.

Other biochemical profiles are more extensive and include the acronyms SMA 24, SMA 18, Chem 18, Chem 24, Chemzyme, and Chemzyme plus. Also, hepatic enzymes and commonly lactate dehydrogenase (LDH), creatinine phosphokinase (CPK), and alkaline phosphatase are determined.

Urinalysis

U/A is a relatively inexpensive and low-risk method to obtain a great deal of information by using a chemical and microscopic examination. The chemical properties determined are color, odor, turbidity, specific gravity, pH, glucose, ketones, blood protein, bilirubin, nitrate, and leukocyte esterase. The microscopic properties determined are presence and types of cells (RBCs, WBCs), casts (WBC, RBC, granular), organisms (bacteria), and crystals (cystine, calcium phosphate, calcium oxalate, uric acid). WBC casts are associated with pyelonephritis, RBC casts with glomerulonephritis, and waxy casts are associated with severe renal damage.

U/A can also be used to determine the presence of a drug or drugs.

Erythrocyte Sedimentation Rate and C-Reactive Protein

The erythrocyte sedimentation rate (ESR, sed rate) is the rate at which RBCs settle in unclotted blood in 1 hour. Inflammation and tissue necrosis result in a change in serum proteins, causing aggregation of erythrocytes and increasing the rate of fall (increased sed rate). The test is, therefore, inherently nonspecific. The ESR may be helpful in diagnosis of occult disease; in differential diagnosis; and to follow the course of an inflammatory process, for example, how rheumatoid arthritis or a respiratory infection responds to treatment. There may be a short delay time between development of a pathologic state and a change in ESR.

Vindicate

Vindicate, in Webster's New Collegiate Dictionary (1981), is defined as "to conform, substantiate; to provide justification or defense for; to set free, deliver; to lay claim to, avenge, exonerate, absolve." These are lofty and worthwhile goals in providing care for the pain patient.

This is especially true because by conservative estimate the chronic pain patient has been seen by an average of five other physicians. The mnemonic VINDICATE PS is a list of etiologies that cause disease that may result in pain. This list of etiologies of disease is cross-indexed with the various organ system(s) suspected as the cause of pain (Box 16–1).

After the comprehensive initial evaluation (history, physical examination, and establishment of a database), other laboratory tests may be indicated. Once again a systematic rather than a random or shotgun approach is used. The VINDICATE PS mnemonic is reviewed and then cross-indexed with the suspected organ system(s) to develop a differential diagnosis. The suspected diagnosis is then confirmed or denied based on selective diagnostic tests.

In summary, the following sequence is recommended for evaluation (initial and ongoing) and treatment of patients with pain-related disorders:

- Perform thorough initial history and physical examination
- Document prior diagnostic workup and therapy
- Confirm that "routine" health care issues are current
- Obtain routine database
- Develop problem list
- Develop differential diagnosis
- VINDICATE PS the patient's differential diagnosis
- Cross-index with the indicated organ system(s)
- Obtain specific diagnostic tests to limit the differential diagnosis (confirm or deny the diagnosis)
- Develop a working diagnosis
- Develop and institute resultant treatment plan in an expeditious manner

Specific laboratory tests based on the VINDICATE PS mnemonic follow.

Viral (Microbial)

This is one example of infection but may encompass other microbes including bacteria and fungi. Viral (microbial) causes are screened with the CBC in the database. Emphasis is placed on the WBC and differential.

Inflammatory

Inflammation can be present for a variety of reasons. These reasons can be divided into primary, secondary, or no microbial infection. Secondary microbial infection can be divided into two other groups: those with evidence of autoimmune disorder and those resulting from trauma.

Neoplastic

Most diagnoses of cancer are based on history and physical examination. It is essential to confirm that the chronic pain patient is current on routine health maintenance, including a chest radiograph for smokers, pelvic and breast examinations for women, and prostate examination for men. Diagnostic tests to confirm the presence of cancer rely on changes in structure.

Degenerative

Degenerative disease is usually cross-indexed or checked against the musculoskeletal system and the nervous system. Within the musculoskeletal system a further subdivision is made between the autoimmune and collagen vascular disease disorders and the degeneration caused by weight bearing and use.

Ischemia

This condition results when tissues receive inadequate oxygen supply, which results in inadequate cellular respiration. Any abnormality in the delivery system (cardiovascular), oxygen-carrying system (hematopoietic), or in the cellular respiratory level can lead to ischemia. Abnormalities in the cardiovascular system are generally defined by electrophysiologic (electrocardiogram, intracardiac conduction) and mechanical flow studies of the coronary arteries, central vessels, and peripheral vessels. Noninvasive flow studies of the larger peripheral vessels are commonly used (Doppler flow).

BOX 16–1 Explanation of VINDICATE PS

V:	Viral/bacterial
I:	Inflammatory
N:	Neoplastic
D:	Degenerative
I:	Ischemia
C:	Congenital/genetic
A:	Autoimmune/collagen vascular disease
T:	Traumatic/mechanical
E:	Endocrine/metabolic
P:	Psychogenic
S:	Secondary gain

Congenital/Genetic

These disorders may result from acquired (prepartum or postpartum) or hereditary causes. Laboratory analysis is less important in this category, but certain disorders do merit special mention. Sickle cell disease is one.[4]

Autoimmune and Collagen Vascular Disease

Serologic tests are the mainstay in confirming the presence or the absence of autoimmune and collagen vascular disease, which include systemic lupus erythematosus (SLE), rheumatoid arthritis (RA), polymyositis/dermatomyositis, ankylosing spondylitis, polymyalgia rheumatica, mixed connective tissue disease, temporal arteritis, and scleroderma. Abnormalities in the database and laboratory work are associated with many of these diseases. Anemia, thrombocytopenia, and elevated ESR are common. Specific tests can help make the definitive diagnosis in many cases.

Traumatic/Mechanical

Few laboratory studies are helpful here. Diagnosis is made with history, physical examination, and imaging studies (usually plain radiographs). However, the cause of the trauma should be considered and may be diagnosed with a laboratory test.

Endocrine/Metabolic

Thyroid disease and diabetes mellitus are the most common metabolic endocrine diseases when considering the pain patient. In addition, many pain patients suffer from an affective component such as dysthymia and depression, which can significantly render a pain treatment program ineffective.

Psychogenic

Laboratory tests can exclude other significant nociceptive or neuropathic causes. They can also confirm compliance with a drug regimen. This is especially important in the dual diagnosis patient—those that have a physical cause of pain but also have psychologic factors that affect their physical condition. Qualitative assays are available for a wide number of substances, and quantitative assays are routinely used for tricyclic antidepressants and anticonvulsants.

Secondary Gain

Few laboratory tests exist in this category to assist the algologist. Lack of objective evidence on physical examination, physical pathologic findings on imaging studies, and normal results on laboratory studies help diagnose by exclusion. Once the diagnosis is made and a treatment plan instituted, laboratory tests can help prevent iatrogenic complications.

References

1. Longmire DR: Tutorial 1: The medical pain history. *Pain Dig* 1:29, 1991.
2. Kennedy LD, Longmire DR: Tutorial 4: Medical/laboratory evaluation of pain patients. *Pain Dig* 1:306, 1992.
3. Wallach JB: *Interpretation of diagnostic tests,* ed 4. Boston, Little, Brown, 1986.
4. Fischbach FF, editor: *A manual of laboratory diagnostic tests,* ed 3. Philadelphia, JB Lippincott, 1988.

1. Laboratory database for a pain patient usually consists of all the following except

   A. Complete blood count
   B. Biochemical profile (renal function, liver function, and electrolytes)
   C. Urinalysis
   D. Thyroid function test

2. The most common endocrine and metabolic disorder seen in a pain patient is

   A. Diabetes mellitus
   B. Parathyroid deficiency
   C. Adrenal insufficiency
   D. Cushing's syndrome

3. Hemoglobin range in the adult women is

   A. 6–10 g/dl
   B. 10–12 g/dl
   C. 12–16 g/dl
   D. 16–20 g/dl

4. Platelets (thrombocytes) are formed in the bone marrow as fragments of megakaryocytes. The platelet lifespan is approximately 8 to 10 days. This becomes important when using nonsteroidal anti-inflammatory drugs (NSAIDs) because of all of the following except

   A. Acetylsalicylates inhibit platelet function
   B. Nonacetyl salicylates do not inhibit platelet function
   C. A bleeding diathesis may occur
   D. Serious sequelae can occur from spinal nerve blocks

5. Serologic tests are the mainstay in confirming the absence or presence of autoimmune and collagen vascular diseases. These diseases include all of the following except

   A. Systemic lupus erythematous (SLE)
   B. Rheumatoid arthritis (RA)
   C. Scleroderma
   D. Complex regional pain syndrome (CRPS)

ANSWERS

1. D
2. A
3. C
4. B
5. D

CHAPTER 17

Psychologic Evaluation

DANIEL M. DOLEYS AND
DENNIS C. DOHERTY

The psychologic and behavioral medicine evaluation of a patient is influenced by several factors:

1. Goal of the assessment. In some cases, the evaluation is carried out only to define the psychologic characteristics or status of the patient. In others, the evaluation may be requested to determine whether the patient is an appropriate candidate to undergo a particular therapy. The use of psychologic testing before and after treatment to determine the effects is yet another goal. Perhaps the most comprehensive goal is the identification of a therapeutic algorithm.
2. Theoretical orientation. Practitioners with a more dynamic or neo-Freudian approach[1] are more likely to direct the interview and interpret the data differently than a behaviorist[2] or a cognitive behaviorist.[3,4] The evaluator must be aware of his or her biases and make them known to those requesting the evaluation. Some evaluators may choose a more eclectic approach.
3. One's definition of *pain*. The International Association for the Study of Pain (IASP) noted that pain includes sensory and affective qualities.[5] Acceptance of this definition clearly dictates evaluation of both factors. Pain can also be defined as a biopsychosocial phenomenon. This orientation necessitates an awareness of, and the ability to assess, the relative contributions of biologic, psychologic, and sociologic factors.

This chapter takes a behavioral approach to the evaluation of the pain patient. Although the assessment empathizes the psychologic and behavioral aspects of the patient, inquiries addressing the biologic, medical, and sociologic-environmental factors are included.

THE INTERVIEW TECHNIQUE

Much more than a collection of facts can be gained from an interview. Although it is important to touch on each area listed in an interview guideline, rigid adherence to a structured list of questions limits both the patient and the evaluator. Patients should be encouraged to tell their story.[6] Embedded in the patient's narrative are the cultural beliefs and experiences that can transcend the patient's experience and existence. Such stories are rich with emotion, experience, expectations, attributions, and behavior and present the thread necessary to weave the facts of the clinician's evaluation into the fabric of pain.

Allowing the patient to express the context in which the pain and behavior are occurring may provide the evaluator with an opportunity to discern themes that may not be covered in the interview outline and may not be identified if the patient only responds to questions. One can only learn answers to questions that are asked. If the clinician wants to know the whole story, he or she may need to provide more latitude to the patient, paying attention to what and how the patient communicates.

Computerized questionnaires, computer interaction, and completion of standardized questionnaires all have a place in the evaluation of the patient with pain. They should, however, supplement rather than replace the interview. Interviewing skills are similar to those needed to perform a physical examination.

THE CLINICAL INTERVIEW

The clinical interview (Box 17–1) can be a valuable source of information.[7–9] It should include the entire process of interacting with the patient and observations made throughout the visit. Office staff can be alerted to note the relative ease or difficulty with which a patient moves about and the presence of posturing, grimacing, or other gestures that occur while the patient is waiting for the interview. It can be beneficial for the interviewer to meet and escort the patient from the waiting room, providing an opportunity to observe the presence or absence of other family members and their interaction patterns. These and other observations help develop a database that can be useful in determining inconsistencies and the presence of nonorganic signs.[10]

We prefer to begin the interview by having the patient fill out a pain drawing, such as that found on the McGill Pain Questionnaire (MPQ),[11,12] to identify areas of pain. Although such drawings do not necessarily correlate with diagnosis or correspond precisely with areas of pain, they can be useful.[13–15]

Noting any difficulties the patient might have in completing the pain drawing may help determine handedness and spatial orientation; all of this is useful information when patients claim upper extremity pain with concomitant weakness or sensory changes.

After the pain drawing is completed, the patient is asked about pain patterns. The MPQ can be helpful in this area. Patients who select multiple descriptors across most categories pose a greater challenge for intervention.

It is important to discuss the details of the patient's complaints at the beginning of the interview. This reassures the patient about the examiner's belief in the authenticity of the

BOX 17–1 Outline for the Clinical Interview

1. Pain
   a. Distribution and pattern
   b. Qualitative and quantitative aspects
   c. Events, activities, and movements that increase or decrease
   d. Anticipatory pain; activity avoidance
   e. Adaptive and maladaptive responses
   f. Sensory and motor abnormality or dysfunction

2. History
   a. Precipitating cause (e.g., work-related injury, gradual onset, disease or illness, surgery)
   b. Evaluation; types and outcomes
   c. Treatments; types and outcomes
   d. Diagnosis and prognosis
   e. Patient's beliefs and comprehension regarding cause
   f. Patient's expectation and goals

3. Financial and legal information
   a. Pending litigation type: Social Security, third party, workers' compensation
   b. Financial and personal losses
   c. Perceived vocational and occupational capabilities and opportunities

4. General medical status
   a. Medical and surgical history
   b. Medications: type, amount, pattern of use, efficacy
   c. Physical status: sleep, weight, appetite, nicotine and caffeine use, sexual function and dysfunction
   d. Mental status examination, including childhood traumas or victimization

5. Psychosocial information
   a. Family background; medical and psychiatric
   b. Education and training
   c. Martial history and status
   d. Detectability of pain and family or significant other response patterns
   e. Daily activity or routine: degree of independence or dependence

complaints. He or she is more likely to be forthcoming and less defensive if complaints of pain are addressed at the outset.

Information regarding what enhances and what relieves the pain can be sought next. The patient who specifies certain work or home activities rather than a particular movement may be more likely to have pain behaviors or complaints that are reinforced by avoidance of activity.

Behavioral and psychologic factors generally have a greater influence in patients reporting pain increases associated with nonpositional or non–activity-related pain, such as the time of day and emotional states.

Events that relieve pain may give clues to positive reinforcing stimuli. For example, patients who report a reduc-

tion in pain produced by medications, activity avoidance, or massage by a family member may be describing consequences that maintain their behavior and enhance their perception of pain.

Obtaining subjective estimates of walking, sitting, and standing tolerances allows comparison to be made with observed data and provides information regarding self-imposed limits, perception of activity tolerance, and tendency toward symptom magnification.

If an on-the-job injury is involved, details are useful, such as how the accident occurred and whether the patient perceives it as avoidable and caused, therefore, by some malfunction, neglect, or inappropriate behavior by a coworker, employer, or machine manufacturer. Depending on this perception, the patient can feel resentful toward or victimized by the accident's perceived perpetrators.

The relationship of job satisfaction to the development of chronic pain is well established[16–18] and should be examined.

The way a patient is treated in the acute and postacute phases can set the stage for recovery or chronicity.[19–21] Having the patient summarize (1) where treatment was sought, (2) the attitude of the treating physician, (3) the outcome of intervention, and (4) the prognosis may reveal the patient's cognitive set and expectations regarding source of pain and estimate of recovery.

Patient expectations contribute heavily to overall satisfaction with postoperative patient-controlled analgesia (PCA).[22] During this time, the patient's approach to rehabilitation may be formulated, because some patients may have been inadvertently provided with rules that are counterproductive.

Another factor to be considered is the impact—real or perceived—of the injury on the patient's life. Suffering can be a major component of chronicity[23,24] and is manifested in many ways. The interviewer's skill and commitment are needed to evaluate when a patient is simply describing circumstances affecting life as part of a pain repertoire, perhaps anticipating a positive consequence (i.e., financial compensation), and when the patient is describing situations and emotional responses to the injury.

Difficulties in obtaining compensation may also contribute to the pain problem. It may be important to consider the patient's status in the process of claim resolution. Those whose claim has been resolved may respond differently from those who are still in litigation. In either case, it may be an overgeneralization to assume that a patient suffering an on-the-job injury and receiving workers' compensation benefits is more or less prone to chronic pain syndrome. One must be careful in evaluating the pain patient to discriminate between speculation, blatant assertion, and fact.

General Medical Status

Obtaining a brief medical history is appropriate in a behavioral medicine and psychologic assessment, yet this step is often ignored or left to someone else. Inquires regarding drug allergies, family history of medical problems, or previous surgery can show that the evaluator is interested in the patient's physical and psychologic state.

Exposure to a parent or family member who has triumphed over adversity is likely to yield a different set of coping strategies than exposure to a parent who has succumbed to an otherwise nonthreatening illness or injury and has become dependent. Individuals who have responded positively to previous surgeries by returning to productivity are likely to have developed more adaptive coping mechanisms.

Medications

A detailed assessment of medication use is crucial, particularly with noncancer pain patients who are suspected of drug misuse. A complete assessment of medication use should be done, which may require interviewing family members, reviewing medical records, and communicating with treating physicians and pharmacies. Although time-consuming, this may yield benefits in patient management.

Behaviors indicating psychologic dependence, physical tolerance, and addiction must be differentiated.[25,26] *Addiction* is defined as a chronic preoccupation with obtaining the substance of choice, misuse or overuse of the substance despite negative consequences, and a propensity for obtaining a substance through illegal means or use of illegal substances to satisfy the needs or craving. A *pseudoaddiction* can be established when the patient is provided with beneficial but inadequate doses of analgesics. This may create relief-seeking rather than drug-seeking behavior.

A history of drug misuse or overuse should cause the examiner to suspect the patient's complaints of pain may be a way of securing habit-forming preparations to satisfy a craving.

Sleep disturbances are commonly reported and may include sleep-onset insomnia, frequent awakening, restless and disturbed sleep, or early morning awakening.[27] Improved sleep patterns through the use of antidepressants may have a positive impact on complaints of pain. Disturbed sleep may also be a symptom of depression.

Although not a standard part of behavioral medicine and psychologic evaluation, a limited review of systems to identify on-going illnesses or diseases helps to obtain an overall impression of the patient's medical status and its role relative to pain. Patients experiencing multiple long-standing problems such as diabetes, obesity, fatigue, or hypertension, which are otherwise not compensable, may be predisposed to increased disability and pain behavior following an on-the-job (compensable) injury.

Sexual difficulties should be addressed. Casual factors for sexual dysfunction may include affective disorder, neurologic impairment from injury or surgery, medication, or medication side effects. A history of marital conflict may increase the likelihood that the pain behavior and complaints are negatively reinforced by reduced sexual demands from an undesirable spouse.

Mental Status and Mood Assessment

A mental status examination should be incorporated into the evaluation.[28] Assessment of memory and concentration may help identify patients suffering from traumatic brain injury coincident with their pain.

The patient's mood can be assessed both during the interview and with psychometric testing. Psychologic states, including depression, anxiety, anger, agitation, irritability, and confusion, can contribute to the perception and experience of pain.[29–31]

Although apparently rare, suicide attempts and completions can occur in response to pain and accompanying depression. The evaluator can assess propensities toward suicide by determining the presence of death wishes, suicidal thoughts, or history of gestures. Patients with a positive personal or family history of psychologic or psychiatric disturbance are more likely to display psychologic symptoms in response to the experience of pain.

A growing body of evidence implicates the role of a history of abuse, molestation, and abandonment as etiologically relevant in the experience of pain.[32–35]

Psychologic History

Many patterns, personality characteristics, expectations, and attitudes are produced by early experiences and family interactions. Obtaining information regarding birth order, parental occupation and background, and presence of parents during childhood can give a general sense of the patient's socioeconomic history. The greater the individual's flexibility, adaptability, and learning capacity, the more likely he or she is to respond to treatment and to be able to consider alternatives, whether vocational or avocational. Questions regarding academic difficulties may uncover attention deficit or learning disorders that can affect the patient's coping ability.

Number and duration of marriages, reason for termination, and any criminal history help determine stability of the patient's lifestyle and the possibility of a personality disorder.

Noting how the patient spends time, engages in self-care, and performs activities of daily living (ADLs) and who, if anyone, assists the patient may alert the evaluator to possible and positive reinforcement contingencies.[36] The degree to which assistance in self-care, home care, and other ADLs is available and volunteered may indicate the presence of positive reinforcers for pain behavior. The patient's general psychologic demeanor should be noted throughout the evaluation. Observations between complaints of pain and general presentation should be recorded.

Conclusion

A well-organized and comprehensive interview is a rich source of information. Observational data collected by several sources, including clinicians, assistants, and office staff, become essential. A thoughtful behavioral medicine and psychologic analysis attempts to identify consistencies and inconsistencies across situations and information sources. Pain behavior is no different from any other behavior; it occurs in the context of specific antecedents, whether internal or external or cognitive or affective, and is followed by consequences emanating from a variety of sources occurring continuously or intermittently, with potentially variable effects depending on the complex system of situation. This very dynamic and complex system is infinitely more involved than establishing a simple stimulus-response-consequence relationship existing at a point in time and assumed to be omnipresent. It is more the rule than the exception that one set of circumstances may stimulate the development of a set of behaviors while another maintains it. Occasionally, the behavior may seem functionally autonomous and may appear much like a habit. More often than not, pain behavior and descriptions do not have a one-to-one correlation with identifiable pathologic conditions.

PSYCHOLOGIC TESTING

In general, psychologic testing should be viewed in the broadest context. Emphasis should be placed on providing descriptive characteristics of the patient meaningful to the development of appropriate treatment strategies or assessment of overall psychologic and behavioral status. Test data should be used in a synergistic fashion with information obtained on interview.

Psychologic testing can and should aid in unraveling response tendencies or biases, degree or magnitude of psychopathology, level of psychologic distress, and personality characteristics as they interact with and influence the patient's perception and experience of pain. Therefore, psychologic data, whether collected by interview, testing, or both, should help render statements referring to Axis I and Axis II diagnoses (see reference 37). Issues concerning the meaning and stability of personality remain[38] and should not be taken lightly.

Personality Tests
Minnesota Multiphasic Personality Inventory

The usefulness of personality tests, such as the Minnesota Multiphasic Personality Inventory (MMPI), in regard to chronic pain patients continues to be debated,[39,40] with valid arguments on each side of the issue. Part of the dilemma may be the questions asked of such tests. We find tests such as the MMPI most useful in our attempt to gain an overall picture of the patient's general psychologic status. Understanding the patient's personality may reveal certain response tendencies. Rather than ask the test to predict global events such as treatment outcome, it seems more productive to use the data in combination with other information to reveal patient characteristics that may require modification of the treatment protocol.

The importance of evaluating personality styles, especially the presence of a personality disorder, lies in the way such behavior patterns declare themselves under sustained stress, such as that created by chronic pain.[41,42] More harm than benefit is derived by stigmatizing or labeling patients with a psychiatric diagnosis, particularly that of personality disorder, until or unless the relationship to and influence on perceived pain and response to treatment have been established.

The MMPI[43] and its more modernized version, the MMPI-2,[44] remain widely used. Depending on the version administered, patients may be required to answer as few as 180 or as many as 576 true-false questions. Various scoring mechanisms exist, ranging from the use of templates for hand scoring to more sophisticated computer-based programs that provide multiple subscale analyses.

Pain Assessment Index

The Pain Assessment Index (PAI) was developed by Smith and Durksen.[45] The PAI combines MMPI scales in an effort to predict surgical outcome in patients with chronic low back pain.

Personality Assessment Inventory

The Personality Assessment Inventory is a multidimensional, self-report measure of personality traits developed as an alternative to the MMPI.[46] It contains approximately 344 items rated on a 4-point scale. The response choices for each question include "false," "slightly true," "mainly true," and "very true." It is felt that the availability of four choices rather than two, as found on the MMPI, may provide a better ability to detect and determine differences among individuals.

Symptom Checklist-90

The Symptom Checklist-90 (SCL-90) and its revised version (SCL-90-R)[47] screen for psychologic symptoms and overall levels of distress. This multidimensional symptom checklist is composed of 90 items describing a physical or psychologic symptom. Patients respond to the 5-point scale ranging from "not at all" to "extremely," indicating the degree to which they have been bothered by a particular item over the past week.

The inventory assesses levels of distress on nine scales, including somatization, obsessive-compulsive tendencies, interpersonal sensitivity, depression, anxiety, hostility, phobic anxiety, paranoid ideation, and psychoticism.

The SCL-90-R has recently been used to evaluate psychologic distress in chronic pain patients,[48] especially those with whiplash[49] and low back pain.[50]

Sickness Impact Profile

The Sickness Impact Profile (SIP) is a self-report measure of the patient's perception of his or her general health status.[51] It is a 136-item scale that measures functioning in areas such as ambulation, mobility, and body care. It appears that scores are sensitive to changes in low back pain patients undergoing intervention.[52]

Millon Behavioral Health Inventory

The Millon Behavioral Health Inventory (MBHI) was developed to specifically address psychologic symptoms in medical populations.[53] It reportedly provides information regarding the patient's personality and style as they relate to medical treatment. The 20 clinical scales can be subsumed under four major categories:

- Basic coping style
- Psychogenic attitudes
- Psychosomatic correlates
- Prognostic indicators

Rorschach Inkblot

Over the last several decades the Rorschach Inkblot test using the Exner scoring method[54] has become more acceptable as a psychometrically sound instrument. It has some utility in investigating personality characteristics, including emotional and intellectual control, capacity to perform social interactions, hostility, depression, anxiety, suicidality, and coping potential in chronic pain patients.[55,56]

Mood States

The contribution of various mood states to the experience of pain is undeniable. The expression and perception of pain appears to be influenced by anger, anxiety, and depression, to name a few. Depression, in particular, is often associated with chronic pain and has been evaluated as a possible risk factor.[57,58] A number of self-report measures have been used to assess depression.

Beck Depression Inventory

The Beck Depression Index (BDI) is one of the most commonly used instruments in the pain literature.[59,60] It is a 21-item, self-report measure of depression in use for 30 years. Responses require the endorsement of one of a series of four statements, rank ordered in severity of content. The scores on each item are tabulated to yield a total depression score. In addition, the first 13 items cover a cognitive-affective subscale and the remaining eight scales the somatic-performance subscale.

Spielberger State-Trait Anxiety Inventory

The Spielberger State-Trait Anxiety Inventory (STAI) is a 40-item, self-report questionnaire that is easy to administer and score.[61] The 40 multiple-choice items have been demonstrated to have good reliability and validity, but there are no validity scales. The measure was designed to provide measures of two aspects of the anxiety construct:

1. Trait anxiety (TA) is perceived to be a stable personality characteristic that describes a person's overall tendency to respond in a rather anxious manner, independent of the specific stimulus.
2. State anxiety (SA) purports to measure anxiety experienced in response to specific conditions.

It is anticipated that TA levels would remain relatively stable across conditions, including those imposed by chronic pain; SA, in contrast, would be expected to show a greater degree of variability and, therefore, may be more useful in evaluating treatment outcomes.

Malingering and Feigning

Malingering is defined as the conscious exaggeration of psychologic or physiologic symptoms for some easily recognized goal or secondary gain resulting from the patient's circumstance and not to personality.[37] It is important to differentiate between symptom exaggeration or magnification that may be secondary to personality characteristics, such as hysteria or conditioning factors, and malingering. The feigning or malingering of psychologic symptoms should not be interpreted as having a one-to-one relationship with faking psychologic symptoms. Several methods have proved sensitive in identifying symptom exaggeration or over-reporting of behavioral and psychologic symptoms.

The difference between the scores on the F and K scales of the MMPI or MMPI-2 can reflect a "fake bad" profile. Variable response inconsistency (VRIN), true response inconsistency (TRIN), and back-page infrequency (Fb) represent validity scales developed for the MMPI-2 and are useful in determining a valid test-taking approach.[44]

The Structured Interview of Reported Symptoms (SIRS) was developed to assess malingering of feigning of psychologic symptoms.[62,63] It is comprised of eight primary scales, which are scored as "honest," "intermediate," "probable feigning," or "definite feigning." Cut-off scores established on normative samples give the probability of feigning symptoms based on the number of scales in the probable feigning range or above. The results, combined with those of the validity scales of the MMPI, may provide a reliable measure of feigning of psychologic symptoms.

The relationship of malingering of psychologic symptoms to malingering of physical symptoms remains unclear. For this reason, data of this type should be combined with other information before any definitive conclusions are drawn.

Perceived Disability and Dysfunction

Disability has been defined as a "disadvantage for a given individual resulting from an impairment or a functional limitation that limits or prevents the fulfillment of a role that is normal . . . for that individual."[64] Although a psychical impairment can be determined more or less objectively, the impact of this impairment on the patient's function is determined in large part by the patient's perceptual effect. Several questionnaires have been developed to evaluate the perception of disability.

Oswesty Low Back Disability Questionnaire

The Oswesty Low Back Disability Questionnaire assesses limitations in ADLs.[65] Ten multiple-choice items cover nine aspects of daily functioning, including personal care, lifting, walking, sitting, standing, sexual activity, and traveling. The patient chooses from among six statements relating to the impact of pain on a particular activity. A percentage score is derived, allowing for the classification of patients ranging from mildly to profoundly impaired.

Sickness Impact Profile

The SIP has found favor as a tool for the evaluation of functioning.[51] This self-reporting measure reveals the patient's perception of general health status in areas such as ambulation, mobility, body care, and social activity. A 136-item scale yields an overall percentage of perceived health-related disabilities.

Roland and Morris Disability Questionnaire

The Roland and Morris Disability Questionnaire[66] is a shorter version of the SIP and has been applied in the evaluation of treatment outcome.[67]

Pain Disability Index

The Pain Disability Index (PDI)[68] provides a rating of 0 (no disability) to 10 (total disability) in seven areas:

- Family-home responsibility
- Recreation
- Social activity
- Occupation
- Sexual behavior
- Self-care
- Life support activities

Multidimensional Pain Inventory

The Multidimensional Pain Inventory (MPI) was developed to assess multiple aspects of pain and functioning.[69] It contains 56 items scored on a 7-point scale. Nine clinical scales include ratings of pain severity, interference of pain, life control, affective distress, social support, punishing responses by significant others, distracting responses by significant others, and general activity level. Probabilities are developed for the patient matching one of the three profile types:

1. Dysfunctional. Characterized by high pain level, decreased activity level and sense of control, high interference of pain with ADLs, and increased emotional distress.
2. Interpersonally distressed. Patients perceiving themselves as lacking in support from family and friends.
3. Adaptive coper. Patients characterized by reporting a low level of pain interference and interpersonal distress along with high levels of activity and interpersonal support.

Coping Strategies Questionnaire

The Coping Strategies Questionnaire (CSQ) has been used to evaluate strategies applied by patients in an effort to manage their pain.[70] These strategies include catastrophizing, reinterpreting pain sensation, praying and hoping, ignoring pain sensation, and distraction.

Pain Cognition Questionnaire

The Pain Cognition Questionnaire evaluates the tendency to apply strategies such as passive optimism, denial of problems, irritability, and helplessness.[71] A patient's beliefs and expectations have been shown to contribute to the experience of pain and outcome of treatment manipulation.[72,73] Four factors were derived from factor analytical techniques:

- Pain constancy
- Pain permanence
- Pain as a mastery
- Self-blame

Medical Outcomes Survey

The Medical Outcomes Survey (MOS), a 36-item Short-Form Health Survey (SF-36), is a 36-item generic questionnaire that yields scores on eight health scales relating to physical, social, and emotional factors.[74,75]

Among the scales measured are:

- Limitation in physical activity resulting from health problems
- Limitation in social activities because of physical and emotional problems
- Limitation in usual role-activity resulting from physical health problems
- General mental health
- Limitation in role activities because of emotional problems
- Vitality
- General health perceptions

Other Scales

Other measures include the Chronic Illness Problem Inventory[76] and the Waddell Disability Instrument.[77]

Subjective Pain Report

The subjective nature of pain demands that some effort be made to quantify the individual's overall experience of pain. Instruments have been designed to assess various dimensions of pain, including intensity, location, and affective or distressed qualities. Numerical pain ratings, Visual Analogue Scale (VAS) scores, verbal rating scales, pain diaries, and pain mapping have each found their place in the assessment scheme.

Conclusion

Adequate evaluation of pain patients should include a battery of assessment tools. Some measure of personality style is useful in determining premorbid adaptation and current tendencies. In this regard, the MMPI-2 is one of the most frequently used measures. The MMPI-2 also provides evidence of affective disturbance.

Specific measures of depression and anxiety may be useful. Both the BDI and the STAI have been shown to be reliable and valid. The patient's perceived level of coping and disability should be assessed. The MPI and Oswesty Disability Scale suffice. Information on social support and family interactions can also be obtained from the MPI.

Suspicion of feigning psychologic or psychiatric symptoms can be addressed with the SIRS. Obtaining a pain diary with hourly records of activity level, medication use, pain intensity, and mood over 3 to 7 days adds information not readily available from other instruments. The use of a comprehensive battery of this type can help determine the appropriate course of treatment and provide a baseline against which to measure outcome.

PSYCHOPHYSIOLOGIC ASSESSMENT

Psychophysiology involves the study of interrelationships between the physiologic and psychologic aspects of behavior.[78] The principles and fundamental strategies have been enumerated.[78,79] Philosophical, practical, and technical developments have resulted in wider application than ever before. Unfortunately, this aspect of assessment is often overlooked.

The use of psychophysiologic methods provides an opportunity to demonstrate the effects of maladaptive, behavioral, and personality patterns on physical processes. The patient can witness these dysfunctions firsthand. Psychophysiologic retraining techniques, such as neuromuscular retraining, biofeedback, and self-regulation strategies, can provide a sense of control. Application of such therapeutic methods also encourages the patient to develop a sense of responsibility regarding management of symptoms, decreasing the dependent attitude that easily develops when the patient is a passive recipient of treatment.

Inadequate evaluation of muscular contributions in carpal tunnel syndrome and back pain may result in unnecessary surgery. When surgical intervention is required, addressing the muscular contributions may improve the likelihood of a positive outcome. Patients weary of interpretations of psychologic factors contributing to their pain problems can appreciate the physiologic factors and be less resistant to relevant interventions.

References

1. Grzesiak RC, Ury GM, Dworkin RH: Psychodynamic psychotherapy with chronic pain patients. In Gatchel RJ, Turk DC, editors: *Psychological approaches to pain management: A practitioner's handbook.* New York, Guilford, 1996.

2. Fordyce WE: *Behavioral methods for chronic pain and illness.* St. Louis, Mosby, 1976.

3. Bradley LA: Cognitive-behavioral therapy for chronic pain. In Gatchel RJ, Turk DC, editors: *Psychological approaches to pain management: A practitioner's handbook.* New York, Guilford, 1996.

4. Turk DC, Meichenbaum DH: A cognitive-behavioral approach to pain management. In Wall PD, Melzack R, editors: *Textbook of pain.* New York, Churchill Livingstone, 1989.

5. Mersky H, Bogduk N, editors: *Classification of chronic pain: Descriptions of chronic pain syndromes and definition of pain terms,* ed 2. Seattle, IASP Press, 1994.

6. Morris DB: The plot of suffering (abstract). Proceedings of the meeting of the American Pain Society, October 1997, New Orleans, p 52.

7. Doleys DM, Klapow JC, Hammer M: Psychological evaluation in spinal cord stimulation therapy. *Pain Rev* 4:186, 1997.

8. Deyo RA, Rainville J, Kent DL: What can the history and physical examination tell us about low back pain? *JAMA* 268:760, 1992.

9. Feuerstein M, Beattie P: Biobehavioral factors affecting pain and disability in low back pain: mechanisms and assessment. *Phys Ther* 75:267, 1995.

10. Waddell G, McCulloch JA, Kummel E et al: Nonorganic physical signs of low back pain. *Spine* 5:111, 1980.

11. Melzack R: The McGill Pain Questionnaire: Major properties and scoring methods. *Pain* 1:277, 1975.

12. Melzack E, editor: The McGill Pain Questionnaire. In *Pain measurement and assessment.* New York, Raven Press, 1983.

13. Mann NH 3rd, Brown MD, Hertz DB et al: Initial-impression diagnosis using low-back pain patient pain drawings. *Spine* 18:41, 1993.

14. Parker II, Wood PL, Main CL: The use of the pain drawing as a screening measure to predict psychological distress in chronic low back pain. *Spine* 20:236, 1995.

15. Ransford AO, Cairns D, Mooney V: The pain drawing as an aid to the psychologic evaluation of patients with low-back pain. *Spine* 1:127, 1976.

16. Bigos SJ, Battie MC, Spengler DM et al: A longitudinal perspective study of industrial back injury reporting. *Clin Orthop* 279:21, 1992.

17. Holmstrom EB, Lindell J, Moritz U: Low back and neck/shoulder pain in construction workers: Occupational workload and psychosocial risk factors. Part 2: Relationship to neck and shoulder pain. *Spine* 17:672, 1992.

18. Skovron ML, Szpalski M, Nordin M et al: Sociocultural factors and back pain. A population-based study in Belgian adults. *Spine* 19:129, 1994.

19. Phillips HC: Avoidance behavior and its role in sustaining chronic pain. *Behav Res Ther* 25:273, 1987.

20. Doleys DM, Gochneaur KS: Behavioral management. In Tollison CD, Kriegel MS, editors: *Interdisciplinary rehabilitation of low back pain.* Baltimore, Williams & Wilkins, 1989.

21. Dolce JJ, Crocker MF, Doleys DM: Prediction of outcome among chronic pain patients. *Behav Res Ther* 24:313, 1986.

22. Jamison RN, Taft K, O'Hara JP et al: Psychosocial and pharmacologic predictors of satisfaction with intravenous patient-controlled analgesia. *Anesth Analg* 77:121, 1993.

23. Chapman CR, Gavrin J: Suffering and its relationship to pain. *J Palliat Care* 9:5, 1993.

24. Loeser JD: Perspectives on pain. In Turner P, editor: *Proceedings of first world congress on clinical pharmacology and therapeutics.* London, Macmillan, 1980.

25. Portenoy RK: Opioid therapy for chronic nonmalignant pain: Current status. In Fields HL, Liebeskind JC, editors: *Progress in pain research and management,* vol 1. Seattle, IASP Press.

26. Krames E: Implantable pain management: An overview. *Phys Ther Forum* XII(3):4, 1993.

27. Dement WC, Mitler M: Commentary: It's time to wake up to the importance of sleep disorders. *JAMA* 269:1548, 1993.

28. Crum RM, Anthony JC, Bassett SS et al: Population-based norms for the Mini-Mental State Examination by age and educational level. *JAMA* 269:2386, 1993.

29. Coste J, Paolaggi JB, Spira A: Classifications of nonspecific low back pain: I. Psychological involvement in the low back pain: A clinical, descriptive approach. *Spine* 17:1028, 1992.

30. Gatchel RJ, Polatin PB, Mayer TG et al: Psychopathology and the rehabilitation of patients with chronic low back pain disability. *Arch Phys Med Rehabil* 75:666, 1994.

31. Krause SJ, Wiener RL, Tait RC: Depression and pain behavior in patients with chronic pain. *Clin J Pain* 10:122, 1994.

32. Blair JA, Blair RS, Rueckett P: Pre-injury emotional trauma and chronic back pain: An unexpected finding. *Spine* 19:1144, 1994.

33. McMahon MJ, Gatchel RJ, Polatin PB et al: Early childhood abuse in chronic spinal disorder patients. A major barrier to treatment success. *Spine* 22:2408, 1997.

34. Schofferman J, Anderson D, Hines R et al: Childhood psychological trauma and chronic refractory low-back pain. *Clin J Pain* 9:260, 1993.

35. Schofferman J, Anderson D, Hines R et al: Childhood psychological trauma correlates with unsuccessful lumbar spine surgery. *Spine* 17:S138, 1992.

36. Lousberg R, Schmidt AJ, Groenman NH: The relationship between mental evidence. *Pain* 51:75, 1992.

37. American Psychiatric Association: *Diagnostic and statistical manual of mental disorders,* revised ed 4. Washington, DC, American Psychiatric Association, 1994.

38. Mischel W: *Introduction to personality.* New York, Holt, Rinehart & Winston, 1971.

39. Helmes E: What types of useful information do the MMPI and MMPI-2 provide on patients with chronic pain? *Am Pain Soc Bull* x:4, 1994.

40. Main CJ, Spanswick CC: Personality assessment and the Minnesota Multiphasic Personality Inventory: 50 years on. Do we still need our security blanket? *Pain Forum* 4:90, 1995.

41. Weisberg JN, Keefe FJ: Personality disorders in the chronic pain population: Basic concepts, empirical findings, and clinical implications. *Pain Forum* 6:1, 1997.

42. Gatchel RJ, Polatin PB, Mayer TG: The dominant role of psychosocial risk factors in the development of chronic low back pain disability. *Spine* 20:2702, 1995.

43. Hathaway M: *Minnesota multiphasic personality inventory manual.* New York, The Psychological Corporation, 1976.

44. Butcher JN: *Minnesota multiphasic personality inventory (MMPI-2): manual for administration and scoring.* Minneapolis, Minn, University of Minneapolis Press, 1989.

45. Smith WL, Durksen DL: Personality and the relief of chronic pain: Predicting surgical outcome. *Clin Neuropsychol* 1:35, 1979.

46. Morley S, Wilkenson L: The pain beliefs and perceptions inventory: A British replication. *Pain* 61:427, 1995.

47. Kinney RK, Gatchel RJ, Mayer TG: The SCL-90-R evaluated as an alternative to the MMPI for psychological screening in chronic low back pain patients. *Spine* 16:940, 1991.

48. Duckro PN, Margolis RB, Tait RC: Psychological assessment in chronic pain. *J Clin Psych* 41:499, 1985.

49. Wallis BJ, Lord SM, Bransley L, Bogduk N: Pain and psychological symptoms of Australian patients with whiplash. *Spine* 21:408, 1996.

50. Bernstein IH, Jaremko ME, Hinkley BS: On the utility of the SCL-90 with low-back pain patients. *Spine* 19:42, 1994.

51. Bergner M, Bobbitt RA, Carter WB et al: The Sickness Impact Profile: Development and final revision of a health status measure. *Med Care* 19:787, 1981.

52. Follick MJ, Smith TW, Ahern DK: The Sickness Impact Profile: A global measure of disability in chronic low back pain. *Pain* 21:61, 1985.

53. Millon T, Green C, Meagher R: *Millon behavioral health inventory manual,* ed 3. Minneapolis, Minn, National Computer Systems, 1982.

54. Exner JE: *The Rorschach: A comprehensive system,* ed 2, vol 1. New York, Wiley, 1985.

55. Acklin W, Rernat E: Depression, alexithymia, and pain prone disorder: A Rorschach study. *J Personal Assess* 51:462, 1987.

56. Carlsson AM: Personality analysis using the Rorschach test in patients with chronic non-malignant pain. *Br J Project Psychol* 32:34, 1987.

57. Faucett JA: Depression in painful chronic disorders: The role of pain and conflict about pain. *J Pain Symptom Manage* 9:520, 1994.

58. Von Korff M, Le Resche L, Dworkin SF: First onset of common pain symptoms: A prospective study of depression as a risk factor. *Pain* 55:251, 1993.

59. Novy DM, Nelson DV, Berry LA et al: What does the Beck Depression Inventory measure in chronic pain? A reappraisal. *Pain* 61:261, 1995.

60. Williams AC, Richardson PH: What does the BDI measure in chronic pain? *Pain* 55:259, 1993.
61. Spielberger CD: Assessment of anger: The state-trait anger scale. In Butcher JN, Spielberger CD, editors: *Advances in personality assessment,* vol 2. Hillside, NJ, Lawrence Erlbaum Associates, 1983.
62. Rogers R, Bagby RM, Dickens SE: *SIRS: Structured interview of reported symptoms: Professional manual.* Odessa, Fla, Psychological Assessment Resources Inc, 1992.
63. Rogers R, Kropp PR, Bagby RM et al: Faking specific disorders: A study of the Structured Interview of Reported Symptoms (SIRS). *J Clin Psychol* 48:643, 1992.
64. Osterweis M, Kleinmar AS, Mechanic D, editors: *Pain and disability.* Washington, DC, National Academy Press, 1987.
65. Fairbank JC, Couper J, Davies JB et al: The Oswestry low back pain disability questionnaire. *Physiotherapy* 66:271, 1980.
66. Roland M, Morris R: A study of the natural history of back pain: Part I. Development of a reliable and sensitive measure of disability and low back pain. *Spine* 8:141, 1983.
67. Deyo RA: Comparative validity of the Sickness Impact Profile and shorter scales for functional assessment of low back pain. *Spine* 11:951, 1986.
68. Pollard CA: Preliminary validity study of the pain disability index. *Precept Motil Skills* 59:974, 1985.
69. Kerns RD, Turk DC, Rudy TE: The West Haven-Yale Multidimensional Pain Inventory (WHYMPI). *Pain* 23:345, 1985.
70. Rosenstiel AK, Keefe FJ: The use of coping strategies in chronic low back pain patients: Relationship to patient characteristics and current adjustment. *Pain* 17:33, 1983.
71. Boston K Pearce SA, Richardson PM: The Pain Cognition Questionnaire. *J Psychosom Res* 34:103, 1990.
72. Dolce JJ, Crocker MF, Moletteire C et al: Exercise quotas, anticipatory concern and self-efficacy expectancy in chronic pain: A preliminary report. *Pain* 24:365, 1986.
73. DeGood DE, Shutty MS: Assessment of pain beliefs, coping, and self-efficacy. In Turk DC, Melzack R, editors: *Handbook of pain assessment.* New York, Guilford, 1992.
74. Ware JE, Sherbourne CD: The MOS 36-item Short-Form Health Survey (SF-36): Conceptual framework and item selection. *Med Care* 30:473, 1992.
75. Ware JE Jr: *SF-36 health survey: Manual and interpretation guide.* Boston, Nimrod Press, 1993.
76. Romano JM, Turner JA, Jensen MP: The Chronic Illness Problem Inventory as a measure of dysfunction in chronic pain patients. *Pain* 49:71, 1992.
77. Waddell G, Main CJ: Assessment of severity in low back disorders. *Spine* 9:204, 1984.
78. Sternbach RA: *Principles of psychophysiology.* New York, Academic Press, 1964.
79. Greenfield NS, Sternbach RA: *Handbook of psychophysiology.* New York, Holt, Rinehart & Winston, 1972.

1. Personality assessment inventory is a self-report measure of personality traits and was developed as an alternative to MMPI. All of the following are true except

   A. It is a multidimensional test
   B. It contains approximately 344 items
   C. It is rated on a 10-point scale
   D. Response to each question requires "false," "slightly true," "mainly true," and "very true"

2. In the SCL-90 and its revised version patients respond to

   A. 3-point scale
   B. 4-point scale
   C. 5-point scale
   D. 6-point scale

3. The MBHI was developed specifically address

   A. Medical symptoms in psychiatric patients
   B. Psychiatric symptoms in medical patients
   C. Medical symptoms only
   D. Psychiatric symptoms only

4. One of the most commonly used instruments for measuring depression is

   A. Rorschach inkblot test
   B. Beck depression inventory
   C. MMPI
   D. Personality assessment inventory

5. A conscious exaggeration of psychologic or physiologic symptoms for physical or psychologic gain is termed

   A. Placebo
   B. Nocebo
   C. Malingering
   D. Noncompliance

ANSWERS

1. C

2. C

3. B

4. B

5. C

CHAPTER 18

Functional Evaluation

ELISE A. TRUMBLE AND MARGARET P. KRENGEL

The role of physical therapy in the management of patients with pain is to evaluate the involved tissue for the stage of healing and possible biomechanical causative factors that contribute to the pathologic condition. Treatment includes evaluation, tissue preparation and pain-relieving modalities, soft tissue mobilization, joint mobilization, therapeutic exercise, postural education, and injury prevention.

INITIAL EVALUATION

History

A complete history should be compiled including the current condition and any previous similar conditions. If a previous similar condition existed, detail the frequency, severity, and character of the previous episodes.

The therapist, who should carefully question whether the pain is constant or intermittent, charts the area and behavior of the pain. Irritating movements, as well as the length of time the activity can be tolerated, should also be noted.[1] Other facts included in a complete history are previous surgeries; treatments used, such as physical therapy; and whether previous methods were effective. Medications, diagnostic tests and results, and the name of the primary treating physician and any other physicians involved in the patient's management are also noted.

Visual Inspection

The visual inspection directs the examiner's attention to a particular area or areas of the system that might be dysfunctional. A thorough visual inspection requires that the involved body part and the joints above and below are completely exposed to the examiner in adequate lighting. The examiner should note any abnormalities of symmetry, muscle tone, atrophy, alignment, skin, body type, and condition. A patient with pain postures himself or herself to relieve painful structures and changes position depending on the irritability of the problem.[2]

Active Movements

Active movements should be tested before passive movements. Assessments of these movements indicates the severity of the disability and guides the examiner in determining how much passive handling the joint or limb will tolerate.[1] The examiner should note the rhythm, range, feel, arc, pattern, and pain behavior.[3] Objective baseline measurement of range of motion is obtained by use of a goniometer, which has been found to be highly reliable.[4,5]

Palpation

On palpation examination, the examiner should note skin temperature and sweating and soft tissue changes. The extensibility and integrity of the superficial to deep myofascial structures are evaluated in a layer method. The superficial palpatory examination includes tissue temperature, moisture, and light touch to determine the extensibility of the superficial connective tissues. Tissue rolling is one technique that is particularly useful. The deep palpatory examination includes compression and shear. Palpable structures are muscle bellies, muscle sheaths, tendons, myotendinous junctions, tenoperiostial junctions, joint capsules, and deep periosteal layers of tissue. The examiner should note any tissue texture abnormalities and restrictions.[6]

Joint Mobility

Testing joint mobility by palpation involves techniques that are used for evaluation and treatment. The test seeks not only range of motion but also "end feel" of the range, the behavior of the pain throughout the range, and the quality of any resistance or muscle spasm that may be present.[1]

Functional Tolerances

Physical therapists often include functional tolerances in their initial assessments. The examiner who asks the right questions in this regard can obtain many benefits and information such as:

1. A functional baseline that is meaningful to both the therapist and patient
2. Direct assessment of irritability of the affected tissue
3. Lifestyle pattern and sleep disturbances
4. Active participation of patients in their programs as they note increases or decreases in tolerances
5. Prescription of an exercise program for reconditioning or work

TREATMENTS

Heat and Cold

Stages, signs, symptoms, and suggested appropriate rehabilitation treatments are shown in Table 18–1. Vasudevan and colleagues[7] performed an exhaustive review of the thermal modalities in 1992. Generally the modalities are used more during the acute stage when reduction of inflammation and pain and increased circulation are important.

TABLE 18–1 Stages, Signs, Symptoms, and Suggested Appropriate Rehabilitation Treatments

Phase	Times	Signs	Symptoms	Treatments
Inflammatory acute	0–48 hr	Swelling Redness Muscle spasm	Constant, severe pain Guarding No movement	Education Inflammation-reducing modalities, postures Protective splints/braces Activities of daily living
Cellular subacute	2 day–2 wk	Decreased edema Localized pain Pain-free at rest Limited movement	Variable pain	Irritation control Pain-free range of motion Isometrics Stretching Gentle soft tissue mobilization Light functional activities
Proliferative settled	2 wk–6 wk	Movement patterns Muscle shortening Scar formation	Stiffness	Educational Weaning from splints, supporters Modified work simulation Reconditioning Lumbar stabilization Soft tissue mobilization
Maturation progressive	6 wk–3 mo 3–6 mo 6 mo	Weakness Fatigue Increased functional ability Limited end range movement Phase 1, 2, and 3 signs and symptoms		Work simulation Adaptive equipment Reconditioning Job analysis Physical capacity evaluation Med-Ex (special exercise) Pain treatment center

Electrical Modalities

A transcutaneous electrical nerve stimulator (TENS) is a very effective modality in the relief of pain.[8–10] The TENS unit works through neuronal stimulation and peripheral nerve stimulation. The pain signal from the injured tissue is masked by the TENS stimulation, which is less noxious, allowing the patient to carry on with daily activities more comfortably.

Muscle stimulators have become more useful for preventing or retarding disuse atrophy, increasing of local blood supply, maintaining or increasing range of motion, relaxing muscle spasms, and re-educating muscle.[11–14] Muscle stimulators are different from TENS units in that a muscle contraction is achieved by the muscle stimulators.

Soft Tissue Mobilization

Soft tissue mobilization is a primary treatment that can be used in the acute through chronic stages. It is critical for a patient with pain in the structure for 3 to 6 months to be treated by a therapist with strong soft tissue mobilization skills because layers of soft tissue restrictions develop over time.

Soft tissue mobilization techniques can be direct or indirect. The treatment is based on localizing the restriction and moving in the direction of the restriction.[6]

Joint Mobilization

Joint mobilization, another primary technique, can also be applied to the acute through chronic stages. The techniques are gentle, and rhythmic oscillations are performed within or at a limit of range. There are four grades of movements[15]:

1. Grade I is a small-amplitude movement near the starting position of the range.
2. Grade II is a large-amplitude movement that carries well into the range and can occupy any part of the range that is free of stiffness or muscle spasm.

3. Grade III is also a large-amplitude movement but does move into stiffness or muscle spasm.
4. Grade IV is a small-amplitude movement stretching into stiffness or muscle spasm.

Grades of mobilization are selected by the feel at the end of the range of the joint. The techniques are not used in any set pattern but should be varied, modified, and used again until the intention is achieved.

Therapeutic Exercise

The benefits of exercise are not generally disputed in the overall well-being of an individual. Recent studies have found that general fitness plays a role in the prevention of, and recovery from, injuries.[16] Therefore, the focus of the exercise therapist is not only on the strength and endurance of the injured area but also on the general condition of the individual.

Initial Evaluation

The exercise therapist questions patients on their previous perceived physical conditions to establish interests so that the exercises can be enjoyable and transferable to their previous lifestyle. The therapist should address any limitations to exercise such as cardiac or pulmonary limitations, incontinence, or discomfort of the individual.

Stretching and Strengthening Exercise

Stretching and strengthening techniques are essential components of an exercise program. In addition, the concept of stabilization has been developed in recent years. The lumbar stabilization program has filled a void in the rehabilitation of low back pain. The basic theory is that there is one position in which the spine functions optimally.[17] This position varies with different body positions and is, therefore, called the functional position of the spine. This is the position of the spine in which the patient experiences the least amount of pain. Stabilization exercises should be included in the rehabilitation exercise program and instituted during acute stages.

OCCUPATIONAL THERAPY AND MANAGEMENT OF PAIN PATIENTS

Occupational therapy services rendered when pain causes an inability to carry out life tasks include work simplification with emphasis on proper methods of body mechanics, activity assimilation, work simulation, psychologic support, behavior modification, job analysis, and functional capacity assessments.[18]

Evaluation

A thorough history of the patient's work and leisure activities are collected and should include medical history, past surgeries, and therapeutic intervention. Patients are asked to fill out a personal inventory questionnaire describing their level of independence in activities of daily living. When reviewed by the therapist, this information reveals the patient's perceptions of how limited they are by the pain or injury.

An assessment of activities of daily living and body mechanics is given to the patient and examined by the therapist. This part of the evaluation allows the therapist to match function with perceived limitations. Also, the body mechanic evaluation can be videotaped and used as part of the treatment to educate the patient in the correct posture to have while performing activities of daily living.

Nonverbal pain behavior adds dimensions to be assessed such as facial expressions, contortions, moaning, and also excessive rubbing of a body part that is painful.[19,20] Impaired function is further assessed by measuring range of motion and decreased mobility, avoidance of occupation, and impaired personal relationships.[19,20]

When asking a patient to describe pain, there are several methods available:

1. Body diagrams
2. McGill Pain Questionnaire[21]
3. Visual Analogue Scale (VAS)[22–24]

Objective Evaluation

The objective of measuring range of motion is to provide data regarding the quality of available active range of motion, passive range of motion, or total range of motion at a specific joint.[25] The initial evaluation is used to establish a baseline for comparison when changes occur over time.

Davidoff and colleagues[26] suggested a specific method of measuring joint pain by palpation using a 4-point scale:

0 = No pain
1 = Mild pain to deep palpation
2 = Severe pain to deep palpation
3 = Severe pain to mild palpation
4 = Hyperesthesia

This scale provides an objective means of measuring joint pain; however, the reliability and validity may be reduced because of varying pain thresholds and anticipated pain among patients.

Manual muscle testing is performing on general muscle groups. The therapist looks for functional movement patterns and muscles working in synergistic balance. It is a way to establish gross muscle function. It should not be used as a sole means of evaluation but should be used in conjunction with other extremity evaluation tools and techniques.[27] Strength can be compared between left and right hands using the Jamar dynamometer,* and this comparison can determine maximal effort exerted and inconsistency.

In a study by Bechtol,[28] in which normal subjects were tested, scores from five handles produced a slightly skewed bell-shaped curve, with the highest strengths occurring in the second and third handle positions. The bell-shaped curve is the expected result when the patient is giving a consistent effort. A less sincere effort can produce a flat curve according to Stokes[29] (Fig. 18–1).

When the evaluation process is completed, the occupational therapist should be able to identify specific areas in which therapeutic intervention can restore or improve independence in activities of daily living, mobility, communication, and pain management skills.

Treatment

Body Mechanics and Activities of Daily Living

When training the patient in body mechanics, it is essential to educate the patient in how the body works and how gravity acts on the body. Gravity acts on a mass as if all the mass were concentrated at one point, the center of gravity.[30] The center of gravity has been determined to be just anterior to the second sacral vertebra if the subject is in the anatomic position.[30] As soon as the individual changes position, the center of gravity also changes its location. This principle is applicable in all activities of work or daily living. When lifting and carrying objects, keeping the object close to the center of gravity is the most relevant factor.

Stages of Healing

The following stages categorize the healing process of an injury according to the stages of recovery.

Stage I

The occupational therapist can treat an injury by understanding its cause. In the case of cumulative trauma, during the first 48 hours after tendinitis, sprains, or strains, it is recommended to try to rest the affected part.[31] Custom splints or manufactured braces can be applied to immobilize the injured body part. Also the application of inflammation-reducing modalities such as ice or electrical stimulation is used. The patient should be educated on how posture or work habits can aggravate the condition.

Stage II

In stage II, the pain has somewhat subsided, and movement through range of motion can be attempted. Early movement is important to reduce scar tissue and muscular and soft tissue shortening and to increase circulation.

The patient then progresses to light functional activities with application of body mechanics. This early intervention

---

*Available from Preston, Inc., Clifton, NJ.

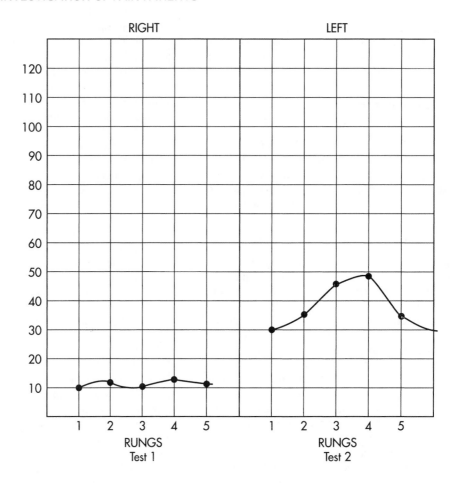

FIG. 18–1 Jamar Dynamometer five handle grip test.

restores patients' confidence and allows them to gain some control of self-care without increased pain. Work restrictions are also entailed and recommended by the treating physician.

Therapeutic modalities such as heat are applied at this stage to relieve pain and relax the muscles before or after activity. External supports are worn to restrict or avoid activities that cause pain to the injured area.[31] Three problem areas must be considered when using external supports:

1. Inactivity can weaken muscle.
2. Long periods of inactivity can cause loss of normal range of motion in the supported joints.
3. If the worker with a splint or brace is assigned jobs that require major movements of the supported area, these motions may be even more stressed with the splint than without it.[31]

Stage III

In stage III, the occupational therapist focuses on increasing the patient's activity level by increasing range of motion and strength. Patients are carefully weaned from supportive devices and are gradually prepared to return to work. Education in body mechanics is reinforced and pacing and

work simplification techniques are discussed. Therapeutic modalities are continued to control pain flair-ups, but they are used less frequently.

Stage IV

At 6 weeks the patient should be experiencing less pain, increased range of motion and strength, and the ability to sustain activity. A job analysis should be performed by the occupational therapist that includes a method for measuring the worker's exposure to each of the major biomechanic risk factors: force, posture, and repetition.[32]

Work Capacity Evaluation

As defined by Matheson and Niemayer,[33] a work capacity evaluation is a systematic process of measuring and developing an individual's capacity to dependably sustain performance in response to broadly defined work demands. The actual evaluation process can be combined with rehabilitation in a work hardening program.

Matheson defined a work-tolerance screening as an intensive (usually 1 day) evaluation that focuses on major physical tolerance abilities related to musculoskeletal strength, endurance, speed, and flexibility. The information from this type of evaluation is usually marketed to the vocational rehabilitation community, and data are used to determine employability.[33]

Components of a physical capacity evaluation include[19]:

1. Lifting and carrying
2. Pushing and pulling
3. Reaching
4. Grasping and handling
5. Manipulating
6. Standing, sitting, and walking
7. Kneeling, crouching, crawling, and stooping
8. Endurance
9. Sequential testing for consistency and maximum effort

Work Hardening and Transition

Matheson and Niemayer[33] defined work hardening as:

1. A prescriptive productivity development program
2. A highly structured productivity-oriented treatment program that uses the injured worker's involvement in real or simulated work activities as its principal means of treatment
3. An individualized, work-oriented treatment process involving the client in simulated or actual work tasks that are structured and graded to progressively increase physical tolerances, stamina, endurance, and productivity.[34]

Work hardening is especially useful with patients who are primarily limited by their pain. They can be taught to control their symptoms while performing a job. Patients may continue to report no change in pain level, while they demonstrate and experience a major improvement in functional capacity.[33] The primary goal of the occupational therapist when treating a patient with pain is to teach the patient how to function in everyday life in spite of the pain.

References

1. Maitland GD: *Vertebral manipulation,* ed 5. Boston, Butterworth, 1986.
2. Charnley J: Orthopedic signs in the diagnosis of the disc protrusion. *Lancet* 1:186, 1951.
3. Cyriax J: *Textbook of orthopedic medicine,* ed 8, vol 2. London, Baltimore, Balliere Tindall, 1982.
4. Riddle DL, Rothstein JM, Lamb RL: Goniometric reliability in a clinical setting: Elbow and knee measurements. *Phys Ther* 67(5):668, 1987.
5. Youdas JW, Carey JR, Garrett TR: Reliability of measurements of cervical spine range of motion—Comparison of three methods. *Phys Ther* 71:98, 1991.
6. Cantu RI, Grodin AJ: *Myofascial manipulation, theory, and clinical application.* Aspen, Colo, Aspen Publications, 1992.
7. Vasudevan S, Hegmann K, Moore A et al: Physical methods of pain management. In Raj PP, editor: *Practical management of pain,* ed 2. St. Louis, Mosby, 1992.
8. Barr JO, Nielsen DH, Soderberg GL: Transcutaneous electrical nerve stimulation characteristics for altering pain perception. *Phys Ther* 66:1515, 1986.
9. Bending G: TENS in a pain clinic. *Physiotherapy* 75:292, 1989.
10. Paris PM: No more pain: Transcutaneous nerve stimulation. *Emerg Med* 18:57, 1986.
11. Currier DP, Mann R: Muscular strength development by electrical stimulation in healthy individuals. *Phys Ther* 63(6):915, 1983.
12. Fulbright JS: Electrical stimulation to reduce chronic toe-flexor hypertonicity: A case report. *Phys Ther* 64:523, 1984.
13. Gould N, Donnermeyer D, Gammon GG et al: Transcutaneous muscle stimulation to retard disuse atrophy after open meniscectomy. *Clin Orthop* 178:190, 1983.
14. Liu HI, Currier DP, Threlkeld AJ: Circulatory response of digital arteries associated with electrical stimulation of calf muscles in healthy subjects. *Phys Ther* 67(3):340, 1987.
15. Grieve GP: *Common vertebral joint problems.* Edinburgh, Churchill Livingstone, 1980.
16. Nachemson AL: Exercise, fitness, and back pain. In Pavi Nurmi, editor: *Congress book—Advanced European course on sports medicine.* Abo, Finland, The Finnish Society of Sports Medicine, 1989.
17. Morgan D: Concepts on functional training and postural stabilization for the low back injuries. *Top Acute Care Trauma Rehab* 2:8, 1988.
18. Hopkins HL, Smith HD: *Willard and Spackman's occupational therapy,* ed 5. Philadelphia JB Lippincott, 1978.
19. Fredrickson LW, Lynd RS, Ross J: Methodology in the measurement of pain. *Behav Ther* 9:486, 1978.
20. Keeke FJ: Behavioral assessment and treatment of chronic pain: Current status and future directions. *J Consult Clin Psychol* 50:896, 1982.
21. Melzack R: The McGill Pain Questionnaire: Major properties and scoring method. *Pain* 1:227, 1975.
22. Downie WW, Downie WW, Leatham PA et al: Studies with pain rating scales. *Ann Rheum Dis* 37:378, 1978.
23. Jenson MP, Karoly P, Brover S: The measurement of clinical pain intensity: A comparison of six methods. *Pain* 27:117, 1986.
24. Michlovitz S: *Thermal agents in rehabilitation,* ed 2. Philadelphia, FA Davis, 1990.
25. Adams LS, Greene LW, Topoozian E: *Clinical assessment recommendations,* ed 2. Chicago, The American Society of Hand Therapists, 1992.
26. Davidoff G, Morey K, Amann M et al: Pain measurement in reflex sympathetic dystrophy syndrome. *Pain* 32:27, 1988.
27. Kienan LS: *Clinical assessment recommendations,* ed 2. Chicago, The American Society of Hand Therapists, 1992.
28. Bechtol CD: Grip test: use of a dynamometer with adjustable handle spacing. *J Bone Joint Surg Am* 36A:820, 1954.
29. Stokes HM: The seriously uninjured hand: Weakness of grip. *J Occup Med* 25:683, 1983.
30. Schenek JM, Cordova DF: *Introduction to biomechanics,* ed 2. Philadelphia, FA Davis, 1980.
31. Fine L: Medical diagnosis and treatment. In Anderson V-P, editor: *Cumulative trauma disorders: A manual for musculoskeletal diseases of the upper limbs.* Bristol, PA, Taylor & Francis, 1992.
32. Anderson V-P, editor: *Cumulative trauma disorders: A manual for musculoskeletal diseases of the upper limbs.* Bristol, PA, Taylor & Francis, 1992.
33. Matheson LW, Niemayer LO: *The work capacity evaluation manual.* 1-2-1-7. Anaheim, Calif, Employment and Rehabilitation Institute of California, 1988.
34. Vocational Evaluation and Work Adjustment Association and American Occupational Therapy Association: *Work hardening guidelines.* The Associations, Bethesda, MD, 1986.

1. The initial evaluation of function consist of all of the following except

   A. History
   B. Visual inspection
   C. Active movements
   D. No touch technique

2. The modalities of treatment in physical therapy include all of these except

   A. Heat and cold applications
   B. Transcutaneous electric nerve stimulation (TENS)
   C. Soft tissue mobilization
   D. Therapeutic exercise

3. Components of physical capacity evaluations include all of the following except

   A. Lifting and carrying
   B. Standing, sitting, and walking
   C. Sequential testing for consistency and maximal effort
   D. Swimming

4. Work hardening is defined as all of the following except

   A. Prescriptive, productivity development program
   B. A randomized exercise program without objective goals
   C. Highly structured productive oriented treatment program with real or simulated activities
   D. Individualized work-oriented treatment process that is structured and graded to increasing physical tolerance, stamina, endurance, and productivity

5. Physical therapy treatments include all of the following except

   A. Soft tissue mobilization
   B. Treatment of depression
   C. Therapeutic exercise
   D. Postural education

ANSWERS

1. D
2. D
3. D
4. B
5. B

CHAPTER 19

Disability Evaluation

SRIDHAR V. VASUDEVAN AND MATTHEW MONSEIN

EVALUATION OF DISABILITY IS A COMPLEX PROCESS

Few physicians treating patients with chronic pain have the training, expertise, and will to learn how to properly apply current rehabilitation medicine knowledge and technology to provide information that may be useful in settling a pending disability claim.[1] To complicate matters, the definition of disability can vary. Often disability is arbitrarily defined by the administrative policy of respective agencies within the broad context of established laws. Many chronic pain rehabilitation programs set goals to return patients to gainful employment. To be effective in this complex task, it is necessary for the physician and other team members to recognize the needs of third-party payers and be familiar with the definitions and conceptual basis of disability.

CONCEPTUALIZATION OF DISABILITY

Despite the classification proposed by the World Health Organization (WHO),[2] society tends to view disability in different ways. Disability can best be conceptualized as "an inability to perform a task." Although the definition appears very simple, the different systems involved in disability determination tend to define disability in much looser terms in some situations and much more stringent terms in others.

The Social Security Administration's definition of disability is significantly more restrictive than the definitions accepted in some commercial disability insurance policies. It is, therefore, essential for the physician working with the chronic pain patient to recognize the different views on disability and to have a personal working system in which the clinician can best conceptualize disability.

Melvin and Nagi[3] provide one of the best overviews of a conceptual basis of disability. Briefly, the following definitions are key to understanding this conceptual framework:

1. Active pathology. Pathology is altered anatomy and physiology. This may follow traumatic injury, a metabolic disorder, or an infectious process and includes an aggravation of a previous chronic problem or the development of a new acute problem. An example is repetitive heavy lifting, causing degenerative disk disease that may be aggravated by a specific episode of lifting at work.
2. Impairment. Impairments are defined as anatomic, physiologic, or psychologic abnormality or loss. It is essential to understand that impairments are "objective." The WHO uses similar language in its definition.[2] Impairments may

be temporary while the actual pathology is still present, or, despite the appropriate and maximal treatment of the acute pathology, impairments may persist. Examples are decreased lumbosacral mobility following a lumbar disk herniation, altered reflexes and decreased strength and sensation despite successful surgical removal of the extruded disk, or an abnormal electromyographic study in someone with radiculopathy.
3. Functional limitation. Functional limitation, which results from impairment, can be described as the lack of ability to perform an activity in the manner or within the range considered normal for that human being.[3] The WHO uses the term *disability* to describe functional limitations[2]; therefore, these are task-specific inabilities. An example of a functional limitation is the inability of someone with lumbar disk disease to lift more than 20 pounds.
4. Disability. The inability to perform one's usual activities and assume one's usual obligation is viewed as disability.[4] Permanent disabilities are presumed to be present if an individual's actual or presumed ability to engage in gainful activity is reduced or absent because of impairment, which in turn may or may not be combined with other factors.[4,5] The ability to engage in gainful employment or work is affected by many nonmedical conditions such as age, sex, education, and economical and social environment, in addition to the definite medically determinable permanent impairment.

Thus, disability can be viewed as a disadvantage for a given individual resulting from an impairment, whereas functional limitation limits or prevents a fulfillment of the role that is "normal" for the individual. The WHO uses the term *handicap* to describe this state.[2]

Examples of disability in this conceptual model include those activities that limit an individual's fulfillment of a role in life such as that of a father, mother, student, or worker. Thus, disability is not only task specific but also role specific.

The conceptual basis of disability provided previously is important for the physician to be aware of, not only for the assessment of the disability but also for the development of treatment strategies for the different stages of the disability process. Physicians may be able to treat the pathologic condition or the disease process, evaluate impairments and treat some of these impairments by specific therapies, alter the functional limitation by provision of adaptive equipment, or alter disability through comprehensive psychosocial and vocational interventions. Disability can also be viewed as a behavioral response to continued impairment that limits a performance of normal function.[3] The American Medical Association (AMA) provides a guideline for evaluating both mental and physical impairment.[6] The AMA differentiates between permanent impairment and permanent disability. Impairment is defined as purely a "medical condition," whereas permanent disability is felt to occur when an individual's ability to engage in gainful activity is reduced or absent because of impairment.

The AMA also takes a strong position that physicians alone are competent to perform impairment assessment, and that disability assessment is an administrative, not medical, responsibility and function. Although this distinction may appear to be somewhat semantic, the determination of one's abilities and disabilities should be performed by a physician. Only with adequate data from the physician can a system award the proper disability and assist the individual in rehabilitation toward overcoming these disabilities.

SYSTEMS OF DISABILITIES

There are many social systems involved in determining disability, each with its own specific definition and expectations of the physician in the assessment of the disability. These include the following:

1. Veteran's Administration (VA) Benefits Program
2. Social Security Disability System
3. Workers' Compensation System

The VA Benefits Program

The VA defines total impairment or disability as "… any disability that is sufficient to render it impossible for the average person to follow a substantial gainful occupation, but only if it is reasonably certain that such disability will continue toward the life of the disabled person."[6]

This definition also includes "… any disease or disorder determined by the administration to be of such a nature or extent, as to justify a determination that the person suffering therefrom is permanently and totally disabled."[6] Disability benefits under the VA program are classified as service-connected and nonservice-connected.

The service-connected program is an entitlement program, under which there is no means test, and the impairment is sustained in the course of military service. In this program there is no requirement for the inability to work, the compensation depends on the percentage of disability, and the percentage of disability is determined by the VA process.

Nonservice-connected disability includes pension programs under which benefits are payable for impairments sustained after military service, payable only if the veteran meets the definition of being totally and permanently disabled. Under this system, the veteran should be at least 60% disabled, according to the VA definition, to be considered totally disabled.

Thus, the service-connected program is a compensation program and the nonservice-connected program is a pension program. The service-connected program is an entitlement program, but eligibility is limited to veterans of the armed forces. In contrast to the Social Security Disability Program, in which there is an "all or none" rule, the VA provides compensation for partial disability. A rating board determines whether disability is service-connected and the percentage of the disability. Therefore, service-connected disability is established regardless of the veteran's inability to engage in substantial gainful activity.

Pain and the VA System

In considering the role of pain, the VA does not consider pain in and of itself disabling. When evaluating a disorder that includes pain, the physician evaluating the disability is instructed to request the veteran to describe the pain; any limitation of function that results from the pain; and the duration of pain and other findings with pain, such as fatigue, weakness, and swelling. Findings in the presence of pain, as well as the limitation that pain imposes, are features in determining the percentage of the disability. Finally, disability can be found to be caused by pain as long as there is an adequate underlying pathologic condition, but pain in excess of an underlying disorder is not considered independently.[6,7]

Social Security Disability Program

The Social Security Administration has responsibility for the administration of two disability programs: (1) the Social Security Disability Insurance program and (2) the Supplemental Social Security Income program.[6,7]

The Social Security Disability Program defines disability as "… the inability to engage in any substantial gainful activity by reason of medically determinable physical or mental impairments, which can be expected to result in death or have lasted, or can be expected to last, a continuous period of not less than 12 months."[8]

Pain and Disability in the Social Security System

In general, an individual's statement as to pain or other symptoms shall not be conclusive evidence for disability as defined. There must be medical signs and findings established by medically acceptable clinical or laboratory techniques that show the existence of medical impairment that results from anatomic, physiologic, or psychologic abnormalities that could reasonably be expected to produce pain or other alleged symptoms and that when considered with all the evidence required would lead to a conclusion that the individual is under a disability.

Workers' Compensation System

Workers' compensation laws have made it necessary for every physician in practice not only to treat patients coming under this act but also to play a significant and important role in assisting the injured employee's return to work. Therefore, the physician involved with patients with acute and chronic pain plays a very important role with the workers' compensation system.

Workers' compensation systems were organized with the following objectives:

1. To provide adequate and prompt medical benefits and income replacement to work accident victims or financial benefits to their dependents regardless of fault
2. To restore the individual's earning capacity and ability to return to productive employment

3. To provide the only means of recovery and eliminate expensive, wasteful, and time-consuming litigation
4. To help prevent or reduce industrial accident injuries

Important elements of the workers' compensation system include the following principles:

1. The negligence of the employer need not be proven.
2. Injury should occur as it relates to work.
3. Injury could be physical or mental injury or illness.
4. The physician plays an important role in determining the stages of disability and in determining permanent disability.

There are four stages of disability under this system:

1. Temporary total disability. This period is soon after the injury while healing is occurring. This stage of disability applies during the time when the injured employee is under active medical treatment. If the employer is unable to provide restricted work, the temporary total disability is continued. During this time, loss of wages payments are made. This is usually two thirds of the regular wages but varies significantly from state to state.
2. Temporary partial disability. This occurs when the employee is able to return to work part time. Inability to work full time should be caused by the effects of the work-related injury. A percentage of the temporary total benefits is paid.
3. Permanent partial disability. This is determined at the time when the "healing period has ended." The healing period is defined as the time when no further treatment will substantially alter the state of the individual's illness or disease and the condition is stable. The permanent partial disability is an assessment of permanent impairment based on whether it is a "scheduled" or "nonscheduled" injury. The compensation rate of permanent partial disability is fixed. Scheduled injuries are fixed in weeks and relate to injuries to the extremities, vision, or hearing. Nonscheduled injuries are due to injuries to the torso, head, abdomen, and thorax and are described as a percentage of the total body, which is 100%. Several states provide rough guidelines for physicians to use when determining a person's disabilities.[9]
4. Permanent total disability. Under this status an individual is "completely disabled" and unable to return to work. This entitlement, when awarded, consists of weekly benefits for life, the amount of which is adjusted yearly by the legislature of each state.

Pain and the Workers' Compensation System

Under most workers' compensation systems the focus is not the continued presence of pain but stabilization of the underlying impairment. Although there is a diversity of workers' compensation programs and their approach to the evaluation of pain of unknown etiology, there is little chance of receiving workers' compensation for pain alone. However, when the allegations of substantial pain are associated with a demonstrable pathologic condition capable of producing the pain, consideration is given to the disabling effects of the alleged pain.

DISABILITY EVALUATION: MEDICAL VERSUS LEGAL PROCESS

It is very important for the physician involved in the process of rehabilitating the patient with chronic pain to recognize the medical and legal perspectives in the process of disability evaluation. Grossman[10] identifies the problems in disability determination by pointing out that "disability" is a concept viewed differently by various professionals that participate in its formulation. He compares the disability evaluation process to the fable of the three blind men asked to describe an elephant, each having touched only one aspect of the elephant's anatomy and, thus, viewing it extremely differently. Grossman reviews the subjectivity of the symptom of pain and emphasizes that the treating doctor's testimony concerning the patient's pain is, at times, not admissible in courts, whereas testimony from doctors not treating the patient is often admissible.

Goodman[11] discusses the incompatibility of medicine and law. He emphasizes that law students are taught to study and solve problems through the "inductive or Socratic method," wherein they are taught to generalize from a single case. On the other hand, physicians are taught to use "deductive or Aristotelian logic." This involves generalization of the plan of care through deductive reasoning. This theory has to be deduced from a multitude of prospective and retrospective case studies. The conclusions must be proven by studies that are reproducible and statistically significant. Thus, Goodman emphasizes that physicians and attorneys involved in the disability process have difficulty with communication because of differing backgrounds.[11]

A MORE OBJECTIVE DETERMINATION OF DISABILITY

Disability is a multifaceted entity that is not only determined by the underlying medical impairment but also influenced by complex interaction between nonmedical issues such as age, education, work opportunities, and other social and cultural factors. Because of the complexity in defining disability, no universally accepted method of objectively measuring it exists.

A commonly held assumption is that the physical examination is an objective and consistent method of assessing impairment that is "medically determinable"; however, studies have demonstrated poor reproducibility between physicians in the evaluation of back pain patients, especially regarding non-neurologic findings such as muscle spasm and guarding.[12,13]

Because pain is a subjective experience and literally the only one experiencing the sensation or feeling is the person, an objective and reliable instrument that measures the subjective aspects of disability based on the patient's perception would be more desirable (in addition to information supplied to the physician by the patient).

Over the years, many pain assessment instruments have been developed.[14,15] Perhaps the most thoroughly studied is the Sickness Illness Profile. This has been used in many studies to demonstrate the effect of a variety of treatment methods in patients with pain. The Sickness Illness Profile has demonstrated satisfactory internal consistency, good test-retest reliability, and construct validity.[14]

Another instrument is the IMPATH, a multidimensional, self-report assessment instrument consisting of 400 yes-no, multiple-choice questions that appear on a computer screen. Patients can directly enter the answers into the computer. The data are analyzed and a printout is generated. The information provided includes medical history; review of symptoms: a list of psychologic, behavioral, cognitive, and social factors that may be contributing to the expression of severity of pain; and the lifestyle disruption and potential for rehabilitation.[16]

PHYSICAL CAPACITIES EVALUATION

In many centers, physical capacities evaluation or functional capacities assessment is a battery of tests done by physical and occupational therapists that provide a measure of the patient's functional abilities and inabilities. Some of these are structured into 8-hour activities and provide a more objective gauge of the patient's ability to perform a task. When properly used, they assist in supporting some limitations the physician may impose on an individual because of an underlying pathologic condition. However, it should be emphasized that physical capability evaluations and functional capacity assessments do not provide a very objective system.

EVALUATION OF DISABILITY—HOW TO WRITE A REPORT

Few physicians treating patients with chronic pain have the training to provide a disability evaluation report.[1] As a consequence, medical reports rarely address the question raised by an agency that is interested in determining disability. By denying the patient an assessment of disability, there is continuation of illness behavior, therefore, reinforcing the disabled role. Because of this difficulty, disability assessment is often performed by independent medical examiners who work outside the interdisciplinary pain team. A well-trained pain-management team and the physician director are in an optimal position to determine the disability of an individual. However, it is essential that the physician have a good conceptual basis of the disability process.

The treating physician or the physician who has been asked to perform an independent medical examination to assess disability should be very meticulous in obtaining a very detailed history. This history should include the symptoms and emphasize the details of the history, how the injury happened, and where and when it happened. Reading through the history, one should be able to conceptualize the actual mechanism of injury so that a relationship between the episode and injury or illness (causation) can be determined. The physician should describe in detail the symptoms of pain and the effect of pain on physical, psychosocial, and vocational functioning.

Evaluation of the impairment of the musculoskeletal system should take into consideration assessment of both active and passive range of motion; gait; muscle strength; and areas of tightness, weakness, and tenderness. Tenderness should be examined repeatedly, looking for consistently reproducible areas that are anatomically identifiable with a consistent degree of pressure. Electromyographic and other neurophysiologic changes may be present in the peripheral and central nervous system. Thus, the evaluation of impairment, which is a function of the physician alone, should be done by appropriate physical examination and additional laboratory, radiologic, electrophysiologic (EP), and psychologic studies.

The next step is to identify those areas of function that are limited by impairments. Physicians must extrapolate their own knowledge of the pathologic condition or disease process and the resulting permanent impairments in assessing those limitations of function that may result from it. At times, additional information is obtained from evaluation by the interdisciplinary team working in the chronic pain center. Knowledge regarding previous education, previous and currently held jobs, and specific tasks for the job is needed. Evaluation of permanent impairment and the extent that it affects the person's ability in one or more activities of daily living (e.g., self-care, communication, ambulation, traveling, and nonspecialized hand activities) is a role of the physician.

The main objective of the physician is to provide an opinion regarding the following:

1. Causation of the injury and the relationship of injury to impairment
2. Identification of the appropriate anatomic, physiologic, and psychologic impairments
3. Identification of those functional limitations that are imposed by the impairments
4. Relationship of functional limitations to work activities and other recreational activities
5. Suggestions for future treatment and rehabilitation
6. Permanency of impairments and statement as to whether the impairments are expected to last 12 months or permanently

SUMMARY

Physicians involved in managing those with chronic pain are often involved in the process of determining and certifying disability. The physician must be objective and thorough to clearly understand the conceptual basis of disability. It has been emphasized throughout this chapter that evaluation of impairment is a medical responsibility and usually objectively determinable. There is no clear and consistent relationship between impairment and the degree of disability.

Pain, although a subjective symptom, is a highly complex phenomenon. Chronic pain syndrome, although helpful as a clinical term, does not in itself constitute a disability. Symptoms of pain alone do not, therefore, justify an award of disability. One of the major objectives of pain rehabilitation programs is not to "cure pain" but to "alter disability." Pain clinics and pain rehabilitation programs indicate the occurrence of a significant alteration of the disability status, although pain may not be changed.

If there are medically determinable impairments that reasonably explain the symptoms of pain, they should be documented. Therefore, the physician involved in the care of those with chronic pain should address the effects of pain and its effect on future physical and vocational functions of the individual.

Assisting in disability determination should be an integral part of the physician's role in the management of those individuals and families with chronic pain.

References

1. Brena SS, Turk DC: Vocational disability: A challenge to pain rehabilitation programs. In Aronoff GM, editor: *Pain centers—A revolution in health care.* New York, Raven Press, 1988.
2. World Health Organization: *Constitution of World Health Organization.* Geneva, Switzerland, World Health Organization, 1964.
3. Melvin JL, Nagi SZ: Factors in behavioral responses to impairments. *Arch Phys Med Rehabil* 51:552, 1970.
4. Melvin JL: *When is permanent permanent? Trial techniques: The medical issue.* Columbus, Ohio, Ohio Legal Center Institute, 1966.
5. American Medical Association Committee on Rating of Mental and Physical Impairment: *Guides to evaluation of permanent impairment.* Chicago, American Medical Association, 1988.
6. *Report on the Commission on Evaluation of Pain.* US Department of Health and Human Services No. 64-031. Washington, DC, US Government Printing Office, 1987.
7. Osterweis M, Kleinman A, Mechanic D: *Institute of Medicine's committee on pain, and disability and chronic illness behavior, pain, and disability: Clinical, behavioral and public policy perspectives.* Washington, DC, National Academy Press, 1987.
8. *Disability evaluation under Social Security—A handbook for physicians.* Washington, DC, US Department of Health, Education, and Welfare, Social Security Administration, HEW Publications, August 1979.
9. *A guide for physicians relative to industrial injuries, state of Wisconsin.* Wausau, Wis, Employers Insurance of Wausau.
10. Grossman HI: A new concept of disability. *J Rehabil* 45:41, 1979.
11. Goodman RS: The incompatibility of medicine and law. *Orthopaedics* 8:10, 1978.
12. Nelson MA, Allen P, Clamp SE et al: Reliability and reproducibility of clinical findings in low back pain. *Spine* 4:97, 1979.
13. Waddell G, Main CJ, Morris EW et al: Normality and reliability in the clinical assessment of backache. *Br Med J* 284:1519, 1982.
14. Deyo RA: Measuring the functional status of patients with low back pain. *Arch Phys Med Rehabil* 69:1044, 1983.
15. Melzack R: The McGill Pain Questionnaire: Major properties and scoring methods. *Pain* 1:277, 1975.
16. Friction JR, Nelson A, Monsein M: IMPATH: Microcomputer assessment of behavioral and psychological factors in craniomandibular disorders. *J Craniomandib Pract* 5:373, 1987.

1. The Social Security Administration's definition of disability includes all of the following except

   A. Inability to engage in any substantial gainful activity
   B. Physical or mental impairment that can be expected to result in death
   C. An impairment that can be expected to last continuously for a period to last for not less than 12 months
   D. An impairment that can be expected to last for 6 months

2. Workman's Compensation System has all of the following stages of disability except

   A. Temporary total disability
   B. Temporary partial disability
   C. Total disability
   D. Permanent partial disability

3. Physical capacity evaluations or functional capacity evaluations are done by

   A. Physical or occupational therapist
   B. Nurses
   C. Physicians
   D. Social worker

4. A treating physician or a physician that has been asked to perform a disability examination should do all of the following except

   A. Quickly obtain a summarized medical history
   B. Obtain a history that includes symptoms and how, where, and when the injury happened
   C. Conceptualize the actual mechanism of injury
   D. Describe in detail the symptoms of pain and their effect on physical, psychosocial, and vocational functioning

5. The main objective of the physician to provide an opinion in a disability case is all of the following except

   A. To determine causation of injury and relation of injury to impairment
   B. To identify nonanatomic, physiologic, and psychologic impairment
   C. To determine the relationship of functional limitation to work activities
   D. To make suggestions for future treatment and rehabilitation

ANSWERS

1. D
2. C
3. A
4. A
5. B

CHAPTER 20

Pain Measurement

MARC A. VALLEY

Modern medicine is based on the treatment of disease processes; treatment is guided by the appropriate interpretation of test results. This is true in the evaluation and treatment of patients with pain syndromes. However, patients with pain also often have concurrent psychologic overlays, either secondary to or in conjunction with the pain syndrome. These psychologic overlays affect both the selection and interpretation of tests used to evaluate pain.

PATIENT SELF-REPORT USING A SINGLE DIMENSION PAIN SCALE

The most commonly used assessment tools for pain are based on patient self-reporting and involve only a single dimension (Box 20–1). These single dimension pain scales are easy for the patient to use and understand and are relatively inexpensive. The primary limitations of the single dimension scales are that they risk oversimplifying a patient's pain syndrome and can potentially lose validity with haphazard and careless administration.

Verbal Descriptor Scales

Verbal descriptor scales use a standard set of five to seven words as pain descriptors. Melzack and Torgerson[1] introduced the following five-word scale that is often used: "mild, discomforting, distressing, horrible, excruciating." The major concern with this test was that it was open-ended. The problem was remedied when Aitken[2] added defined endpoints, "no pain" and "unendurable." This type of scale allows for standardized descriptors and correlates with the visual analog scale (VAS) in many situations,[3] while potentially more useful than VAS in experimental pain situations.[4]

The disadvantages of the verbal descriptor scale include the limited number of possible responses and the noncontinuous scale (nonparametric statistics are required for analysis), which potentially make this scale weaker than the VAS.[5]

Numerical Pain Scales

The numerical pain scale is an ordinal method of assessing pain using an 11-point scale in which 0 = "no pain" and 10 = "most excruciating pain imaginable." The advantages of this scale are that no special training is required to administer it, it gives consistent and reproducible measurements, it allows for interpatient assessment and the changes within a patient during treatment,[6,7] and this scale may be a better assessment of remembered chronic pain.[8]

BOX 20–1 Single Dimension Pain Scales

1. Verbal descriptor scale:
   Instructions: From the list below, choose the word that best describes your present pain level.
   ( ) Mild
   ( ) Discomforting
   ( ) Distressing
   ( ) Horrible
   ( ) Excruciating
2. Behavioral rating scale (BRS-6):
   ( ) No Pain
   ( ) Pain present, but can be ignored
   ( ) Pain present, cannot be ignored but does not interfere with everyday activities
   ( ) Pain present, cannot be ignored, interferes with concentration
   ( ) Pain present, cannot be ignored, interferes with all tasks excepting taking care of basic needs such as toileting and eating
   ( ) Pain present, cannot be ignored, rest or bed rest required
3. Simple numerical rating scale:
   Instructions: Choose a number from 0 to 10 to indicate how strong your pain is right now.
   0 = No pain at all 1 2 3 4 5 6 7 8 9 10 = Worst pain imaginable
4. Numerical rating scale (NRS-101):
   Instructions: Indicate on the line below the number between 0 and 100 that indicates how strong your pain is right now. A zero (0) would mean "no pain" and a hundred (100) would mean "worst pain imaginable."

   ---

5. Point box scale (BS-11):
   Instructions: Zero (0) means "no pain" and ten (10) mean "worst pain imaginable" on this scale of 1 to 10. Place an "X" through the number that best represents your pain level.
   0 1 2 3 4 5 6 7 8 9 10
6. Visual analog scale (VAS):
   Instructions: Place a mark on the following line to show the intensity of pain that you are feeling.
   no pain_____worst pain
7. Pain relief scale:
   Instructions: Make a mark on the line below to indicate the amount of relief you feel from your pain right now as compared to yesterday.
   no relief _____complete relief

A disadvantage of the numerical pain scale is that it can be statistically weak because of the required nonparametric analysis; however, this is probably clinically insignificant.

Visual Analog Scale

The VAS is a progression of the numerical pain scale that allows for continuous data analysis and uses a 10-cm line with 0 ("no pain") on one end and 10 ("worst pain") on the other end. Patients are asked to place a mark along the line to denote their level of pain.

The primary advantage of the VAS is that it can give valid data for chronic and experimental pain that can be assessed parametrically.[9–11] However, other studies have questioned its validity when it is used to measure retrospective pain scores[12] or assess treatment efficacy.[13] A second concern is that some patients, especially older adults, may not be able to complete the scale. A third concern is that the VAS can be derived from other scores or that the VAS can be modified to a 5-m scale to somehow facilitate its use.

Other Single Dimension Pain Scales

Numerous variations of the numeric scale exist: the 11-point box scale (the numbers 0 through 10 are placed in individual boxes and patients are instructed to mark out the box that best corresponds to their pain), the 101-point numerical rating scale (patients are instructed to write the number between 0 and 100 that best describes their pain), and the 4-point and 5-point verbal rating scale. These methods are similar in accuracy and validity to the VAS.[14] A problem common to all numerical and descriptive pain scales is that they rely on the intact language skills of an intelligent patient. Facial drawings (Fig. 20–1) are reliable markers of pain designed specifically for use with children, the mentally handicapped, or patients with poor language skills.[15]

PATIENT SELF-REPORTING USING A MULTIDIMENSIONAL PAIN SCALE

Single dimension pain evaluation is probably the most commonly used method of evaluation in the pain clinic. However, if more than one dimension is desired, patients should be blinded to their previous VAS ratings,[13] or the data obtained are suspect. In addition, pain has a motivational-affective dimension that may not be appropriately measured on a single dimension assessment scale.[16] To overcome this limitation, multidimensional assessment tools were created to simultaneously evaluate multiple pain parameters.

McGill Pain Questionnaire

The McGill Pain Questionnaire (MPQ)[17] (Fig. 20–2) was developed in 1975 by Melzack and colleagues at the McGill University in an attempt to organize pain descriptors into a comprehensive evaluation tool.[18,19] It consists of three major measures: (1) pain rating index, which is based on the numerical score assigned to the descriptors; (2) total number of words chosen; and (3) the present pain intensity, which is a modification of the single dimension, 5-point verbal descriptive scale that is used to evaluate the intensity of pain at the time of completing the questionnaire.

The major strength of the MPQ is the pain rating index. This index is an organized list of words divided into subcategories of related words, which are rated on a common-intensity scale.[1] By evaluating the patient's responses (the number of words chosen) and the total score based on each subclass's intensity scale, it is possible to compare diagnosis and treatment in patients with varied pain syndromes.

The major sections in the pain rating index are designed to assess the three components of pain postulated by the gate control theory: the sensory, the affective, and the evaluative

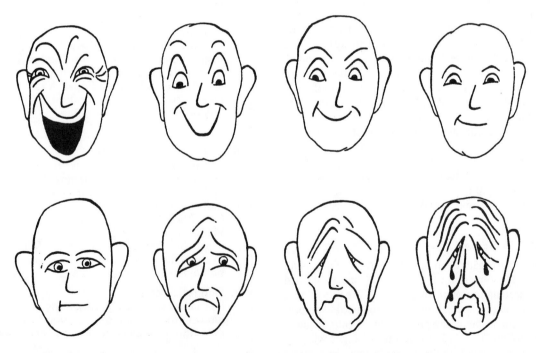

FIG. 20–1 Facial pain expressions. *(From Frank AJM, Moll LMH, Hort JF: A comparison of three ways of measuring pain.* Rheumatol Rehabil *21:211, 1982).*

McGill-Melzack
PAIN QUESTIONNAIRE

Patient's name _____ Age _____

File No. _____ Date _____

Clinical category (e.g. cardiac, neurological, etc.):

_____

Diagnosis: _____

_____

Analgesic (if already administered):

1. Type _____
2. Dosage _____
3. Time given in relation to this test _____

Patient's intelligence: circle number that represents best estimate

1 (low)　　　2　　　3　　　4　　　5 (high)

****

This questionnaire has been designed to tell us more about your pain. Four major questions we ask are:

1. Where is your pain?
2. What does it feel like?
3. How does it change with time?
4. How strong is it?

It is important that you tell us how your pain feels now. Please follow the instructions at the beginning of each part.

© R. Melzack, Oct. 1970

Part 1.　Where is your Pain?

Please mark, on the drawings below, the areas where you feel pain. Put E if external, or I if internal, near the areas which you mark. Put EI if both external and internal.

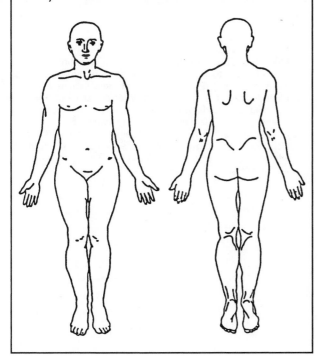

Part 2. What Does Your Pain Feel Like?

Some of the words below describe your present pain. Circle ONLY those words that best describe it. Leave out any category that is not suitable. Use only a single word in each appropriate category—the one that applies best.

1	2	3	4
Flickering	Jumping	Pricking	Sharp
Quivering	Flashing	Boring	Cutting
Pulsing	Shooting	Drilling	Lacerating
Throbbing		Stabbing	
Beating		Lancinating	
Pounding			
5	**6**	**7**	**8**
Pinching	Tugging	Hot	Tingling
Pressing	Pulling	Burning	Itchy
Gnawing	Wrenching	Scalding	Smarting
Cramping		Searing	Stinging
Crushing			
9	**10**	**11**	**12**
Dull	Tender	Tiring	Sickening
Sore	Taut	Exhausting	Suffocating
Hurting	Rasping		
Aching	Splitting		
Heavy			
13	**14**	**15**	**16**
Fearful	Punishing	Wretched	Annoying
Frightful	Grueling	Blinding	Troublesome
Terrifying	Cruel		Miserable
	Vicious		Intense
	Killing		Unbearable
17	**18**	**19**	**20**
Spreading	Tight	Cool	Nagging
Radiating	Numb	Cold	Nauseating
Penetrating	Drawing	Freezing	Agonizing
Piercing	Squeezing		Dreadful
	Tearing		Torturing

Part 3. How Does Your Pain Change With Time?

1. Which word or words would you use to describe the pattern of your pain?

1	2	3
Continuous	Rhythmic	Brief
Steady	Periodic	Momentary
Constant	Intermittent	Transient

2. What kind of things relieve your pain?

3. What kind of things increase your pain?

Part 4. How Strong Is Your Pain?

People agree that the following 5 words represent pain of increasing intensity. They are:

1	2	3	4	5
Mild	Discomforting	Distressing	Horrible	Excruciating

To answer each question below, write the number of the most appropriate word in the space beside the question.

1. Which word describes your pain right now? _____
2. Which word describes it at its worst? _____
3. Which word describes it when it is least? _____
4. Which word describes the worst toothache you ever had? _____
5. Which word describes the worst headache you ever had? _____
6. Which word describes the worst stomach-ache you ever had? _____

FIG. 20–2　The McGill Pain Questionnaire. *(From Melzack R: The McGill Pain Questionnaire: Major properties and scoring methods. Pain 1:277, 1971).*

dimensions. The subclasses of the pain rating index have been found to be reliable and valid measures of pain under diverse conditions.[18–20]

A major modification of the MPQ occurred when the short form MPQ[21] was introduced by Melzack in 1987 (Fig. 20–3). The major advantage of this questionnaire was its simplicity and ease of use while it correlated with the full MPQ.

Other Multidimensional Pain Scales

Numerous multidimensional inventories have been created to assess general chronic pain patients and specific pain syndromes. These inventories are, in general, modifications of MPQ or Minnesota Multiphasic Personality Inventory (MMPI) and possess the strengths and weaknesses of those inventories. Table 20–1 lists a representative sample of these inventories and their uses.

PSYCHOLOGIC AND BEHAVIORAL ASSESSMENT TOOLS

A major premise in the evaluation of pain is the assumption that pain can be evaluated using a disease process model.

With this model, the patient's cognitive assessment of pain is consistent with physical findings and single dimension or multidimensional self-assessment tools are used for pain measurement. However, this premise may not be valid in all patients. In situations in which the physical findings are absent or are insufficient to explain the extent of the patient's pain syndrome, behavioral analysis is indicated.[22]

Observation of the Pain Patient

The most common method of determining the behavioral component of a patient's pain is direct observation. A primary requirement for behavioral observation is a consistent examination that considers the potential psychologic pathology of the patient[22] and potential future therapeutic interventions.[23]

The physician typically assesses the history and physical examination and then categorizes the patient by using a rank ordered scheme such as no pain or minimal, mild, or severe pain. Other physicians classify patients using a four category system,[24] in which Class 1 consists of patients with low organic and high behavioral determinants, Class 2 patients have low organic and low behavioral determinants, Class 3 patients have high organic and high behavioral determi-

---

Short-form McGill Pain Questionnaire
Ronald Melzack

Patient's name: _____   Date: _____

	None	Mild	Moderate	Severe
Throbbing	0) ___	1) ___	2) ___	3) ___
Shooting	0) ___	1) ___	2) ___	3) ___
Stabbing	0) ___	1) ___	2) ___	3) ___
Sharp	0) ___	1) ___	2) ___	3) ___
Cramping	0) ___	1) ___	2) ___	3) ___
Gnawing	0) ___	1) ___	2) ___	3) ___
Hot-burning	0) ___	1) ___	2) ___	3) ___
Aching	0) ___	1) ___	2) ___	3) ___
Heavy	0) ___	1) ___	2) ___	3) ___
Tender	0) ___	1) ___	2) ___	3) ___
Splitting	0) ___	1) ___	2) ___	3) ___
Tiring-exhausting	0) ___	1) ___	2) ___	3) ___
Sickening	0) ___	1) ___	2) ___	3) ___
Fearful	0) ___	1) ___	2) ___	3) ___
Punishing-cruel	0) ___	1) ___	2) ___	3) ___

PPI   No pain |————————————————————| Worst possible pain

0 No pain   ___
1 Mild   ___
2 Discomforting ___
3 Distressing   ___
4 Horrible   ___
5 Excruciating   ___

© R. Melzack, 1984

FIG. 20–3 The short form McGill Pain Questionnaire. Descriptors 1 to 11 represent the sensory dimension of pain experience, and 12 to 15 represent the affective dimension. Each descriptor is ranked on an intensity scale of 0 = none, 1 = mild, 2 = moderate, and 3 = severe. The Present Pain Intensity of the standard long from McGill Pain Questionnaire (LF-MPQ) and visual analog scale (VAS) are also included to provide overall intensity scores. *(From Melzack R: The short form McGill Pain Questionnaire. Pain 30:191, 1987).*

nants, and Class 4 patients have a predominantly organic component to their pain.

Pain Diary

To assess pain behavior outside the clinical setting, various types of pain diaries have been used. Diaries assess nocturnal variation of the pain, factors that may aggravate or diminish it, and the effect of pain on activity and mobility. A potential weakness of the pain diary is that it may not correspond to what the medical staff observes.[25]

Pain Drawing

A major source of information in assessing pain is the patient's graphical depiction of the pain (Fig. 20–4). These drawings help identify the location of the pain and the type of pain perceived at the various locations of the body. Pain drawings have been extensively used in patients with back pain.[26]

Medication Use

Another method of monitoring patient behavior is to document medication use either with the aid of the patient or by enlisting the patient's family or a member of the medical staff.

SPECIAL CONSIDERATIONS

Guidelines for Test Instrument Selection

Before discussing specific pain situations, it is important to have an organized approach to the measurement of pain. Almost all patients can use at least one of the single-dimension pain measurement tools. These tools are easily understood by the patient, are easily administered by pain clinic staff, display appropriate reliability and validity, and produce results that can be used in assessing analgesic efficacy. Most patients can also understand the multidimensional tests, but their administration can be more time consuming than single-dimension tests. Behavioral testing is appropriate in many patients, especially those with a possible functional component to their pain. A sample algorithm[27] for pain evaluation is presented in Figure 20–5.

Laboratory Methods of Pain Management

Pain management in the laboratory consists of giving defined, readily controlled stimuli. This stimulus should be conveniently applied, produce minimal tissue damage, closely associate with changes that cause pain, and reproduce

TABLE 20–1 Multidimensional Pain Assessment Inventories

Name	Comments
Pain Disability Index[a]	Modified numeric pain scale, which includes category-defining activity. Useful in assessing patient's function.
Neck Disability Index[b]	Modification of the pain disability index.
Dallas Pain Questionnaire[c]	16-item VAS with items describing activity, personal relationships, and emotional status. Used in assessing back pain.
West Haven-Yale Multidimensional Pain Inventory (WHYMPI)[d]	Psychometric inventory including personal assessment, perceptions of significant others' attitudes toward the patient, and responses to defined activities.
Illness Behavior Questionnaire (IBQ)[e]	Similar to MMPI, with seven scales: hypochondriasis, disease conviction, psychologic perception of illness, affective inhibition, affective disturbance, denial, and irritability. Useful in assessing functional pain.
Western Ontario and McMaster (WOMAC) Osteoarthritis Index[f]	Specifically designed to assess osteoarthritis patients, this inventory consists of five dimensions: pain, stiffness, physical function, social function, and emotional function.
Descriptor Differential Scale (DDS)[g]	12-descriptor items (faint to extremely intense) for each dimension studied. Subject then marks on a 10-point scale whether perception is greater or less than each of the descriptors. This allows for easier scaling and intersubject evaluation. Usable for any chronic pain syndrome.
Wisconsin Brief Pain Questionnaire (WBPQ)[h]	Modified numeric pain scale measuring pain and therapy efficacy. Specifically designed for cancer pain but can be used for any chronic syndrome.
Sickness Impact Profile[i,j]	Assesses functional status and correlates well with MMPI regarding emotional and affective condition of patient.
Abu-Saad Pediatric Pain Assessment Tool[k]	A modified MPQ for children. Written in Dutch.

[a]Taff RC, Chibnall JT, Krause S: The Pain Disability Index: Psychometric properties. *Pain* 49:171, 1980.
[b]Vernon H, Mior S: The neck disability index: A study of reliability and validity. *J Manipulative Physiol Ther* 14:409, 1991.
[c]Lawlis GF, Cuencas R, Selby D et al: The development of the Dallas Pain Questionnaire: An assessment of the impact of spinal pain on behavior. *Spine* 14:511, 1989.
[d]Kerns RD, Turk DC, Rudy TE: The West Haven-Yale Multidimensional Pain Inventory (WHYMPI). *Pain* 23:345, 1985.
[e]Pilowsky I, Spence N, Cobb J et al: The Illness Behavior Questionnaire as an aid to clinical assessment. *Gen Hosp Psychiatry* 6:123, 1984.
[f]Bellamy N: Pain assessment in osteoarthritis: Experience with the WOMAC Osteoarthritis Index. *Semin Arthritis Rheum* 18:14, 1989.
[g]Gracely RH, Kwilosz J: The Descriptor Differential Scale: Applying psychophysical principles to clinical pain assessment. *Pain* 35:379, 1988.
[h]Daut RL, Cleeland CS, Flanery RC: Development of the Wisconsin Brief Pain Questionnaire to assess pain in cancer and other diseases. *Pain* 17:197, 1983.
[i]Bergner M, Bobbitt RA, Carter WB et al: The Sickness Impact Profile: Development and final revision of a health status measure. *Med Care* 19:787, 1981.
[j]Follick MJ, Smith TW, Ahern DK: The Sickness Impact Profile: A global measure of disability in chronic low back pain. *Pain* 21:67, 1985.
[k]Abu-Saad HH, Kroonen E, Halfens R: On the development of a multidimensional Dutch pain assessment tool for children. *Pain* 43:249, 1990.
MMPI, Minnesota Multiphasic Personality Inventory; MPQ, McGill Pain Questionnaire; VAS, visual analog scale.

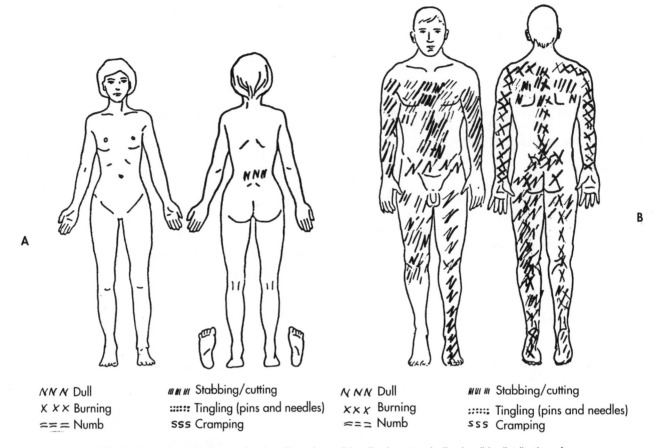

⋀⋀⋀ Dull	⫽⫽⫽ Stabbing/cutting	⋀⋀⋀ Dull	⫽⫽⫽ Stabbing/cutting
X X X Burning	∷∷∷ Tingling (pins and needles)	X X X Burning	∷∷∷ Tingling (pins and needles)
≈≈≈ Numb	sss Cramping	≈≈≈ Numb	sss Cramping

FIG. 20–4 *A,* An organic pain drawing. Note the well-localized, anatomically plausible distribution of pain. *B,* A nonorganic pain drawing. Note the widespread, poorly defined pattern of pain distribution. *(From Udén A, Åströmm M, Bergenudd, H: Pain drawings in chronic back pain. Spine 13:389, 1988).*

the quantitative measurements of the pain threshold under the same conditions.[28] The major differences between laboratory and clinical pain measurement are:

1. Laboratory pain is usually acute; therefore, the psychologic overlays present in patients with chronic pain do not play a major role.
2. The subject understands that the pain will be limited and can be terminated at any time.

Furthermore, these differences make direct comparisons between laboratory data and clinical scenarios difficult.

Cancer Pain

Cancer pain may have an insidious onset and is often due to many factors. In addition, the characteristics and intensity of the pain are dependent on the type of pain (bone, musculoskeletal, neuropathic, or visceral). Often the patients are on narcotics and other medications that may affect their ability to communicate. Verbal rating scales, VAS, and the MPQ have been used, but each has specific weaknesses.[29] Verbal rating scales and VAS only rate pain intensity and are not affective components; yet MPQ is often misunderstood by the elderly and debilitated patients who make up this population.

A major problem in the treatment of cancer patients remains in the lack of correlation between the patient's self-reporting and the assessment of clinical staff.[30,31]

Psychiatric Pain

The psychiatric assessment of pain is an important but complicated part of the evaluation. The diagnosis of functional pain should be entertained if there is disparity between the patient's VAS and the present pain intensity section of the MPQ.[32] Also, certain psychiatric diseases may present with pain.

Geriatric Pain

A recent study found that approximately 80% of patients in nursing homes complain of pain.[33] The assessment of pain in this population can be complicated by communication difficulties resulting from stroke or dementia and confusion with the instructions for the commonly used assessment tools.[34]

Pediatric Pain

It is now known that even neonates experience pain.[15] A child's perception of pain is based on the following factors: sex, age, cognitive level, previous experience of pain, family learning, and culture. Before understanding and completing a VAS, observed behavior (crying, nervousness, grimacing, etc.) is the major assessment tool. Older children can be tested with the modified MPQ and the VAS. For younger children, the faces pain scale is used (see Fig. 20–1),[35,36] which is a modification of the numerical rating scale.

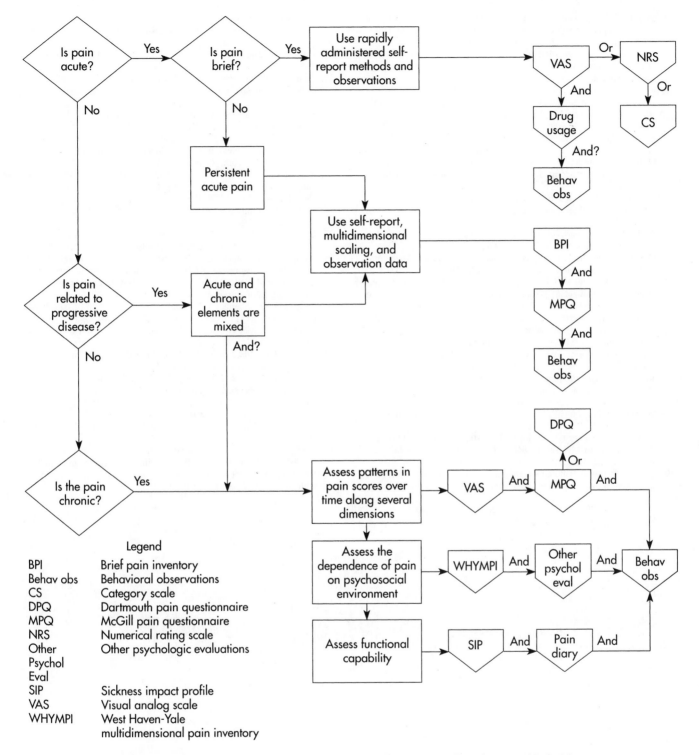

FIG. 20–5 Algorithm for selection of pain measurement instruments. *(From Chapman CR, Syrjala KL: Measurement of pain. In Bonica JJ, editor: The management of pain, ed 2. Philadelphia, Lea & Febiger, 1990).*

Legend

BPI	Brief pain inventory
Behav obs	Behavioral observations
CS	Category scale
DPQ	Dartmouth pain questionnaire
MPQ	McGill pain questionnaire
NRS	Numerical rating scale
Other Psychol Eval	Other psychologic evaluations
SIP	Sickness impact profile
VAS	Visual analog scale
WHYMPI	West Haven-Yale multidimensional pain inventory

SUMMARY

Pain ratings per se cannot be used as an endpoint; clinical correlation and individualized treatment must be used. The clinician should remember to act on what is learned; this is really what matters.

References

1. Melzack R, Torgerson WS: On the language of pain. *Anesthesiology* 34:50, 1971.
2. Aitken RC: Measurement of feelings using visual analog scales. *Proc R Soc Med* 62(10):989–93, 1969.
3. Woodfore JM, Merskey H: Correlation between verbal scale and visual analogue scale and pressure algometer. *J Psychom Res* 16:173, 1971.

4. Duncan GH, Bushnell MC, Lavigne GJ: Comparison of verbal and visual analogue scales for measuring the intensity and unpleasantness of experimental pain. *Pain* 37:295, 1989.

5. Ohnhaus EE, Adler R: Methodological problems in the measurement of pain: A comparison between the verbal rating scale and the visual analog scale. *Pain* 1:379, 1975.

6. Ferraz MB, Quaresma MR, Aquino LR et al: Reliability of pain scales in the assessment of literate and illiterate patients with rheumatoid arthritis. *J Rheumatol* 17:1022, 1990.

7. Joos E, Peretz A, Beguin S et al: Reliability and reproducibility of visual analog scale and numeric rating scale for therapeutic evaluation of pain in rheumatic patients [Letter]. *J Rheumatol* 18:1269, 1991.

8. Linten SJ, Götesam KG: A clinical comparison of two scales: Correlation, remembering chronic pain, and a measure of compliance. *Pain* 17:57, 1983.

9. Price DD, McGrath PA, Rafii A et al: The validation of visual analog scales as ratio scale measures for chronic and experimental pain. *Pain* 17:45, 1983.

10. Phillip BK: Parametric statistics for evaluation of the visual analog scale [Letter]. *Anesth Analg* 71:708, 1990.

11. Flandry F, Hunt JP, Terry GC et al: Analysis of subjective knee complaints using visual analog scales. *Am J Sports Med* 19:112, 1991.

12. Lui WHD, Aitkenhead AR: Comparison of contemporaneous and retrospective assessment of postoperative pain using the visual analog scale. *Br J Anaesth* 67:768, 1991.

13. Carlsson AM: Assessment of chronic pain: I. Aspects of the reliability and validity of the visual analog scale. *Pain* 16:87, 1983.

14. Jensen MP, Karoly P, Braver S: The measurement of clinical pain intensity: A comparison of six methods. *Pain* 27:117, 1986.

15. Frank AJM, Moll LMH, Hort JF: A comparison of three ways of measuring pain. *Rheumatol Rehabil* 21:211, 1982.

16. Melzack R: Concepts of pain measurement. In Melzack R, editor: *Pain measurement and assessment.* New York, Raven Press, 1983.

17. Melzack R: The McGill Pain Questionnaire: Major properties and scoring methods. *Pain* 1:277, 1975.

18. Prieter EJ, Geisinger KF: Factor-analytic studies of the McGill Pain Questionnaire. In Melzack R, editor: *Pain measurement and assessment.* New York, Raven Press, 1983.

19. Melzack R: The McGill Pain Questionnaire. In Melzack R, editor: *Pain measurement and assessment.* New York, Raven Press, 1983.

20. Reading AE: The McGill Pain Questionnaire: An appraisal. In Melzack R, editor: *Pain measurement and assessment.* New York, Raven Press, 1983.

21. Melzack R: The short-form McGill Pain Questionnaire. *Pain* 30:191, 1987.

22. Fordyce WE: The behavioral analysis of pain. In Fordyce WE, editor: *Behavioral methods for chronic pain and illness.* St. Louis, Mosby, 1976.

23. Keefe FJ, Gil KM: Behavioral concepts in the analysis of chronic pain syndromes. *J Consult Clin Psychol* 54:776, 1986.

24. Hammonds W, Brenna S: Pain classification and vocational evaluation of chronic pain states. In Melzack R, editor: *Pain measurement and assessment.* New York, Raven Press, 1983.

25. Kremer EF, Block A, Gaylor MS: Behavior approaches to treatment of chronic pain: The inaccuracy of patient self-report measures. *Arch Phys Med Rehabil* 62:188, 1981.

26. Udún A, Åströmm M, Bergenudd H: Pain drawings in chronic back pain. *Spine* 13:389, 1988.

27. Chapman CR, Syrjala KL: Measurement of pain. In Bonica JJ, editor: *The management of pain,* ed 2. Philadelphia, Lea & Febiger, 1990.

28. Wolff BB: Laboratory methods of pain measurement. In Melzack R, editor: *Pain measurement and assessment.* New York, Raven Press, 1983.

29. Deschamps M, Band P, Coldman AJ: Assessment of adult cancer pain: Shortcomings of current methods. *Pain* 32:133, 1988.

30. Grossman SA, Sheidler VR, Swedeen K: Correlation of patient and caregiver ratings of cancer pain. *J Pain Symptom Manage* 6:53, 1991.

31. Cleeland CS: Measurement and prevalence of pain in cancer. *Semin Oncol Nurs* 1:87, 1985.

32. Perry F, Heller PH, Levine JD: A possible indicator of functional pain: Poor pain scale correlation. *Pain* 46:191, 1991.

33. Roy R, Thomas MR: A survey of chronic pain in the elderly population. *Can Fam Physician Med Fam Can* 32:513, 1986.

34. Herr KA, Mobily PR: Complexities of pain assessment in the elderly: Clinical considerations. *J Gerontol Nurs* 17:12, 1991.

35. McGrath PA: Evaluating a child's pain. *J Pain Symptom Manage* 4:198, 1989.

36. Bieri D, Reeve RA, Champion GD et al: The faces pain scale for the self-assessment of the severity of pain experienced by children: Development, initial validation, and preliminary investigation for ratio scale properties. *Pain* 41:139, 1990.

1. The visual analog scale is characterized by all of the following except

    A. It is a progression of the numerical pain scale
    B. It uses a 10-cm line with 0 on one side and 10 on the other
    C. It is a multidimensional pain scale
    D. The patient is asked to place a mark along the line to denote the level of pain

2. The major strength of the McGill Pain Questionnaire (MPQ) is that it is organized as a list of words, which are rated on a common intensity scale. It is possible to compare diagnosis and treatment with various pain syndromes by calculating the score obtained by the patients' responses. All of the following are part of the evaluation except

    A. The number of words chosen
    B. The total score based on each subclass intensity scale
    C. Rating of the common intensity scale
    D. Rating of the patient's depression scale

3. To assess pain behavior outside the clinical setting, various types of pain diaries have been used. Diaries assess all of the following except

    A. Nocturnal variation of the pain
    B. Effect of the pain on activity and mobility
    C. Correlation with medical staff observations
    D. Serial documentation of day to day pain intensity

4. The laboratory methods of pain management have all of the following characteristics except

    A. Measurement is usually for acute pain
    B. Psychologic overlay of the patients are usually not determined
    C. Subject may not understand that the pain will be limited
    D. Pain can be terminated at any time

5. Approximately 80% of patients in nursing homes complain of pain. The assessment of pain in this population can be complicated due to all of the following except

    A. Communication difficulties
    B. Dementia
    C. Arthritis
    D. Alzheimer's disease

ANSWERS

1. C
2. D
3. C
4. C
5. C

CHAPTER 21

Diagnostic Tools Available for Pain Management

BERNARD M. ABRAMS, HOWARD J. WALDMAN,
VALERIE R. ECKARD, SOLOMON BATNITZKY,
DONALD ECKARD, ALON P. WINNIE,
AND KENNETH D. CANDIDO

ELECTROMYOGRAPHY

Electromyography (EMG) as an extension of the clinical examination is a useful adjunct in the diagnosis and management of pain. EMG is a method of testing both the physiologic state and the anatomic integrity of lower motor neuron structures, their sensory components, and some spinal and brainstem reflex pathways.[1] Conditions in which EMG may be of use include painful peripheral neuropathies, entrapment neuropathies, traumatic nerve injuries, radicular and multiradicular problems, lumbar spinal stenosis, arachnoiditis, and painful myopathies.

The problems inherent in applying electrodiagnostic techniques to pain diagnosis and management are no different from those encountered in history taking, physical examination, radiologic evaluation, and therapeutic diagnostic testing. Pain is a subjective experience, often without an objective "litmus test."

Electrodiagnosis is an extremely useful investigative technique in evaluating the patient with pain because it satisfies two fundamental steps[2] in the assessment of neuropathic pain syndrome, before any attempt at therapy:

1. Rigorously establishing the presence or absence of a peripheral nervous system lesion
2. Determining the relevance of an established peripheral neuropathic lesion to the subjective clinical complaint

In brief, electrodiagnosis techniques may occasionally be helpful for central nervous system (CNS) disorders[3] but are more useful in disorders of the nerve roots, plexus lesions, neuropathies, and disorders of the peripheral nerves and less often in painful myopathies.

Electrical Testing of Nerves and Muscles

Brief History

Lord Adrian performed the first experimental work with EMG in 1925. In 1928, Proebster first described the presence of "spontaneous irregular action potentials in denervated muscle."[4] In its progression to clinical application, EMG made a major step forward with the use of the cathode ray oscilloscope, as well as with the concentric needle electrode and loudspeaker.[5] Vast numbers of nerve injuries in World War II and later conflicts added further impetus to the study of nerve and muscle by electrodiagnostic technique.

The Electrodiagnostic Method

There are four components to an electrical diagnostic measurement system[6]:

1. Electrodes
2. Stimulator
3. High-gain differential amplifier
4. Recording display or central processing device

The EMG apparatus amplifies and displays biologic information derived from surface or needle electrodes. Electrical information may be recorded from muscles, nerves, or other nervous system structures and is displayed on an oscilloscope. A permanent recording may be made, audio amplification may allow it to be heard over a loudspeaker, and analog-digital analysis of signals may be used. Electrical nerve stimulation is used to stimulate nerves to measure nerve conduction.

For nerve conduction studies, skin surface electrodes are used to record compound muscle or nerve action potentials. For needle EMG, needle electrodes are used with a strong trend toward disposable needles. For sensory testing, ring electrodes are used for measurement.

Precautions for testing include extra care with patients who are taking coumadin or other blood thinners, who have hemophilia or other blood dyscrasias, whose status is positive for HIV, or who have a cardiac pacemaker or transcutaneous stimulator.[1]

Physiology

Physiologic Mechanisms in the Production of Muscle Potentials

When an impulse arrives at the region of the junction between nerve and muscle, the entire muscle fiber is thrown into an almost simultaneous contraction. This is brought about by a wave of excitation that moves rapidly along the fiber surface and stimulates the contractile substance as it passes over the fiber. The stimulus is transmitted along the fiber by an excitable membrane that surrounds the muscle fiber. The action potential results from the breakdown of the surface membrane potential, which is associated with critical changes in ionic permeability. In the resting muscle fiber, the potential difference across the surface membrane is 90 mV, with negative inside and positive outside. During excitation, the resting potential temporarily reverses to 40 mV, negative outside.

In recording extracellularly, as in EMG, the electrode picks up the action potential as it is conducted through the medium that surrounds the active fiber. The impedance of the external medium is small compared with the impedance of the fiber interior. The functional unit in reflex or voluntary activity is the motor unit; the group of muscle fibers innervated by a single anterior horn cell.

Conduction along the fine intramuscular branches of the anterior horn cell axon occurs so rapidly that all muscle fibers in a motor unit are activated nearly simultaneously. The number of muscle fibers per motor unit varies considerably from muscle to muscle. The motor unit is various muscles covering differing areas of muscle cross-section. The distribution of fibers is such that fibers from several different motor units are intermingled, which is why four to six motor units can be identified by EMG from the same intramuscular recording point. In normal muscle, these single motor unit potentials can be differentiated only during weak voluntary effort.[7,8]

The potentials from different motor units are recognized by their frequency of discharge, which varies from each motor unit. Moreover, the various potentials often differ in appearance because of the differential distance of the recording electrode from the individual fibers of the activated motor units and the differential distribution of the motor end plates in the several units within range of a concentric or single needle electrode in one position in the muscle. An upward deflection on the oscilloscope is considered electrically negative, and a downward deflection is considered electrically positive. In the immediate vicinity of a potential, there is an upward or a negative deflection.

Physiology of Nerve Conduction

The cell membrane of a nerve axon separates the intracellular axoplasm from the extracellular fluid.[9] The unequal distribution of ions between these fluids produces a potential difference across the cell membrane. When a nerve fiber is stimulated, it causes a change in the membrane potential; a rapid but brief flow of sodium ions occurs through ionic channels inward across the cell membrane, giving rise to an action potential.

The way in which an action potential is conducted along an axon depends on whether the axon is myelinated or unmyelinated.[10] In a *myelinated* fiber, the action potential is regenerated only at the nodes of Ranvier, so that the resulting action potentials jump from node to node, yielding saltatory conduction. The velocity of nerve conduction depends on the diameter of the myelinated fiber. Small myelinated fibers may conduct as slowly as 12 m/sec, whereas large motor and sensory fibers conduct at a rate of 50 to 70 m/sec. In an *unmyelinated* fiber, the conduction is about 2 m/sec.

Several factors affect conduction velocity other than whether or not the axon is myelinated[9,11]:

1. Temperature of the limb
2. Age of the patient
3. Height of the patient

Basic Examination

EMG must be combined with the clinical examination of the patient by the electromyographer. This includes a grading of muscle strength. It is of prime importance for the electromyographer to personally correlate clinical data and the data obtained by EMG. Each examination must be planned individually. The electromyographer determines the segment or segments of the peripheral nervous system to either substantiate or invalidate the presumptive clinical diagnoses.

Conducting the Examination

The needle examination is designed to determine:

1. Integrity of muscle and its nervous system
2. Location of any abnormality
3. Any abnormalities of the muscle

The electrodes may be monopolar or concentric. The examination proceeds through the following steps[7,12]:

1. Determination of activity of the muscle in the relaxed state
2. Evaluation of any insertional activity that arises
3. Assessment of the activity seen on weak voluntary effort
4. Determination of the pattern seen on the maximum voluntary effort, known as the interference pattern

Needle Findings in Normal Muscle

Insertional Activity

When the needle is inserted into a normal muscle, it evokes a brief burst of electrical activity that lasts no more than 2 to 3 msec, a little longer than the actual movement of the needle.[3] This activity is described as insertional activity and is generally 50 to 250 mV (Fig. 21–1*A*). These insertional potentials are believed to represent discharges from muscle fibers produced by injury, mechanical stimulation, or irritation.

Spontaneous Activity

When the needle is stationary and the muscle is relaxed, there is no electrical activity present in normal muscle (except when the needle is in the area of the end plate). Two types of end-plate "noise" are normal (see Fig. 21–1*C*):

1. Low-amplitude and undulating
2. High-amplitude intermittent discharges

Any other spontaneous activity is abnormal. An increase in duration of insertional activity may be seen in loss of innervation or primary disease of muscle fiber.[3] Reduction may occur in myopathies or more advanced degeneration in which muscle tissue has been replaced by fat or fibrous connective tissue.[13]

Voluntary Activity

Voluntary activity of the muscle is analyzed after the muscle is studied at rest (see Fig. 21–1*D*). Electrical activity, or *motor unit action potential,* is noted. The force of contraction determines the number of motor units brought into play.[7,8] This begins with a single motor unit that fires and can be identified on the screen by its distinctive morphology. As the effort increases, other motor units come into play. As the contraction increases, the firing rate of each individual motor unit action potential increases, and the action potential is subsequently joined by other motor unit action potentials whose firing rates also increase. This phenomenon is known as *recruitment* (see Fig. 21–2*A* to *C*). In normal muscles, the strength of a voluntary muscle contraction is directly related to the number of individual motor units that have been recruited and their firing rate.[8,14] Analysis of motor units includes:

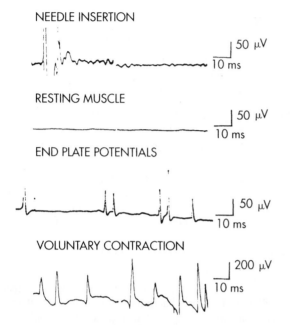

FIG. 21–1 *A*, Trace shows normal insertional activity. *B*, No spontaneous activity in a normal muscle at rest. *C*, Spontaneous end-plate potentials. *D*, Normal biphasic and triphasic motor unit potentials during weak voluntary contraction.

1. Waveform
2. Amplitude
3. Interference patterns

Waveform

Most units are biphasic or triphasic. The number of phases is determined by the "baseline crossings." Motor units that cross the baseline or have more than five phases are called polyphasic motor units. Polyphasic potentials are a measure of fiber synchrony.

Amplitude

The amplitude depends on the number of fibers in the motor unit and the type of EMG needle used. Normal amplitude ranges from 1 to 5 mV.

Interference Patterns

With maximum voluntary effort a large number of motor units are brought into play and their firing rate increases. They tend to interfere with each other, and they are not recognized further as individual units. This gives rise to the situation that is called an interference pattern (see Fig. 21–2*A* to *C*). In a normal muscle, there is a "full" interference pattern.

Various abnormalities may occur that indicate the presence of total denervation—neurogenic paresis, peripheral type, or neurogenic pareses, anterior horn cell type. In addition, myogenic pareses may be detected. The following are needle abnormalities in abnormal muscles:

1. Insertional activity
2. Spontaneous activity
3. Abnormalities of voluntary motor activity, especially recruitment
4. Abnormal motor unit morphology

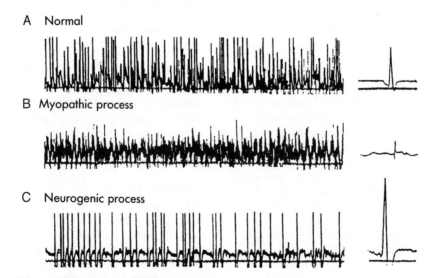

FIG. 21–2 *A*, Full interference pattern on maximum effort in a normal muscle. *B*, Full interference pattern in a myopathic muscle on submaximal effort. *C*, Reduced interference pattern in a denervated muscle on maximal effort resulting from the loss of motor units.

Nerve conduction studies are of value in the following cases:

1. Determining whether a disease of nerve is present
2. Determining the distribution of a neuropathy
3. Determining at what point in a nerve there is conduction block and locating an entrapment site
4. Studying the progress of disease of a peripheral nerve
5. Seeing whether there is reinnervation of a previously sectioned nerve
6. Establishing in a disease of the myoneural junction that conduction along the nerve is adequate or normal

Conduction velocity studies are carried out by the insertion of a needle electrode into a muscle innervated by the nerve under study or by the use of surface electrodes over that muscle. Textbooks of stimulation points and pick-up points are readily available.[8,15] Normal values are usually established for each nerve in individual laboratories, but normal values for commonly tested sensory and motor nerves are generally available (Table 21–1). Median nerve stimulation is comparable to ulnar nerve stimulation.

F-Wave

Definition

Motor conduction velocity along the whole axon, including proximal portions, can be studied by eliciting the F-wave response, which is a small, late muscle response that occurs from backfiring of anterior horn cells.[16–18] F-waves may be obtained from almost any mixed nerve that can be stimulated, but the median, ulnar, peroneal, and posterior tibial nerves are the most commonly used. If standard distal motor conduction velocities are normal but the F-wave value is prolonged, slowing must be occurring somewhere more proximal to the distal normal segment. Limb temperature and arm or leg length also may be important to know. A comparison with the opposite limb may be most helpful if that limb is asymptomatic.

Pitfalls and Comments

In addition to the variability of F-waves, many electromyographers overuse the F-wave study when proximal slowing in a nerve or nerve root is not even in the differential diagnosis.

Hoffman Reflex (H-Reflex)

Definition

The H-reflex is obtained by electrostimulation of the posterior tibial nerve in the popliteal space at a slow rate with long duration and submaximal electrical shock; it is recorded with surface electrodes over the gastrocnemius-soleus. The impulse travels up the sensory fibers to the spinal cord, synapses with the alpha motor neuron, and returns down the motor fibers to the calf muscle. H-reflex latencies are, therefore, long, in the range of 40 to 45 msec. To determine a delay or an asymmetry, one should always study the opposite leg for comparison.[19–22]

Pitfalls and Comments

The H-reflex is somewhat more useful than the F-wave, but the main reason for the study can be seen in the evaluation of a suspected S1 radiculopathy. Usually when an absent H-reflex is noted, suggesting a problem with S1 nerve root conduction, an absent or depressed ankle reflex has already been noted in the physical examination, so the study is redundant. Pitfalls occur when the opposite leg is not studied to show normal H-reflex as a contrast. Older patients often do not have good H-reflexes as a normal finding. In addition, a unilaterally absent H-reflex with normal needle EMG examination does not indicate when the injury occurred.

Quantitative Sensory Testing (Pseudomotor Axon Reflex Test)

Quantitative sensory testing takes various forms, including the quantitative somatosensory thermotest using a controlled ramp of ascending or descending temperature through a Peltier device.[23] Certain abnormal patterns are characteristic of dysfunction of small-caliber peripheral nerve afferents.[24] To obtain maximal information from a quantitative somatosensory thermotest, it is necessary to test for cold, pain, and heat sensations, mandatory in the evaluation of painful syndromes.[25] Quantitative sensory testing performed at different sites along an extremity in cases of polyneuropathy yields useful information about staging of the pathologic process along the extremity.

The quantitative pseudomotor axon reflex test (Q-sart) is a quantitative thermoregulatory sweat test. It has been used to detect postganglionic pseudomotor failure in neuropathies[26,27] and preganglionic neuropathies with presumed trans-synaptic degeneration.[28]

Clinical Correlations

Clinical correlations can be based on a careful history, clinical examination, and electrodiagnostic studies. Electrodiagnostic

---

TABLE 21–1 Normal Values for Commonly Tested Sensory and Motor Nerves

Nerves	Amplitude (Avg.)	Distal Latency inmilliseconds (Avg.)*	Conduction Velocity in meters/sec (Avg.)
Median (sensory)	10–85 µV (20)	2.0–3.7 (3.2)	
Ulnar (sensory)	5–70 µV (15)	1.6–3.2 (2.8)	
Radial (sensory)	10–60 µV (18)	1.7–2.8 (2.4)	
Median (motor)	5–25 mV (8)	2.0–4.0 (3.3)	48–69 (54)
Ulnar (motor)	5.5–20 mV (8)	1.6–3.1 (2.6)	50–69 (55)
Sural (sensory)	3–38 mV (8)		2.3–4.6 (4.1)
Peroneal (motor)	2.5–18 mV (4)	2.3–6.0 (4.1)	41–61 (46)
Posterior tibial (motor)	4–38 mV (11)	2.1–6.0 (4.3)	41–58 (45)

*Distal latencies are based on standard distance: 13 cm for median (S); 11 cm for ulnar (S); 10 cm for radial (S); 14 cm for sural (S); 4 to 6 cm for median (S) and ulnar (M); 6 to 8 cm for peroneal (M); 8 to 12 cm for the posterior tibial (M) nerves.

M, Motor; MV, millivolt; S, sensory; µV, microvolt.

studies are best for separating neuropathy from myopathy and determining if a neuropathy is generalized axonal, demyelinating, mixed, or focal. Furthermore, nerve trauma can be follow up serially to determine recovery.

Nerve Trauma

Often after injury, the nerve is completely severed. At rest, denervation potentials are recorded in the muscles supplied by that nerve in the form of positive sharp waves of fibrillation potentials, and, on EMG, no motor unit action potentials are seen.

Neurapraxia

Neurapraxia is the mildest form of nerve injury. It consists of conduction loss without associated axonal structural changes. This form of conduction block often occurs with compressive or ischemic nerve injuries. In neuropraxic injuries, focal demyelination occurs. Serial nerve conduction determinations along the course of the nerve enable one to locate the conduction block.

Axonotmesis

In axonotmesis, a more severe form of nerve injury, the axon is disrupted in its myelin sheath. The neural tube, consisting of the endoperineurium and epineurium, remains intact. The nerve undergoes wallerian degeneration, with fragmentation of the axon distal to the site of injury. Motor and sensory paralysis occurs with associated atrophy of supplied muscle and loss of reflexes.

Neurotmesis

Neurotmesis is the most severe form of nerve injury and consists of severe disruption or transection of the nerve. Nerve regeneration and recovery are often incomplete and may require surgical reanastomosis. Neuromas may form and are commonly associated with pain.

Nontraumatic Neuropathies

In a patient with a nontraumatic neuropathy, segmental demyelination is generally associated with slowing of nerve conduction velocities and temporal dispersion of evoked responses. With axonal degeneration, however, reduction of the evoked response amplitudes with mild or minimal slowing of nerve conduction velocities is typical.

Polyneuropathy

EMG and nerve conduction evaluation are useful in diagnosing polyneuropathy and in determining whether a pathologic process is axonal and demyelinating. A diagnosis of polyneuropathy is made when abnormal nerve conduction and EMG findings are bilateral and symmetric.

Generalized peripheral neuropathies often associated with pain are noted in Box 21–1.[29–34] Electrodiagnostic findings characteristic of axonal neuropathy are as follows:

1. Abnormally low or absent sensory nerve action potentials and compound muscle action potential amplitudes
2. Normal distal latencies
3. Near-normal motor and sensory conduction velocities

If a disease process affects the large-diameter axons, some slowing of conduction occurs; the velocity is seldom reduced by more than 20% to 20% of normal. In contrast, diffuse demyelinating neuropathy is characterized by reduction of conduction velocities, usually more than 40% of the normal range. In a pure demyelinating neuropathy, there is no denervation of muscle fibers.

Once it has been determined electromyographically whether a neuropathy is primarily axonal or demyelinating, one can then consider clinically which neuropathies are diffusely axonal and which are demyelinating. Subacute and chronic diffuse axonal types include most toxic and nutritional neuropathies, uremia, diabetes, hypothyroidism, HIV infection, and Lyme disease. Demyelinating polyneuropathies include hereditary motor and sensory neuropathies, types 1 and 3; Refsum's disease; multifocal leukodystrophy; and Krabbe's disease. Acute nonuniform demyelinating diseases include Guillain-Barré syndrome, diphtheria, and acute arsenic intoxication, whereas chronic versions include inflammatory demyelinating peripheral neuropathy, idiopathic disease, and neuropathies accompanying HIV.[35]

Mononeuropathies and Entrapment Neuropathies

With an entrapment neuropathy, the most commonly involved nerves are the median, ulnar, radial, common peroneal, and tibial. Entities such as trauma, vasculitis, diabetes mellitus, leprosy, and sarcoidosis can affect any nerve in the body.

Median Nerve

The median nerve is commonly entrapped at the wrist as it passes through the carpal tunnel. The diagnosis of carpal tunnel syndrome is made by demonstrating localized slowing of sensory and motor conductions across the wrist as evidenced by prolonged sensory and motor distal latencies.[1]

Pronator Teres and Anterior Interosseous Syndromes

The pronator teres and anterior interosseous syndrome are proximal compression or entrapment neuropathies of the median nerve.[36]

Ulnar Nerve

The ulnar nerve is usually injured at the elbow but occasionally at the wrist in the canal of Guyon or deep in the

---

BOX 21–1 Generalized Peripheral Neuropathies

Diabetes mellitus
Polyneuropathy associated with insulinoma
Polyneuropathy associated with nutritional
  deficiency
Alcohol-nutritional deficiency polyneuropathy
Vasculitis-associated neuropathy
Amyloidosis
Toxic (arsenic and thallium)
HIV-related distal symmetric polyneuropathy
Fabry's disease
Guillain-Barré syndrome
Cryptogenic sensory or sensorimotor neuropathy
Polyneuropathy resulting from neoplasm,
  including paraneoplastic syndromes

palm. When the lesion is in the wrist at the canal of Guyon, usually both sensory and motor fibers are involved and the amplitude of the sensory nerve action potential and muscle action is reduced. With a lesion in the deep palmar branch, there is no sensory abnormality and all of the changes are in the motor distribution distal to the lesion. When the abnormality is at the elbow, there may be localized slowing of conduction velocity across the elbow.[37-39]

Radial Nerve

The radial nerve is usually involved at the spiral groove of the humerus, often secondary to a humeral fracture. With a lesion at the spinal groove, the triceps muscle is spared on EMG, but all of the exterior muscles of the forearm are involved.

Posterior Interosseous Syndrome

The posterior interosseus nerve syndrome occurs from entrapment of this radial nerve branch at the arcade of Frohse between the two heads of the supinator. EMG shows involvement of the exterior carpi ulnaris, exterior digitorum longus, extensor pollicis longus, and extensor indicis while sparing the more proximal supinator and extensor carpi radialis longus and brevis.[40]

Posterior Tibial Nerve at the Ankle

The posterior tibial nerve is derived from L4 through S3 roots and may be compressed in the tarsal tunnel. Nerve conduction studies show prolongation of the distal motor and sensory latency of the tibial nerve.[41-43]

Other Neuropathies

Some other neuropathies include those of the common peroneal nerve and the sciatic nerve. More uncommon mononeuropathies include those involving the long thoracic nerve, dorsal scapular nerve, suprascapular nerve, musculocutaneous nerves, and axillary nerves in the shoulder girdle and upper extremity.

Radiculopathies

Radiculopathies are disease of the nerve roots and must be differentiated from plexopathies as well as from complex individual nerve root lesions. Roots are commonly involved by compression, especially in the cervical and lumbar regions. Motor and sensory nerve conductions are rarely useful because the lesion in a radiculopathy is proximal to the dorsal root ganglion and motor conduction studies are usually normal. Because most limb muscles are supplied by more than one nerve root (Tables 21–2 and 21–3), a normal study does not exclude the diagnosis of radiculopathy.

Plexopathies

In plexopathies, motor conduction studies are useful in excluding a peripheral nerve lesion; otherwise, findings are normal except that amplitudes of compound muscle action potentials may be reduced. Sensory nerve conductions are usually helpful in excluding other causes.

Anterior Horn Cell Disease

Disorders of the anterior horn cell do not cause pain except for acute poliomyelitis.

Disorders of the Central Nervous System

EMG findings are almost always normal in diseases of the CNS.

Primary Muscle Disorders

One of the clearest applications of EMG is in differentiating myopathies from neuropathic processes. In myopathy, the potentials are reduced in amplitude and may be very polyphasic, recruit paradoxically, and are accompanied by marked signs of irritability. In *polymyositis* and *metabolic muscle disorders,* sensory nerve conductions are always normal. The compound muscle action potential amplitude may be low, but otherwise motor conduction results are normal.

Usefulness and Limitations of Electromyography

EMG and nerve conduction studies are useful in localizing neuromuscular disease sites and in providing information about the nature of the process but cannot give the cause. Figure 21–3 presents a summary of EMG findings in various conditions. In addition, a normal result does not mean the patient does not have pain. Sympathetic and small unmyelinated nerve fiber functions are not evaluated by quantitative

TABLE 21–2 Segmental Innervation of Commonly Tested Muscles in the Upper Extremity

Muscle	Spinal Segment	Nerve Supply
Cervical paraspinal	C2 to C8	Corresponding cervical root
Trapezius	C2, C3, C4	Spinal accessory
Supraspinatus	C5, C6	Subscapular
Infraspinatus	C5	Subscapular
Deltoid (circumflex)	C5, C6	Axillary
Biceps brachii	C5, C6	Musculocutaneous
Brachioradialis	C6, C7	Radial
Flexor carpi radialis	C6, C7, C8	Median
Pronator teres	C6, C7	Median
Triceps brachii	C7, C8	Radial
Extensor digitorum communis	C7, C8	Radial
Extensor indicis	C7, C8	Radial
Flexor carpi ulnaris	C8, T1	Ulnar
Abductor pollicis brevis	C8, T1	Median
First dorsal interosseus	C8, T1	Ulnar
Abductor digiti minimi manus	C8, T1	Ulnar

TABLE 21–3　Segmental Innervation of Commonly Tested Muscles in the Lower Extremity

Muscle	Spinal Segment	Nerve Supply
Lumbosacral paraspinal	L1 to S1	Corresponding roots
Iliacus	L2, L3, L4	Femoral
Adductors of thigh	L2, L3, L4	Obturator
Quadriceps femoris	L2, L3, L4	Femoral
Tibialis anterior	L4, L5	Deep peroneal
Gluteus medius	L4, L5, S1	Superior gluteal
Gluteus maximus	L5, S1	Inferior gluteal
Peroneus longus	L5, S1	Superficial peroneal
Biceps femoris-long head	L5, S1	Sciatic
Biceps femoris-short head	L5, S1	Sciatic
Flexor digitorum longus	L5, S1	Posterior tibial
Tibialis posterior	L5, S1	Posterior tibial
Extensor digitorum brevis	L5, S1	Deep peroneal
Gastrocnemius-lateral	L5, S1	Posterior tibial
Gastrocnemius-medial	S1, S2	Posterior tibial
Abductor hallucis	S1, S2	Posterior tibial
Abductor digiti quinti	S1, S2	Posterior tibial
Tensor fasciae latae	L5, S1	Superior gluteal

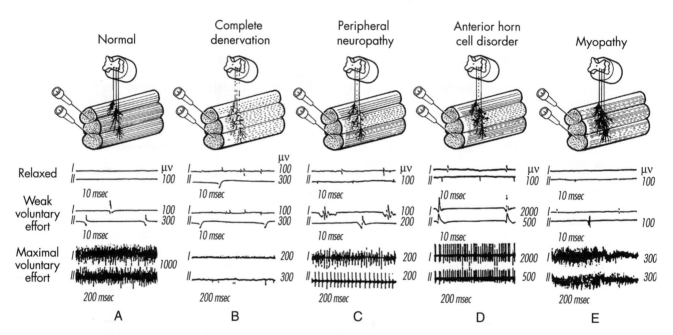

FIG. 21–3　Summary of electromyographic findings in various conditions. Diagrams show electromyograms from normal muscle and from muscle paresis of neurogenic and myogenic origin with a schematic presentation of the muscle fibers from three motor units (*marked solid circle, open circle, or x; affected fibers are dotted*). Two recording electrodes I and II and the corresponding recordings I and II. Up is negative. *A*, Normal. *At rest:* no action potentials. *Weak voluntary effort:* single motor unit potentials. *Maximal voluntary effort:* interference pattern; no synchronization. *B*, Total denervation. Diffuse atrophy of muscle fibers. *At rest:* diphasic and positive denervation potentials. *Voluntary effort:* no motor unit potentials. *C*, Peripheral neurogenic paresis. Patchy loss of muscle fibers. *At rest:* denervation potentials. *Voluntary effort:* often with increased action potential duration; polyphasic potentials. Pattern of single motor unit potentials or mixed pattern during maximal voluntary effort. No synchronization between various leads. *D*, Neurogenic paresis in diseases of the anterior horn cells. Patchy loss of muscle fibers. *At rest:* denervation potentials. *Voluntary effort:* increased action potential duration and voltage; polyphasic potentials. Single motor unit potentials with maximal voluntary effort, often synchronous in different leads. *E*, Myogenic paresis. Diffuse atrophy of muscle fibers. *At rest:* spontaneous discharges of short duration (in severe cases). *Voluntary effort:* diminished action potential duration, diminished action potential voltage, polyphasic potentials. Interference pattern with maximal effort; a short duration of the single spike potentials is often seen. *(From Buchthal F: An introduction to electromyography. Copenhagen, Scandinavia University Books, 1957).*

sensory testing. The timing of the EMG in relation to injury or onset of symptoms may be very important. Cost-containment issues have become extremely important, and Medicare and other insurers have developed guidelines for when it is appropriate to test for various conditions.

EVOKED POTENTIALS

Evoked potentials (EPs) are electrical responses of the nervous system to external sensory stimuli. It has been known for decades that these responses are present; however, their clinical usefulness did not become possible until the development of computerized averaging and advanced signal processing in the late 1960s.[44] Since then, the importance of EPs in diagnosing diseases of the peripheral nervous system and the CNS has undergone exponential growth.

The utility of EPs is based on their ability to provide objective and reproducible data concerning the status of the sensory nervous system. EP testing can demonstrate abnormalities of the sensory system when clinical signs and symptoms are ambiguous. In addition, evidence of clinically unsuspected lesions may be provided when the history and physical examination are normal. EP testing may help delineate the anatomic distribution of nervous system lesions and help monitor their progression or regression; this testing may be used to demonstrate integrity of nervous system pathways placed at risk during surgery.[44,45]

General Principles

EP responses have very low amplitude (0.1 to 20 mV); consequently, they are obscured by random noise consisting primarily of spontaneous electroencephalographic activity, muscle artifact, and environmental interference. Extraction of the EP response is accomplished by signal averaging. This process summates the "time-locked" EP response, which occurs at the same interval after the stimuli and minimizes unwanted noise.

Although EPs can be elicited by a wide variety of stimuli, the most commonly used stimuli are visual, auditory, and somatosensory.[46] This gives rise to the *visual evoked potential* (VEP) test, the *brainstem auditory evoked potential* (BAEP) test, and the *somatosensory evoked potential* (SEP) test. In each of these tests, the EP response consists of a sequence of upward and downward deflections. The characteristics to be evaluated are presence or absence, polarity, configuration, amplitude, latency, and interval between individual peaks (*interpeak latency* [IPL]).

Equipment

Most laboratories use commercially available EP equipment that should meet the standards established by the American Association of Electrodiagnostic Medicine and by the American Electroencephalographic Society.[47–49] In simplest terms, recording the EP consists of attaching electrodes to the patient over specific areas of the extremities, spine, and scalp, depending on the type of test being performed. After the electrodes are attached to record the EP signals, repetitive stimuli timed with recording process are presented to the patient. The EP signal is collected by the recording electrodes and amplified, filtered, averaged, and displayed for evaluation, printing, and storage.

Specific Tests of Evoked Potentials

The three tests of EPs that are used most often measure the visual, brainstem auditory, and somatosensory pathways. Testing of cognitive function and transcranial,[47] magnetic stimulation to determine central motor conduction may also be performed. In the patient with pain, SEP testing generally offers the greatest clinical utility.

Somatosensory Evoked Potentials

SEPs are evoked responses to stimulation of sensory nerves. Allowing assessment of somatosensory pathway function, SEPs have been obtained by stimulating sensory and mixed nerves in the upper and lower extremities, dermatomal sensory areas of the skin, and cranial nerves. Recording of the SEP response depends on stimulation of large, fast-conducting sensory fibers in the peripheral nerve. From the peripheral nerve, the SEP pathway enters the spinal cord through the dorsal root ganglion, ascending in the ipsilateral dorsal columns. The pathway crosses at the medial lemniscus, traveling to the contralateral ventroposterolateral nucleus of the thalamus and then on to the primary sensory cortex.

Methodology

Numerous methods have been described to record SEPs, with attempts at standardization occurring only recently.[50–52] Consequently, recording technique, waveform nomenclature, and normal values may vary between investigators.[53,54] However, certain general principles apply to most studies. The stimulus of choice for the SEP is electrical and consists of a square wave pulse delivered to the patient by surface or, less commonly, by needle electrodes. Stimulus duration is usually 100 to 200 msec at a rate of 3 to 7 stimuli per second. Stimulus intensity is adjusted to the point of producing an observable muscle twitch for mixed nerves or 2.5 to 3 times sensory threshold for sensory nerve stimulation. When properly applied, the stimulus generally is not painful.

Unilateral stimulation is used routinely to permit lateralization of abnormalities, with bilateral stimulation often reserved for intraoperative monitoring.[45] The site of the stimulation depends on the nerve being studied.

The ascending SEP response is recorded by placing pairs of recording electrodes at different locations along the somatosensory pathway being studied.

Upper Extremity SEP

Sites for recording electrodes to study nerves in the upper extremity generally include Erb's point in the supraclavicular fossa, the cervical spine, and the contralateral scalp overlying the area of the primary sensory cortex. Also, a reference electrode is placed on the forehead (Fz) and a ground electrode is placed proximal to the stimulation site. A noncephalic reference electrode may also be used to allow better visualization of subcortical potentials.

The median nerve has been the most extensively studied extremity nerve and is prototypical of an upper extremity SEP.[50,51] When the median nerve is stimulated at the wrist, expected responses are recorded at each electrode site (Fig. 21–4):

1. At Erb's point, a negative peak with a latency of about 9 msec (designated N9)

2. From the cervical spine, a negative peak at about 13 msec (designated N13)

3. From the scalp, a negative peak at about 20 msec (designated N20), followed by a positive peak at around 23 msec (designated P23)

Lower Extremity SEP

Recording the SEP from nerve situated in the lower extremity generally includes placement of recording electrodes on the lumbar spine over the L3 spinous process, on the lower thoracic spine at T12, and on the scalp over the primary sensory cortex (Cz). In studies of the extremity, SEP responses are difficult to record above the thoracic spine; thus, cervical spine recording sites are usually not included.

As in the upper extremity SEPs, a reference electrode and ground electrode are necessary. Like the median nerve in the upper extremity, the tibial nerve provides a characteristic SEP of the lower extremity.[51,55] When the tibial nerve is stimulated at the ankle, expected responses include the following (Fig. 21–5):

1. A negative peak with an approximate latency of 19 msec recorded at L3 (designated L3S)

2. At T12, a negative peak at about 21 msec (designated T12S)

3. At the scalp, a positive peak at approximately 37 msec (designated P37), followed by a negative peak with a latency of about 45 msec (designated N45)

Interpretation

Interpretation of SEP results depends on the presence or absence of expected waves and, when present, their absolute time and the latency time between each individual wave (IPLs). Latencies beyond 2.5 to 3 standard deviations from the mean are considered abnormal. If the SEP is considered a wave traveling from the stimulation site at the peripheral nerve and ascending proximally through the various record-

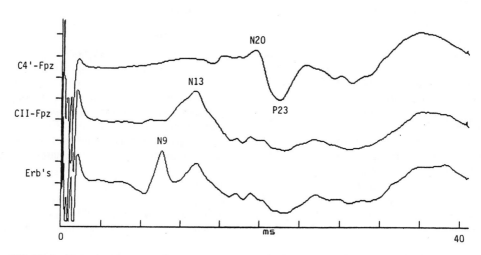

FIG. 21–4 Normal upper extremity somatosensory evoked potential (SEP) response from stimulation of the left median nerve. Responses were recorded from Erb's point (N9), the second cervical vertebra (N13), and the cortex (N20-P23).

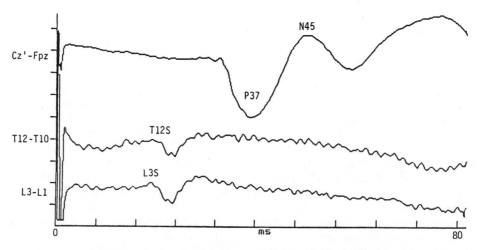

FIG. 21–5 Normal lower extremity somatosensory evoked potential (SEP) response from stimulation of the left posterior tibial nerve. Responses were recorded from the third lumbar vertebra (L3S), the twelfth thoracic vertebra (T12S), and the cortex (P37-N45).

ing sites on its way to the cortex, it can be seen that a lesion along the ascending somatosensory pathway results in normal responses distal to the lesion and abnormal responses proximally. Thus, if the brachial plexus response (N9) is normal and the cervical spine potential (N13) is delayed or absent, a lesion is located central to the brachial plexus but below the lower medulla in the cervical root or cord. Because diseases of the peripheral nerves that cause slowing of conduction velocity prolong the latencies of all peaks proximal to the nerve, IPLs are useful to confirm normal conduction through the CNS despite abnormal peripheral nerve abnormalities.[56]

Indications

Peripheral Nerve Disease

The occurrence of CNS amplification of the peripheral nerve volley permits cortical SEPs to be recorded when sensory nerve responses are unrecordable by conventional techniques.[57–59] Therefore, in cases of severe peripheral nerve disease in which conventional determination of nerve conduction is impossible, nerve conduction velocities may be calculated by stimulating a peripheral nerve at two sites and subtracting the latencies of the corresponding scalp-recorded SEPs.

Radiculopathy

Much has been published on the use of SEPs in the diagnosis of radiculopathy.[58,60–70] These studies have shown that SEPs recorded from nerves derived from several nerve roots have limited value in diagnosing radiculopathies because abnormalities in a single root would be overshadowed by contributions from uninvolved roots supplying that nerve. To circumvent this problem, techniques to derive SEPs from single nerve roots have been investigated.

Despite the problem, some consensus exists regarding the usefulness of SEPs in diagnosing radiculopathies. They are purportedly useful in radiculopathies in which sensory symptoms predominate and diagnosis by other diagnostic techniques (e.g., EMG) is difficult.[58,61,64,71] Nevertheless, EMG remains the "gold standard" for the electrodiagnostic evaluation of radiculopathies.

Thoracic Outlet Syndrome

Although ulnar nerve SEPs are controversial, they have been used in an attempt to identify thoracic outlet syndrome. In patients with suspected thoracic outlet syndrome who demonstrate no objective signs of neurologic involvement, ulnar nerve SEPs are generally normal.[72] In neurogenic thoracic outlet syndrome, SEP abnormalities included prolonged, attenuated, or absent N9 or N13 peaks or both and an increased N9 to N3 IPL.

Brachial Plexopathy

Studies have shown that SEPs may provide useful information for the management of patients with brachial plexopathies.[56,58] The ability to record SEPs helps confirm axonal continuity and may help determine whether lesions are preganglionic or postganglionic. SEPs are limited, in that they test the sensory portions of nerves, allowing only inference concerning motor function.

Lumbar Spinal Stenosis and Cervical Spondylosis

SEPs have been useful in the diagnosis of lumbar and cervical spine stenosis, with dermatomal SEPs reported to be superior to EMG in central and lateral recess lumbar stenosis.[73–75] SEP abnormalities have improved after surgical decompression of these lesions.[76]

Spinal Cord Lesions

SEPs are often abnormal in spinal cord lesions affecting the posterior columns. Intramedullary and extramedullary tumors, traumatic spinal cord injury, and vascular lesions may produce these abnormalities. Complete spinal cord lesions generally abolish all recordable SEP responses above the lesion.

Trigeminal Nerve Lesions

SEPs recorded from the trigeminal nerve are reported are to be abnormal in approximately 41% of patients with idiopathic and multiple sclerosis related trigeminal neuralgia. In patients undergoing retrogasserian injection of glycerol, alteration in SEP waveforms correlated well with successful treatment measured by pain relief.

Lesions of the Brainstem and Cerebral Hemisphere

Tumors, infarcts, and hemorrhages involving the somatosensory pathway of the brainstem and cerebrum generally produce SEP abnormalities.[44,77,78] SEPs may be particularly useful in patients with thalamic pain in whom abnormalities of N20 and P23 have been reported following median nerve stimulation.

Multiple Sclerosis

SEPs are used frequently in conjunction with VEPs and AEPs to evaluate patients with suspected multiple sclerosis. The incidence of SEP abnormalities runs higher in patients with sensory symptoms. Furthermore, SEP abnormalities are more frequent in the lower extremities.[78–80]

Other Uses

SEP abnormalities have been found in various degenerative, hereditary, and metabolic disorders, including Friedreich's and other ataxias.

Motor Evoked Potentials

Because of the inability of conventional nerve conduction studies to evaluate anatomically deep structures, alternate techniques were sought. An extension of conventional nerve conduction studies, motor EPs allow assessment of motor pathways in peripheral neuronal structures. Unlike conventional nerve conduction studies, assessment of central motor conduction pathways may also be performed. Stimulation may be electrical or magnetic, although magnetic stimulation is the most commonly used form because it is relatively painless.

Motor EPs have found their greatest usefulness in determining central conduction through the motor structures of the brain and spinal cord. By recording from distant sites, one can determine motor conduction throughout the entire motor pathway.

Clinical Utility

Motor EPs have found wide clinical utility in the diagnosis of disorders that affect central or peripheral motor pathways.

Abnormalities of motor EPs have been described in multiple sclerosis, Parkinson's disease, cerebrovascular accident, myelopathy in the cervical and lumbar spines, plexus lesions, and motor neuron disorders.[57,81-85] Cortical hyperexcitability has been demonstrated in migraine patients with transcranial magnetic stimulation.[86]

Event-Related Potentials

Unlike the previously discussed EPs, which are recorded from simple sensory or motor stimuli, event-related potentials record cortical activity evoked by a stimulus with cognitive significance. Various techniques have been developed to access temporal aspects of cognitive processing. The most common technique uses the presentation of randomly occurring stimuli of a different type. The subject is instructed to attend only to the infrequent stimuli, which results in an evoked waveform called the P300 response. Prolongation of the P300 response is associated with disorders that impair cognition, such as dementia and neurodegenerative disorders.[44,77]

RADIOLOGY

Radiologic imaging is often a useful tool in both the diagnosis and management of the patient with pain. The key to successful management and diagnosis involves good communication between the radiologist and the consulting physician. The radiologist not only provides the service of interpreting the films but also recommends the most appropriate study. When choosing the most appropriate test, one must consider the patient's symptomatology and the clinician's presumed diagnosis as well as the cost-benefit ratio, the patient's ability to tolerate the examination, and the urgency of diagnosis.

Plain X-ray Films

Plain x-ray films can often provide an accurate diagnosis and can do so in the most efficient and cost-effective manner possible.

Thoracic Disorders

A common complaint among patients in both clinics and emergency departments is chest pain. Chest pain may be the result of either acute or chronic disease. Acute causes of chest pain can be life threatening, as in cases of myocardial infarction, tension pneumothorax, acute aortic dissection, or pulmonary hemorrhage. In the case of aortic rupture resulting from trauma, the chest x-ray film may demonstrate widening of the mediastinum secondary to mediastinal hematoma, displacement of mediastinal structures, irregularity of the thoracic aorta, or hemothorax and apical capping.

Musculoskeletal Disorders

Most fractures are adequately evaluated by plain x-ray film (Figs. 21-6 and 21-7). Occasionally, additional imaging is required for further evaluation. Examples include evaluation of the intra-articular extent of a fracture; chronicity of a fracture, as with compression deformities of the spine; or simply exclusion of the presence of a fracture in a severely osteopenic patient. Soft tissue pathology, including joint effusions, hematomas, and tendinous calcifications, can also be visualized adequately on plain x-ray film (Fig. 21-8), as can the presence or absence of infection, such as osteomyelitis (Fig. 21-9) or diskitis, or inflammatory disease, such as rheumatoid arthritis or collagen vascular disease. Primary and secondary bone tumors are also well demonstrated on plain film radiography.

Conventional Tomography

Tomography can be used in the evaluation of joint spaces where the anatomic features are complex and are often obscured by overlying structures. Examples include exclusion of an odontoid fracture in the patient who is unable to cooperate for the open-mouth view or for a more detailed examination of a tibial plateau fracture. Conventional tomography can further aid in the evaluation of solitary bone lesions, healing fractures, arthrodeses, and osteotomies.

Computed Tomography

Computed tomography (CT) is the appropriate study of choice in the evaluation of many intrathoracic and intra-abdominal processes. Other indications include the preliminary assessment for trauma; the search for abscess or other nidus of infection or inflammation; and evaluation of aortic aneurysm or dissection, primary neoplasm, metastases, lymphadenopathy, or interstitial lung disease. CT also provides valuable information regarding patency of vascular structures, perfusion of organs, and the anatomy of the surrounding subcutaneous tissues.

There must be approximately a 5% or greater variance in absorption of x-rays to distinguish differences between various soft tissues on plain x-ray films.[87] With CT technol-

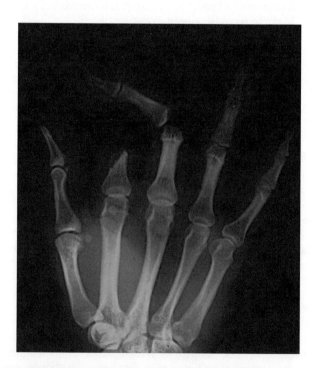

FIG. 21-6 Fracture-dislocation and traumatic amputation. Fracture-dislocation of the proximal interphalangeal joint of the third finger and traumatic amputation of the index finger through the midshaft of the proximal phalanx.

ogy, however, only a 0.5% variance between soft tissues is required. This rate of variance allows the radiologist to detect much more subtle differences in soft tissues and, subsequently, provides drastically improved diagnostic capabilities.

Magnetic Resonance Imaging

Magnetic resonance imaging (MRI) has been the premier development in imaging technology in the last two decades. Like CT, MRI is also a computer-based imaging modality that allows cross-sectional imaging with superb anatomic detail. Unlike CT, MRI has no spinal restriction; images can be generated in any plane.

Advantages

In comparisons of imaging modalities, MRI has numerous advantages. First, there are no known adverse biologic effects. In addition, the patient receives no ionizing radiation in MRI. MRI demonstrates significantly better tissue contrast than any other imaging modality available. Next MRI images can be obtained in multiple planes without the need for patient repositioning. Although coronal CT images of the head or an extremity can be acquired directly, this acquisition often comes at the cost of great discomfort to the patient.

Contraindications

MRI is contraindicated for patients with a pacemaker, ferromagnetic cerebral aneurysm clips, cochlear implants, and metallic foreign bodies in or around the orbits. Relative contraindications include external fixation devices and pain control units, which can cause local thermal burns.

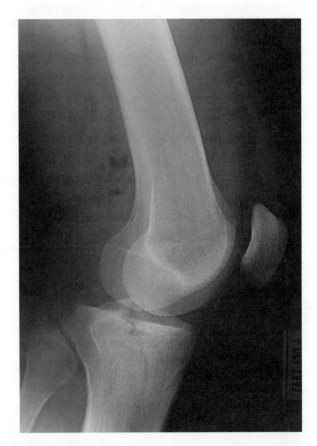

FIG. 21–8 Tibial plateau fracture with lipohemarthrosis. Lateral view of the knee demonstrating tibial plateau fracture and ancillary soft tissue findings of a fat-fluid level in the suprapatellar bursa.

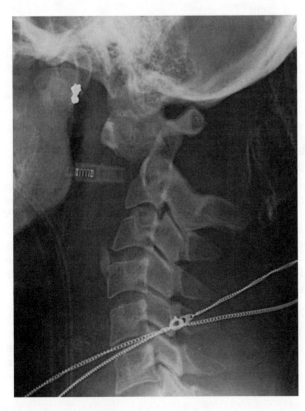

FIG. 21–7 Atlantoaxial dislocation. Lateral view of the cervical spine showing complete atlantoaxial dislocation. This patient died of respiratory arrest in the emergency department following a high-speed motorcycle accident.

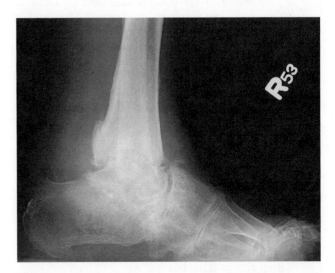

FIG. 21–9 Chronic osteomyelitis. Lateral radiograph of the foot in a patient with chronic foot pain demonstrates cortical destruction, volume loss, and sclerosis of the talus, calcaneus, distal tibia, and proximal row of tarsal bones. Chronic bilateral osteomyelitis developed following *Escherichia coli* septicemia.

Arthrography

Arthrography may be used in conjunction with conventional tomograms, CT, or MRI. The joint spaces most often evaluated with this procedure are the wrist, shoulder, hip, knee, and elbow. The procedure involves the administration of a small amount of contrast medium into the joint space under fluoroscopic guidance, followed by manipulation of the joint to disperse the contrast.

Myelography

A myelography procedure involves introducing a small amount of nonionic contrast into the thecal sac following a lumbar puncture. Imaging is then performed in multiple projections, allowing the contrast to delineate the subarachnoid space, spinal cord, and the nerve root sleeves.[88–90]

The advent of MRI has seen a significant decrease in the number of myelograms performed in most institutions. MRI is considered to be superior in both specificity and sensitivity in the evaluation of the spinal cord. However, myelography is still advantageous when:

1. MRI or CT provides no diagnoses despite continued patient symptomatology.
2. The abnormality detected on MRI or CT does not correlate with the clinical picture.
3. The patient is unable to tolerate MRI or CT secondary to pain, claustrophobia, or body habitus.

Coronary and Pulmonary Arteriography

Coronary arteriography remains the procedure remains the procedure of choice for documentation of the presence and severity of atherosclerotic disease.[91]

Pulmonary arteriography has long been the standard for diagnosis of pulmonary embolus.[92] It is most commonly employed when ventilation-perfusion scintigraphy returns a low or intermediate probability for embolus in patients for whom the clinician has high index of suspicion and who are candidates for anticoagulant therapy. Pulmonary arteriography is also indicated for patients classified as likely to undergo embolectomy or venous occlusion and for those in the high-probability group who are considered poor candidates for anticoagulation therapy.

Despite its benefits, pulmonary angiography is a highly invasive procedure that carries considerable mortality and morbidity.[92] It is crucial that the referring physician weigh the costs and benefits and assess the possible effects on patient management before proceeding with pulmonary angiography.

Venography

Venography is often used for evaluation for the absence or presence or the extent of thrombosis in an extremity vein, the pelvic veins, or the inferior vena cava. Iodinated contrast material is injected through a peripheral intravenous line in the hand or foot, and digital imaging is performed. Venography is widely regarded as the standard for evaluation of deep venous thrombosis.

Skeletal Scintigraphy

The bone scan is the study with which referring physicians are the most familiar. The scan can be used either alone or in conjunction with other imaging procedures as either the initial or a follow-up examination.

There are many indications for skeletal scintigraphy:

1. Assessment of bone or joint pain when plain x-ray films are nondiagnostic or normal
2. Detection of osseous metastatic disease
3. Ligamentous injury
4. Detection of stress fractures or occult fractures
5. Evaluation for osteomyelitis
6. Evaluation of avascular necrosis
7. Evaluation for suspected loose or injection joint prosthesis
8. Primary bone tumor
9. Diagnosis and assessment of Paget's disease
10. Determination of biopsy sites
11. Assessment of viability of bone graft

Most fractures pose no serious diagnostic dilemma and can be easily identified on plain radiographs. Occasionally, however, a hairline fracture that is elusive on plain x-ray film can easily be detected on a bone scan.

Bone scintigraphy can also be used to estimate the age of a fracture, as with compression deformities of the vertebral bodies. Elderly, osteopenic patients often complain of back pain; plain x-ray films might show compression fractures of the spine but provide no clues as to the age of the fracture. In 95% of patients younger than 65 years, an increase in bone remodeling is evident by 48 hours; by 72 hours after injury, almost all patients show radionuclide uptake. Lack of uptake or normal activity in a collapsed vertebra is sufficient evidence that the fracture is not an acute event.[93]

Bone scanning is also helpful in the evaluation of a stress fracture. Plain radiograph findings in stress fractures can be extremely subtle, comprising a thin line or radiodensity, or they may not be apparent at all. Stress fractures may be the result of the overuse of normally mineralized bone, as with the classic march fracture of the third metatarsal described in military recruits, or they may be insufficiency fractures caused by normal use of inadequately mineralized bone.

Regional Diagnosis

Headache and Facial Pain

Severe and sudden-onset headaches are most efficiently and effectively evaluated by CT to exclude subarachnoid hemorrhage or other intracranial hemorrhage as the cause.[87,89,94] Facial pain that is presumed to originate from sinusitis is best assessed with CT; facial bone fractures are also best evaluated in this manner. Panorex studies and MRI imaging of the temporomandibular joint are also appropriate for the evaluation of orofacial pain.[95,96]

Chest and Abdomen

Chest and abdominal pain is often addressed by the emergency department physician or primary care physician. Complaints resulting from gastroesophageal reflux disease, angina, peptic ulcer disease, pancreatic disease, prostate disease, or renal abnormalities are a few examples from a host of disorders that are not seen by the pain physician until they have become chronic.

In the initial evaluation of chest and abdominal pain, plain x-ray films can be advantageous in ruling out processes such as pneumothorax; congestive heart failure; free intraperitoneal air from ruptured viscus; or calcifications in a distribution, which suggests cholelithiasis or urolithiasis. In the absence of findings on plain x-ray film or other diagnostic studies, such as echocardiography or electrocardiography (ECG), CT, ultrasound, or gastrointestinal contrast examinations are the next recommended course of action.

Neck and Upper Extremity

Causes of neck and upper extremity pain and discomfort are multiple. Pain can originate from soft tissues, spinal cord or nerve roots, or musculoskeletal structures, or it can be referred from viscera. Naturally, degenerative disease of the cervical spine and herniated or bulging disks are the culprits behind most complaints, causing nerve root compression with resultant neck and upper extremity numbness, weakness, and pain.

Following initial plain x-ray films, MRI is the study of choice for further evaluation. It is superior in demonstrating not only disk disease and cervical spondylosis but also primary or metastatic lesions within the spinal cord. Joint pain of the upper extremity is also best evaluated with MRI to follow up the initial plain x-ray films.

Low Back Pain

Low back pain is known to affect 80% of adults during their lifetime.[97] Spinal disorders represent the most common cause of disability among workers in the United States and account for the chief medical condition on which health care dollars are spent.[98]

MRI has advantages over both CT and myelography in the evaluation of degenerative disk disease.[99] The multiple terms commonly used to describe degenerative disk disease are often poorly understood and used incorrectly. For example, the terms *bulging disk* and *herniated disk* cannot be used interchangeably. Furthermore, the distinction has considerable effect on patient treatment[99]:

- A bulging disk extends past the cortical margins of the adjacent vertebral bodies.
- In a herniated disk, defect in the annulus fibrosis allows extension of the nucleus pulposus through this defect producing a focal extension of the margin of the disk. The herniated nucleus pulposus is still attached posteriorly by some uninterrupted fibers.
- In an *extruded disk,* no annular fibers remain intact. The nuclear material bulges into the spinal canal or intervertebral foramen.
- A *sequestered disk* describes disk material that is no longer contiguous with the remaining nuclear material. This fragment can be located anterior or posterior to the posterior longitudinal ligament.

Failed Back Surgery Syndrome

Failed back surgery syndrome (FBSS), by definition, is the persistence of back or leg symptoms following lumbar surgery. Any patient with multiple previous low back surgeries should be evaluated using a systematic and uniform approach to differentiate between low back pain and leg symptomatology.

First, there must be a differentiation between mechanical causes of FBSS. *Mechanical* lesions, such as spinal stenosis, recurrent disk, or spinal instability, can cause compression of the adjacent cord or nerve root. These problems can often be corrected with an additional surgical procedure.[100] *Nonmechanical* lesions include epidural fibrosis or arachnoiditis, psychosomatic pain, and system medical illness; these entities are not amenable to treatment by additional surgery.[100]

Causes and prevalence of FBSS include[100–104]:

- Recurrent disk herniation (12% to 16%)
- Stenosis not identified in the preoperative period (central spinal stenosis, 7% to 40%; lateral recess stenosis, 50%)
- Epidural fibrosis (6% to 8%)
- Arachnoiditis (6% to 16%)

DIFFERENTIAL NEURAL BLOCKADE IN THE DIAGNOSIS OF PAIN MECHANISMS

Differential neural blockade is the selective blockade of one modality without blocking the others and represents an extremely useful diagnostic tool.

Two clinical approaches can be used:

1. The *anatomic* approach is based on having sufficient anatomic separation of sympathetic and somatic fibers, so that the injection of local anesthetic to block one modality does not block the others.
2. The *pharmacologic* approach is based on the presumed difference in the sensitivity of the various types of nerve fibers to local anesthetics, so that the injection of different concentrations of local anesthetics can selectively block different types of fibers.

Differential neural blockade is controversial, however. The two main reasons are:

1. The changes in our understanding of the factors that determine the process of nerve conduction and blockade are believed by some to invalidate the procedure.
2. Our new-found understanding of the complexities of chronic pain may limit the diagnostic utility of the blockade.

Techniques of Differential Neural Blockade

Pharmacologic Approach

A differential spinal block is the simplest pharmacologic approach with the most discrete end points. Fiber diameter determines the modalities subserved by the fiber.

A fibers are subdivided into four subclasses—alpha, beta, gamma, and delta (Table 21–4). A-alpha fibers subserve motor function and proprioception, A-beta fibers subserve touch and pressure, and A-gamma fibers subserve muscle spindle tone. A-delta fibers subserve pain and temperature sensations as well as nociception (tissue damage).

The myelinated B fibers are thin, preganglionic, autonomic axons, and the nonmyelinated C fibers subserve pain and temperature transmission as well as nociception. C fibers are thinner than the myelinated fibers and have a much lower conduction velocity than even A-delta fibers.

Conventional Sequential Differential Spinal Block

After informed consent is obtained from the patient, an intravenous infusion is started and prehydration with crystalloid is begun as with any spinal anesthesia. All customary monitors are applied and baseline values are recorded.

Four solutions (Table 21–5) are prepared. After the usual preparation and draping of the back, a 25- to 27-gauge spinal needle is introduced into the lumbar subarachnoid space at the L2-3 or L3-4 interspace. The patient is shown the four syringes, which all appear the same. The patient is told that each of the solutions will be injected sequentially at 10- to 15-minute intervals. The patient is instructed to notify the physician regarding which, if any, of the solutions relieves the pain. (The solutions are referred to as A through D so that they can be discussed in front of the patient without referring to the word *placebo*.)

- Solution A: contains no anesthetic (placebo)
- Solution B: contains 0.25% procaine
- Solution C: contains 0.5% procaine
- Solution D: contains 5.0% procaine

The conventional sequential differential spinal block is interpreted as follows:

Psychogenic pain. If the patient's pain is relieved after solution A (which is the placebo), the patient's pain is tentatively classified as psychogenic. If the pain relief is prolonged or permanent, the pain is probably truly psychogenic in origin; however, if the pain relief is transient and self-limiting, the response is probably a placebo reaction.

Sympathetic pain. If the patient does not obtain relief from the placebo, but does obtain relief from the 0.25% procaine injection, the mechanism subserving the patient's pain is considered to be sympathetic pain.

Somatic pain. If the 0.25% procaine does not provide relief, but the 0.5% concentration does, this usually indicates that the patient's pain is subserved by A-delta and/or C fibers and is classified as somatic (provided the patient did exhibit signs of sympathetic blockade

after the previous injection of 0.25% procaine and the onset of pain relief is accompanied by the onset of analgesia or anesthesia). This is important because if a patient has an elevated C_m for B fibers, pain relief from 0.5% procaine might be due to a sympathetic block rather than to a sensory block.

Central pain. If pain relief is not obtained by any of the preceding injections, 5% procaine is injected to block all modalities. If the 5% concentration does relieve pain, the mechanism is still considered to be somatic and it is presumed that the patient has an elevated C_m for A-delta and C fibers. However, if the patient does not obtain pain relief with the 5% concentration, the pain is classified as central in origin. See Table 29–4.

There are disadvantages to the previously discussed technique:

1. It is time-consuming.
2. Sometimes a patient's C_m for sympathetic blockade is greater than 0.25%; therefore, when relief is produced by 0.5% procaine, one might conclude that this is somatic pain rather than sympathetic pain, which it really represents.
3. Each injection with this technique deposits increasing amounts of procaine in the subarachnoid space, so that after the final injection when all the modalities are blocked, a considerable period is required for full recovery of function.
4. With this technique, the needle remains in place throughout the entire procedure, so the patient must lie in the lateral position throughout the test. This requirement occasionally poses a serious problem when it involves patients who experience pain only in a position that the needle in situ disallows.

Modified Differential Spinal Block

To overcome the disadvantages of the conventional technique mentioned previously, sometimes the modified

TABLE 21–4 Classification of Nerve Fibers on the Basis of Fiber Size (Relating Fiber Size to Fiber Function and Sensitivity to Local Anesthetics)*

Fiber Group/ Subgroup	Diameter (μm)	Conduction Velocity (m/sec)	Modality Subserved	Sensitivity to Local Anesthetics (%)†
A (myelinated)				
A-alpha	15–20	80–120	Large motor, proprioception	1.0
A-beta	8–15	30–70	Small motor, touch and pressure	↓
A-gamma	4–8	30–70	Muscle spindle, reflex	
A-delta	3–4	10–30	Temperature, sharp pain, nociception	0.5
B (unmyelinated)	3–4	10–15	Preganglionic autonomic	0.25
C (unmyelinated)	1–2	1–2	Dull pain, temperature, nociception	0.5

*Vertical arrow in column 5 indicates intermediate values in descending order.
†Subarachnoid procaine.

TABLE 21–5 Preparation of Solutions for Conventional Sequential Differential Spinal Blockade

Solution	Preparation of Solution	Yield	Blockade
D	To 2 ml of 10% procaine, add 2 ml of normal saline	4 ml of 5% procaine	Motor
C	To 1 ml of 5% procaine, add 9 ml of normal saline	10 ml of 0.5% procaine	Sensory
B	To 5 ml of 0.5% procaine, add 5 ml of normal saline	10 ml of 0.25% procaine	Sympathetic
A	Draw up 10 ml of normal saline	10 ml of normal saline	—

differential spinal block is the best choice. As with the conventional technique, after informed consent has been obtained, an infusion is started and the monitors are applied. The back is prepared and draped. A small-bore spinal needle is used to enter the subarachnoid space. Normal saline (2 ml) is injected and the observations are made as in the conventional technique. If the patient obtains no relief or only partial relief from the placebo injection, 2 ml of 5% procaine is injected, the needle is removed, and the patient is returned to the supine position.

Because the injected 5% procaine is hyperbaric, the position of the table may have to be manipulated to obtain the desired level of anesthesia. Once this is done, the same observations are made as after the previous injection (Table 21–6).

The modified differential spinal block is interpreted as follows:

If the patient's pain is relieved after the injection of normal saline solution, the interpretation is the same as when pain relief is provided by the placebo in the conventional differential spinal block.

If a patient does not obtain pain relief after the injection of the 5% procaine, the diagnosis is considered to be the same as when the patient does not obtain relief following the injection of all of the solutions with the conventional technique (Table 21–7).

If the patient obtains complete pain relief after the injection of 5% procaine, the pain is considered to be organic in nature.

If the pain returns when the patient again appreciates pinprick as sharp (recovery from analgesia), the mechanism is considered to be somatic (to be subserved by A-delta and/or C fibers).

If the pain relief persists for a prolonged period after recovery from analgesia, the mechanism is considered to be sympathetic.

Differential Epidural Block

More than 20 years ago, Raj[105] suggested the use of a sequential differential epidural block instead of a conventional sequential differential spinal to obviate the possibility of spinal headache after the procedure. With his proposed technique, solution A was still to be the placebo, but solution B was 0.5% lidocaine, which was presumed to be the mean sympatholytic concentration of lidocaine in the epidural space. Solution C was 1% lidocaine, presumed to represent the mean sensory blocking concentration in the epidural space; and solution D was 2% lidocaine, a concentration sufficient to block all modalities. In short, the technique proposed was virtually identical to the technique used in carrying out a conventional differential spinal block, except that the local anesthetic was lidocaine, it was injected directly into the epidural space, and the concentrations were modified as already described.

There were two problems with the technique Raj proposed:

1. Because of the slower onset of blockade of each modality after the injection of local anesthetic into the epidural space, a longer time would be required between injections. Thus, the overall procedure time was lengthened.
2. Also, if local anesthetics occasionally fail to give discreet end points when injected into the subarachnoid space, they do so even more often when injected into the epidural space.

However, the second problem can be overcome with a slight modification of the technique.

TABLE 21–6   Observations Following Each Injection

Sequence	Observation
1	Blood pressure and pulse rate
2	Patient's subjective evaluation of the pain at rest
3	Reproduction of patient's pain by movement
4	Signs of sympathetic block (temperature change, psychogalvanic reflex)
5	Signs of sensory block (response to pinprick)
6	Signs of motor block (inability to move toes, feet, legs)

TABLE 21–7   Anatomic Approach: Procedural Sequence for Differential Diagnostic Nerve Blocks

Site of Pain	Saline	Solutions To Be Injected Local Anesthetic	Local Anesthetic
Head	Placebo block	Stellate ganglion block	Block of C2 Block of trigeminal I, II, III (or block of specific nerve)
Neck	Placebo block	Stellate ganglion block	Cervical plexus block (or block of specific nerve)
Arm	Placebo block	Stellate ganglion block	Brachial plexus block (or block of specific nerve)
Thorax*	Placebo block	Thoracic paravertebral sympathetic block	Lumbar paravertebral somatic block
Abdomen†	Placebo block	Celiac plexus block	Paravertebral somatic or intercostal block
Pelvis†	Placebo block	Superior hypogastric plexus block	Paravertebral somatic or intercostal block
Leg	Placebo block	Lumbar paravertebral sympathetic block	Lumbosacral plexus block (or block of specific nerve)

*In our opinion, thoracic paravertebral sympathetic blocks carry such a high risk of pneumothorax that a pharmacologic approach should be used.
†Because of the simplicity of intercostal blocks compared with celiac plexus and superior hypogastric plexus blocks, the procedural sequence is altered for abdominal pain (somatic before sympathetic).

Differential Brachial Plexus Block

When using this technique, two sequential injections are made into the perivascular compartment using an approach appropriate for the site of the patient's pain. One injection consists of normal saline solution; the other injection consists of 2% chloroprocaine. The same observations should be made as those following differential spinal blocks.

If the patient obtains pain relief from the saline solution, the pain is considered psychogenic. If the pain disappears after the injection of chloroprocaine, the pain is labeled organic. If the pain returns as soon as the sensory block dissipates, the mechanism is somatic. If the pain relief persists for a prolonged period after recovery of the sensory block, the mechanism is presumed to be sympathetic. If the pain does not disappear, even when the arm is fully anesthetized, the diagnosis is central pain.

Anatomic Approach

To obviate the problems inherent in high spinal anesthesia, it is occasionally safer to use an anatomic approach to differential neural blockade. After injection of a placebo, the sympathetic and then the sensory and/or motor fibers are blocked sequentially by injecting a local anesthetic at points where one modality can be blocked without blocking the other. The procedural sequences by which differential nerve blocks are carried out for pain in the various parts of the body using this approach are presented in Table 21–7.

Role of Differential Neural Blockade

Human limitations being what they are and pain being the complex process that it is, no one ever acquires sufficient experience or expertise to make the correct diagnosis 100% of the time. Differential neural blockade provides an objective means of confirming a diagnosis when the patient's pain appears obvious. More important, however, differential neural blockade provides a means of establishing a diagnosis when there appears to be no demonstrable cause.

References

1. Roongta S: Electromyography. In Raj P, editor: *Practical management of pain,* ed 2. St. Louis, Mosby, 1992.
2. Verdugo R, Ochoa JL: *Use and misuse of conventional electrodiagnosis, quantitative sensory testing, thermography, and nerve blocks in the evaluation of painful neuropathic syndromes.* American Association of Electrodiagnostic Medicine, International Symposium on Neuropathic Pain, October 18, 1992, Charleston, SC.
3. Waldman HJ: Neurophysiologic testing in the evaluation of the patient in pain. In Waldman SD, Winnie AP, editors: *International pain management.* Dannemiller Memorial Educational Foundation. Philadelphia, WB Saunders, 1996.
4. McDermott JF, Modaff WL, Boyle RW: Electromyography. *GP* 27, January 1963.
5. Norris FH: *The EMG.* New York, Grune & Stratton, 1963.
6. Longmire D: Tutorial 10: Electrodiagnostic studies in the assessment of painful disorders. *Pain Dig* 3:116, 1993.
7. Kimura J: *Electrodiagnosis in diseases of nerve and muscle: Principles and practice.* Philadelphia, FA Davis, 1983.
8. Wiechers DO: Normal and abnormal motor unit potentials. In Johnson EW, editor: *Practical electromyography,* ed 2. Baltimore, Williams & Wilkins, 1988.
9. Oh SJ: *Clinical electromyography: Nerve conduction studies,* ed 2. Baltimore, Williams & Wilkins, 1993.
10. Waxman SG: Conduction in myelinated, unmyelinated and demyelinated fibers. *Arch Neurol* 34:585, 1977.
11. Bolton CF, Carter K, Koval JJ: Temperature effects on conduction studies of normal and abnormal nerve. *Muscle Nerve* 5:S145, 1982.
12. Brown WF, Bolton CF: *Clinical electromyography,* ed 2. Boston, Butterworth-Heinemann, 1993.
13. Ball RD: *Basics of needle electromyography: An AAEE workshop.* Rochester, Minn, American Association of Electrodiagnosis and Electromyography, October 1985.
14. Jablecki C: *Physiologic basis of electromyographic activity: Standard needle electromyography of muscles.* American Association of Electrodiagnosis and Electromyography, 11th Annual Continuing Education Course, San Diego, October 1988.
15. Dumitru D: *Electrodiagnostic medicine.* Philadelphia, Hanley and Belfus, 1995.
16. Kimura J: F-wave velocity in the central segment of the median and ulnar nerves: A study in normal subjects and in patients with Charcot-Marie-Tooth disease. *Neurology* 24:539, 1974.
17. Mayer RF, Feldman RG: Observations on the nature of the F wave in man. *Neurology* 17:147, 1967.
18. Magladery JW, McDougal DB: Electrophysiological studies and reflex activity in normal man: Identification of certain reflexes in the electromyogram and conduction velocity of peripheral nerve fiber. *Bull Johns Hopkins Hosp* 86:265, 1950.
19. Hoffmann P: *Untersuchungen uber Bie Eigenreflexe (Sehnenre flexe) Nenschlicher Muskeln.* Berlin, Springer, 1922.
20. Braddom RL, Johnson EW: Standardization of H reflex and diagnostic use in S1 radiculopathy. *Arch Phys Med Rehabil* 55:161, 1974.
21. Braddom RL, Johnson EW: H-reflex: Review and classification with suggested clinical uses. *Arch Phys Med Rehabil* 55:412, 1974.
22. Schuchmann JA: H reflex latency in radiculopathy. *Arch Phys Med Rehabil* 59:185, 1978.
23. Fruhstorfer H, Lindblom U, Schmidt WG: Method for quantitative estimation for thermal thresholds in patients. *J Neurol Neurosurg Psychiatry* 39:1071, 1976.
24. Verdugo RJ, Ochoa JL: Quantitative somatosensory thermotest: A key method for functional evaluation of small caliber afferent channels. *Brain* 115:893, 1992.
25. American Diabetes Association: Report and recommendations of the San Antonio Conference on Diabetic Neuropathy. *Diabetes Care* 11:592, 1988.
26. Low PA, Caskey PE, Tuck RR et al: Quantitative pseudomotor axon reflex test in normal and neuropathic subjects. *Ann Neurol* 14:573, 1983.
27. Low PA, Zimmerman BR, Dyck PJ: Comparison of distal sympathetic with vagal function in diabetic neuropathy. *Muscle Nerve* 9:592, 1986.
28. Cohen J, Low P, Fealey R et al: Somatic and automatic function in progressive autonomic failure and multiple system atrophy. *Ann Neurol* 22:692, 1987.
29. Schaumburg HH, Berger AR, Thomas PK: *Disorders of peripheral nerves,* ed 2. Contemporary Neurology Series. Philadelphia, FA Davis, 1992.
30. Barohn RJ: Approach to peripheral neuropathy and neuronopathy. *Semin Neurol* 18:7, 1998.
31. Ropper AH, Gorson KC: Neuropathies with paraproteinemia. *N Engl J Med* 338:1601, 1998.
32. Cornblath DR, Mellits ED, Griffin JW et al: Motor conduction studies in Guillain-Barré syndrome: Description and prognostic value. *Ann Neurol* 23:354, 1988.
33. Pourmand R, Maybury B: *Paraneoplastic sensory neuronopathy.* American Association of Electrodiagnostic Medicine, case report no. 31. Rochester, Minn, The Association, December 1996.
34. Albers JW, Donofrio PD, McGonagle TK: Sequential electrodiagnostic abnormalities in acute inflammatory demyelinating polyradiculopathy. *Nerve Muscle* 8:528, 1985.
35. Bromberg MB: Comparison of electrodiagnostic criteria for primary demyelination in chronic polyneuropathy. *Nerve Muscle* 14:968, 1991.
36. Rosenbaum RB, Ochoa JL: *Carpal tunnel syndrome and other disorders of the median nerve.* Boston, Butterworth-Heinemann, 1993.
37. Kincaid JC, Phillps LH 2nd, Daube JR: The evaluation of suspected ulnar neuropathy at the elbow: Normal conduction values. *Arch Neurol* 43:44, 1986.
38. Miller RG: The cubital tunnel syndrome: Diagnosis and precise localization. *Ann Neurol* 6:56, 1979.
39. Ebbling P, Gilliatt RW, Thomas PK: A clinical and electrical study of ulnar nerve lesions in the hand. *J Neurol Neurosurg Psychiatry* 23:1, 1960.

40. Stuart JV: The radial nerve. In Stewart JV, editor: *Focal peripheral neuropathy,* ed 2. New York, Raven Press, 1993.
41. DeLisa JA, Sead MA: *The tarsal tunnel syndrome.* American Association of Electrodiagnosis and Electromyography: Case report no. 8. *Muscle Nerve* 6:664, 1983.
42. Keck C: The tarsal tunnel syndrome. *J Bone Joint Surg* 44:180, 1992.
43. Oh SJ, Sarala PK, Kuba T et al: Tarsal tunnel syndrome, electrophysiological study. *Ann Neurol* 5:327, 1979.
44. Chiappa K: *Evoked potentials in clinical medicine.* New York, Raven Press, 1985.
45. Nuwer MR: *Evoked potential monitoring in the operating room.* New York, Raven Press, 1986.
46. Starr A: *Natural forms of somatosensory stimulation that can evoke cerebral, spinal, peripheral nerve potentials in man.* American Association of Electrodiagnosis and Electromyography International Symposium on Somatosensory Evoked Potentials, Rochester, Minn, 1984.
47. American Electroencephalography Society: Clinical evoked potential guidelines. *J Clin Neurophysiol* 1:6, 1984.
48. American Association of Electrodiagnosis and Electromyography: *Guidelines for somatosensory evoked potentials.* Rochester, Minn, The Association, 1984.
49. Gitter AJ, Stolov WC: *AAEM minimonograph no. 16: Instrumentation and measurement in electrodiagnostic medicine.* Rochester, Minn, American Association of Electrodiagnostic Medicine, 1995.
50. Eisen A, Stevens J: *Upper limb somatosensory evoked potentials.* American Association of Electrodiagnosis and Electromyography workshop. Rochester, Minn, undated monograph.
51. Kimura J: *Somatosensory evoked potentials to median and tibial nerve stimulation and electrodiagnosis somatosensory evoked potentials.* Sixth Annual Continuing Education Course, Rochester, Minn, 1983.
52. Halliday A: *Current status of SEP.* American Association of Electrodiagnosis and Electromyography International Symposium on Somatosensory Evoked Potentials, Rochester, Minn, 1984.
53. Branddom R: Somatosensory, brain stem, and visual evoked potentials. In Johnson E, editor: *Practical electromyography,* ed 2. Baltimore, Williams & Wilkins, 1988.
54. Celesia G: *Somatosensory evoked potentials: Nomenclature.* American Association of Electrodiagnosis and Electromyography International Symposium on Somatosensory Evoked Potentials, Rochester, Minn, 1984.
55. Baran E, Daube J: *Lower extremity somatosensory evoked potentials.* American Association of Electrodiagnosis and Electromyography workshop. Rochester, Minn, 1984.
56. Jones S: *Clinical applications of somatosensory evoked potentials: Peripheral nervous system.* American Association of Electrodiagnosis and Electromyography International Symposium on Somatosensory Evoked Potentials. Rochester, Minn, 1984.
57. Kanda M, Fujiwara N, Xu X et al: Pain-related and cognitive components of somatosensory evoked potentials following CO_2 laser stimulation in man. *Electroencephalogr Clin Neurophysiol* 100:103, 1996.
58. Eisen A: SEP in the evaluation of disorders of the peripheral nervous system. In Cracco R, Bodis-Wollner I, editors: *Evoked potentials.* New York, AR Liss, 1986.
59. Aminoff M, Cutler J, Brant-Zawadzki M: The sensitivity of MR imaging and multimodality evoked potentials in the evaluation of patients with suspect multiple sclerosis. In Barber C, Blum T, editors: *Evoked potentials III.* Boston, Butterworth, 1987.
60. Aminoff M, Goodin DS, Parry GJ et al: Electrophysiologic evaluation of lumbosacral radiculopathies: Electromyography, late responses, and somatosensory evoked potentials. *Neurology* 35:1514, 1985.
61. Perlik S, Fisher MA, Patel DV et al: On the usefulness of somatosensory evoked responses for the evaluation of lower back pain. *Arch Neurol* 43:907, 1986.
62. Aminoff M, Goodin DS, Barbaro NM et al: Dermatomal somatosensory evoked potentials in unilateral lumbosacral radiculopathy. *Ann Neurol* 17:171, 1985.
63. Katifi H, Sedgwick E: Dermatomal somatosensory evoked potentials in lumbosacral disk disease: Diagnosis and results of treatment. In Barber C, Blum T, editors: *Evoked potentials II.* Boston, Butterworth, 1987.
64. Katifi HA, Sedgwick EM: Evaluation of the dermatomal somatosensory evoked potential in the diagnosis of lumbo-sacral root compression. *J Neurol Neurosurg Psychiatry* 50:1204, 1987.
65. Eisen A, Hoirch M, Moll A: Evaluation of radiculopathies by segmental stimulation and somatosensory evoked potentials. *Can J Neurol Sci* 10:178, 1983.
66. Machida M, Asai T, Sato K et al: New approach for diagnosis in herniated lumbosacral disc. Dermatomal somatosensory evoked potentials (DSSEPs). *Spine* 11:380, 1986.
67. Rodriguez A: Somatosensory evoked potentials from dermatomal stimulation as an indicator of L5 and S1 radiculopathies. *Arch Phys Med Rehabil* 6:366, 1987.
68. Scarff R, Dallmann D, Roleikis J: Dermatomal somatosensory evoked potentials in the diagnosis of lumbosacral root entrapment. *Surg Forum* 32:489, 1981.
69. Schmid U, Hess C, Ludin H: Somatosensory evoked potentials following nerve and segmental stimulation do not conform cervical radiculopathy with sensory deficit. *J Neurol Neurosurg Psychiatry* 51:182, 1988.
70. Seyal M, Palma GA, Sandhu LS et al: Spinal somatosensory evoked potentials following segmental sensory stimulation: A direct measure of dorsal root function. *Electroencephalogr Clin Neurophysiol* 69:390, 1988.
71. Dumitru D, Dreyfuss P: Dermatomal/segmental somatosensory evoked potential evaluation of L5/S1 unilateral/unilevel radiculopathies. *Muscle Nerve* 19:442, 1996.
72. Komanetsky RM, Novak CB, Mackinnon SE et al: Somatosensory evoked potentials fail to diagnose thoracic outlet syndrome. *J Hand Surg* 21:662, 1996.
73. Oh SJ: *Clinical electromyography: Nerve conduction studies.* Baltimore, University Park Press, 1984.
74. Stolov W, Slimp J: *Dermatosensory evoked potentials in lumbar spinal stenosis.* American Association of Electrodiagnosis and Electromyography/American Electroencephalographic Society joint symposium of somatosensory evoked potentials and magnetic stimulation, Rochester, Minn, 1988.
75. Yiannikas C, Shahani B, Young R: Short-latency somatosensory evoked potentials from radial, median, ulnar, and peroneal nerve stimulation in the assessment of cervical spondylosis. *Arch Neurol* 43:1264, 1986.
76. Gonzales E: Lumbar spinal stenosis: Analysis of pre- and post-operative somatosensory evoked potentials. *Arch Phys Med Rehabil* 66:11, 1985.
77. Dorfman LJ, Robinson LR: *AAEM minimonograph no. 17: Normative data in electrodiagnostic medicine.* Rochester, Minn, American Association of Electrodiagnostic Medicine, 1997.
78. Oken B, Chiappa K: Somatosensory evoked potentials in neurological diagnosis. In Cracco RQ, Bodis-Wollner J, editors: *Evoked potentials.* New York, AR Liss, 1986.
79. Hume AL, Waxman SG: Evoked potentials in suspected multiple sclerosis: Diagnostic value and prediction of clinical course. *J Neurol Sci* 83:191, 1988.
80. Aminoff M: *American Association of Electrodiagnosis and Electromyography minimonograph no. 22: The clinical role of somatosensory evoked potential studies: A critical appraisal.* Rochester, Minn, American Association of Electrodiagnosis and Electromyography, 1984.
81. Eisen AA, Shtybel W. *AAEM minimonograph 35: Clinical experience with transcranial magnetic stimulation.* Rochester, Minn, American Association of Electrodiagnostic Medicine, 1990.
82. Chiappa KH: Transcranial motor evoked potentials. *Electromyogr Clin Neurophysiol* 34:15, 1994.
83. Kalita J, Misra UK: Motor and sensory evoked potential studies in brainstem strokes. *Electromyogr Clin Neurophysiol* 37:379, 1997.
84. Andersson T, Siden A, Persson A: A comparison of motor evoked potentials and somatosensory evoked potentials in patients with multiple sclerosis and potentially related conditions. *Electromyogr Clin Neurophysiol* 35:17, 1995.
85. Salerno A, Carlander B, Camu W et al: Motor evoked potentials (MEPs): Evaluation of the different types of responses in amyotrophic lateral sclerosis and primary lateral sclerosis. *Electromyogr Clin Neurophysiol* 36:361, 1996.
86. Van der Kamp W, Maassen VA, Ferrari MD et al: Interictal cortical hyperexcitability in migraine patients demonstrated with transcranial magnetic stimulation. *J Neurol Sci* 139:106, 1996.
87. Batnitzky S, Eckard DA: The radiology of brain tumors: General considerations and neoplasms of the posterior fossa. In Morantz RA, Walsh JW, editors: *Brain tumors: A comprehensive text.* New York, Marcel Dekker, 1994.

88. Grossman RI, Youssem DM: *Neuroradiology: The requisites.* St. Louis, Mosby, 1994.

89. Osborne AG: *Diagnostic neuroradiology.* St. Louis, Mosby, 1994.

90. Batnitzky S: Intraspinal disorders. In Sarwar M, Azar-Kia B, Batnitsky S, editors: *Neuroradiology.* St. Louis, Warren Green, 1983.

91. Higgins CB, Lipton MJ: Chest pain. In Eisenburg Rl, editor: *Diagnostic imaging: An algorithmic approach.* Philadelphia, JB Lippincott, 1988.

92. Early PH, Sodee DB: *Principles and practice of nuclear medicine.* St. Louis, Mosby, 1995.

93. Alazaki MP, Mishkin FS: *Fundamentals of nuclear medicine.* New York, Society of Nuclear Medicine, 1984.

94. Sadato N, Numaguchi Y, Rigamonti D et al: Bleeding in ruptured posterior fossa aneurysms: A CT study. *J Comput Assist Tomogr* 15:612, 1991.

95. Katzberg RW: Temporomandibular joint imaging. *Radiology* 170:297, 1989.

96. Helms CA, editor: Temporomandibular joint. In *MRI of the musculoskeletal system,* ed 2. New York, Raven Press, 1990.

97. Nachemson A: The lumbar spine: An orthopedic challenge. *Spine* 1:59, 1976.

98. Burton CV: High resolution CT scanning: The present and future. *Orthop Clin North Am* 14:539, 1983.

99. Modic MT, Masaryk TJ, Ross JS: *Magnetic resonance imaging of the spine.* Chicago, Year Book Medical Publishers, 1989.

100. Boden SD, editor: The multiply operated low back patient. In *The aging spine: Essentials of pathophysiology, diagnosis, and treatment.* Philadelphia, WB Saunders, 1991.

101. Ross JS, Jueftle MG: Postoperative spine. In Modic MT, Masaryk TJ, Ross JS, editors: *Magnetic resonance imaging of the spine.* Chicago, Year Book Medical Publishers, 1989.

102. Teplick JG: The postoperative lumbar spine. In *Lumbar spine: CT and MRI.* Philadelphia, JB Lippincott, 1992.

103. Burton CV, Kirkaldy-Willis WH, Yong-Hing K et al: Causes of failure of surgery on lumbar spine. *Clin Orthop* 157:191, 1981.

104. Ross JS, Masaryk TJ, Modic MT et al: Lumbar spine: Postoperative assessment with surface-coil MR imaging. *Radiology* 164:851, 1987.

105. Raj PP: *Sympathetic pain mechanisms and management.* Second Annual Meeting of the American Society of Regional Anesthesia. Hollywood, Fla, 10–11, 1977.

1. The following are the components of an electrical diagnostic measurement except

   A. Electrodes
   B. Stimulator
   C. High-speed differential amplifier
   D. Blood pressure monitor

2. The cell membrane of a nerve axon separates the intracellular exoplasm from the extracellular fluid. This produces a potential difference between the cell membranes. When the nerve fiber is stimulated it causes a change in membrane potential by

   A. Rapid but brief flow of sodium ions through the ionic channels inward
   B. Rapid but brief flow of potassium ions through the ionic channels outward
   C. Rapid but brief flow of calcium ions through the ionic channels inward
   D. Rapid but brief flow of magnesium ions through the ionic channels inward

3. In myogenic paresis, all of the following are needle abnormalities in abnormal muscles except

   A. Insertional activity
   B. Spontaneous activity
   C. Abnormalities of voluntary motor activities
   D. Normal motor unit morphology

4. Reflex obtained by stimulation of the posterior tibial nerve in the popliteal space and characterized by slow rate and long duration is termed

   A. Babinski reflex test
   B. Pseudomotor axon reflex test
   C. F-wave
   D. H-reflex (Hoffman's reflex)

5. The advantages of magnetic resonance imaging (MRI) is all of the following except

   A. Patient receives no ionizing radiation
   B. MRI has significantly superior tissue contrast than any other imaging technique
   C. MRI images can be obtained in multiple planes without patient repositioning
   D. The cost of this procedure is cheaper than other imaging techniques

ANSWERS

1. D
2. A
3. D
4. D
5. D

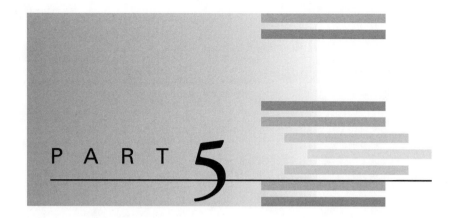

PART 5

Modalities
of Pain Management

Pharmacologic Techniques

NELSON HENDLER

The pharmacotherapy of chronic pain is complex because it requires knowledge of psychopharmacology as well as the effects of vasoactive drugs, nonsteroidal anti-inflammatory drugs (NSAIDs), opioids, antidepressants, tranquilizing agents, and hypnotics. No single formula is applicable to all chronic pain states because the origins of chronic pain are both multiple and as varied as the individuals who have the problem. Therefore, to choose from among the various medications effectively, one must understand the mechanism of action of each drug. In addition, drug interactions, synergy, antagonism, and side effects are important considerations in pharmacotherapy.

Among the other problems that attend pharmacotherapy in chronic pain patients are the psychologic factors that accompany the chronic pain problem. The goal of any drug therapy program must be elimination of drug dependancy,[1] treatment of depression and anxiety,[2] correction of sleeplessness,[3] and use of appropriate doses of analgesics.[4]

NEUROCHEMISTRY OF PAIN TRANSMISSION PATHWAYS

To understand the mechanism of pharmacotherapy for chronic pain patients, one must know the neurochemistry of the pain transmission pathways. From 2% to 5% of the neurotransmitters in the central nervous system (CNS) are biogenic amines.[5] These are indolamines, such as serotonin and catecholamines, including norepinephrine, epinephrine, dopamine, and dopa. The hypothalamus contains 90% biogenic amine neurosynaptic transmitters, but these types of transmitters are also found in the median forebrain bundle, the periventricular area of the hypothalamus, and the reticular activating system. All of these anatomic locations are components of the limbic system and are directly associated with emotion and with physiologic functions such as temperature regulation, sex, eating, drinking, and behavior, as well as pain perception. Neurosynaptic transmitters also include a number of peptides such as enkephalins and pentapeptides or β-endorphins.[1] Many of the receptors specific for these naturally produced morphine-like substances are in the same anatomic locations as the biogenic amine receptors.[6,7]

High levels of enkephalin are found in the periaqueductal and periventricular gray matter. Electrically stimulating these areas can produce analgesia that, according to some but not all investigators, can be blocked using naloxone, a morphine antagonist. Electrical stimulation probably causes the release of morphine-like substances into the surrounding brain.[8]

DRUGS MODIFYING PAIN PERCEPTION

Indolamines

One of the most useful categories of drugs for modifying pain perception is the indolamines. These are derived from L-tryptophan, which is converted to 5-hydroxytryptophan and then becomes 5-hydroxytryptamine. This indole ring structure occurs with a six-member carbon ring attachment by members of the ring structure. Most indolamines in the body are serotonin and related compounds. When serotonin is added to the CNS directly via the ventricle, it accumulates in the periventricular area. This increases the effectiveness of morphine analgesia.[9] Other researchers have found that augmenting serotonin by giving precursors that cross the blood-brain barrier or inhibiting the presynaptic reuptake with a variety of antidepressant drugs enhances serotonin-mediated activities such as sleep, raised threshold to pain, antidepressant activity, and antianxiety activity. Conversely, depletion of serotonin increases the perception of pain by lowering the pain threshold (Table 22–1).

Catecholamines

Catecholamines consist of a single six-member carbon ring with an ethyl amide chain and various substitutions. The prototypical catecholamine is levodopa (L-dopa), which is converted to dopamine, then to norepinephrine, and finally to epinephrine. Reducing norepinephrine levels in the ventricular system increases analgesia as a result of electrical stimulation that raises the pain threshold and increases morphine effectiveness.

Drugs with Anti-inflammatory Activity

A number of drugs have anti-inflammatory activity or inhibit prostaglandin synthesis:

- Acetaminophen: blocks prostaglandin synthesis centrally, which accounts for its antipyretic effect; however, it does not act on prostaglandins peripherally, so it cannot block local inflammation.
- Salicylates: have antipyretic and analgesic effects as well as anticoagulant and anti-inflammatory actions. Theoretically, these actions result from the antiprostaglandin activity, both centrally and peripherally.
- NSAIDs: have been well reviewed by Klipper and Kolodny.[10] They list nine major categories:
- Pyrazolines
- Indoleacetic acids
- Idene acetic acids
- Pyrrole acetic acids

TABLE 22–1   Effects of Synaptic Transmitters on Pain Perception

	Reduce Pain Perception	Heighten Pain Perception
Deplete or Block		
Norepinephrine	*	
Dopamine		*
Serotonin		*
L-Dopa		(?)
Augment or Mimic		
Norepinephrine		+(?)
Dopamine	*	
Serotonin	*	
L-Dopa	*	

*Effect.
Modified from Hendler N, Cimini C, Ma T et al: A comparison of cognitive impairment due to benzodiazepines and to narcotics. *Am J Psychiatry* 137:828, 1980.

TABLE 22–2   Mechanism of Action of Newer Antidepressants

Name	Dose Range	Presynaptic Mechanism of Action	Postsynaptic Mechanism
Mirtazapine (Remeron)	15–45 mg	Stimulates norepinephrine and serotonin release	Blocks 5-HT$_2$ and 5-HT$_3$ receptors
Fluoxetine (Prozac)	20–80 mg	Inhibits serotonin reuptake	
Paroxetine (Paxil)	20–50 mg	Inhibits serotonin reuptake	
Sertraline (Zoloft)	50–200 mg	Inhibits serotonin reuptake	
Venlafaxine (Effexor)	37.5–375 mg	Inhibits serotonin and norepinephrine reuptake	
Nefazodone (Serzone)	37.5–375 mg	Inhibits serotonin and norepinephrine reuptake	Blocks 5-HT$_2$ receptor
Bupropion (Wellbutrin)		Inhibits serotonin and dopamine reuptake	
Fluvoxamine (Luvox)		Inhibits serotonin and norepinephrine reuptake	

- Phenylacetic acids
- Propionic acids
- Anthranilic acids
- Benzothiazine group
- Quinazolinones

All NSAIDs inhibit the production of prostaglandin G, leading to gastric irritation. Because prostaglandin G protects the gastric mucosa, the addition of NSAIDs creates a different type of gastric irritation than excessive acid secretion. In effect, normal acid secretion in the absence of prostaglandin G can produce gastritis and ulcer disease.

A new category of drugs may supplement the NSAIDs. Collectively, drugs in this group are called *aspirin alternatives,* or APHs. In some animal studies, these drugs have been 60 times more powerful than aspirin for pain relief but produce none of the side effects of anticoagulation, gastric ulcers, and bleeding.

Antidepressants

Antidepressants for the treatment or control of chronic pain perception have been well studied. This type of drug may be divided into four broad categories:

1. Drugs that inhibit neurosynaptic transmitter reuptake
2. Drugs that have direct receptor stimulation
3. Drugs that produce receptor blockade
4. Drugs that inhibit the activity of enzymes such as monoamine oxidase

From a practical prospective, most antidepressants used for chronic pain fall into the first category, the neurosynaptic transmitter reuptake inhibitors.

Tricyclic antidepressant drugs, as well as some newer bicyclic and tetracyclic drugs, all work by inhibiting neurosynaptic transmitter reuptake. This mechanism of action on the catecholamines, as well as the indolamines, provides both antidepressant and antianxiety properties. These drugs also regulate sleep mechanisms and, if more sedative is used, can assist the patient to sleep at night. The ratio between the inhibition of norepinephrine and serotonin reuptake is discussed in Table 22–2. A thorough study of synaptic reuptake effects is shown in Table 22–3.[11]

A new class of antidepressant has been developed, the selective serotonin reuptake inhibitors (SSRIs). Drugs in this class are fluoxetine, sertraline, and paroxetine.

In the treatment of pain patients with chronic pain, all tricyclic antidepressants share the abilities to help the patient sleep, reduce anxiety and depression, and raise the pain threshold. Apparently, whatever mechanism of action they exhibit helps the chronic pain patient tolerate pain better, theoretically by inhibiting serotonin reuptake. Thus, the use of antidepressants in chronic pain has great practical significance. Table 22–4 gives effective dose ranges of tricyclic antidepressants, and Table 22–5 lists the effective dose ranges for some of the newer antidepressants.

Phenothiazines, Butyrophenones, and Other Anxiolytics

Anxiety commonly complicates chronic pain states. Most patients have been treated with a benzodiazepine. These may be effective as acute antianxiety agents, but their long-term use is contraindicated because they reduce biogenic amine activity.

TABLE 22–3 Antidepressant Potencies for Blockade of Neurotransmitter Uptake into Rat Brain Synaptosomes

Blockade of Norepinephrine		Blockade of Serotonin		Blockade of Dopamine	
Drug	**Potency**	**Drug**	**Potency***	**Drug**	**Potency***
Desipramine	++++	Clomipramine	++++	Bupropion	++
Protriptyline	++++	Fluoxetine	++++	Fluoxetine	+
Nortriptyline	+++	Imipramine	+++	Nortriptyline	+
Amoxapine	+++	Amitriptyline	+++	Clomipramine	+
Maprotiline	+++	Trazodone	++	Protriptyline	+
Imipramine	++	Nortriptyline	+	Amoxapine	+
Doxepin	++	Doxepin	+	Amitriptyline	+
Amitriptyline	++	Protriptyline	+	Maprotiline	+
Clomipramine	++	Desipramine	+	Trimipramine	+
Fluoxetine	+	Amoxapine	+	Imipramine	=
Trimipramine	+	Trimipramine	=	Desipramine	=
Bupropion	=	Maprotiline	=	Doxepin	=
Trazodone	=	Bupropion	0	Trazodone	0
Reference Compounds					
D-Amphetamine	++				++++
Cocaine	+				+++

*10 x 1/K where K is inhibitor constant in molarity. Data can be compared both vertically and horizontally across the table to find the most potent drug for a specific property and to find the most potent property of a specific drug.

++++, most potent; +++, potent; ++, moderately potent; +, =, weak effect; 0, no effect.

From Richelson G: Side effects of old and new generation antidepressants: a pharmacological framework. *J Clin Psychiatr Monogr* 9:13, 1991.

TABLE 22–4 Effective Dose Range of Tricyclic Antidepressants

Drug	Dose Range
Nortriptyline (Pamelor, Aventyl)	50–150 mg
Imipramine (Tofranil)	50–300 mg
Desipramine (Norpramin)	50–250 mg
Amitriptyline (Elavil)	25–250 mg
Protriptyline (Vivactil)	10–60 mg
Doxepin (Sinequan)	50–300 mg

TABLE 22–5 Effective Dose Range of Selective Serotonin Reuptake Inhibitors (SSRIs) and Other Mixed Action Drugs

Drug	Dose Range
SSRI	
Sertraline (Zoloft)	25–300 mg
Fluoxetine (Prozac)	10–80 mg
Paroxetine (Paxil)	10–80 mg
Others (Mixed Action)	
Venlafaxine (Effexor)	37.5–375 mg
Bupropion (Wellbutrin or Zyban)	75–450 mg
Fluvoxamine (Luvox)	50–300 mg
Mirtazapine (Remeron)	15–45 mg
Nefazodone (Serzone)	200–600 mg

TABLE 22–6 Equivalent Doses of Major Tranquilizers against 100 mg of Chlorpromazine (Thorazine) Standard*

Fluphenazine (Prolixin)	5 mg
Haloperidol (Haldol)[†]	5 mg
Perphenazine (Trilafon)	8 mg
Trifluoperazine (Stelazine)	5 mg
Thiothixene (Navane)*[†]	5 mg
Loxapine (Loxitane)*[†]	10 mg
Molindone (Moban)*[†]	25 mg
Thioridazine (Mellaril)	100 mg

*Based on clinical experience.
[†]Not a phenothiazine.
From Hendler N, Cimini C, Ma T et al: A comparison of cognitive impairment due to benzodiazepines and to narcotics. *Am J Psychiatry* 137:828, 1980.

Combinations of tricyclic mood elevators and phenothiazine tranquilizers of the sedative class have been used effectively in treating post-therapeutic neuralgia and intractable cancer pain. Their effectiveness may result from their antidepressant and antianxiety effects or because they actually alter the perception of pain.

There are at least three mechanisms by which a phenothiazine or butyrophenone tranquilizer produces reduced pain perception: (1) antianxiety, (2) postsynaptic blockade of noradrenergic receptors, and (3) inhibition of enkephalin-hydrolyzing enzymes. A practical guide to the use of these drugs is given in Table 22–7.

Benzodiazepines

The benzodiazepines are the largest group of prescribed drugs in the United States today (Table 22–8). These drugs have created a major problem for physicians involved in pain therapy because many patients like them, just as they like alcohol, and they resist withdrawal. Seizures caused by benzodiazepine withdrawal have been reported, and approximately 70% of the patients, either iatrogenically addicted or

The other compounds that have been used effectively to treat chronic pain are the phenothiazine tranquilizers (Table 22–6). One group is the sedative tranquilizers such as chlorpromazine. These drugs block dopamine postsynaptically but also block norepinephrine and have strong atropine-like action.

Another group of tranquilizers in the phenothiazine class, comprising fluphenazine, trifluoperazine, and perphenazine, blocks dopamine but has less effect on norepinephrine blockade and less atropine-like action.

TABLE 22–7   Guide to Use of Phenothiazines and Butyrophenone

Generic Name (Trade Name)	Equivalent Dose (Against 100 mg Chlorpromazine)	Usual Daily Dose	Common Side Effects
Phenothiazines			
Chlorpromazine (Thorazine)	100 mg	50 mg qid	Drowsiness, orthostasis, hypotension, atropine effects, tardive dyskinesia
Thioridazine (Mellaril)	100 mg	50 mg qid	As above, plus impotence
Fluphenazine (Prolixin)	5 mg	2 mg tid	Parkinsonian side effects, akathisia, tardive dyskinesia
Butyrophenone			
Haloperidol (Haldol)	5 mg	2 mg tid	As above, plus oculogyric crisis, torticollis, other dystonias

TABLE 22–8   Antianxiety Drugs Used for Pain

Generic Name	Trade Name
Clorazepate	Azene
Lorazepam	Ativan
Flurazepam	Dalmane
Chlordiazepoxide	Librium
Oxazepam	Serax
Clorazepate	Tranxene
Prazepam	Centrax
Diazepam	Valium
Temazepam	Restoril
Halazepam	Paxipam
Alprazolam	Xanax

self-addicted to these drugs, have changes of 15 to 25 cycles per second on electroencephalographic (EEG) examination, which is usually indicative of a sedative effect.

The benzodiazepines have three mechanisms of action[12]:

1. They act on benzodiazepine receptors to reduce anxiety.
2. They act on the glycine receptor to reduce muscle spasm.
3. They act on the γ-aminobutyric acid (GABA) receptors, which then reduces the turnover of biogenic amines by inhibiting presynaptic release of these transmitters.

The use of benzodiazepines to help patients sleep has created problems because normal sleep results in part from the accumulation of serotonin in the dorsal median raphe nuclei of the reticular activating system. A drug that decreases serotonin levels clearly alters natural sleep (Table 22–9). Serotonin, an indolamine, is responsible for producing natural sleep and increasing pain tolerance, and it has antidepressant qualities. Its release is inhibited by benzodiazepines. Dopamine, a catecholamine, is needed for morphine analgesia and also increases pain tolerance (Table 22–10). Its release is inhibited by benzodiazepines.

Opioids

Clinically, a physician may divide pain into three broad categories:

- Acute pain
- Chronic pain
- Pain of malignant origin

These distinctions are not beneficial because there are different physiologic mechanisms as well as different psychologic responses associated with the three different types of pain.

Certainly, no one would object to the use of opioids in patients with acute pain, nor would one object to similar use in patients with malignant pain problems. It is in the area of chronic pain of nonmalignant origin that problems arise. Opioids can produce tolerance with failure to obtain pain relief even if the drug dose is escalated. In these instances, opioids for chronic pain states of nonmalignant origins might be contraindicated.

Acute pain can be well controlled with the use of opioids, but one should be aware of the half-life of the individual agent to avoid severe peaks and valleys of relief and pain.

For nonmalignant pain, some physicians have advocated the use of opioids as needed, with a fixed number being given for a set time. Alternatively, very fixed schedules of administration with careful control can be used.

Legal issues influence opioid prescription more than medical concerns. Most state laws regarding chronic opioid prescriptions are similar to laws of Texas and California, sharing the following tenets:

1. The patient should have consulted another physician.
2. A clear-cut diagnosis must be established.
3. Previous nonopioid treatment must have been tried and must have failed.
4. Use of the opioid helps the patient function better than he or she would without the opioid.

Unusual Drugs

The use of several drugs employed in pain therapy cannot be validated through controlled studies, although anecdotal reports suggest they may be helpful and are worthy of additional trials. Drugs that fall under this category are:

- L-Dopa
- Propranolol
- Phentolamine
- Valproic acid
- Gabapentin
- Carbamazepine
- Diamox
- Mexiletine
- Antabuse

Muscle Relaxants

Muscle relaxants are a useful adjunct in the treatment of patients with chronic and persistent pain. There are a number of categories in muscle relaxants, but one may

TABLE 22–9 Effects of Drugs on Central Nervous System Synaptic Transmitters

	L-Dopa	Dopamine	Norepinephrine	Serotonin	Acetylcholine
Imipramine	0	0	++	++	− −
L-Dopa	+++	(+++)	++	++	0
Amitriptyline	0	0	+	++++	− − − −
Desipramine	0	0	++++	++	0
Chlorpromazine	− −	− − − −	− − − −	− −	− − − −
Diazepam	0	0	− −	− − −	−
Dextroamphetamine	+	++++	+++	0	0

0, no effect; +, augmentation; −, inhibition.
From Hendler N, Cimini C, Ma T et al: A comparison of cognitive impairment due to benzodiazepines and to narcotics. *Am J Psychiatry* 137:828, 1980.

TABLE 22–10 Drug that Exert Hypnotic Effects

	Serotonin	Rapid Eye Movement (REM) Sleep*	Effect On Stages 3 and 4 (Slow-Wave) Sleep
Doxepin	++++	+	+++
Amitriptyline	++++	+	+++
Imipramine	+++	+	++
Phenobarbital	− −	− − −	−
Flurazepam	− −	0	− − −
Diazepam	− − −	− −	− −
Chlorpromazine	0	+++	0
Desipramine	0	+++	0

0, no effect; +, augmentation; −, inhibition (Augmentation effects range from mild, +, to strong, + + + +; inhibition effects range from mild, −, to strong,− − − −.)
*REM sleep required acetylcholine and norepinephrine.
†Serotonin is needed to produce slow-wave (stages 3 and 4) sleep.
From Hendler N, Cimini C, Ma T et al: A comparison of cognitive impairment due to benzodiazepines and to narcotics. *Am J Psychiatry* 137:828, 1980.

broadly divide them into (1) centrally acting muscle relaxants and (2) peripherally acting muscle relaxants.

Tricyclic Antidepressant/Analgesic Interactions

An early report suggest that tricyclic antidepressants may enhance the intensity and duration of morphine sulfate analgesia in rats, as measured by behavioral tests.[13] More important, the chronic administration of desipramine led to higher circulating levels of unmetabolized morphine. Four possible explanations for this synergism are offered:

1. An additive central anticholinergic effect takes place because morphine reduces acetylcholine release in brain tissue, and some tricyclic antidepressants exert a postsynaptic blockade of central muscarinic sites.
2. To a varying degree, tricyclic antidepressants block the presynaptic reuptake of serotonin, which enhances morphine analgesia and prolongs its action.
3. After long-term administration, tricyclic antidepressants may interfere with opioid biotransformation, thereby leading to higher levels of opioid by interfering with the cytochrome P-450 system or by decreasing *N*-demethylation.[14]
4. Another tricyclic antidepressant-analgesic reaction may exist for the naturally occurring morphine-like substance enkephalin.

It is by these four mechanisms that tricyclic antidepressants enhance analgesia and exert their direct effect on enhancing sleep and reducing anxiety and depression; however, there are also negative antidepressant analgesic drug interactions. These interactions have been classified in two broad categories[15]:

1. Pharmacokinetic interactions involving the absorption, distribution, metabolism, or clearance of drugs
2. Pharmacodynamic interactions that occur directly at the site of action or indirectly by interfering with physiologic mechanisms

Because many chronic pain patients receive multiple drugs from a variety of drug categories, these patients have a heightened risk for unplanned and deleterious drug interactions. Understanding drug metabolism may help predict some of these problems. The coadministration of opioids and antidepressants requires close attention to the possibility of drug interaction.

Unless one is a pharmacologically skilled psychiatrist, the best rule is as follows:

1. Select one antidepressant for a patient.
2. Slowly escalate the dose until a desired effect is achieved (or until side effects intervene).
3. Taper the medication slowly.
4. Recognize that because many of the newer antidepressants have half-lives of 2 weeks or more, any new antidepressant or any other type of antidepressant will have to be started at a lower dose.

References

1. Bennett JP, Logan WJ, Snyder SH: Amino acids as central nervous system transmitters: The influence of ions, amino acid analogues, and ontogeny on transport systems for L-glutamate and L-aspartic acids and glycine into the central nervous synaptosomes of the rat. *J Neurochem* 21:1533, 1973.

2. Birmbaumer LG: Proteins in signal transduction. *Annu Rev Pharmacol Toxicol* 30:675, 1990.

3. Colclough G, Carter A, Ackerman WE 3rd: Mexiletine for chronic pain [letter]. *Lancet* 342:1484, 1993.

4. Depoortere H, Zivkovic B, Lloyd KG et al: Zolpidem, a novel nonbenzodiazepine hypnotic: I. Neuropharmacological and behavioral effects. *J Pharmacol Col Exp Ther* 237:649, 1986.

5. Hokfelt T, Jonssson G, Linbrink P: Electron microscope identifications of monoamine nerve ending particles in rat brain homogenates. *Brain Res* 22:147, 1970.

6. Pert C, Snyder S: Opiate receptor: Demonstration in nervous tissue. *Science* 179:1011, 1973.

7. Snyder SH: The opiate receptor and morphine-like peptides in the brain. *Am J Psychiatry* 135:645, 1978.

8. Hosobuchi Y, Adams JE, Linchitz R: Pain relief by electrical stimulation of the central gray matter in humans and its reversal by naloxone. *Science* 197:183, 1977.

9. Sewell RDE, Spencer PSJ: Modification of the antinociceptive activity of narcotic amines in mice. *Br J Pharmacol* 51:140, 1974.

10. Klipper A, Kolodny AL: Nonsteroidal anti-inflammatory drugs. In Hendler N, Long D, Wise T, editors: *Diagnosis and treatment of chronic pain.* Littleton, Mass, Wright-PSG, 1982.

11. Richelson G: Side effects of old and new generation antidepressants: A pharmacological framework. *J Clin Psychiatr Monogr* 9:13, 1991.

12. Hendler N: Benzodiazepines: Mechanism of action and appropriate use. In Day S, editor: *Life stress: A companion to the life sciences,* vol 3. New York, Van Nostrand Reinhold, 1982.

13. Goldstein FJ, Mojaverian P, Ossipov MH et al: Elevation in analgetic effect and plasma levels of morphine by desipramine in rats. *Pain* 14:279, 1982.

14. Melzack R: A tragedy of needless pain. *Sci Am* 262:27, 1990.

15. Steffens DC, Krishnan AB, Ranga R, Doraiswamy PM: Psychotropic drug interactions. *Biol Psychiatry* 4:24, 1997.

Questions • Pharmacologic Techniques

1. Serotonin and catecholamines are biogenic amines that are present in the central nervous system. These are called

   A. Neurosynaptic transmitters
   B. Opioids
   C. Anti-inflammatory drugs
   D. Endorphins

2. When serotonin is added to the central nervous system directly via the ventricles, it accumulates in

   A. The spinal cord
   B. The cerebral cortex
   C. Periaqueductal gray
   D. Periventricular area

3. Nonsteroidal anti-inflammatory drugs come from the following categories except

   A. Pyrazolines
   B. Propionic acids
   C. Benzothiazine
   D. Butyrophenones

4. Drugs that inhibit neurosynaptic transmitter uptake and inhibits the activity of monoamine oxidase are called

   A. Antidepressants
   B. Anti-inflammatory agents
   C. Opioids
   D. Muscle relaxants

5. Because many chronic pain patients receive multiple drugs, these patients have a heighten risk for deleterious drug reactions. The administration of opioids and antidepressants require all of the following except

   A. Select one antidepressant for the patient
   B. Taper the medication slowly
   C. Recognize that the newer antidepressants have effects on receptor sites of 2 weeks or more
   D. Escalate the dose quickly to achieve desired effects

ANSWERS

1. A

2. D

3. D

4. A

5. D

CHAPTER **23**

Interventional Techniques

PATRICK M. MCQUILLAN, RONNY KAFILUDDI, AND MARC B. HAHN

SUBARACHNOID BLOCK

Spinal anesthesia is produced by injection of a local anesthetic solution into the lumbar subarachnoid space. Its use for surgical procedures was first described in 1899 by Augustus Bier, a German surgeon who successfully produced spinal anesthesia for lower limb orthopedic procedures by injecting cocaine into the subarachnoid space. Interestingly, the first description of a postdural puncture headache was reported at this time. Spinal anesthesia rapidly gained widespread acceptance, primarily because it was easily performed, effective, and inexpensive. Despite a decrease in popularity during the middle of the 20th century, spinal anesthesia is now the most commonly used regional anesthetic technique worldwide.

Anatomy

Bony Elements and Ligaments

The vertebral column consists of 7 cervical, 12 thoracic, and 5 lumbar vertebrae. Each vertebra consists of a vertebral body and a bony arch. The arch consists of two pedicles anteriorly and two laminae posteriorly. The junction of the pedicles and laminae forms the transverse processes, and the spinous processes are formed posteriorly at the junction of the laminae. The lumbar region is of the most interest in spinal anesthesia. The lumbar vertebrae have the largest and most massive bodies, and the bony elements form a triangular vertebral foramen (Fig. 23A–1). The laminae are broad and short and do not overlap. The spinous processes of lumbar vertebrae are thick, broad, and hatchet-shaped.

Spinal Cord and Meninges

The spinal canal extends from the foramen magnum to the sacral hiatus. It contains the spinal cord and its coverings: the pia, arachnoid, and dura mater. The spinal cord is approximately cylindrical. It is continuous with the medulla oblongata of the brain at the foramen magnum and terminates in the tapered conus medullaris at the lower border of the first or second lumbar vertebra (Fig. 23A–2). Whereas the spinal cord ends at the L1 or L2 level, the lower lumbar and sacral nerves extend for some distance in the spinal canal as the cauda equina.

The spinal cord is enclosed in three covering layers. The *dura mater* is the outermost covering. It is a long, tubular sheath of dense, white fibrous and elastic connector tissue extending from the foramen magnum to the level of the second sacral vertebra. The spinal *arachnoid membrane* continues with the same layer investing the brain. It follows completely the limits of the spinal dura mater, separate from it only by the minute subdural space. The spinal *pia mater* is the intimate connector tissue covering of the spinal cord that enmeshes its blood vessels. At the conus medullaris, or ending of the substance of the spinal cord, the pia mater continues into the filum terminale, gradually replacing all of the nervous elements within it.

Spinal Nerves

Attached to the spinal cord are 31 pairs of nerves—8 cervical, 12 thoracic, 5 lumbar, 5 sacral, and 1 coccygeal. Each nerve is formed from the union of the dorsal and ventral roots, which remain separated within the subarachnoid space. They form a mixed nerve only after becoming ensheathed by the dura-arachnoid distal to the dorsal root ganglion. Each spinal nerve supplies a specific region of skin and skeletal muscle.

Blood Supply

The blood supply of the spinal cord originates from the spinal branches of the vertebral, deep cervical, intercostal, and lumbar arteries. These spinal branches divide into anterior and posterior radicular arteries that travel along the nerve routes to reach the cord and divide to form a plexus of arteries in the pia mater. Usually one radicular artery is much larger than the rest and is responsible for supplying most of the blood to the lower two thirds of the cord.

Cerebrospinal Fluid

Cerebrospinal fluid (CSF) is a clear, colorless ultrafiltrate of blood formed by the choroid plexuses in the ventricle of the brain. CSF passes through the interventricular foramen of Monro into the third ventricle, then through the cerebral aqueduct to the fourth ventricle. It exits the fourth ventricle by way of the lateral and median foramina of Luschka and Magendie to reach the subarachnoid space. CSF is then

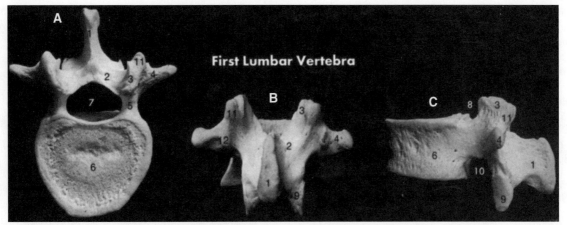

FIG 23A–1 Lumbar vertebra demonstrating comparative anatomy. *A,* Superior view. *B,* Posterior view. *C,* Left lateral view of the first lumbar vertebra. 1, Spinous process; 2, lamina; 3, superior articular process; 4, transverse process; 5, pedicle; 6, vertebral body; 7, vertebral foramen; 8, superior vertebral arch; 9, inferior articular process; 10, inferior vertebral notch; 11, mamillary process; 12, accessory process. *(From Hogan Q: Spinal anatomy. In Hahn MB, McQuillan PM, Sheplock GJ, editors:* Regional anesthesia: an atlas of anatomy and technique. *St. Louis, Mosby, 1996.)*

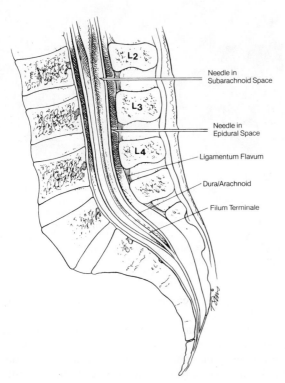

Needle in Subarachnoid Space

Needle in Epidural Space

Ligamentum Flavum

Dura/Arachnoid

Filum Terminale

FIG. 23A–2 Sagittal section showing needle placement in the subarachnoid and the epidural space. *(From Raj PP, Pai U, Rawal N: Techniques of regional anesthesia in adults. In Raj PP, editor:* Clinical practice of regional anesthesia. *New York, Churchill Livingstone, 1991.)*

absorbed by arachnoid villi that project from the subarachnoid space.

Technique

Equipment

Spinal anesthesia's initial popularity came almost to an abrupt halt in 1954 following the Wooley and Roe cases in which two patients were permanently paralyzed after spinal injections. These catastrophes were determined to be the result from sterilization procedures used at the time. Fortunately, there are many disposable spinal anesthesia trays on the market that are supplied with the essential items and customized to each practitioner's needs.

Spinal needles vary in length and inside and outside diameters. The latter affects the size and shape of the hole made in the dura as well as the speed with which CSF appears in the hub after dural puncture. The incidence of postdural puncture headache appears to be directly related to the size of needle used and the orientation of the needle in performing spinal anesthesia. A spinal needle oriented parallel to the dura separates the fibers rather than cutting them, as a perpendicularly oriented needle does, and produces a smaller defect in the dura.

All spinal needles come with a removable stylet, which must be close fitting to prevent coring of the skin and the resultant obstruction of the needle and contamination of spinal space with epidermal tissue and skin bacteria.

The commonly used spinal needle with a cutting point is the Quincke-Babcock, which has a short bevel with cutting edges and a rounded heel. The cutting-point spinal needles appear to be associated with a high incidence of postspinal headache even when smaller needles are used.

Position

Spinal anesthesia can be performed with the patient in the lateral decubitus, sitting, or prone position. The lateral or sitting position affords the greatest patient comfort. In the lateral position, the line of spinous processes is oriented parallel to the floor. The normal slope from pelvis to shoulder usually orients the patient with a slight head-down position, so reorientation of the table in slight reverse Trendelenburg position is often required to ensure this parallel relationship. To "open" spinal interspaces, the patient flexes his or her back by drawing the knees to the chest and flexing the neck, so the chin rests on the chest.

The sitting position encourages flexion and facilitates recognition at the midline, particularly in obese patients. In the sitting position, the CSF pressure is elevated and the lumbar sac is distended, facilitating placement of the needle tip within the subarachnoid space by promoting free flow of CSF.

The prone position is used primarily for personal procedures that use a hypobaric local anesthetic solution. Subarachnoid block in this position is technically more difficult because of limited flexion, low CSF pressure, and a contracted dural sac.

Interspace Selection and Approach to the Subarachnoid Space

Spinal anesthesia is usually instituted with a needle inserted at an easily palpable interspace below L2. Depending on the patient's individual anatomic features, the second, third, or fourth lumbar interspace may be selected. After the most prominent point of the iliac crests is located, an imaginary line is drawn between them (Tuffier's line), which usually crosses the L4 spinous process or the L4-L5 interspace (Fig. 23A–3). As with any other invasive procedure, strict aseptic technique should be observed; the area of skin over the insertion site is prepared with an antiseptic solution. Routine cardiopulmonary monitoring is also required.

With the midline approach, the spinal needle transverses the skin, the supraspinous ligament, the interspinous ligament, the ligamentum flavum, and the epidural space before entering the subarachnoid space (Fig. 23A–4). A skin wheal of local anesthetic is raised with a small-gauge needle. Subsequently, the spinal needle is inserted at this site, parallel or slightly cephalad, and directed to the spinous processes. With the operator's nondominant hand straddling the interspace selected to fix the tissues and act as a "gun site," the needle is advanced at a slightly cephalad angle until it is firmly engaged in the supraspinous ligaments. After the ligaments are engaged, it is no longer possible to change the direction of the needle tip. As the operator continues to advance the spinal needle it traverses the ligamentum flavum and punctures the dura. This is often realized by a subtle release through the ligamentum flavum or a slight pop as the needle passes through the dura mater. Correct needle placement is confirmed by the appearance of CSF at the hub of the spinal needle after the stylet has been removed.

In the lateral approach, the needle passes through the skin, subcutaneous fat, lumbar aponeurosis, paravertebral muscles, ligamentum flavum, and epidural space before entering the subarachnoid space.

Contact with bone with any approach usually means that the lamina or spinous process has been encountered. This can be distinguished by the relative depth of the needle when contact has been made; a shallow depth reaches the spinous process, whereas a deeper depth reaches the lamina. If bone has been contacted, a small change in needle direction is required. The needle must be withdrawn into the introducer or withdrawn to a depth at which the ligaments no longer have purchase on the needle.

When the spinal needle is determined to be positioned in the subarachnoid space, by free flow of CSF once the stylet of the needle is removed, the appropriate dose of local anesthetic is injected, preceded and followed by aspiration of CSF (Table 23A–1).

After the needle has been removed, the patient is turned to the desired position. Spread of local anesthetic is determined either by pinprick or by loss or change of sensation to ice or alcohol. Usually, no further spread of local anesthetic is seen after 15 to 20 minutes.

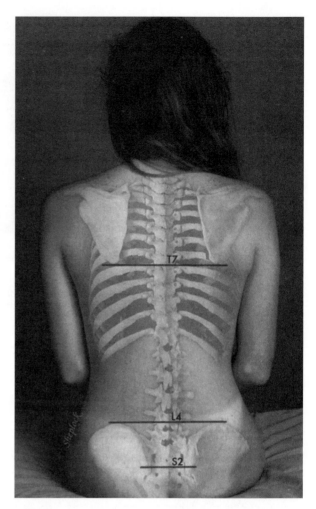

FIG. 23A–3 Computer-enhanced image of the vertebral column superimposed over the surface anatomy. T7 spine is approximately at a vertical line through the scapulae tips, L4 is approximately at a vertical line through the iliac crests, and S2 is approximately at a vertical line through the posterior superior iliac spines. *(From Hogan Q: Spinal anatomy. In Hahn MB, McQuillan PM, Sheplock GJ, editors:* Regional anesthesia: an atlas of anatomy and technique. *St. Louis, Mosby, 1996.)*

Factors Affecting Spread of Local Anesthetics

Once some local anesthetic solution has been injected in the subarachnoid space, onset of a block is relatively rapid, and the patient should be placed in the appropriate position immediately. Factors affecting the spread of local anesthetic include (1) baricity of the local anesthetic, (2) position of the patient after injection, (3) level of injection, (4) speed of injection, (5) dose and volume of the local anesthetic used, and (6) a technique known as barbotage. Of these, the two with the greatest influence are the baricity of the local of the local anesthetic and the position of the patient. The specific gravity of the local anesthetic solution may be adjusted with

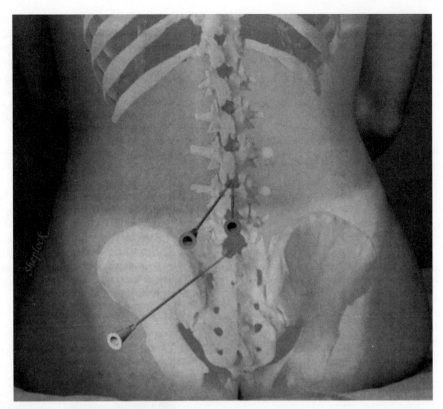

FIG. 23A–4 Computer-enhanced image of the spine and bony landmarks superimposed over the surface anatomy to demonstrate the point of needle insertion for a midline, a paramedian, and a Taylor approach to the subarachnoid space. *(From Drasner K: Subarachnoid space. In Hahn MB, McQuillan PM, Sheplock GJ, editors:* Regional anesthesia: an atlas of anatomy and technique. *St. Louis, Mosby, 1996.)*

TABLE 23A–1   Dosing for Subarachnoid Blockade (Adult)

		Dose (mg) to Achieve			Duration (min)	
		L4	**T10**	**T4**	**With Epinephrine**	**Without Epinephrine**
Lidocaine	Hyperbaric	50	50–75	75–100	60–90	60–90
	Isobaric		50		60–90	60–90
Bupivacaine	Hyperbaric	7.5	10–12	15	9–150	9–150
	Isobaric		10		9–150	9–150
Tetracaine	Hyperbaric	5	8–10	12–15	180–270	120–180
	Isobaric		10–12		180–270	120–180
	Hypobaric	5–10			180–270	120–180

From Drasner K: Subarachnoid. In Hahn MB, McQuillan PM, Sheplock GS, editors: *Regional anesthesia: An atlas of anatomy and technique.* St. Louis, Mosby, 1996.

the addition of water, normal saline solution, or glucose to make it hypobaric, isobaric, or hyperbaric in relationship to CSF.

A *hyperbaric solution* has higher specific gravity than CSF so that it moves to low-lying parts of the subarachnoid space. A *hypobaric solution* has a lower specific gravity than CSF and spreads to higher-lying areas within the subarachnoid space. An *isobaric solution,* with a specific gravity matching that of CSF, tends to remain at the injection point, irrespective of position changes after injection.

Factors affecting the duration of spinal anesthesia include (1) drug used, (2) dose injected, (3) spread achieved, (4) addition of vasoconstrictors, and (5) age and general condition of the patient.

Side Effects and Complications

Immediate adverse effects of spinal anesthesia occur as a direct result of the physiology of neural blockade often associated with a "high spinal." These include nausea, vomiting, hypotension, and bradycardia. Delayed adverse effects or complications of spinal anesthesia range from relatively minor problems, such as headache, backache, and urinary retention, to rare but severe complications, such as arachnoiditis, cauda equina syndrome, transient radicular irritation, and, in some instances, paralysis.

Potential causes of major neurologic sequelae are numerous, including infection, trauma, ischemia, and neurotoxic reactions.

EPIDURAL BLOCK

Historical Background

The first use of epidural anesthesia has often been attributed to James Leonard Corning, a neurologist whose intentions were to treat some neurologic disorders by using cocaine "spinally."[1]

In the early 1990s, French urologists Cathelin and Sicard were the first to accurately document the application of epidural anesthesia using the sacral route. Edwards and Hingson[2] were the first to report on the application of continuous caudal epidural anesthesia in 1942. The earliest use of epidural injections for low back pain secondary to sciatica was described by Viner in 1925.[3] Box 23A–1 lists the various applications for epidural administration.

Applied Anatomy

Understanding both surface anatomy and the anatomy of the spinal canal and surrounding structures is essential to the successful performance of any epidural procedure. Knowledge of surface anatomic landmarks is important in determining the level of needle insertion. The most commonly used landmarks (see Fig. 23A–3) from the cranial to caudal are as follows:

1. The C7 spinous process, also known as the vertebral prominence, is the most prominent spinous process when the neck is flexed.
2. The T7 vertebral body is approximately at the cross section of the spinous process and an imaginary line between the inferior angles of the scapulae.
3. L1 is found by imaging a line between the distal margins of the right and left 12th rib.
4. A line between the superior aspects of the iliac crest crosses L4.
5. S2 is at a horizontal line through the posterosuperior iliac spines.

Once the level of entry of the epidural needle has been determined, the anesthesiologist must decided whether to approach the epidural space via a midline or a paramedian technique. Either technique can be used in the thoracic or lumbar region. The midline approach is commonly used in the cervical area. Because of the perpendicular orientation of the cervical and lumbar spinous processes (Fig. 23A–5), a midline needle must enter at an angle approximately 90 degrees with respect to the skin. Thoracic spinous processes between T4 and T9 are angulated and even overlap in places (see Fig. 23A–5). Because of this angulation, some clinicians prefer a paramedian approach in the thoracic region.

After the clinician identifies the level and angulation, the epidural needle encounters the following structures from superficial to deep, assuming a midline approach: skin, subcutaneous tissue, supraspinous ligament, interspinous ligament, ligamentum flavum, and epidural space. Some of these structures can be missed, which can result in failure or possible complications if the clinician does not clearly identify the midline.

BOX 23A–1 Applications of Epidural Administration

Acute Pain Syndromes
Intraoperatively
Postoperative/post-trauma
Obstetrics
Pancreatitis
Frostbite
Acute herpes zoster
Ischemic pain syndromes
Renal colic

Chronic Pain Syndromes
Low back pain
Postherpetic neuralgia
Complex regional pain syndromes
Chronic malignancy
Phantom limb pain
Diagnostic/prognostic blocks
Epidural electrical stimulation
Epiduroscopy

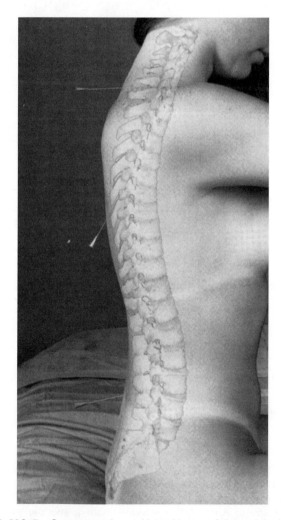

FIG. 23A–5 Computer-enhanced lateral image of the vertebral column superimposed over the surface anatomy, demonstrating the angle needed for needle placement at the cervical, thoracic, and lumbar regions. *(From Hogan Q: Spinal anatomy. In Hahn MB, McQuillan PM, Sheplock GJ, editors: Regional anesthesia: an atlas of anatomy and technique. St. Louis, Mosby, 1996.)*

Physiozlogic Effects of Epidural Blockade

The physiologic effects of epidural blockade depend on the level and number of spinal segments involved. The effects on the respiratory, cardiovascular, and gastrointestinal systems are secondary to sympathetic or somatic motor blockade following epidural administration of local anesthetic agents.

Respiratory Effects

It is conceivable that a high thoracic or cervical block may impair respiratory function by affecting sensory function, motor function, and sympathetic function. Sympathetic block may diminish pulmonary blood flow and ventilation-perfusion (V/Q) mismatch. All these changes have the potential to lead to airway closure, atelectasis, decreased blood flow, and diminished functional reserve capacity, causing V/Q mismatch and hypoxemia.

Cardiovascular Effects

The effect of epidural anesthesia on the cardiovascular system depends on the extent and degree of sympathetic blockade. This sympathectomy may lead to alterations in cardiac rhythm, heart rate, myocardial contractility, and vascular tone. The principal cardiovascular consequences of extensive epidural blockade are hypotension and bradycardia. The extent of sympathetic blockade, however, correlates very poorly with the sensory level. The amount of sympathetic denervation and sensory blockade might be larger than the classically taught two levels.

Extensive sympathetic blockade from epidural or subarachnoid nerve block may result in hypotension caused by preganglionic sympathetic blockade, affecting predominately (1) heart rate, (2) venous return by changing both mean systemic pressure (P_{MS}) and resistance to venous return (R_V), and (3) contractility.

Gastrointestinal Effects

The gastrointestinal tract is innervated by both the sympathetic and parasympathetic systems. Visceral afferent parasympathetic fibers transmit sensations of satiety, distention, and nausea (but not pain). Parasympathetic efferent outflow increases tonic contraction, sphincter tone, peristalsis, and secretions. Pain is mediated via sympathetic afferents, whereas sympathetic efferent fibers inhibit peristalsis and gastric secretions, constrict vasculature, and increase sphincter tone. Sympathetic denervation of the gastrointestinal tract may lead to generalized contraction of the bowel secondary to unopposed parasympathetic efferent outflow.

Technique

Cervical Epidural Blockade

Cervical epidural blockade using steroids is often employed to treat chronic cervical pain caused by nerve root irritation secondary to conditions such as herniated cervical disk and spinal stenosis. Cervical epidural anesthesia can also be used for pain control in the perioperative period for carotid, thyroid, or breast surgery. Epidural blocks can be performed with the patient seated, in a lateral decubitus position, or prone.

No matter which position is selected, it is important to flex the spine maximally to open the intervertebral spaces. A soft roll under the chest or hips is required to flex the spine for prone patients. The most frequently used space is the C7-T1 interspace. The vertebral prominence (C7) is easily palpated and moves anterior and posterior on extension and flexion of the neck, respectively.

The most common method of identifying the epidural space is the loss-of-resistance technique. A syringe containing saline solution or air is attached to the needle anchored in the interspinous ligament.

It is said that control of the advancing needle is what makes epidural blockade a challenge. One way to control the needle is to hold the index finger of the noninjecting hand against the patient's back, which acts as a resistance to the sudden forward movement. The thumb and middle finger hold the needle hub. Another way is the "Bromage" grip (Fig. 23A–6). The needle is firmly gripped between the thumb and index finger of the nondominant hand. The dorsum of the wrist is placed against the patient's back. The needle is advanced by extension of the wrist while the dominant hand provides intermittent or constant pressure on the plunger, depending on whether one uses the loss-of-resistance technique to air or to saline solution, respectively.

After optimizing the position, one can perform the block using either a midline approach to the epidural space or a paramedian technique, depending on (1) location, (2) degree of calcification of the ligamentous structures, or (3) acquired or congenital deviation of the spine.

For a midline approach in the cervical area, a 27-gauge, 3.2-cm needle is used to make a skin wheal midway between the spinous process after the site is prepared with antiseptic solution and sterilely draped. This needle can also be used to infiltrate local anesthetic in the ligamentous structures and to explore the subcutaneous tissues down the base of the spinous process. The skin may be nicked with an 18-gauge, 3.8-cm needle before insertion of the epidural needle.

The epidural needle is inserted about 3 to 4 cm in adults and anchored into the interspinous ligament. The stylet is withdrawn, and either a drop of fluid is placed in the needle hub or a syringe containing either air or saline solution is attached to the syringe. The needle should be redirected (caudally or cephalad) if one encounters bony structures at 2 to 4 cm. The use of fluoroscopy for anteroposterior (AP) and lateral views makes it easier to approach the epidural space because bony structures are well visualized.

Needle placement in the epidural space after loss of resistance to air or saline solution can be confirmed fluoroscopically by injection of 3 to 5 ml of radiopaque nonionic contrast medium. An AP view is used to identify needle depth. The lateral view is helpful when the use of contrast medium is contraindicated and when one suspects a false loss of resistance.

A paramedian approach is easier to perform if the patient is placed in a left or right lateral position with the head and neck well flexed. The skin is prepared with antiseptic solution, and sterile drapes are placed around the site. The same interspace (C7-T1 or C6-C7) is identified, and a skin wheal is made 1 cm lateral to the midline; a 25-gauge, 3.8-cm needle with 1% lidocaine is used to perform deeper infiltration of the subcutaneous tissue. A nick in the skin can be

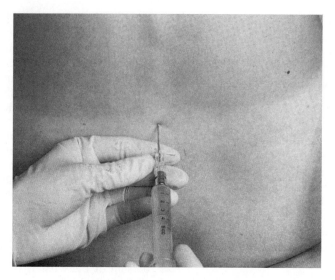

FIG. 23A–6 Lumbar epidural blockade performed via a midline approach with the patient sitting. Needle placement is accomplished through the loss of resistance to saline technique. The "Bromage" grip is used to advance the needle in a controlled fashion. Continuous pressure is applied on the plunger of the syringe by the dominant hand while the needle is advanced slowly by the nondominant hand. A loss of resistance to the syringe plunger occurs when ligamentum flavum is pierced. *(From Hogan Q: Epidural. In Hahn MB, McQuillan PM, Sheplock GJ, editors:* Regional anesthesia: an atlas of anatomy and technique. *St. Louis, Mosby, 1996.)*

made with an 18-gauge, 3.8-cm needle before the 18- to 20-gauge epidural needle is inserted. The epidural needle is then directed toward the midline at a 15- to 20-degree angle to the sagittal plane.

After the needle is inserted 2 to 3 cm, the stylet is removed and a syringe with either air or saline solution is attached to the epidural needle. Loss of resistance to air or saline injection signifies entry of the epidural space.

Thoracic Epidural Blockade

Thoracic epidural blocks can be performed via a midline or paramedian technique. The paramedian technique is simpler to perform in the thoracic area.

The overlying skin is prepared with antiseptic solution and draped. A skin wheal is made 1 to 1.5 cm lateral to the interspace between two spinous processes with a 25-gauge, 3.8-cm needle (Fig. 23A–7). The needle is then introduced perpendicular to the skin, and 1% lidocaine is infiltrated into the deeper structures until the lamina is encountered. Contacting lamina is the most important landmark with this technique.

The 25-gauge needle is withdrawn, and a skin nick is made with an 18-gauge needle before insertion of an 18- to 20-gauge epidural needle. The epidural needle is advanced perpendicular to the skin until the lamina is encountered. After the epidural needle is withdrawn approximately 0.5 cm, the stylet is removed and a syringe with air or saline solution is attached to the hub of the epidural needle. The epidural needle is now redirected 45 degrees in the parasagittal plane and 15 to 20 degrees in the axial plane (see Fig. 23A–7).

Each time the needle contacts the lamina, it is withdrawn 0.5 cm and walked off the lamina in a medial and cephalad direction until a clear pathway to the epidural space is created. The epidural space is identified using loss of resistance to air or saline solution.

Lumbar Epidural Blockade

The patient may be in either the sitting or the lateral position for a midline approach to the lumbar epidural space. The prone position is chosen if fluoroscopy is used.

The overlying skin is prepared with either alcohol or povidone-iodine solution, and the area is draped sterilely. A skin wheal is made midway between the chosen spinous processes with a 25-gauge, 3.8-cm needle and 1% lidocaine. It is helpful to identify the caudal spinous process with the 25-gauge needle if no bony landmarks are identifiable. The skin is then nicked with an 18-gauge needle. The 18- to 20-gauge epidural needle is inserted until it is anchored in the interspinous process.

Once the spinous process is identified, the epidural needle is withdrawn 0.5 cm, directed more cephalad in the sagittal plane, and walked off the spinous process until a clear pathway is identified. The stylet is removed after the needle is anchored into the interspinous process. At this point, a syringe with air or saline solution is attached to the hub of the needle. The epidural needle is advanced using the two-handed intermittent or the Bromage technique. The epidural space is identified using the loss-of-resistance to air or saline technique. Once the epidural space is identified, aspiration should be negative for heme or CSF to avoid injecting drugs intravascularly or intrathecally, respectively.

The paramedian approach can be performed with the patient sitting, lateral, or prone. The overlying skin is prepared with antiseptic solution and draped sterilely.

A skin wheal is made 1.5 cm lateral to the caudal edge of the spinous process below the space in which the epidural puncture is to be made with a 25-gauge, 3.8-cm needle and 1% lidocaine. Deeper tissue is infiltrated along the intended pathway. The skin is nicked with an 18-gauge needle before an 18- to 20-gauge epidural needle is inserted. The epidural

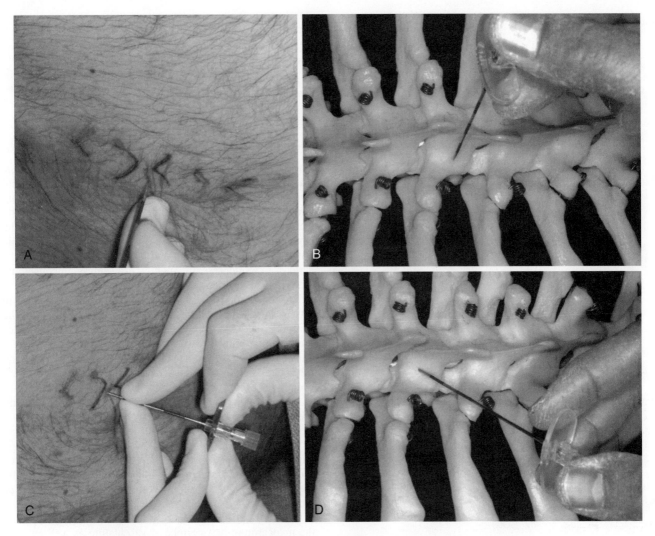

FIG. 23A–7   Thoracic epidural blockade with the patient in the left lateral decubitus position for a right thoracotomy. A left paramedian technique is used to enter the T4-T5 epidural space (the arrow tips medial to the needle represent the inferior and superior borders of T4 and T5, respectively). After the skin has been infiltrated with 1% lidocaine, a Weiss (winged) 17-gauge epidural needle is used to enter the skin perpendicularly, approximately 1 to 1.5 cm lateral to the interspinous space of T4 and T5 (*A* and *B*). The needle is advanced until the lamina of T5 is encountered (*B*). The needle is subsequently withdrawn for 2 cm and redirected at a 45-degree angle in the sagittal plane and 15 degrees in the axial plane (*C* and *D*). The angle of approach is changed once resistance is met. This probably indicates that the needle contacts either laminae of T4 or T5 or the spinous process of T4. Once the pathway is clear, the needle is advanced until loss of resistance to air or saline occurs.

needle is advanced cephalad and medially so that it makes a 15-degree angle to the sagittal plane.

After the needle is advanced 3 to 4 cm, the stylet is removed and a syringe containing air or saline solution is attached to the hub of the needle. Loss-of-resistance to air or saline solution identifies the epidural space.

Caudal Blockade

Theoretically, the caudal block can be used for any indication recommended for lumbar epidural block. This technique is, however, reserved for procedures requiring blockade of the sacral and lumbar nerves, because it is often difficult to obtain a high enough level of local anesthetic block (Fig. 23A–8). The sacral route is also used for epidurography and lysis of epidural adhesions in patients with

low back pain and radicular symptoms following spinal surgical intervention.

The sacral hiatus is most easily identified with the patient lying in the prone or lateral position. A pillow is placed under the pelvis when the patient is prone. Firm pressure is used to identify the coccyx with the nondominant index finger. The first pair of bony protuberances in moving cephalad are the two cornua, surrounding the sacral hiatus.

The skin is prepared with antiseptic solution and draped sterilely. A skin wheal is raised using a 25-gauge, 3.8-cm needle with 1% lidocaine. The skin is nicked with an 18-gauge needle before insertion of an epidural needle. This can be either a 20-gauge epidural needle or a 21-gauge, short-bevel (2.5-cm) needle. The needle is introduced through the skin wheal and nick in the skin at about a

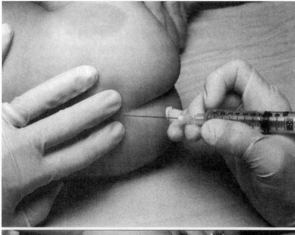

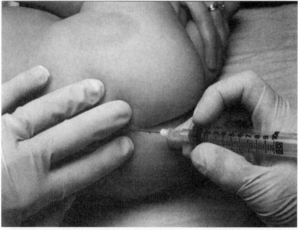

FIG. 23A–8 Caudal blockade of a pediatric patient in the lateral decubitus position. *(From Rice LJ: Caudal. In Hahn MB, McQuillan, PM, Sheplock GJ, editors:* Regional anesthesia: an atlas of anatomy and technique. *St. Louis, Mosby, 1996.)*

120-degree angle to the back. The bevel of the needle should be facing anteriorly to minimize the chance of piercing the anterior sacral wall.

When the needle is advanced, a distinct "snap" is felt on piercing of the sacrococcygeal membrane. At this point, the needle is lowered to an angle of 160 degrees and advanced an additional 5 to 7 mm. The needle should not be advanced more than 1.5 cm, because the dural sac ends at the S2 level in adults. The dural sac ends even more caudally in children, and the epidural needle should, therefore, be advanced only 0.5 cm into the sacral epidural space.

Complications

Any invasive procedure is associated with complications. The complications associated with epidural blockade can be drug related and technique related.[3] Drug-related complications result primarily from the systemic absorption of local anesthetic compounds that are accidentally injected into a vein of the rich epidural venous plexus. It is conceivable that systemic toxicity might occur because of the relatively large doses of local anesthetic required to achieve pharmacologic or surgical effectiveness. Intravascular injection leads to a rapid rise in plasma level. Unintentional injection into epi-

dural veins results in plasma levels similar to those obtained after an intravenous injection.

Four systems are affected by high plasma levels of local anesthetics:

- Central nervous system (CNS)
- Cardiovascular system
- Hematologic system
- Immune system

Central Nervous System

The earliest symptoms of CNS toxicity are lightheadedness, tinnitus, perioral numbness, numbness of the tongue, and blurred vision. Signs include generalized CNS excitation, such as shivering, muscular twitches, confusion, and tremors of the facial muscles, followed by tremors of the extremities. These may progress to generalized tonic-clonic convulsions. The excitatory signs are then followed by a state of CNS depression, such as drowsiness, unconsciousness, respiratory depression, and arrest.

The excitatory effect of local anesthetics in the brain involves the selective blockade of inhibitory pathways in the cerebral cortex. Inhibition of inhibitory pathways facilitates unopposed excitatory activity. At higher doses of the local anesthetic, both inhibitory and excitatory pathways become inhibited, leading to generalized state of CNS depression. Treatment of the CNS toxicity should be directed toward maintaining an adequate airway, supporting ventilation, and preventing hemodynamic collapse.

Cardiovascular Complications

High systemic levels of local anesthetics can produce profound effects on the cardiovascular system. In general, the cardiovascular system is more resistant to the toxic effects of these agents than is the CNS.

Cardiovascular toxicity results from direct actions on the myocardium and peripheral vasculature as well as indirect effects involved with the CNS. All local anesthetics exert a dose-dependent negative inotropic action in vitro, using isolated myocardial tissue,[4,5] as well as in situ, using open-chest myocardial canine preparations.[6] In terms of their myocardial depressant effect, local anesthetics can be divided into three groups according to their anesthetic potency:

1. Highly potent agents (tetracaine, bupivacaine, and etidocaine) depress cardiac contractility at very low concentrations.
2. Agents of moderate anesthetic potency (mepivacaine, prilocaine, lidocaine, and cocaine) are intermediate cardiodepressants.
3. Agents of lowest potency (chloroprocaine and procaine) are the least cardiodepressant.[5,7]

The cardiovascular effects of local anesthetics can be summarized as follows. At low, nontoxic blood levels, local anesthetics may slightly increase blood pressure, related to a mild increase in cardiac output and heart rate that results from enhancement of sympathetic activity and direct vasoconstrictor action. Concentrations that produce CNS toxicity result in marked increases in heart rate, cardiac output, peripheral resistance, and blood pressure. A further increase in dose leads to severe hypotension and cardiovascular collapse secondary to decreased cardiac output and peripheral vascular dilatation.

Hematologic Complications

High doses of prilocaine and benzocaine can result in methemoglobinemia. Benzocaine is used only topically and would require enormous doses to cause side effects. However, hydroxylated orthotolidine, a metabolite of prilocaine, may cause clinically significant methemoglobinemia when doses in the excess of 600 mg are administered epidurally.

The signs of methemoglobinemia include central cyanosis, which is treated with intravenous administration of methylene blue of 1% solution.

Immune System

Allergic reactions to local anesthetics are extremely rare. Signs and symptoms include pruritus, dermatitis, urticaria, anaphylactoid reactions, and bronchospasms. The local anesthetics most commonly implicated in hypersensitivity or allergic reactions are the amino esters.

Other Complications

Subdural Injection

The subdural space is a potential space between dura and arachnoid mater. Injection of drugs into this space can cause extensive and erratic spread. Moreover, a profound patchy sensory block with mild motor block may develop.

Postdural Puncture Headache

A headache after puncture of the dura during an epidural injection has typical characteristics. These headaches are positional and are associated with diplopia, vertigo, tinnitus, nystagmus, hearing loss, photophobia, nausea, and vomiting. A major factor in the cause of these headaches is the size of the needle used. The pain is thought to be cause by traction on pain-sensitive intracranial blood vessels following the loss of intracranial CSF.

Back Pain

The incidence of back pain after a dural block is approximately 10%. One major factor is the size of the needle used. The mechanism is usually secondary to injury involving musculoskeletal structures of the spine. The pain is self-limiting and is treated with nonsteroidal anti-inflammatory drugs, acetaminophen, or hot compression.

Epidural Hematoma

Trauma to the epidural veins occurs frequently (10%). This, however, does not lead to a large hematoma unless the patient had received anticoagulants, is coagulopathic or thrombocytopenic, or has a functional platelet defect. A large hematoma acts like a space-occupying lesion and can cause cord compression, ischemia, or myelopathy, leading to mild sensory or motor deficit or to paraplegia and incontinence.

Epidural Abscess

As with hematomas, abscesses can cause severe, sudden neurologic deficits. Patients present with back pain, radiculopathy, lower extremity weakness, decreased sensation and deep tendon reflexes, and bladder and bowel incontinence. Other signs are pyrexia, leukocytosis with a leftward shift, and an elevated erythrocyte sedimentation rate. Epidural abscesses most likely occur secondary to bacteremia with colonization of an epidural hematoma.

Adhesive Arachnoiditis

Adhesive arachnoiditis starts initially as a minimal cellular inflammatory response after a wide variety of circumstances involving all meningeal components. It may follow trauma; surgery; tumors; infections; hemorrhage; or the intrathecal administration of various compounds such as iophendylate, potassium chloride, thiopental sodium, parenteral nutrition, or povidone-iodine. It leads to clumping and thickening of the nerve roots and progresses to collagenous adhesions.

Meningitis

Meningitis following neuroaxial block may be infectious or aseptic. Aseptic meningitis results from injection of an irritant into the subarachnoid space after spinal anesthesia or an unintentional dural puncture from an attempted epidural block. Symptoms include fever, headache, lethargy, confusion, and nuchal rigidity.

Spinal Cord and Nerve Root Injury

The spinal cord or a single spinal nerve may be injured by direct needle trauma, following the injection of chemicals directly into the nerve or spinal cord, or after damage to the blood supply to the cord. Table 23A–2 summarizes the neurologic complications, clinical presentations, and outcome associated with epidural anesthesia.

TABLE 23A–2 Various Types of Neurologic Damage Following Epidural Blockade

Pathology	Cause	Onset	Clinical Features	Outcome
Spinal nerve neuropathy	Needle trauma	0–2 days	Pain during insertion of needle and injection, paresthesias, pain, numbness over distribution of spinal nerve	Recovery in 1–12 weeks
Anterior spinal artery syndrome	Arteriosclerosis, hypotension	Immediate	Painless paraplegia	Painless paraplegia
Adhesive arachnoiditis	Irritant injectate	0–7 days	Pain on injection, variable degree of neurologic deficit; often progressive with pain and paraplegia	May progress to severe disability
Hematoma or abscess	Coagulopathy	0–2 days	Severe backache with progressive paraplegia	Requires immediate surgery

From Covino BK, Scott DB: *Handbook of epidural anaesthesia and analgesia.* Orlando, Fla, Grune & Stratton, 1985.

References

1. Corning JL: Spinal anesthesia and local medication of the cord with cocaine. *N Y Med J* 42:483, 1885.
2. Edwards WB, Hingson RA: Continuous caudal anesthesia in obstetrics. *Am J Surg* 57:169, 1942.
3. Mackey DC, Carpenter RL, Thompson GE et al: Bradycardia and asystole during spinal anesthesia: A report of three cases without morbidity. *Anesthesiology* 70:866, 1989.
4. Block A, Covino BG: Effect of local anesthetic agents on cardiac conduction and contractility. *Reg Anesth* 6:55, 1982.
5. Feldman HS, Covino BM, Sage DJ: Direct chronotropic and inotropic effects of local anesthetic agents in isolated guinea pig atria. *Reg Anesth* 7:149, 1982.
6. Stewart DM: Effects of local anesthetic on the cardiovascular system of the dog. *Anesthesiology* 24:621, 1963.
7. Covino BG, Scott DB: *Handbook of epidural anaesthesia and analgesia.* Orlando, Fla, Grune & Stratton, 1985.

CHAPTER *23*

Interventional Techniques

MARK ROMANOFF, PAUL J. KUZMA, AND MARK D. KLINE

SOMATIC NERVE BLOCKS OF THE HEAD AND NECK

There are many indications for performing somatic nerve blocks of the head and neck:

1. They may be required for surgical procedures to provide complete analgesia in the awake patient or as a supplement to a general anesthetic.
2. They can be used for postoperative pain management.
3. In patients suffering from chronic pain syndromes, they are used for diagnostic or therapeutic purposes. Identifying the nerve involved in the pain by selective blockade can ensure an appropriate diagnosis. This information can then be applied to educate the patient and to direct further therapy.
4. Nerve blocks can be employed to reduce inflammation and entrapment of a nerve or neuroma or to "break the cycle of pain."
5. Recalcitrant pain syndromes may warrant neurolysis of the nerve or surgical ablation (neurectomy). All treatment decisions are predicted on the information derived from the selective blockade of these somatic nerves.

Trigeminal Nerve/Gasserian Ganglion Block

Indications

Trigeminal neuralgia is the most common indication for a gasserian ganglion block. Other indications include cancer-related pain, cluster headaches, and atypical facial pain. Often a neurolytic block or neurodestructive lesion is required for long-term pain relief in these patients.

Anatomy

The gasserian ganglion receives sensory information from the scalp, face, nasal areas, oral mucosal membranes, and teeth (Fig. 23B–1). Proprioceptive information from the muscles of mastication and extraocular muscles also terminates there. The ganglion is located in the middle cranial fossa.

The ganglion is shaped like a crescent moon. The convex side is aimed anterolaterally. The posterior border of the ganglion includes the dura of Meckel's cave and cerebrospinal fluid (CSF). The peripheral branches of the ganglion form the ophthalmic, maxillary, and mandibular nerves (Table 23B–1).

Technique

The gasserian ganglion block combines a technically challenging procedure with possible life-threatening side effects. Intra-arterial or CSF injections occur frequently because of the ganglion's location. This maneuver must be done with x-ray or fluoroscopic guidance to confirm needle position.

The patient is placed supine with the cervical spine extended. A sterile preparation of the face is performed, carefully avoiding the eye. Local anesthetic infiltration is done approximately 2.5 cm lateral to the corner of the mouth, at the midpupillary line. A 10- to 15-cm, 22- or 20-gauge needle is directed almost perpendicular to the skin above and lateral to the molars at that point. The direction of travel should be superior and toward the medial aspect of the external auditory meatus (Fig. 23B–2*A* and *B*). The needle is advanced until it touches the base of the skull. The needle is gently repositioned into the foramen ovale. A mandibular nerve paresthesia is common. If it occurs, the needle should be redirected until no paresthesia occurs.

X-ray guidance should be used throughout this procedure to confirm needle placement but especially before injection. An aspirate that is negative for blood and CSF is also mandatory before injection. Only small quantities of local anesthetic (1 to 3 ml) are necessary for a successful block. The local anesthetic should be given in small divided doses (0.25 ml) until the desired amount or therapeutic endpoint is reached. Thermocoagulation, radiofrequency coagulation, phenol (6%), glycerol, and absolute alcohol have been used successfully to perform neurolytic gasserian ganglion blockade. Thermocoagulation and radiofrequency coagulation are techniques of choice because they avoid the difficulties inherent in chemical neurolysis.

Concerns

The gasserian ganglion block is technically challenging and is usually painful. These two factors mandate conscious sedation or a general anesthetic. Local anesthetic can be

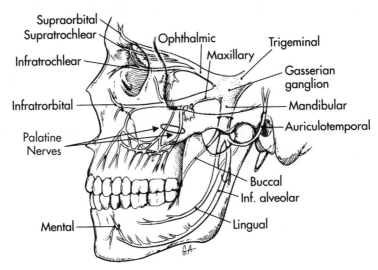

FIG. 23B–1   Anatomy of the trigeminal nerve.

TABLE 23B–1   Trigeminal Nerve Branches and Innervation

Name	Sensory Area, Motor Function	Name	Sensory Area, Motor Function
Ophthalmic Nerve		**Facial Location**	
Lacrimal nerve	Skin of upper eyelid, lacrimal gland	Infraorbital nerve	
		Palpebral nerve	Skin of lower eyelid
Frontal Nerve		Nasal nerve	Skin on side of nose and septum
Supraorbital nerve	Lateral skin of forehead and scalp	Superior labial nerve	Skin of cheek, upper lip, mouth
Supratrochlear nerve	Medial skin of forehead and scalp		
		Mandibular Nerve	
Nasocillary Nerve		Meningeal nerve	Middle cranial fossa dura, mastoid air cells
Anterior ethmoidal nerve	Nasal mucous membranes, septum, skin of external nose	Medial pterygoid nerve	Medial pterygoid muscle
Long ciliary nerves	Cornea		
Infratrochlear nerve	Skin of medial eyelid and side of nose	**Anterior Trunk**	
Posterior ethmoidal nerve	Ethmoid and sphenoid sinuses	Buccal nerve	Posterior aspect of buccal surface of gum
Maxillary Nerve		Masseteric nerve	Innervates masseter muscle and TMJ
		Deep temporal nerves	Innervates temporalis muscle
Cranial Location		Lateral pterygoid nerve	Innervates lateral pterygoid muscle
Meningeal nerve	Middle cranial fossa dura		
		Posterior Trunk	
Pterygopalatine Location		Auriculotemporal nerve	Skin of tragus, helix of ear, tympanic membrane, parotid gland, skin of temporal region, TMJ
Ganglionic nerve	Sphenopalatine ganglion; nasal, palate, and pharyngeal mucous membranes		
Zygomatic nerve	Skin of temple	Lingual nerve	Mandibular gums, floor of mouth, anterior two thirds of tongue
Posterior superior alveolar nerve	Maxillary sinus, maxillary molar teeth, gum	Inferior alveolar nerve	
		Mylohyoid nerve	Innervates mylohyoid and anterior belly of digastric muscles
Infraorbital Canal Location		Premolar, molar nerves	Mandibular premolar and molar teeth and gums
Middle superior alveolar nerve	Maxillary premolar teeth		
Anterior superior alveolar nerve	Maxillary incisor and canine teeth	Incisive nerve	Incisor and canine teeth and gums
		Mental nerve	Skin of chin and lower lip

TMJ, Temporomandibular joint.

injected into the CSF because of the proximity of the ganglion to Meckel's cave and the trigeminal cistern (see Fig. 23B–2*C*). A CSF injection can occur despite an aspiration that is negative for CSF. The most severe complications include loss of consciousness, cardiac arrest, and apnea resulting from this "high spinal" blockade.

Vascular trauma may take the form of hematoma or ecchymosis at the needle insertion site or around the cheek area. As a consequence of this block, the oculomotor and abducens nerves may be anesthetized. If a neurolytic agent is injected into the CSF, other cranial nerves may be affected permanently.

Ophthalmic Nerve Block

Indications

Retrobulbar blocks are used to provide surgical anesthesia for intraocular surgery, strabismus "squint" surgery, or facial

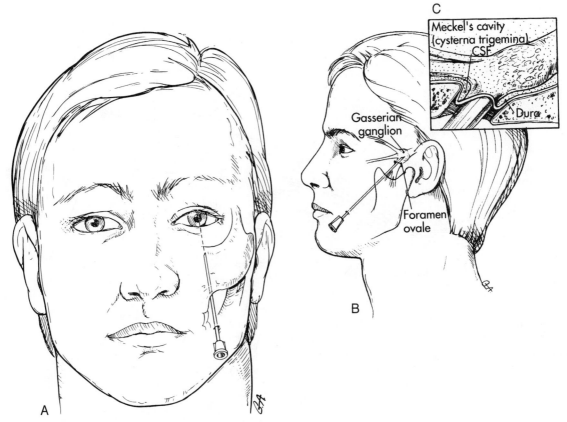

FIG. 23B–2 Anatomy of gasserian nerve block. *A,* Needle direction in anteroposterior view. *B,* Needle direction in lateral view. *C,* Enlargement of Meckel's (trigeminal) cave.

repairs. In refractory cases of eye pain, this block can be performed initially as a diagnostic procedure.

Anatomy

The ophthalmic nerve, a sensory nerve, is the superior and smallest division of the trigeminal nerve. It travels anteriorly in the cavernous sinus laterally; then enters the superior orbital fissure; and continues in the orbit as the frontal, lacrimal, and nasociliary nerves (Fig. 23B–3). It supplies sensation to the eye, lacrimal gland, conjunctiva, and a portion of the nasal mucous membranes as well as the skin of the scalp, forehead, eyelid, and nose (see Table 23B–1).

Technique

The ophthalmic nerve block involves an injection on the temporal side of the orbit (Fig. 23B–4*A*). The sterile preparation must be done carefully to avoid the eye. The needle (27-gauge, 20 to 31 mm) is inserted into the skin at the inferior and lateral aspects of the orbit perpendicular to the skin. The needle is advanced until its tip is lateral to the globe. It is then redirected superiorly and nasally, aimed for a point behind the proximal iris (see Fig. 23B–4*B*).

The needle is advanced approximately 25 to 30 mm. It should lie in the anterior intracone space near the ciliary ganglion (see Fig. 23B–4*C* and *D*). From 2 to 4 ml of 2% lidocaine or 0.5% bupivacaine is injected slowly after an aspiration that is negative for blood and CSF. Pupillary dilation and paralysis of the extrinsic muscles should occur after the block, depending on the volume injected.

Concerns

Because CSF injection can result in loss of consciousness, cardiac arrhythmias, and respiratory compromise as with the gasserian ganglion block, appropriate resuscitative equipment must be present.

Eye damage can result from needle entry into the sclera. Optic nerve damage has also been reported. Bleeding can occur and may cause retinal detachment or ischemia of the eye. Long-term extraocular muscle weakness or damage has been reported with high concentrations of local anesthetic and can result in permanent ptosis.

Supraorbital and Supratrochlear Nerve Blocks
Indications

Supraorbital and supratrochlear neuropathies can be identified and treated with local anesthetic alone or with corticosteroids. Migraine headaches may be triggered by these neuropathies. Common causes of neuropathy include trauma, postsurgical damage, and idiopathic conditions. Localized trigeminal neuralgia or postherpetic neuralgia above the eye or in the scalp may also be seen, especially in patients in the seventh decade of life.

Anatomy

The large supraorbital and smaller supratrochlear nerves are the final terminations of the frontal branch of the ophthalmic nerve. The supraorbital nerve exits through the supraorbital foramen and supplies sensation to the upper eyelid, lateral forehead, and scalp. The supratrochlear nerve

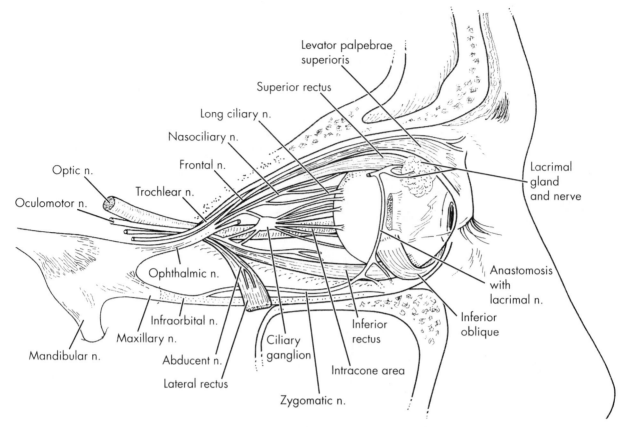

FIG. 23B–3 Anatomy of the orbit, globe, and nerves in the lateral view.

exits the orbit medial to the supraorbital foramen and supplies sensation to the upper eyelid, the medial forehead, and scalp.

Technique

The patient is placed in semi-Fowler's position. A 3- to 4-cm, 25-gauge needle is inserted into the skin perpendicular to the supraorbital foramen, which is located at the superior orbital rim above the pupil. The needle is advanced until (1) bone is encountered, (2) the foramen is entered, or (3) a paresthesia is elicited. From 2 to 5 ml of local anesthetic is injected there and just lateral and medial to this point. If the supratrochlear nerve is also to be blocked, the needle is advanced subcutaneously and medially approximately 2 to 3 cm and the same volume is injected (Fig. 23B–5).

Concerns

Hematoma formation or ecchymosis at the needle site can occur but with less frequency than at the infraorbital location. The supraorbital artery can be lacerated.

Maxillary Nerve Block

Indications

Indications for maxillary nerve block include the treatment of trigeminal neuralgia in the maxillary distribution or other neuropathic processes of the maxillary nerve and analgesia for surgery of the upper jaw, teeth, gums, hard or soft palate, and cheek. Atypical facial pain may be related to any of the

terminal branches of the maxillary nerve. Some of these branches are inaccessible to specific blockade but can be anesthetized by a maxillary nerve block.

Anatomy

The maxillary nerve is a purely sensory nerve that begins at the gasserian ganglion and travels anteriorly and inferiorly along the cavernous sinus through the foramen rotundum. It extends to the superior aspect of the pterygopalatine fossa along the inferior portion of the orbit in the infraorbital fissure and exits through the infraorbital foramen. The branches of the maxillary nerve supply sensation to the dura, upper jaw, teeth, gums, hard and soft palates, and cheek as well as parasympathetic fibers.

Technique

The patient is placed supine with the head turned toward the contralateral side. The mandibular notched is identified. A 22-gauge, 7.5- to 8-cm needle is then placed perpendicular to the skin at the posterior and inferior aspects of the notch (Fig. 23B–6). The needle is advanced until it encounters the lateral pterygoid plate. The needle is then withdrawn and redirected anteriorly and superiorly at about a 45-degree angle toward the eye. The needle is again advanced until a paresthesia is obtained. To minimize the risk of injection into the CSF, the needle should not be advanced farther than 1.5 cm past the lateral pterygoid plate.

From 3 to 5 ml of local anesthetic is injected. Neurolytic procedures can be done with 6% phenol or absolute alcohol.

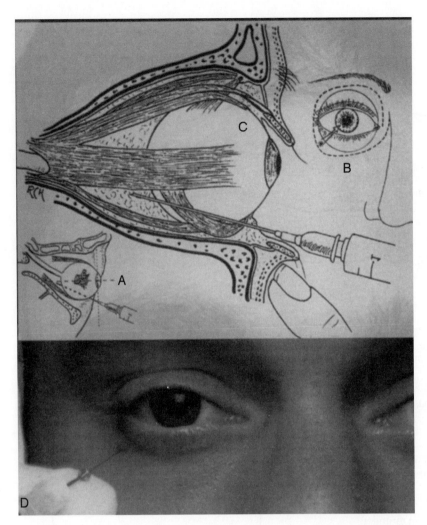

FIG. 23B–4 Anatomy of retrobulbar block of the ophthalmic nerve. *A,* Needle direction in anteroposterior view. *B,* Needle direction viewed from the superior aspect of orbit. *C,* Needle direction viewed from the lateral aspect of orbit. *D,* Needle in final position. *(A to C, Courtesy of Gimbel Educational Services. D, From Hamilton RC: Ophthalmic nerve (retrobulbar blockade). In Hahn MB, McQuillan PM, Sheplock GJ, editors: Regional anesthesia: an atlas of anatomy and techniques. St. Louis, Mosby, 1996.)*

A maximum volume of 1 to 1.5 ml delivered in 0.1-ml divided does is recommended.

Concerns

Injection into the CSF with the complications noted previously can occur. The close proximity of the orbit to this nerve makes it likely to be involved in a complication. Orbital swelling, anesthesia of the orbital tissues, ophthalmoplegia, loss of visual acuity, or diplopia can occur if the local anesthetic or neurolytic solution enters the infraorbital fissure. Damage to vascular structures can cause hemorrhage into the orbit, and blindness can occur. Because the maxillary nerve is close to many blood vessels, hematoma formation is common.

Infraorbital Nerve Block

Indications

The primary indications for an infraorbital nerve block include the treatment of localized trigeminal neuralgia and the treatment of infraorbital neuropathies.

Anatomy

The infraorbital nerve is the terminal branch of the maxillary division. It exits the cranium through the infraorbital foramen. It supplies sensation to the cheek from the lower

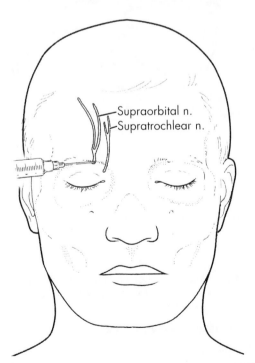

FIG. 23B–5 Needle insertion for supraorbital and supratrochlear nerve blocks.

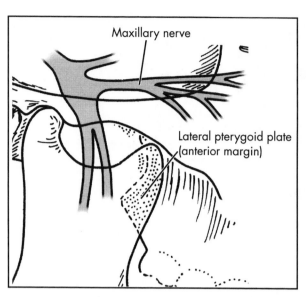

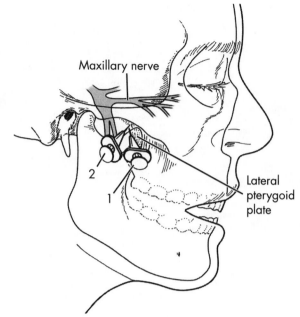

FIG. 23B–6 Maxillary nerve block in the lateral view. Initial needle direction (*1*) and redirection of needle (*2*) after it encounters the pterygoid plate are shown. *Inset* shows detailed anatomy.

eyelid to the upper lip as far medially as the nasal ala and laterally to the midzygoma region.

Technique

There are two approaches to the infraorbital nerve: the extraoral (the most common) and the intraoral.

Extraoral Approach

The infraorbital foramen can be palpated 1 to 1.5 cm under the inferior edge of the orbit at the midpupillary line. The skin is prepared, and a 22- to 25-gauge, 1- to 3-cm needle is inserted at a 30-degree angle to the skin, with the needle directed toward the eye (Fig. 23B–7). If a paresthesia is obtained, the needle should be withdrawn 2 mm to avoid an intraneural injection.

The needle can sometimes be advanced into the canal. It should not be advanced more than 2 to 3 mm into the canal to avoid a neuropraxia of the nerve and also to prevent anesthetizing more proximal branches of the maxillary nerve (see Fig. 23B–1 and Table 23B–1). After an aspiration that is negative for blood and CSF, injection of 2 to 5 ml of local anesthetic solution produces a block.

Intraoral Approach

In the intraoral approach, the upper lip is retracted. A 25-gauge, 3- to 4-cm needle is inserted into the alveolar area above the teeth at the junction of the buccal mucosal membranes of the lip. The needle is then directed toward a point 1 cm below the infraorbital foramen. The neurovascular bundle lies in this area. From 2 to 5 ml of anesthetic solution is injected after an aspiration that is negative for blood and CSF.

Concerns

Hematoma formation or ecchymosis at the needle site can result from damage to the relatively large infraorbital artery

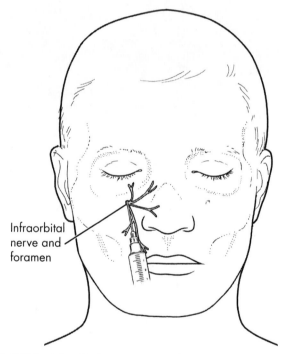

FIG. 23B–7 Infraorbital nerve block with needle direction in the anteroposterior view.

or vein. A paresthesia is often encountered when performing this block. It is important to withdraw the needle slightly to avoid damaging the nerve.

Greater Palatine Nerve Block

Indications

Indications for the greater palatine nerve block include surgical anesthesia of the hard and soft palates and maxillary molars. This block can control pain resulting from acute ulceration of the palate.

Anatomy

The greater palatine is a branch of the maxillary nerve. It originates in the superior aspect of the greater palatine canal and is adjacent to the sphenopalatine ganglion. Fibers run inferiorly with the lesser palatine nerves and nasal branches of the maxillary nerve. The greater palatine nerve continues and exits the greater palatine foramen (see Fig. 23B–1).

Technique

The technique is identical to that used for a sphenopalatine ganglion block by the intraoral route. The patient is placed in a semi-Fowler's position and the mouth is opened wide. A 25- or 27-gauge, 5- to 7.5-cm needle should be bent gently in the middle at a 75-degree angle to allow insertion into the canal. A dental or three-ring syringe is helpful, but the block can be done with a typical syringe. The second molar is identified. The foramen can often be palpated 1 cm lateral to the molar on the hard palate.

The anesthesiologist directs the needle into the canal perpendicular to the palate by grasping the needle with the other hand to stabilize it. Often, the hard palate is encountered after approximately 5 to 10 mm. The needle should be withdrawn and redirected into the canal. The needle should then be advanced 5 mm into the canal. After an aspiration that is negative for blood and CSF, no more than 2 ml of local anesthetic should be injected.

Concerns

If more than 2 ml of local anesthetic solution is used, the sphenopalatine ganglion can be blocked as well. Localized bleeding is seen but easily controlled with pressure. Injection into the mucosa of the palate instead of the foramen is common.

Mandibular Nerve Block

Indications

Indications for mandibular nerve block include treatment of trigeminal neuralgia in the mandibular distribution or other neuropathic processes of the mandibular nerve and analgesia for surgery of the lower jaw, teeth, gums, or cheek.

Anatomy

The mandibular nerve is the inferior and largest division of the gasserian ganglion. It has motor and sensory functions. The nerve exits the foramen ovale, runs inferiorly and medially to the lateral pterygoid muscle, and then branches into anterior and posterior trunks. There are multiple nerve terminations of these trunks (see Table 23B–1). The mandibular nerve receives sensory information from the skin from the temporal area to the chin, the lower teeth and gums, and mucous membranes of the mouth floor and anterior two thirds of the tongue. The motor fibers innervate the temporalis, masseter, and pterygoid muscles.

Technique

The approach is essentially identical to that of the maxillary nerve procedure. The difference lies in the direction of the

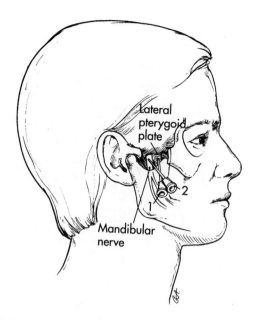

FIG. 23B–8 Mandibular nerve block in the lateral view. Initial needle direction (*1*) and redirection of needle (*2*) after it encounters the pterygoid plate are shown.

needle once the pterygoid plate is encountered. For a mandibular nerve block, the needle is directed inferiorly and posteriorly if a mandibular distribution paresthesia is not encountered. A paresthesia is necessary for a successful block (Fig. 23B–8). The local anesthetic and neurolytic solution requirements are the same as for the maxillary nerve block.

Concerns

Concerns are similar to those of the maxillary nerve block.

Auriculotemporal Nerve Block

Indications

Indications for the auriculotemporal block include neuralgia of the auriculotemporal nerve and atypical facial pain in the appropriate sensory dermatome.

Anatomy

The auriculotemporal nerve is derived from the posterior trunk of the mandibular nerve and travels under the lateral pterygoid muscle, lateral to the temporomandibular joint (TMJ) near the apex of the parotid gland. It becomes superficial just posterior to the superficial temporal artery and anterior to the external auditory meatus. It then runs vertically to the temporal area. It receives sensory input from the TMJ, parotid gland, external auditory meatus, tympanic membrane, skin over the temporal area, and tragus of the ear.

Technique

The patient is placed supine with the head turned toward the contralateral side. The superficial temporal artery is palpated posterior to the external auditory meatus. A 25-gauge, 1- to 2-cm needle is inserted perpendicular to the skin midway between the artery and the meatus. The needle is advanced until bone is encountered. The needle is withdrawn 2 mm,

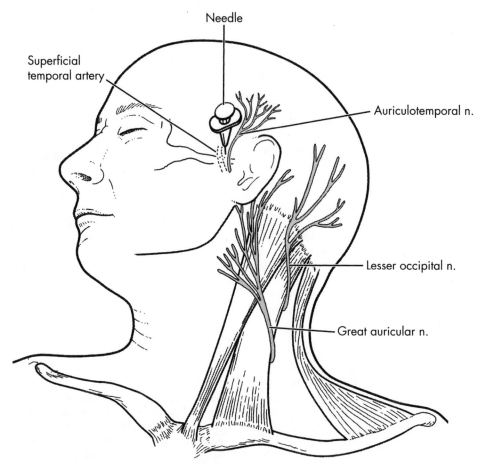

FIG. 23B–9 Needle direction for auriculotemporal nerve block in the lateral view.

and 2 to 3 ml of local anesthetic solution is injected after negative aspiration (Fig. 23B–9). A subcutaneous infiltration of 2 to 3 ml at the insertion site is sometimes necessary to ensure skin analgesia in the temporal area.

Concerns

If the needle is placed too far posteriorly, it advances into the space adjacent to the cartilage of the auditory canal. The injection can be made there but often anesthetizes only the auditory meatus. A hematoma can occur if the needle is placed too far anteriorly and if the superficial temporal vessels are damaged.

Mental Nerve Block

Indications

Indications for the mental nerve block include surgical analgesia, mental nerve neuralgia, atypical facial pain in the appropriate sensory dermatome, and numb chin syndrome.

Anatomy

The mental nerve is the terminal branch of the inferior alveolar nerve of the mandibular nerve. It exits the mental foramen and innervates the skin of the chin and mucous membranes of the lower lip.

Technique

There are extraoral and intraoral approaches to the mental nerve.

Extraoral Approach

The mental foramen is palpated on the mandible. It is located along the midpupillary line (Fig. 23B–10). A 22- or 25-gauge, 1- to 4-cm needle is inserted perpendicular to the foramen. If no paresthesia is elicited, the needle should be advanced until the mandible is encountered. It is then withdrawn 2 mm. After an aspiration that is negative for blood and CSF, 2 to 5 ml of local anesthetic solution can be injected.

Intraoral Approach

The lower lip is pulled away from the teeth. The foramen can be palpated on the mandible just lateral and inferior to the first premolar tooth. A 25-gauge, 3- to 4-cm needle is inserted into the alveolar mucosa at the level of the foramen. The needle is directed almost perpendicular to the bone and angled slightly inferiorly. The injection is performed as described for the extraoral route.

Concerns

To avoid damage to the nerve, the needle should not enter the foramen. There is some evidence that the intraoral approach is less painful and has a higher degree of success.

Greater Occipital Nerve Block

Indications

Greater occipital neuralgia is a common cause of headaches. Many tension-type headaches in the occipital region or

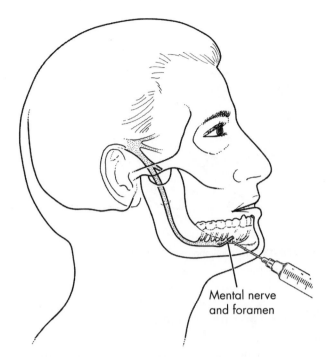

FIG. 23B–10 Needle direction for mental nerve block in the lateral view.

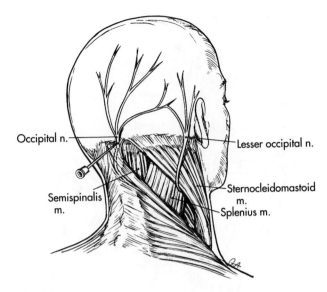

FIG. 23B–11 Needle direction for greater occipital nerve block in the posteroanterior view.

whiplash injuries are related to irritation or compression of these nerves. Migraine headaches may also be triggered by an occipital neuralgia.

Anatomy

The medial branch of the second cervical dorsal root travels between the semispinal and inferior oblique muscles of the head and emerges at the superior level of the cervical trapezius muscle insertion. It runs vertically with the occipital artery up to the vertex of the skull. It supplies the skin of the scalp in the occipital area.

Technique

The occipital artery can often be palpated at the superior nuchal line approximately 4 cm lateral to the midline (Fig. 23B–11). A 22-gauge, 3- to 4-cm needle is inserted perpendicular to the skin, just medial to the artery pulsations. The needle is advanced until a paresthesia or bone is encountered and then withdrawn 2 mm. From 2 to 5 ml of local anesthetic solution is injected after an aspiration that is negative for blood and CSF.

Concerns

Few complications of this injection are noted, although an intravascular injection is possible.

Glossopharyngeal Nerve Block
Indications

A glossopharyngeal nerve block can be used for the evaluation of atypical facial pain, the treatment of glossopharyngeal neuralgia, and the treatment of intractable pain caused by pharyngeal cancer. Refractory hiccups have also been treated successfully.

Anatomy

The ninth cranial nerve has both sensory and motor fibers. It arises from the medulla and runs anteriorly under the temporal bone. It exits the skull through the jugular foramen and runs between the internal carotid artery and the internal jugular vein posterior to the styloid process. It then proceeds anteriorly into the pharyngeal muscles. It receives sensory information from the posterior third of the tongue, soft palate, tonsils, pharynx, and auditory canal.

Technique

There are extraoral and intraoral approaches to this nerve.

Extraoral Approach

The patient is placed supine. The styloid should lie midway between the mastoid process and the angle of the jaw. A 22-gauge, 4-cm needle is inserted at the site perpendicular to the skin and angled slightly superiorly. The needle is then advanced until the styloid process is encountered. Next, the needle is redirected (Fig. 23B–12). The glossopharyngeal nerve can be encountered either anteriorly or posteriorly at this point because it is almost horizontal in this area. The needle is advanced 1 to 2 cm, and after negative aspiration, 3 to 5 ml of local anesthetic solution is injected.

Intraoral Approach

The patient is placed supine or in a semi-Fowler's position. The mouth is opened wide, and a tongue depressor is used to improve the view of the tonsillar area. A 25-gauge, 7.5-cm needle is directed to the tonsillar pillar at the 7 o'clock position (Fig. 23B–13). The needle can be bent at a 45-degree angle 1.5 cm from the tip to help obtain the correct position within the confines of the mouth. The needle is advanced 5 mm deep, and after an aspiration that is negative for blood and CSF, 3 to 5 ml of local anesthetic is injected.

Concerns

Intravascular injection can occur into a carotid artery or internal jugular vein. An intravascular injection of less than

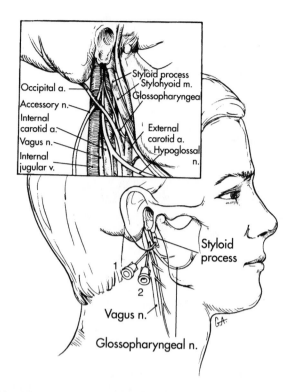

FIG. 23B–12 Needle direction for glossopharyngeal nerve block in the lateral view. The initial needle direction (*1*) and the redirection of needle posteriorly (*2*) are shown. *Inset* shows anatomy detail.

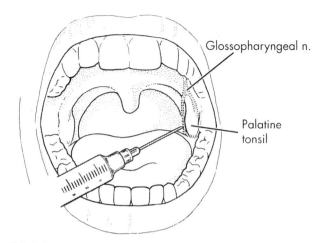

FIG. 23B–13 Intraoral approach to glossopharyngeal nerve block.

0.5 ml of local anesthetic solution into the carotid artery can cause a seizure or cardiovascular compromise. Unintentional blockade of other cranial nerves can occur. Difficulties with swallowing and hoarseness can result from the glossopharyngeal and vagus nerve blocks, respectively.

Vagus Nerve Block

Indications

The vagus nerve block is useful in the treatment of atypical facial pain and pharyngeal pain, including cancer-related pain.

Anatomy

The 10th cranial nerve has both sensory and motor functions. It originates in the medulla and exits through the jugular foramen. The nerve travels inferiorly through the neck in the carotid sheath. The vagus nerve is located just posterior and deep to the glossopharyngeal nerve between the internal carotid and the internal jugular vein at the level of the styloid process. As the nerve continues down the lower aspect of the thyroid gland, the route taken to the thorax differs on the right and left.

Technique

The vagus nerve is blocked in the same way as in the extraoral approach to the glossopharyngeal nerve (see Fig. 23B–12).

Concerns

The complications are similar to those accompanying the glossopharyngeal nerve block.

Superior Laryngeal Nerve Block

Indications

Blockade of the superior laryngeal nerve is performed to obtain supplemental analgesia for the upper airway for laryngoscopy or to prevent the hemodynamic responses to laryngoscopy. It can also supplement surgical anesthesia for bronchoscopy, endoscopy, or tracheal procedures.

Anatomy

The superior laryngeal nerve is a branch of the vagus nerve and travels along the pharynx, initially deep and then medial to the internal carotid artery. There are two branches: (1) the external laryngeal nerve innervates the cricothyroid muscle and (2) the internal laryngeal nerve receives sensory input from the mucous membranes of the pharynx, epiglottis, arytenoid cartilage, and vestibule of the larynx.

Technique

The patient is placed supine. The upper neck is palpated and the cornu of the thyroid cartilage is identified. A 22- to 25-gauge, 2-cm needle is inserted into the skin angled 45 degrees superiorly and medially (Fig. 23B–14*A*). The needle is advanced approximately 5 mm between the thyroid cartilage and the hyoid bone. After an aspiration that is negative for blood and CSF, 3 to 5 ml of local anesthetic solution is injected.

Concerns

Intravascular injection can occur. The internal carotid artery lies just lateral to the needle insertion site and should be located before injection. The superior laryngeal artery may be entered during this procedure.

Recurrent Laryngeal Nerve Block

Indications

Recurrent laryngeal nerve block can provide supplemental analgesia for the trachea for laryngoscopy or to prevent the hemodynamic responses to laryngoscopy as well as supplemental surgical anesthesia for bronchoscopy or tracheal procedures.

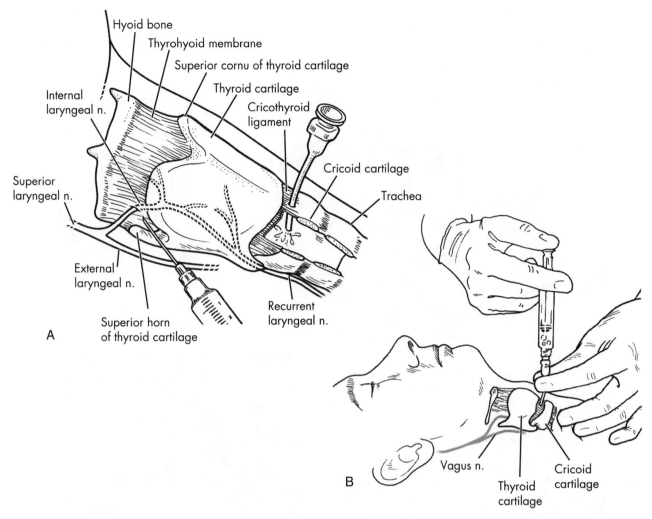

FIG. 23B–14 Anatomy of superior laryngeal and recurrent laryngeal nerve blocks. *A,* Needle direction in anteroposterior view. *B,* Approach to recurrent laryngeal nerve block.

Anatomy

The recurrent laryngeal nerve, a vagal branch, supplies sensation to the trachea below the vocal cords. The transtracheal approach anesthetizes the mucous membranes cutaneously, preserving recurrent laryngeal nerve function elsewhere.

Technique

The cricothyroid membrane is identified between the thyroid and the cricoid cartilage. A 20- to 22-gauge, 4-cm intravenous (IV) catheter with an attached syringe filled with 3 to 5 ml of 2% lidocaine is inserted perpendicular to the skin. The syringe must have enough room remaining to allow for aspiration. The catheter system is advanced during aspiration. The trachea is entered when air is aspirated into the syringe (see Fig. 23B–14*A* and *B*). The catheter system should be advanced another 2 mm to ensure that the catheter, and not just the needle, is in the lumen. The needle should be removed and the injection made with only the catheter in place.

Concerns

A needle can be used for this block, but the needle must be stabilized before injection. Forceful coughing and move-

ment of the patient usually occur during the injection, and tracheal puncture can occur.

Spinal Accessory Nerve Block

Indications

Indications for spinal accessory nerve blockade include torticollis and refractory muscle spasm of the trapezius and sternocleidomastoid (SCM) muscles.

Anatomy

The 11th cranial nerve has a spinal root originating from the spinal nucleus. It passes through the jugular foramen and travels posteriorly, deep to the internal jugular vein and medial to the styloid process. It then enters the superior aspect of the SCM muscle. It exits superior to the middle of the muscle posteriorly and continues across the posterior triangle of the neck. It continues caudally and enters the trapezius muscle 5 cm above the clavicle.

Technique

The patient is placed in semi-Fowler's position with the head slightly toward the contralateral side. The patient is asked to

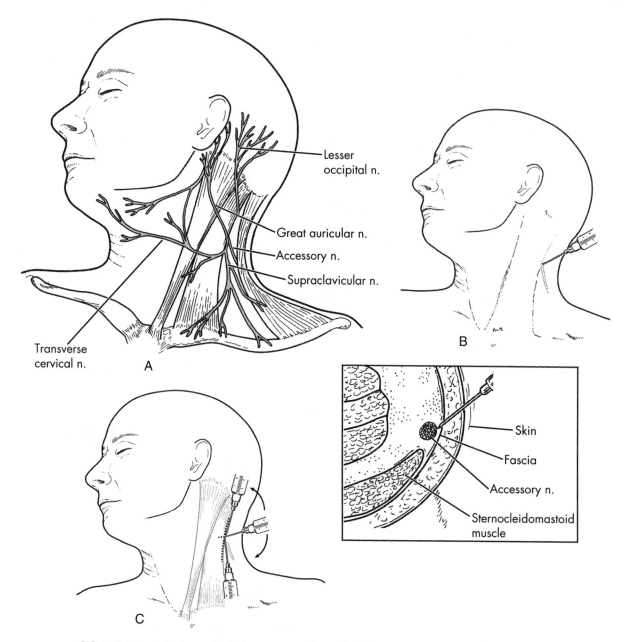

FIG. 23B–15 *A,* Anatomy of spinal accessory and superficial cervical plexus blocks. *B,* Needle direction for spinal accessory nerve block. *Inset,* Shows anatomic detail. *C,* Needle directions (*curved arrows*) for superficial cervical plexus block.

lift the head. Between the middle and upper thirds of the posterior aspect of the muscle, a 22-gauge, 4-cm needle is inserted perpendicular to the skin with a slightly caudal angle (Fig. 23B–15). The needle is advanced 1 to 2 cm. After aspiration that is negative for blood and CSF, 5 to 10 ml of local anesthetic solution is injected.

Concerns

If the needle is advanced too deeply, the stellate ganglion is blocked and Horner's syndrome occurs. The vagus nerve may also be anesthetized, which causes hoarseness and difficulty swallowing. Hematoma formation or bleeding can occur if the external jugular vein is not recognized and is entered during the procedure.

Deep Cervical Plexus Block

Indications

Indications for deep cervical plexus blockade include deep analgesia for surgical procedures around the neck, such as carotid endarterectomy and thyroid, parathyroid, or radical neck dissection operations. This block can be used for the treatment of chronic pain of the head and neck, including neuralgias of the nerves that make up the plexus.

Anatomy

The second, third, and fourth cervical spinal nerves form the deep cervical plexus. The plexus lies posterior to the SCM muscle and deep to the internal jugular vein. The plexus is

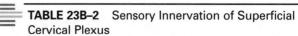

TABLE 23B–2 Sensory Innervation of Superficial Cervical Plexus

Nerve	Sensory Area
Lesser occipital nerve	Skin of neck and scalp behind ear, posterior auricle of the ear
	Communications with greater occipital nerve, greater auricular nerve, facial nerve (auricular branch)
Greater auricular nerve	Skin of face over parotid gland, mastoid process, posterior auricle (lower portion), lateral aspect and concha of the ear
	Communications with lesser occipital nerve, facial nerve (auricle branch), vagus nerve (auricular branch)
Transverse cervical nerve	Skin over anterolateral neck as low as sternum
Suprascapular nerve	Skin over upper posterior shoulder and chest as low as second rib, sternoclavicular joint

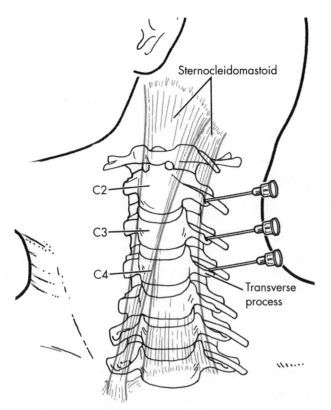

FIG. 23B–16 Needle directions for the deep cervical plexus block in the oblique view.

anterior to the medial scalene muscle and the levator muscle of the scapula. The nerves initially divide and then communicate with the other nerves in the plexus. The deep plexus supplies motor input to the capitus muscles and the longus colli muscle. This plexus also supplies sensation to the deep components of the neck.

Technique

The patient is placed supine with the head slightly turned toward the contralateral side. The mastoid process is identified. The patient is asked to lift the head off the table so that the lateral border of the SCM muscle can be identified. A 22-gauge, 4-cm needle is placed perpendicular to the skin in a slightly inferior direction at these locations (Fig. 23B–16). Each needle is advanced until a paresthesia occurs or the transverse process is encountered. Alternatively, a nerve stimulator can be used. The depth is usually 2 to 4 cm, depending on the size of the patient. All needles should be placed before any injection. If a paresthesia is not obtained and if the needle has encountered bone, it should be compared with the other needles. The most superficial needle is correctly placed on the transverse process; the deeper needle is most likely on the body of the vertebra too far anterior or posterior. After aspiration that is negative for blood and CSF, 3 to 5 ml of local anesthetic is injected at each site.

Concerns

An intrathecal injection of local anesthetic can occur despite an aspiration that is negative for CSF if the needle is in the dural sleeve. If the needle is placed too deeply, the vertebral artery can be entered. Small amounts of local anesthetic can lead to central nervous system symptoms or seizure. Partial or complete anesthetization of the phrenic nerve can lead to respiratory embarrassment in some patients.

Superficial Cervical Plexus Block

Indications

Indications for superficial cervical plexus blockade include skin analgesia for surgical procedures around the neck or thyroid, parathyroid, and neck dissection operations. This blockade also helps in the treatment of chronic pain of the head and neck, including neuralgias of the nerves that make up the plexus.

Anatomy

The plexus is made up of the lesser occipital, greater auricular, transverse cervical, and supraclavicular nerves. They are derived from the anterior branches of the second, third, and fourth cervical nerves and are sensory in nature. All the nerves are initially located at the posterior aspect of the SCM muscle and then travel to their respective destinations. All the nerves of the plexus ascend from the neck to the head except for the supraclavicular nerve. The sensory distribution of each nerve is described in Table 23B–2 and shown in Figure 23B–17.

Technique

The landmarks for this procedure are similar to those used for the spinal accessory nerve block. A 22- to 25-gauge, 7.5- to 9-cm needle is inserted into the skin at the midpoint of the posterior (lateral) aspect of the lateral head of the SCM muscle. Infiltration is performed subcutaneously 5 cm superiorly and the same distance inferiorly along the posterior aspect of the lateral head of the SCM muscle (see Fig. 23B–15C). A total of 10 to 20 ml of local anesthetic solution is used.

Concerns

Because this injection is superficial, there are few complications. As with the spinal accessory nerve block, the location

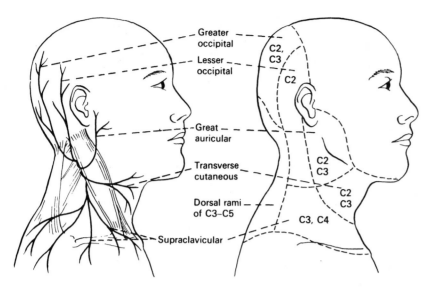

FIG. 23B–17 Sensory areas of the superficial cervical plexus. *(From Bonica JJ, editor: The management of pain, ed 2. Philadelphia, Lea & Febiger, 1990.)*

of the external jugular vein must be noted and the vein avoided.

SOMATIC NERVE BLOCKS OF THE UPPER AND LOWER EXTREMITIES

Regional blockade of the extremities has wide application in providing surgical anesthesia and analgesia as well as in treating chronic pain syndromes involving the extremities. Extremity regional anesthesia has several advantages in the postoperative period compared with general anesthesia, including:

1. Decreased sedation
2. Decreased nausea and vomiting
3. Early discharge from the recovery room
4. A smooth transition to pain control as the block effects gradually dissipate

Continuous infusion of local anesthetic near a peripheral nerve or plexus via percutaneous catheter has become an increasingly common form of postoperative analgesia for painful surgical procedures. Neural blockade of the extremities has both diagnostic and therapeutic value when used for chronic pain conditions. Selective neural blockade may help delineate somatic and sympathetic contributions to chronic pain and can often anatomically localize neural pain generators.

Diagnostic blocks must be used with caution and selectively because multiple factors confound their interpretation. When neural blocks are used therapeutically in chronic pain conditions, patient benefit can be maximized if physical and occupational therapy take place during periods of analgesia from blockade.

Interscalene Brachial Plexus Block

Applications

Interscalene block provides excellent anesthesia for surgical procedures of the shoulder or upper arm. It is ideal for closed reduction of shoulder dislocation. An interscalene block may also be used primarily for postoperative analgesia. They may be used therapeutically for chronic pain conditions of the upper extremity.

Anatomy

Interscalene block is performed at the level of the cervical roots as they course from the transverse processes between the anterior and middle scalene muscles before passing beneath the clavicle and over the first rib (Fig. 23B–18).

Technique

Interscalene block may be performed with the patient supine or sitting. The patient's head is directed away from the injection site at a 45-degree angle. The C6 level is identified by palpation of the cricoid cartilage, and the posterior border of the SCM is identified at this level. The examiner's fingers are then rolled posteriorly off the edge of the SCM to identify the interscalene groove. The external jugular vein often overlies the groove. The groove is accentuated during deep inspiration as the interscalene muscle contracts to elevate the first rib.

A 22-gauge, 1.5-inch needle is inserted medially at a slightly caudal and posterior angle. The needle should be perpendicular to the skin in all planes. The needle is advanced slowly until a paresthesia to the shoulder, arm, or hand is obtained.[1] If a paresthesia is not elicited, the needle augmentation is maintained and new insertion points are chosen in the plane that connects the cricoid cartilage to the transverse process of C6. When a paresthesia is obtained, 40 to 50 ml of anesthetic solution is injected incrementally.

Supraclavicular Brachial Plexus Block

Applications

Supraclavicular brachial plexus block provides anesthesia of the upper extremity with more consistency and more rapid onset than other brachial plexus techniques.

Anatomy

The supraclavicular brachial plexus block relies on the predictable anatomy of the three major trunks of the brachial plexus crossing over the first rib between the insertion of the anterior and middle scalene muscles in a cephaloposterior relation to the subclavian artery. The brachial plexus is most compact at this point, which occurs lateral and posterior to the insertion of the lateral head of the SCM.

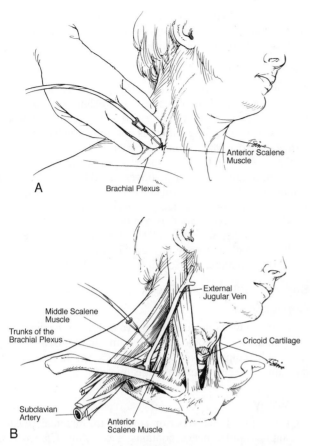

FIG. 23B–18 *A,* Superficial landmarks, site of entry, and position of the needle for the interscalene approach to the brachial plexus. *B,* The needle usually contacts the upper trunk. *(From Raj PP, Pai U, Rawal N: Techniques of regional anesthesia in adults. In Raj PP, editor: Clinical practice of regional anesthesia. New York, Churchill Livingstone, 1991.)*

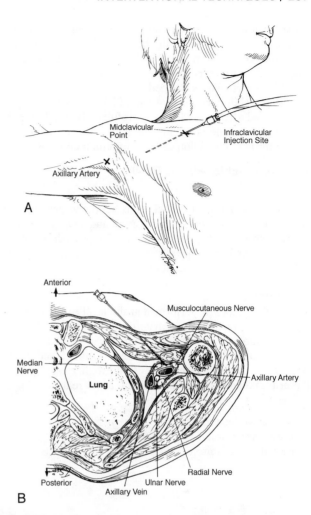

FIG. 23B–19 *A,* Brachial plexus blockade via the infraclavicular approach. *B,* Horizontal section of the axilla showing the lateral direction of the needle from the point of entry. *(From Raj PP, Pai U, Rawal N: Techniques of regional anesthesia in adults. In Raj PP, editor: Clinical practice of regional anesthesia. New York, Churchill Livingstone, 1991.)*

Technique

The classic supraclavicular approach is performed with the patient supine and the head turned away from the side to be blocked. The needle insertion site is approximately 1 cm posterior to the midpoint of the clavicle in the interscalene groove (if palpable). A 22-gauge, 1.5-inch needle is inserted in a caudal direction, parallel to the sagittal plane, until the first rib is contacted. Medial angulation must be must be prevented to avoid pneumothorax. Once bone contact is made, the needle is walked in a sagittal plane between the anterior and posterior angle of the rib until a paresthesia to the forearm or hand is obtained. After an aspiration that is negative for blood and CSF, 40 ml of local anesthetic solution is injected incrementally.

Infraclavicular Brachial Plexus Block

Applications

For the infraclavicular brachial plexus block, a long needle and a nerve stimulator are required.[2] Thus, this technique is not commonly used for surgical anesthesia. Because the infraclavicular approach employs a needle entry site below the clavicle and a long subcutaneous path, a catheter placed with this approach is immobile, easily dressed, and well tolerated by the patient. Infraclavicular catheters are well suited for treatment of patients with chronic pain of the

upper extremity by continuous infusion of local anesthetic solutions over prolonged periods.

Anatomy

The infraclavicular approach blocks the brachial plexus at the level of the formation of the musculocutaneous and axillary nerves high in the axilla, thus providing anesthesia from the shoulder to the hand (Fig. 23B–19). The medial wall of the axilla is formed by the first four ribs. The brachial plexus enters the axilla at the cephalad end of the wall as the neurovascular bundle courses beneath the clavicle and over the lateral edge of the first rib.

Technique

The patient lies supine, with the arm abducted at 90 degrees and the head turned away from the arm. A line is drawn from the C6 tubercle to the brachial artery in the arm, crossing the midpoint of the clavicle. The needle insertion site is 2.5 cm caudal to the midpoint of the clavicle. A 22-gauge, 3.5-inch needle is directed through the insertion site laterally toward the brachial artery at a 45-degree angle to the skin. The needle tip penetrates the pectoralis group of muscles, causing adduction of the shoulder with the nerve stimulator. As the needle approaches the brachial plexus, the forearm and hand are observed carefully for signs of motor stimulation. When appropriate motor stimulation is achieved, needle advancement is stopped.

A single-shot injection of 40 ml of local anesthetic is performed, and a Teflon catheter is carefully advanced over the needle. The needle is withdrawn, and a flexible catheter is placed through the Teflon catheter for continuous infusion.

Axillary Brachial Plexus Block

Applications

Axillary brachial plexus blockade is simple to perform and widely used for surgery of the forearm and hand. It does not reliably provide adequate anesthesia for procedures above the elbow. Axillary blockade may also be used therapeutically for chronic pain conditions.

Anatomy

The axillary block is performed at the level of the terminal nerves of the brachial plexus in the distal axilla (Fig. 23B–20). The musculocutaneous nerve has already separated from the neuromuscular bundle, but the medial, ulnar, and radial nerves are still in close proximity to the axillary artery. With the arm abducted at 90 degrees, the usual relationships of nerves to artery are as follows:

1. Median nerve (superior)
2. Ulnar nerve (inferior and anterior)
3. Radial nerve (inferior and posterior)

The musculocutaneous nerve is posterior and superior to the artery outside the fascial sheath in the groove between the coracobrachialis and biceps muscles.

Technique

Axillary blockade may be successfully achieved with paresthesia, nerve stimulator, or transarterial techniques. The transarterial technique is very simple and associated with a nearly 100% success rate. The patient is positioned supine, with the arm abducted at 90 degrees. The artery is identified as proximal as possible in the axilla, usually just lateral to the border of the pectoralis minor. Two fingers straddle the artery and compress the overlying subcutaneous tissue. A 23-gauge, 1-inch needle, or 22-gauge, 1.5-inch needle, is advanced slowly until arterial blood is aspirated. The needle is then advanced further until the return of blood has just ceased. With the needle correctly positioned and firmly fixed, 40 to 50 ml of local anesthetic solution is injected incrementally.

Suprascapular Nerve Block

Applications

Blockade of the suprascapular nerve is used in the diagnosis and treatment of chronic shoulder pain conditions, as well as to provide temporary relief from muscle spasm or strain in the supraspinatus or infraspinatus muscles.

Anatomy

As a branch of the superior cord of the brachial plexus, the suprascapular nerve contains fibers from C5 and C6

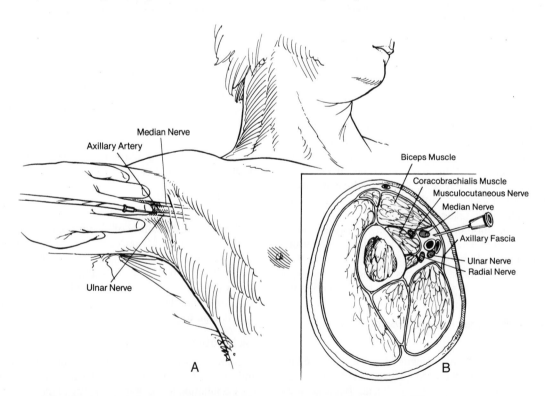

FIG. 23B–20 *A,* Axillary approach to brachial plexus blockade. *B,* The needle is in the neurovascular bundle close to the brachial artery. The musculocutaneous nerve lies in the coracobrachialis muscle, outside the brachial plexus sheath at this site. *(From Raj PP, Pai U, Rawal N: Techniques of regional anesthesia in adults. In Raj PP, editor: Clinical practice of regional anesthesia. New York, Churchill Livingstone, 1991.)*

(Fig. 23B–21). It passes under the transverse ligament of the scapula through the suprascapular notch into the supraspinous fossa, where it supplies motor fibers to the supraspinatus muscle. Another branch proceeds laterally around the neck or the scapula to the infraspinatus fossa to supply the infraspinatus muscle. Sensory fibers innervate portions of the shoulder joint and surrounding soft tissues.

Technique

The spine of the scapula is palpated and marked at its midpoint. The needle insertion point is 2.5 cm lateral and cephalad to this point. A 22-gauge, 2.5-inch needle is inserted at right angles to the skin and advanced until bone is contacted. The needle is then walked medially and laterally until it slides into the suprascapular notch. At this point, 10 ml of local anesthetic is injected.

Ulnar, Median, and Radial Nerve Blocks at the Elbow

Applications

Upper extremity blocks at the elbow may be performed to supplement brachial plexus blockade. Blocks at the elbow are useful for diagnosis and treatment of chronic pain conditions of the hand, wrist, and distal forearm.

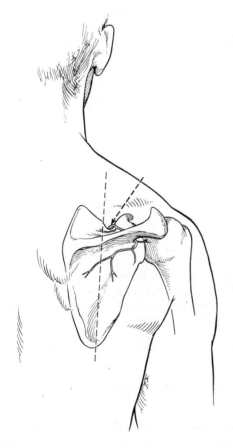

FIG. 23B–21 Suprascapular nerve block. The nerve is blocked in the suprascapular fossa. The spine of the scapula is palpated and marked at its midpoint. *(From Raj PP, Pai U, Rawal N: Techniques of regional anesthesia in adults. In Raj PP, editor: Clinical practice of regional anesthesia.* New York, Churchill Livingstone, 1991.)

Anatomy

The ulnar nerve lies in a dense fascial sheath in the ulnar groove, located between the olecranon process and the medial epicondyle of the humerus (Fig. 23B–22). The median nerve lies medial to the biceps tendon and the brachial artery. The radial nerve lies between the brachialis muscle and the brachioradialis muscle just proximal to the elbow.

Technique

The ulnar nerve block is performed with the forearm flexed on the upper arm to identify the ulnar groove. A line is drawn between the olecranon process and the medial epicondyle of the humerus. The groove is entered with a 22- or 23-gauge needle at a point 1 cm proximal to the line and from 3 to 5 ml of local anesthetic is injected.

The median nerve is located by palpation of the biceps tendon between the medial and lateral epicondyles of the humerus. The brachial artery pulse is palpated medially to the biceps tendon. The needle is inserted perpendicular to the skin medial to the brachial pulse, and 3 to 5 ml of local anesthetic solution is injected.

The radial nerve block is also preformed on a line between the medial and lateral epicondyles of the humerus. The brachioradialis muscle is palpated, and a 22- or 23-gauge needle is inserted just medial to the muscle perpendicular to the skin. A fan-like injection of 5 to 8 ml of local anesthetic solution is carried out.

Ulnar, Median, and Radial Nerve Blocks at the Wrist

Applications

Nerve blocks at the wrist may be used for the diagnosis and treatment of chronic pain conditions in the hand and digits.

Anatomy

The ulnar nerve lies medial to the ulnar artery and lateral to the tendon of the flexor carpi ulnaris beneath the deep fascia at the palmar crease of the wrist (see Figs. 23B–22 and 23B–23). The medial nerve lies medial to the palmaris longus tendon and lateral to the flexor carpi radialis tendon beneath the deep fascia at the palmar crease of the wrist. The radial nerve has already divided into superficial branches over the lateral aspect of the distal radius.

Technique

For blocks of the median and ulnar nerves, the hand is in the supinated position. The radial block is performed with the hand in the midpronation. For ulnar nerve block, a 22-gauge, 1.5-inch needle is advanced between the ulnar artery and the flexor carpi ulnaris tendon at the palmar crease of the wrist until the needle is felt to penetrate the fascia or until a paresthesia is obtained. The medial nerve block is performed in the same fashion, with needle insertion between the palmaris longus and flexor carpi radialis tendons. For the radial nerve branches, a subcutaneous ring block of the lateral wrist is performed over the distal aspect of the radius with a 27-gauge, 1.5-inch needle.

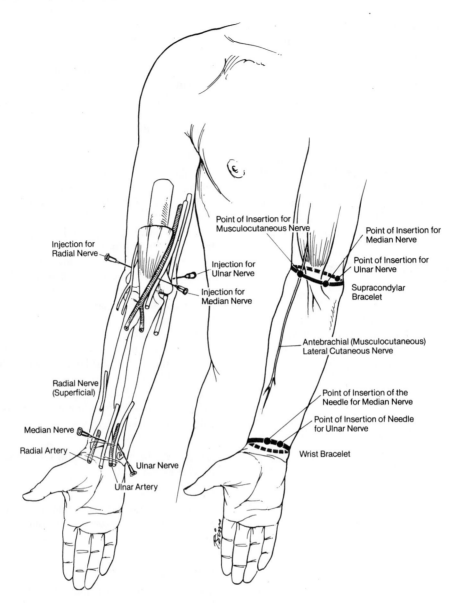

FIG. 23B–22 Anatomy of the median, ulnar, and radial nerves at the elbow and wrist. *(From Raj PP, Pai U, Rawal N: Techniques of regional anesthesia in adults. In Raj PP, editor:* Clinical practice of regional anesthesia. *New York, Churchill Livingstone, 1991.)*

Digital Block

Applications

Digital blocks provide anesthesia to the finger or toe. These injections may be given for procedures such as debridement, foreign body removal, or repair of lacerations.

Anatomy

The digital nerves run along the lateral and medial sides of the fingers as well as the toes. Each digit has two palmar digital nerves and two dorsal digital nerves.

Technique

Blockade is obtained by advancing a 25- or 27-gauge needle along each side of the digit, from the dorsal surface until the needle has just about exited the skin on the palmar surface. Approximately 1 to 2 ml of local anesthetic solution is injec-

ted as the needle is withdrawn, leaving a line of anesthetic on both sides of the digit. Any type of local anesthetic may be given; however, solutions containing vasoconstrictors, such as epinephrine, should be avoided. Epinephrine may result in constriction of blood vessels responsible for distal perfusion, thus leading to necrosis and potential loss of that digit.

Intravenous Regional Anesthesia

Applications

IV regional anesthesia is a simple technique that calls for no particular technical skills other than the insertion of IV catheters. The technique may be used for upper and lower extremity surgery on any portion of the extremity distal to the tourniquet and has also been used with varying success of the treatment of reflex sympathetic dystrophy and causalgia.

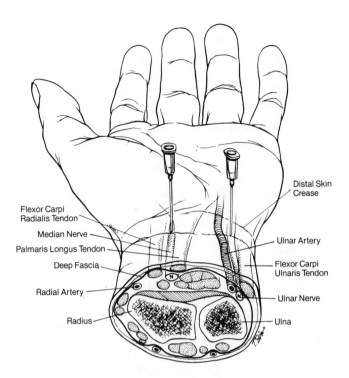

FIG. 23B–23 Blocking technique for the median and ulnar nerves at the wrist. (*From Raj PP, Pai U, Rawal N: Techniques of regional anesthesia in adults. In Raj PP, editor: Clinical practice of regional anesthesia. New York, Churchill Livingstone, 1991.*)

Labels in figure:
- Flexor Carpi Radialis Tendon
- Median Nerve
- Palmaris Longus Tendon
- Deep Fascia
- Radial Artery
- Radius
- Distal Skin Crease
- Ulnar Artery
- Flexor Carpi Ulnaris Tendon
- Ulnar Nerve
- Ulna

Technique

The patient is placed in the supine position, and the IV access is obtained in another extremity. A tourniquet is placed on the operative extremity. A 20- or 22-gauge IV catheter is placed on the dorsal aspect of the operative hand or foot. More proximal cannula locations may be associated with leakage under the tourniquet if the tip of the cannula is too close to the distal edge of the tourniquet. The arm or leg is elevated, and an Esmarch bandage is wrapped tightly around the extremity from the distal end up to the tourniquet for exsanguination. The tourniquet is then inflated to 50 to 100 mm Hg for the leg. The Esmarch bandage is removed, and adequate tourniquet pressure is verified by absence of distal pulses. After the limb is returned to a resting position, local anesthetic solution is injected. From 40 to 50 ml of 0.5% lidocaine is recommended for upper extremity anesthesia, and up to 100 ml of local anesthetic solution may be required for complete anesthesia of the lower extremity.

Lower Extremities

It is possible to provide anesthesia and analgesia for surgery on the lower extremity as well as for the relief of many acute and chronic painful conditions via neural blockade of the somatic nerves to the lower extremity. Whereas central neuraxial blockade is commonly used for many lower extremity procedures and painful conditions, in many instances a more peripheral blockade of the neural structures offers significant benefit. This is particularly true for patients who have significant systemic illnesses or who have taken anticoagulation agents.

Neural Anatomy

The lower extremity derives its innervation from the lumbar and sacral plexuses. The lumbar plexus arises from the ventral rami of the first through the fourth lumbar nerve roots. These roots form the plexus within the body of the psoas muscle. The lumbar plexus then forms the nerves that supply the inguinal and genital region as well as three of the four major nerves to the lower extremity. The lateral femoral cutaneous nerve, the femoral nerve, and the obturator nerve all arise from the lumbar plexus and supply most of the innervation to the anterior portion of the upper leg. The femoral nerve continues below the knee as the saphenous nerve and is the only nerve derived from the lumbar plexus that has a significant area of innervation below the knee.

Paravertebral Nerve Block

Applications

The paravertebral nerve block can provide anesthesia for surgery involving any of the areas innervated by the lumbar plexus. This includes surgery in the inguinal region, such as inguinal herniorrhaphy. It can be combined with blockade of the sciatic nerve to provide anesthesia for surgery on the lower extremity, including the hip. It is also an effective technique for providing anesthesia for total hip and total knee arthroplasties.

Technique

The patient can be positioned in a number of ways (prone, seated, or lying on the opposite side to be blocked). Once the patient is comfortably positioned, the spinous processes of the lumbar vertebrae are identified and marked. The line between the iliac crests can be used to orient the physician, because this generally identifies the fourth lumbar vertebra or the L4-5 interspace. Marks for needle entry are then made approximately 2.5 to 3 cm lateral to the spinous processes on the side to be blocked.

After sterile preparation of the skin, skin wheals can be raised, and a 22-gauge, 10-cm needle is advanced perpendicular to the skin until the transverse process is contacted. The depth of needle insertion is then noted. The needle is redirected slightly caudally until it is walked off the lower border of the transverse process. Next, the needle is advanced 1 to 1.5 cm, and 3 ml of local anesthetic solution is deposited. This process is repeated for each level to be blocked.

Psoas Compartment Block

Applications

The psoas compartment block is another effective method of providing anesthesia and analgesia to the areas innervated by the lumbar plexus. It can be used to provide excellent anesthesia for lower extremity surgery, particularly when it is combined with blockade of the sciatic never. This is an effective technique for providing anesthesia for total hip and total knee arthroplasties.

Technique

The patient can be lying on the side opposite that to be blocked or can be seated. A line is drawn between the iliac crests and along the spinous processes. A second line is drawn 5 cm lateral to the line along the spinous processes. The needle insertion is 3 cm caudal to the line between the iliac crests along the parasagittal line. This entry site is roughly 5 cm lateral to the spinous process of the fifth lumbar vertebra. After sterile preparation of the skin, a 20- or 22-gauge, 15-cm needle is used.

Most often, a nerve stimulator is used. The needle is advanced through the entry site until stimulation of the nerves of the lumbar plexus is obtained. Lumbar plexus stimulation often causes extension of the knee. If stimulation of the sacral plexus is obtained, the needle may be too medial or too caudal, and it should be redirected until lumbar plexus stimulation is obtained. Once adequate stimulation is obtained, 30 ml of local anesthetic solution is injected. The patient should remain in this position for 5 to 10 minutes while the block takes effect.

Inguinal Paravascular Three-In-One Block[3]

Applications

Because the three-in-one technique attempts to block the lumbar plexus by proximal spread of local anesthetic solution from a more distal injection site, it is not as effective at blocking the nerves that arise from the higher portions of the lumbar plexus. As a result, this block is not useful for surgery in the inguinal region.

This technique is easy to perform and can provide good anesthesia for surgery on the lower extremity, particularly if it involves surgery in the distribution of the femoral nerve.

Technique

The patient is placed supine with the groin sterilely prepared. A skin wheal is raised approximately 1 cm lateral to the femoral arterial pulsation just below the inguinal ligament. A 22-gauge, B-bevel needle is inserted with a cephalad angulation. A paresthesia can be sought, or a nerve stimulator can be used. After a paresthesia is obtained or adequate nerve stimulation is achieved, 25 to 30 ml of local anesthetic solution is injected and the needle removed. Distal pressure is held in an effort to facilitate cephalad spread of the anesthetic to the level of the lumbar plexus.

Peripheral Blockade of the Nerves of the Lumbar Plexus

The lumbar plexus divides within the body of the psoas muscle to form a number of peripheral nerves. These nerves can be reliably blocked to provide anesthesia and analgesia to the areas that they supply.

Ilioinguinal and Iliohypogastric Nerve Block

Applications

This block can be used to provide anesthesia and analgesia for surgery in the inguinal region, particularly for inguinal herniorrhaphy and lymph node biopsies. These blocks can also be used as part of a diagnostic evaluation for patients with inguinal pain.

Anatomy

The ilioinguinal and iliohypogastric nerves arise from the L1 ventral nerve root. These nerves then travel along the abdominal wall toward the iliac crest, where they perforate the transversus abdominis muscle. The iliohypogastric nerves lies slightly more cephalad than the ilioinguinal nerve and sends cutaneous branches that innervate the skin over the lower abdominal wall and the groin. The ilioinguinal nerve sends cutaneous branches to the skin and then enters the inguinal canal with the spermatic cord.

Technique

The patient is placed in the supine position, and a mark is placed 3 cm medial to the anterior superior iliac spinous along a line between it and the umbilicus. This mark overlies the course of the iliohypogastric nerve. A second mark 3 cm caudal to the first overlies the ilioinguinal nerve.

After the skin is sterilely prepared, a 5-cm, 22-gauge B-bevel needle is placed through the skin at the upper mark until it pierces the fascia of the internal oblique muscle. This can be appreciated by a tactile "popping" sensation. A dose of 5 to 10 ml of local anesthetic solution is injected. The needle is then inserted through the caudal site, and the process is repeated.

Genitofemoral Nerve Block

Applications

The genitofemoral nerve block can be used in the diagnostic evaluation of patients with inguinal and genital pain. It is often done as part of a series of blocks.

Anatomy

The genitofemoral nerve arises from the L1 and L2 ventral nerve roots, then passes through the psoas muscle. It divides into two terminal branches. The femoral branch supplies innervation to a small area on the upper, inner thigh, and the genital branch innervates the skin over the scrotum in males and the labia majora in females.

Technique

The patient is placed in the supine position, and the groin is sterilely prepared. A 22-gauge, 5-cm B-bevel needle is placed through the skin just lateral to the pubic tubercle. The needle is advanced through the inguinal ligament, and 5 ml of local anesthetic solution is deposited. The genital branch of the genitofemoral nerve can be blocked independently by infiltration around the spermatic cord at its exit from the inguinal canal.

Lateral Femoral Cutaneous Nerve Block

Applications

The lateral femoral cutaneous nerve block provides analgesia for surgery on the lateral thigh. It can be used for harvesting of skin grafts and fascia lata grafts. It can be performed along with blockade of the femoral, obturator, and sciatic nerves for surgery on the lower extremity. This block can also be used in the diagnosis and treatment of patients with meralgia paresthetica.

Anatomy

The lateral femoral cutaneous nerve originates from the ventral rami of the second and third lumbar nerve roots. It exits the lateral aspect of the psoas muscle and travels along the upper edge of the pelvis and enters the thigh just medial and inferior to the anterosuperior iliac spine.

Technique

The patient is placed in the supine position, and a mark is made 2 cm medial and 2 cm caudal to the anterosuperior iliac spine. This mark should be just below the inguinal ligament. A 22-gauge, 5-cm B-bevel needle is inserted until it passes through the fascia lata, at which time a tactile "pop" can be appreciated. Then, 5 to 10 ml of local anesthetic is injected. Because the nerve often divides into branches proximally, it may be useful to inject the local anesthetic solution in a fan pattern to improve the success rate of the block.

Femoral Nerve Block

Applications

The femoral nerve block can be used to provide anesthesia for surgery on the upper and lower leg. It is often combined with blockade of the lateral femoral cutaneous, obturator, and sciatic nerves.

Anatomy

The femoral nerve originates from the ventral rami of the second through the fourth lumbar nerve roots (Fig. 23B–24). It separates from other nerves of the lumbar plexus within the body of the psoas muscle. The femoral nerve exits on the medial aspect of the psoas muscle and enters the thigh under the inguinal ligament, just lateral and somewhat posterior to the femoral artery. Shortly after entering the thigh, the femoral nerve divides into muscular and sensory branches.

Technique

The patient is supine, and the groin is prepared in sterile fashion. A skin wheal is raised approximately 1 cm lateral to the femoral arterial pulsation just below the inguinal ligament. A 22-gauge, B-bevel needle is inserted with a cephalad angulation. After a paresthesia or adequate nerve stimulation is achieved, 15 to 20 ml of local anesthetic solution is injected, and the needle is removed.

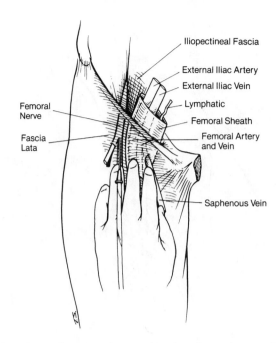

FIG. 23B–24 Technique for blockade of the femoral nerve. *(From Raj PP, Pai U, Rawal N: Techniques of regional anesthesia in adults. In Raj PP, editor: Clinical practice of regional anesthesia. New York, Churchill Livingstone, 1991.)*

Obturator Nerve Block

Applications

The obturator nerve block is often combined with femoral, lateral femoral cutaneous, and sciatic nerve blocks for surgery of the lower extremity.

Anatomy

The obturator nerve originates from the ventral nerve roots of the second through the fourth lumbar nerve roots. It exits on the medial border of the psoas muscle and travels along the lateral edge of the pelvis. The nerve then enters the obturator canal along with the obturator vessels. The obturator nerve then divides into anterior and posterior branches. The anterior branch innervates the adductor muscles of the thigh and the skin over the medial aspect of the upper thigh. The posterior branch also innervates the adductor muscles as well as an area lower down on the medial thigh.

Technique

The patient is supine with the legs slightly separated (Fig. 23B–25). The groin is prepared in sterile fashion. A skin wheal is raised 2 cm lateral and 2 cm caudal to the pubic tubercle. A 22-gauge, 10-cm needle is advanced perpendicular to the skin until bone is contacted. The needle is then redirected laterally and slightly caudally until it walks off the pubic bone. Next, it is advanced 3 cm into the obturator canal, and from 10 to 15 ml of local anesthetic solution is injected.

Saphenous Nerve Block (at the Knee)

Applications

The saphenous nerve block at the knee can be combined with blockade of the sciatic nerve to provide effective analgesia for surgery on the lower leg.

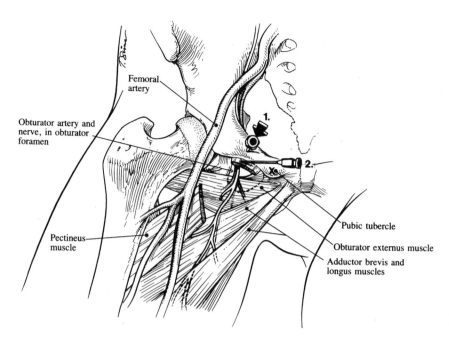

FIG. 23B–25 Technique for blockade of the obturator nerve. *1,* needle position on the superior ramus; *2,* needle position in the obturator foramen. *(From Raj PP, Pai U, Rawal N: Techniques of regional anesthesia in adults. In Raj PP, editor: Clinical practice of regional anesthesia. New York, Churchill Livingstone, 1991.)*

Anatomy

The saphenous nerve is the distal continuation of the femoral nerve and is the only nerve derived from the lumbar plexus that ramifies below the knee. The femoral nerve passes through Hunter's canal and exits as the saphenous nerve on the medial aspect of the lower thigh. The nerve passes along the medial aspect of the knee between the tendons of the gracilis muscle and the sartorius muscle. The nerve then continues down the lower leg to the medial aspect of the ankle and foot along with the great saphenous vein.

Technique

The patient is positioned supine with the legs slightly separated. The skin over the medial aspect of the knee is sterilely prepared. At the level of the patella, a 22-gauge, 5-cm B-bevel needle is placed through the skin between the tendons of the gracilis and sartorius muscles. After the needle passes through the fascia, a paresthesia is sought. Then 5 to 10 ml of local anesthetic solution is injected.

Saphenous Nerve Block (at the Ankle)

For surgery on the foot, the saphenous nerve block is often performed with blockade of distal branches of the sciatic nerve.

Anatomy

After the saphenous nerve passes below the knee, it continues down the medial aspect of the lower leg, approximating the course of the greater saphenous vein. As the nerve reaches the ankle, it passes just anterior to the medial malleolus and supplies sensory innervation to the medial ankle and part of the medial foot.

Technique

The patient is placed supine, and the ankle is sterilely prepared (Fig. 23B–26). A 4-cm, 22-gauge needle is placed through the skin 3 cm anterior to the medial malleolus. The needle is passed subcutaneously toward the medial malleolus until it is just overlying the bone. As the needle is withdrawn, 4 to 5 ml of local anesthetic solution is injected.

Sacral Plexus

The sacral plexus arises from the ventral rami of the fourth lumbar through the third sacral nerve roots (Fig. 23B–27). The branches pass along the pelvis where they form the sciatic nerve. The sciatic nerve comprises two main portions: the tibial nerve and the peroneal nerve. The posterior femoral cutaneous nerve also arises from the sacral plexus and supplies sensation to the posterior gluteal region.

Sciatic Nerve Block (Posterior Approach of Labat)[4]

Applications

The sciatic nerve block is used to provide anesthesia and analgesia for surgery on the lower extremity. It is commonly combined with lateral femoral cutaneous, femoral, and obturator nerve blocks. The sciatic nerve block can be combined with the saphenous nerve block at the knee for lower leg and foot surgery.

Technique

The patient is positioned on the side with the side to be blocked facing up (Fig. 23B–28). A line is drawn between the posterior superior iliac spine and the greater trochanter. The midpoint of this line is identified, and a line is drawn perpendicular (caudally) to the first line. Needle entry is 5 cm caudal to the first line along this perpendicular line. A 22-gauge, 10-cm needle is inserted through the skin and advanced until a paresthesia is obtained.

Sciatic Nerve Block (Anterior Approach)[5]

Technique

The patient is placed in the supine position, and a line is drawn between the anterior superior iliac spine and the pubic

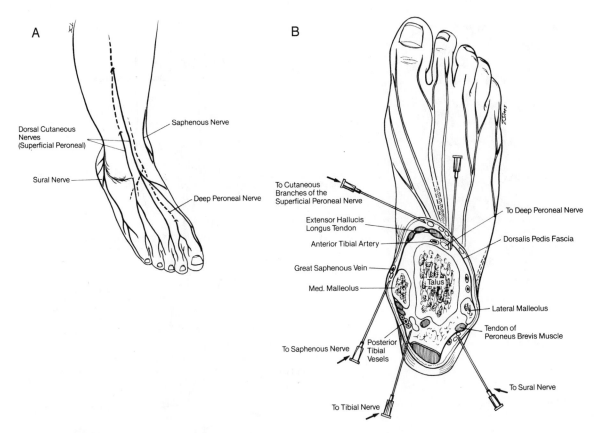

FIG. 23B–26 *A,* Anatomy of the peripheral nerves at the ankle. *B,* Needle placement fir the blockade of the tibial peroneal nerves. *(From Raj PP, Pai U, Rawal N: Techniques of regional anesthesia in adults. In Raj PP, editor:* Clinical practice of regional anesthesia. *New York, Churchill Livingstone, 1991.)*

tubercle (Fig. 23B–29). A second line is drawn parallel to the first line but starting more caudally on the leg at the greater trochanter. The first line is then divided into three equal sections. At the junction of the medial and middle sections, a perpendicular line is drawn caudally until it intersects with the more caudal line. This is the insertion point. A 12-cm, 22-gauge needle is inserted until it contacts the medial aspect of the femur. The needle is then walked off the medial edge of the femur and advanced 5 cm until a paresthesia is obtained, and from 20 to 30 ml of local anesthetic solution is injected.

Sciatic Nerve Block (Lithotomy Approach)[6]

Technique

The patient is placed in the supine position, and the extremity to be blocked is placed in the lithotomy position (Fig. 23B–30). A line is drawn between the greater trochanter and the ischial tuberosity. A 22-gauge, 12-cm needle is placed through the midpoint of this line and is advanced until a paresthesia is obtained. After the nerve is located, 15 to 20 ml of local anesthetic solution is injected.

Popliteal Fossa Block

Applications

Blockade of the branches of the sciatic nerve at the popliteal fossa can be used for surgery on the lower leg and the foot.

Anatomy

The sciatic nerve travels through the posterior aspect of the upper leg until it reaches the upper aspect of the popliteal fossa. Its upper lateral border is the medial aspect of the biceps femoris muscle, and its medial border is the lateral aspect of the semitendinous ligament. Caudally, the two heads of the gastrocnemius muscle border the fossa.

When the sciatic nerve reaches the upper aspect of the popliteal fossa, it divides into two branches: the tibial nerve and the common peroneal nerve. The tibial nerve is larger and passes straight through the popliteal fossa and enters the lower leg between the heads of the gastrocnemius muscle. Then the common peroneal nerve passes more laterally and travels under the biceps femoris muscle. It then wraps anteriorly around the head of the fibula and divides into the deep and superficial peroneal nerves.

Technique

The patient is placed in the prone position, and the popliteal fossa is sterilely prepared. The borders of the popliteal fossa are identified. A line is drawn horizontally across the popliteal fossa at the widest point of the diamond-shaped fossa. This line roughly corresponds to the skin crease that is created by bending the knee. This mark divides the space into a cephalad and a caudal triangle. The caudal triangle is then bisected into two equal triangles by a line drawn vertically from the cephalic point of the upper triangle. A mark

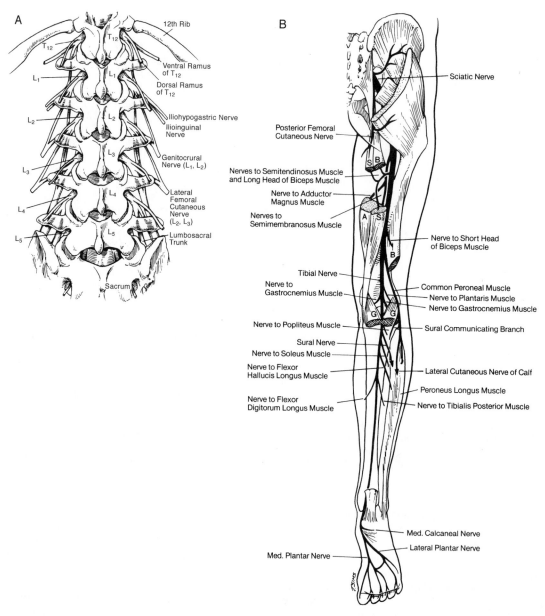

FIG. 23B–27 *A,* Formation of the lumbar and sacral nerve plexi, *B,* Anatomy of the sciatic nerve and its branches. *(From Raj PP, Pai U, Rawal N: Techniques of regional anesthesia in adults. In Raj PP, editor:* Clinical practice of regional anesthesia. *New York, Churchill Livingstone, 1991.)*

is made at a point that is 5 cm superior to the horizontal line along the bisecting line of the cephalad triangle. Needle insertion is 1 cm lateral to this point.

Alternatively, the needle can be inserted at the most cephalad point of the popliteal fossa at the junction of the biceps femoris and semitendinous. A 22-gauge, 4-cm needle is inserted and a paresthesia is sought. After the nerve is identified, 30 to 40 ml of local anesthetic solution is injected.

Deep and Superficial Peroneal Nerve Block (at the Ankle)

Applications

The deep and superficial peroneal nerve block is combined with blockade of the other nerves at the ankle to provide anesthesia for surgery on the foot.

Anatomy

The deep and superficial nerves are the continuation of the common peroneal nerve. They enter the foot anteriorly at the ankle. The deep peroneal nerve lies just medial to the extensor hallucis longus muscle on the anterior aspect of the ankle. It enters the foot and supplies sensation to the skin between the first and second toes.

The superficial peroneal nerve has already divided into several branches when it crosses the ankle. It lies superficially on the anterolateral aspect of the ankle and provides sensation to much of the dorsum of the foot.

Technique

The patient is placed in the supine position, and the ankle is prepared in sterile fashion (see Fig. 23B–26). Having the

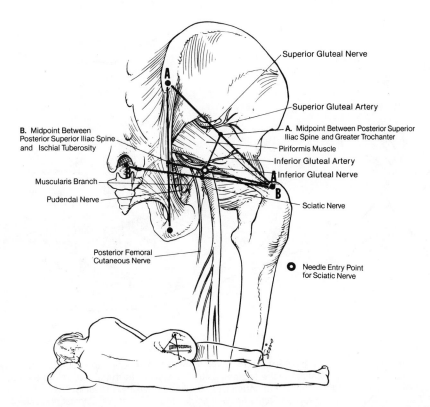

FIG. 23B–28 Technique for blockade of the sciatic nerve via a posterior approach. *(From Raj PP, Pai U, Rawal N: Techniques of regional anesthesia in adults. In Raj PP, editor:* Clinical practice of regional anesthesia. *New York, Churchill Livingstone, 1991.)*

patient dorsiflex the great toe identifies the tendon of the hallucis longus muscle. A 22-gauge, 4-cm needle is inserted through the skin just medial to the tendon until a paresthesia is obtained, and from 5 to 10 ml of local anesthetic is injected. The needle is withdrawn until it is just subcutaneous and is then advanced subcutaneously toward the lateral malleolus. As the needle is withdrawn, 5 to 10 ml of local anesthetic solution is injected to block the superficial peroneal nerve.

Posterior Tibial Nerve Block (at the Ankle)

Applications

The posterior tibial nerve block is combined with blockade of the other nerves at the ankle to provide anesthesia for surgery on the foot.

Anatomy

The tibial nerve travels through the lower leg deep to the soleus muscle. As it approaches the ankle, it travels medially between the Achilles tendon and the medial malleolus. It enters the foot and forms the plantar nerves, which supply sensation to the bottom of the foot.

Technique

The patient is placed in the supine position, and the leg is externally rotated. The skin is sterilely prepared. If the posterior tibial arterial pulsation can be palpated, this can serve as a landmark. A 22-gauge, 4-cm needle is inserted between the medial malleolus and the Achilles tendon. It is advanced through the fascia until paresthesia is obtained, and from 5 to 10 ml of local anesthetic solution is injected.

Sural Nerve

Applications

The sural block is combined with blockade of the other nerves at the ankle to provide anesthesia for surgery on the foot.

Anatomy

The sural nerve is a branch of the tibial nerve that travels between the Achilles tendon and the lateral malleolus to supply sensation to the lateral aspect of the foot.

Technique

The patient is supine with the leg internally rotated. The skin is sterilely prepared. A 4-cm, 22-gauge needle is inserted between the Achilles tendon and the lateral malleolus until it passes through the fascia and 5 to 10 ml of local anesthetic is injected.

A

B

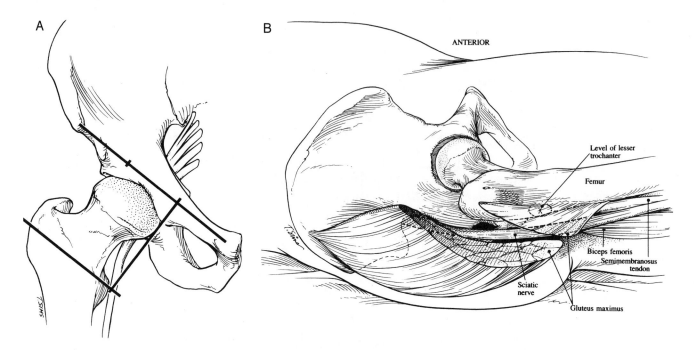

FIG. 23B–29 *A,* Technique for blockade of the sciatic nerve via an anterior approach. *B,* Anatomy of the sciatic nerve with the patient in the supine position as viewed from the side. Note the course of the sciatic nerve behind the femur and anterior to the gluteus maximus muscle. *(From Raj PP, Pai U, Rawal N: Techniques of regional anesthesia in adults. In Raj PP, editor: Clinical practice of regional anesthesia. New York, Churchill Livingstone, 1991.)*

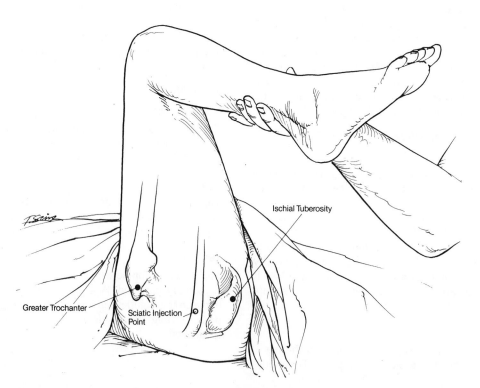

FIG. 23B–30 Technique for blockade of the sciatic nerve via the lithotomy approach. *(From Raj PP, Pai U, Rawal N: Techniques of regional anesthesia in adults. In Raj PP, editor: Clinical practice of regional anesthesia. New York, Churchill Livingstone, 1991.)*

References

1. Roch JJ, Sharrock NE, Neudachin L: Interscalene brachial plexus block for shoulder surgery: A proximal paresthesia is effective. *Anesth Analg* 75:386, 1992.
2. Raj PP, Montgomery SJ, Nettles D et al: Infraclavicular brachial plexus block: A new approach. *Anesth Analg* 52:897, 1973.
3. Winnie AP, Ramamurthy S, Durrani Z: The inguinal paravascular technique of lumbar anesthesia: The "3-in-1 block." *Anesth Analg* 52:989, 1973.
4. Labat G: *Regional anesthesia.* Philadelphia, WB Saunders, 1930.
5. Beck GP: Anterior approach to sciatic nerve block. *Anesthesiology* 24:222, 1963.
6. Raj PP, Parks RI, Watson TD et al: New single position supine approach to sciatic-femoral nerve block. *Anesth Analg* 54:489, 1975.

CHAPTER **23**

Interventional Techniques

RICHARD L. RAUCK, AND
OSCAR A. DE LEON-CASASOLA

HISTORY

Galen's many contributions to the field of anatomy include the earliest history of the sympathetic nervous system.[1] A text published in 1528 describes a nerve trunk along the rib heads that communicates with the spinal cord. He also notes three enlargements along this nerve trunk and described a ganglion at the entrance of the nerve into the abdomen. Although Galen erroneously thought this nerve was a branch of the vagus nerve, he initiated a concept that sympathy or consent existed between different parts of the body.

Later anatomists described the vagus nerve and sympathetic trunk as a single functional entity until Estienne[2] in 1545 correctly identified them as individual anatomic structures. In 1732, Winslow[3] was the first to term the paravertebral chain "the great sympathetic nerve." Later, in 1765, Whytt[4,5] wrote that all sympathy or consent must be referred to the central nervous system (CNS) initially, because it occurred between body parts without interconnecting nerves.

Numerous publications during the 19th century helped to essentially complete the anatomic understanding of the sympathetic nervous system. In 1889, Langley and Dickinson[6] proposed the name *autonomic nervous system* and differentiated the functional effects of the thoracolumbar and craniosacral outflows, subsequently naming the latter system parasympathetic.

The beginning of the 20th century brought extensive research examining the role of sympathetic nerves and the transmission of visceral pain.[7–9]

Whereas Koller first demonstrated the local anesthetic properties of cocaine in 1884, Sellheim used a paravertebral approach in 1905 to inject somatic spinal nerves for surgical anesthesia. Techniques were later refined to allow blocks of parts of the sympathetic nervous system. Kappis and others in 1923 began to use paravertebral sympathetic blocks as a therapeutic measure for severe pain and certain visceral pain syndromes.[10–13]

During the 1920s, Leriche studied the function of the stellate ganglion and subsequently reported superb pain relief from causalgia and reflex sympathetic dystrophy with stellate ganglion blocks in the upper extremities and lumbar sympathetic blocks in the lower extremities.[10–14] A large group of patients injured in World War II with causalgia and reflex sympathetic dystrophy were successfully managed with sympathetic nerve blocks.

Since World War II, refinements have continued in nerve block techniques used in the sympathetic nervous system.

ANATOMY

The autonomic nervous system is divided into the sympathetic and parasympathetic nervous systems, each consisting of preganglionic and postganglionic nerves (Fig. 23C–1*A* to *C*). Preganglionic nerves of the sympathetic system arise from the thoracic and lumbar segments of the spinal cord; parasympathetic nerves also arise from the brainstem and sacral cord. These divisions are termed *thoracolumbar* and *craniosacral,* respectively. Most visceral structures are innervated by both sympathetic and parasympathetic systems, although some structures, such as blood vessels and sweat glands, have only single innervation.

Cell bodies of preganglionic sympathetic nerves exit in the intermediolateral and intermedial columns of the spinal cord and join ventral nerve roots from T2 to L2. Anatomic variations exist, with some preganglionic sympathetic nerves existing from C7 and others from L3 and L4.[8,15–18] More important for the anesthesiologist performing sympathetic blocks are the variations that occur intraspinally. Preganglionic sympathetic nerves travel up to 12 segments intraspinally before exiting the spinal cord.[15] Similarly, axons to thoracic ganglia remain ipsilateral, whereas those to lumbar ganglia take both ipsilateral and contralateral pathways.[19] Finally, preganglionic nerves often travel several segments within the sympathetic chain before synapsing or synapse in ganglia closer to their respective visceral structures.[20,21]

Paravertebral sympathetic ganglia lie on both sides of the vertebral column. In the cervical and thoracic regions, the chain is close to somatic nerves. Cervically, the ganglia can be found just anterior to transverse processes; in particular, the superior cervical ganglion is associated with the upper four cervical levels; the middle ganglion, when present, is related to C5 and C6; and the inferior ganglion comprises

AUTONOMIC INNERVATION
TO THE THORAX

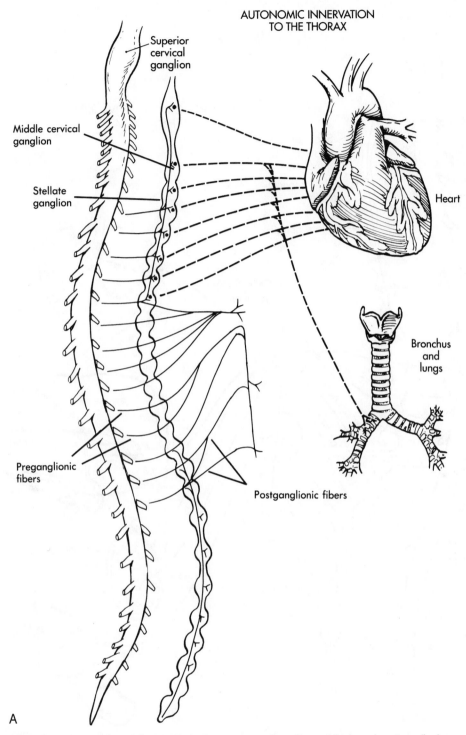

FIG. 23C–1 Innervation of the sympathetic nervous system. Preganglionic and postganglionic fibers are differentiated. *A*, Innervation to thorax.

C6 and C7 output. In 82% of cases, the inferior ganglion is fused with the first thoracic ganglion to form the stellate ganglion.[15,21–24] If not connected, the first thoracic ganglion is labeled as a stellate ganglion.[25]

In the thoracic region, up to 11 ganglia lie near the necks of the ribs. Four ganglia exist in the lumbar and sacral regions, although variations occur commonly. The position of the sympathetic chain and ganglia in the lumbar region differs. It is found at the anterolateral border of the vertebral body, separated from somatic nerves by the psoas muscle and psoas fascia (Fig. 23C–2).

Sympathetic innervation of the abdominal viscera differs from innervation cephalad to the diaphragm, with preganglionic nerves passing through the sympathetic chain. They become the splanchnic nerves and synapse at collateral ganglia around the abdominal aorta, following branches of

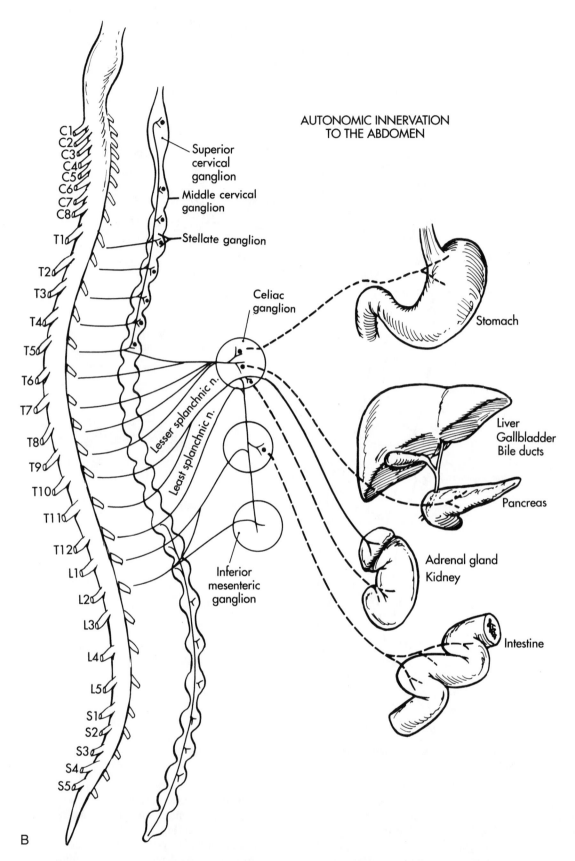

AUTONOMIC INNERVATION TO THE ABDOMEN

C1
C2
C3
C4
C5
C6
C7
C8

Superior cervical ganglion

Middle cervical ganglion

Stellate ganglion

T1
T2
T3
T4
T5
T6
T7
T8
T9
T10
T11
T12

Celiac ganglion

Lesser splanchnic n.

Least splanchnic n.

Inferior mesenteric ganglion

L1
L2
L3
L4
L5

S1
S2
S3
S4
S5

Stomach

Liver
Gallbladder
Bile ducts

Pancreas

Adrenal gland
Kidney

Intestine

B

FIG. 23C–1—cont'd *B,* Innervation to abdomen.

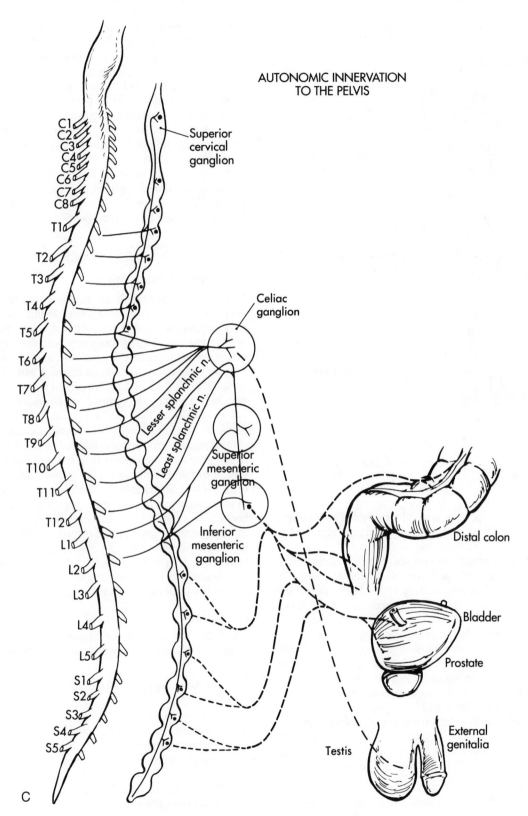

AUTONOMIC INNERVATION
TO THE PELVIS

C1
C2
C3
C4
C5
C6
C7
C8
T1
T2
T3
T4
T5
T6
T7
T8
T9
T10
T11
T12
L1
L2
L3
L4
L5
S1
S2
S3
S4
S5

Superior
cervical
ganglion

Celiac
ganglion

Lesser splanchnic n.

Least splanchnic n.

Superior
mesenteric
ganglion

Inferior
mesenteric
ganglion

Distal colon

Bladder

Prostate

External
genitalia

Testis

C

FIG. 23C–1—cont'd   *C,* Innervation to pelvis.

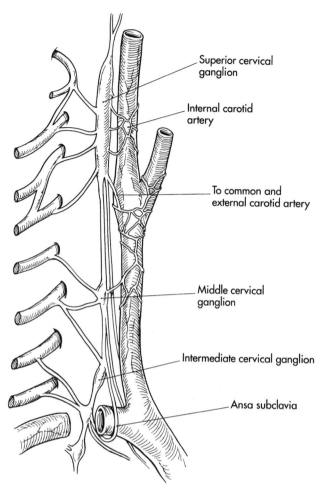

Superior cervical ganglion

Internal carotid artery

To common and external carotid artery

Middle cervical ganglion

Intermediate cervical ganglion

Ansa subclavia

FIG. 23C–2 Schematic diagram of upper thoracic and cervical sympathetic chain.

the aorta to each respective visceral structure. These collateral ganglia are diffuse and more appropriately represent a plexus of nerves called the *celiac plexus.*

Preganglionic sympathetic nerves exit the spinal cord with ventral nerve roots and connect to the sympathetic chain by the white communicating rami. These fibers are myelinated, thus giving the whitish appearance to the nerve bundle. Postganglionic nerves form a sympathetic chain and also communicate with the spinal nerve en route to the periphery. These are unmyelinated and grayish and are called the gray communicating rami. Each presynaptic fiber may synapse with as many as 30 postsynaptic nerves; this diffuse aspect allows for the stress response seen when the sympathetic system is activated.[7,15,26]

Blockade of the sympathetic nervous system can be achieved at several levels. Sympathetic fibers pass through deep fascial planes and can be considered more inaccessible than somatic nerves. Blockade can be performed at the sympathetic nerves by:

- Interruption of the somatic nerve, which blocks the corresponding sympathetic fibers
- Perivascular infiltration
- Intravenous (IV) regional anesthesia
- Intraspinal block

Although any of these techniques theoretically can produce successful sympathetic block, monitoring and documentation of a success block must always be performed because alternative and diffuse sympathetic pathways may exist.

The most appropriate site for blockade depends on each patient's clinical status. A patient can have signs and symptoms suggesting sympathetically mediated pain, but the diagnosis may be inconclusive. In these cases, a diagnostic sympathetic block should be performed.

The best location for a diagnostic block is the sympathetic chain. A block at this level affects only sympathetic nerves, and, if pain is relieved, one can be satisfied that the sympathetic system is responsible for the pain experienced.

An alternative location is the differential intraspinal (epidural or intrathecal) block. However, a differential intraspinal block will not characteristically differentiate sympathetic pain from other sources of pain.

STELLATE GANGLION BLOCK

Anatomic Considerations

Cell bodies for preganglionic nerves originate in the anterolateral horn of the spinal cord; fibers destined for the head and neck originate in the first and second thoracic spinal cord segments, whereas preganglionic nerves to the upper extremity originate at segments T2 to T8 and occasionally T9. Preganglionic axons to the head and neck exit with the ventral roots of T1 and T2 and then travel as white communicating rami before joining the sympathetic chain and passing cephalad to synapse at the inferior (stellate), middle, or superior cervical ganglion. Postganglionic nerves either follow the carotid arteries (external and internal) to the head or integrate as the gray communicating rami before joining the cervical plexus or upper cervical nerves to innervate neck structure (Fig. 23C–3). To achieve successful sympathetic denervation of the head and neck, one should block the stellate ganglion, because all preganglionic nerves either synapse here or pass through on their way to more cephalad ganglia. Blockade of the middle or superior ganglia misses the contribution of sympathetic fibers traveling from the stellate ganglion to the vertebral plexus and, ultimately, to the corresponding areas of the cranial vault supplied by the vertebral artery.[7]

Indications

The following clinical conditions have been treated with sympathetic block of the cervicothoracic chain:

1. Pain
   a. Reflex sympathetic dystrophy
   b. Causalgia
   c. Herpes zoster
   d. Postherpetic neuralgia, early
   e. Phantom limb pain
   f. Paget's disease
   g. Neoplasm
   h. Postradiation neuritis
   i. Pain from CNS lesions
   j. Intractable angina pectoris
2. Vascular insufficiency
   a. Raynaud's disease
   b. Frostbite

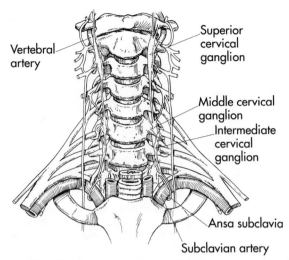

FIG. 23C–3 Cervical sympathetic ganglia and stellate ganglion. Note the relationship of structures to the respective ganglia.

c. Vasospasm
d. Occlusive vascular disease
e. Embolic vascular disease
f. Scleroderma
3. Other
a. Hyperhidrosis
b. Ménière's disease
c. Shoulder/hand syndrome
d. Stroke
e. Sudden blindness
f. Vascular headaches

Some of these indications remain controversial, and reports of efficacy are based largely on case reports instead of large studies with good study design. In particular, treatment with stellate ganglion block for phantom limb pain, postherpetic neuralgia, vascular occlusion of large vessels, stroke, and Ménière's disease has yielded questionable results. Other conditions, such as angina pectoris, require blockade of the upper five thoracic sympathetic ganglia, in addition to the stellate ganglion, to provide relief.[10]

Technique

Patient Preparation

Proper preparation of the patient for the initial block ideally begins at the visit before the procedure. Patients are much more likely to remember discharge instructions and expected side effects if these are explained during a visit when they are not apprehensive about an impending procedure.

Conversations about realistic expectations of sympathetic blockade should be held before any procedures. The goals of blockade and the number of blocks in a given series differ with each specific pain syndrome, and these should be discussed when possible at visits before the blockade. Patients are much less likely to experience frustration or despair if they understand beforehand what can be expected.

Informed consent must be obtained whenever sympathetic blockade is anticipated. Potential risks, complications, and side effects that may occur should be explained in detail.

An IV line placed before the block is not considered mandatory at all pain clinics. Its placement facilitates the use of IV sedation, when indicated, and provides access for the administration of resuscitative drugs should a complication occur. In skilled hands, a stellate ganglion block can be performed quickly and relatively painlessly.

Anterior Approach

1. The patient is asked to lie supine with the head resting flat on the table, without the use of a pillow.
2. A folded sheet or thin pillow is placed under the shoulder of most patients to further facilitate extension of the neck and make palpation of bony landmarks easier (Fig. 23C–4).
3. The patient keeps the head midline with the mouth slightly open to relax the tension on the anterior cervical musculature.
4. The site of needle entry is at the C6 level (Chassaignac's tubercle), which can be most readily identified by first locating the cricoid cartilage (Fig. 23C–5).
5. To ensure proper needle location, one should correctly identify the C6 tubercle by using firm pressure with the index finger.
6. To perform the procedure most easily, one can attach the syringe before needle placement. The skin is prepared antiseptically and the needle is inserted posteriorly, penetrating the skin at the tip of the clinician's index finger.
7. One should use a 23-gauge needle, 4- to 5-cm long, to puncture the skin directly downward (posteriorly).
8. The needle passes through the underlying tissue until it contacts either the C6 tubercle or the junction between the C6 vertebral body and the tubercle.
9. If the needle contacts the medial aspect of the transverse process at a depth somewhat greater than expected, the clinician should be prepared to withdraw the needle 0.5 cm to avoid injection into the longus colli muscle.
10. Once bone is encountered, one should maintain pressure with the palpating finger, withdraw the needle 2 to 5 mm, and inject the medication. Alternatively, once bone is met, one should release the palpating hand and fix the needle by grasping its hub.
11. The injection of medication is performed in a routine and systematic fashion. If the aspiration results are negative for CSF and blood, the clinician should give 0.5 to 1.0 ml of solution and ask the patient to raise his or her thumb to indicate that there are no adverse symptoms.
12. The clinician should maintain verbal contact by asking the patient to point a thumb or finger upward during the procedure.
13. After the initial test dose, one should inject the remainder of the solution, carefully aspirating after each 3 to 4 ml.

The total volume of the solution necessary depends on the block desired.[10] If placed properly, 5–10 ml of solution blocks the stellate ganglion.

Evidence of Block

Sympathetic nerve interruption to the head, which is supplied by the stellate ganglion, can be easily documented by the presence of Horner's syndrome: myosis, ptosis, and enophthalmos. Associated findings include conjunctival injection, nasal congestion, and facial anhidrosis.

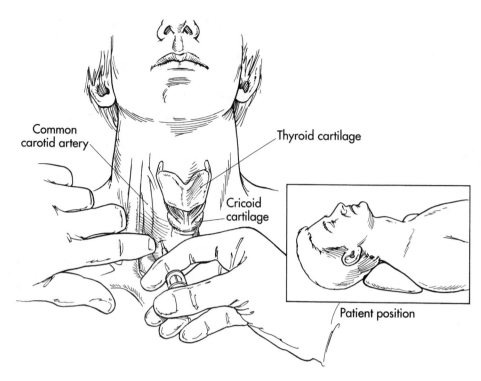

Common carotid artery

Thyroid cartilage

Cricoid cartilage

Patient position

FIG. 23C–4 Stellate ganglion block. The C6 anterior tubercle is directly beneath the operator's index finger. The carotid artery is retracted laterally when necessary. The needle is perpendicular to all skin planes and is inserted directly posteriorly. *Inset,* The patient is positioned for stellate ganglion block. A pillow or roll should be between the shoulder to extend the neck, bring the esophagus midline, and facilitate palpation of Chassaignac's tubercle.

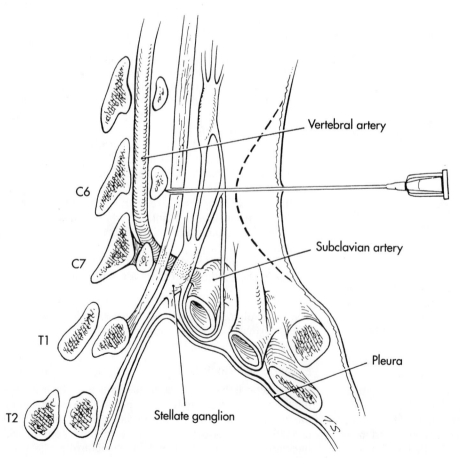

Vertebral artery

C6

C7

Subclavian artery

T1

Pleura

T2

Stellate ganglion

FIG. 23C–5 Sagittal view of the sympathetic chain. The stellate ganglion is positioned directly posterior to the vertebral artery. The longus colli muscle separates the ganglia from the bone at the C6 level. The needle is superior to the stellate ganglion. Dashed line represents compression effect of the finger on subcutaneous tissue.

Evidence of sympathetic blockade to the upper extremity includes visible engorgement of the veins on the back of the hand and forearm, psychogalvanic reflex, plethysmography, thermography, and a positive result on a sweat test. A rise of skin temperature also occurs, provided that the preblock temperature has not exceeded 33°C to 34°C.

Efficacy of Block

Findings[27] support the work of Malmqvist and colleagues[28] who showed that stellate ganglion blocks performed at C6 do not reliably denervate sympathetic activity to the upper extremity. These findings also indicate that many patients derive excellent relief with one stellate ganglion block but ineffective relief with a subsequent block despite a noticeable Horner's syndrome and, possibly, temperature elevations with each procedure. Future work should examine more reliably effective methods to sympathetically denervate the upper extremity.

Neurolysis

Many clinicians avoided performing neurolysis of the stellate ganglion because of the fear of producing a permanent Horner's syndrome. One must be extremely cautious not to produce any brachial plexus block with this technique or to allow any drug into the epidural or subarachnoid space. Careful positioning of the needle with image intensification and contrast injection is recommended.

Alternatively, radiofrequency (RF) denervation has been done at the level of the stellate ganglion. To diminish the likelihood of a permanent Horner's syndrome, it is advantageous to place the needle into the inferior aspect of the ganglion. A 5- to 10-mm active tip is recommended using a 70°C, 60-second cycle to produce the lesion.

Side Effects and Complications

Most unpleasant side effects result from the Horner's syndrome and include ptosis, myosis, and nasal congestion.

Common complications occur from the diffusion of local anesthetic solution onto nearby nervous structures. These include the recurrent laryngeal nerve with complaints of hoarseness, feeling of a lump in the throat, and sometimes a subjective shortness of breath. Bilateral stellate blocks are rarely advised, because bilateral blocking of the recurrent laryngeal nerve can result in respiratory compromise and loss of laryngeal reflexes. Blockade of the phrenic nerve results in temporary paralysis of the diaphragm and can cause respiratory embarrassment in patients whose respiratory reserve is already severely compromised. Partial brachial plexus block can also be secondary to spread along the prevertebral fascia[29] or a needle location that is too posterior.

The two most feared complications from a stellate ganglion block are an intraspinal injection and seizures from an intravascular injection. The risk of pneumothorax also exists with the anterior approach.

Alternative Approach: C7 Anterior

The anterior approach to the stellate ganglion at C7 is similar to the approach describe at C6. Unlike the C6 tubercle, C7 has only a vestigial tubercle, which is very difficult to palpate. To identify C7, one should first find Chassaignac's tubercle (C6), then move one finger-breadth caudad from the inferior tip. The patient is positioned with a pillow under the shoulder to extend the cervical spine and to help make the tubercle more superficial.

The advantage of blockade at C7 is the lower volume of local anesthetic necessary to provide complete interruption of the upper extremity sympathetic innervation: 6 to 9 ml of solution suffices. The bothersome side effect of a recurrent laryngeal nerve block is less frequent with this approach. The technique carries two disadvantages: (1) the less pronounced landmarks make needle positioning less reliable and (2) the risk of pneumothorax increases because the dome of the lung is in close proximity.

Posterior Approach

The case of performing a stellate ganglion block by the anterior approach has rendered the posterior approach unnecessary except for specific indications.[10,30] One should use the posterior approach if a Horner's syndrome develops with an anterior approach but no other signs of sympathetic denervation to the upper extremity are present. If this occurs despite repetitive, well-placed blocks, the patient may have a fascial tissue barrier preventing caudal diffusion of the drug. The posterior approach at the T2 or T3 level provides sympathetic interruption to the upper extremity.

Patients selected for chemical sympathectomy of the upper extremity also should undergo blockade with the posterior approach. Although dilute solutions of phenol have been injected by the anterior approach at C6, the smaller volume used for the posterior approach may prevent diffusion to the stellate ganglion.[30] The posterior approach can often avoid a Horner's syndrome. A major disadvantage to sympathetic block by posterior approach is the high risk of pneumothorax (Fig. 23C–6).

Anatomic Considerations

The sympathetic chain lies close to the neck of the ribs in the thoracic space. Unlike the cervical and lumbar regions, where the longus colli muscle and psoas muscles, respectively, separate the sympathetic chain from somatic nerves, no muscular separation exists in the thoracic region. The risk of intravertebral diffusion of drug during this block necessitates that the patient be closely monitored. The pleura also abut the sympathetic chain in the thoracic region, making precise needle location essential to avoid a pneumothorax.

Technique

The posterior approach can be performed with the patient either prone or lateral with the side to be blocked uppermost.[7,31] This block was classically taught with needles inserted 6 cm from the midline. Entry at this point makes it extremely difficult to localize the needles properly along the vertebral body without passing through the pleura or parenchymal tissue (see Fig. 23C–6).

A distance of 3 to 4 cm from the midline allows proper alignment; the needle shaft should pass from the lamina and should be parallel with the sagittal plane. The clinician should direct the needle laterally, beyond the perpendicular plane. If the needle continues to contact lamina after repositioning to the perpendicular plane, a new skin wheal is raised 1 cm lateral to the original wheal and the process is retraced.

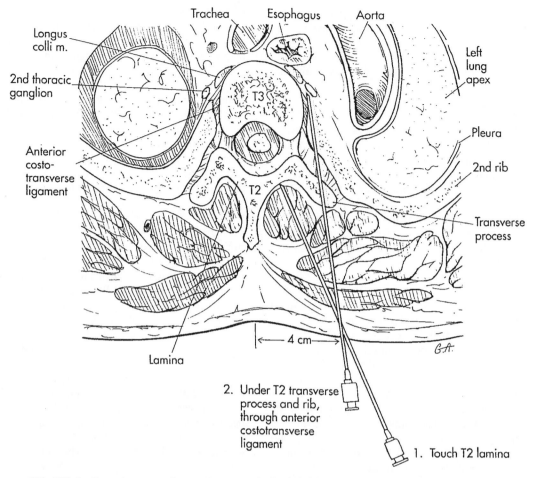

FIG. 23C–6 Posterior approach to upper sympathetic chain block. The needle is introduced 4 cm from midline, then walked off the T2 lamina. The needle should always be directed medially.

The space lateral to the T1 spinous process can be used if local anesthetic solution is injected. If a neurolytic procedure is anticipated, one should identify either the T2 or T3 spinous process. After preparing and draping the area, a skin wheal is raised 3 to 4 cm lateral to the spine. One should use a 22-gauge, 8- to 10-cm needle to contact to ipsilateral lamina. Then the needle is positioned laterally of the lamina until it passes through the anterior costotransverse ligament. This can be done by loss-of-resistance technique, similar to that described for epidural location. Alternatively, a skin marker is placed after contact with the lamina. At this point, 2 to 3 ml of radiocontrast material is injected. Proper spread is characteristically seen. If dye cannot be visualized, pleural or intravascular injection is likely. If neurolysis is anticipated, the clinician should inspect the intraspinal space closely for any back-diffusion of dye before injecting a neurolytic agent. Once proper location is verified with contrast, one should inject 2 to 3 ml of local anesthetic or neurolytic slowly with repeated aspiration.

Neurolysis

Neurolysis of the upper thoracic sympathetic chain by the posterior approach should be performed only when one of the image intensifiers is used, preferably computed tomo-graphy (CT). Needles can be positioned erroneously with disastrous results if a neurolytic agent is injected.

For neurolysis, use the T2 or T3 spinous process. Although a Horner's syndrome may be avoided by this approach, the risk remains, and the patient must understand and accept this possible occurrence.

Alternatively, RF denervation of the upper thoracic sympathetic chain has been performed. Image intensification with either CT or fluoroscopy is advised. Positioning of the needle at the upper aspect of the T2 vertebral body as seen in the anteroposterior projection and at the midvertebral body level as seen on lateral view is recommended.

Complications

The two main complications after neurolysis are pneumothorax and intraspinal injection; a third possible complication is a persistent Horner's syndrome. A pneumothorax can be avoided with careful placement of the needle; the clinician should ensure that the needle angulation is never lateral and that the advancement through the costotransverse ligaments is controlled and slow and uses the loss-of-resistance technique. Intraspinal injection most commonly occurs by diffusion through the intervertebral foramen, and one can avoid this by initially injecting a water-soluble contrast dye and checking location by x-ray examination.

INTERPLEURAL APPROACH TO SYMPATHETIC DENERVATION

Injection of local anesthetic into the interpleural space may produce a Horner's syndrome.[32] This result occurs by diffusion of drug medially to the paravertebral thoracic chain and cephalad to the stellate ganglion. If this approach could reliably produce sympathetic denervation to the upper extremity, one could place a catheter and leave it for days with repeated bolus injections or infusions of local anesthetics and continuous sympathetic denervation.

Technique

The patient is prepared in sterile fashion. The patient is draped in the prone position, with the arms hanging from the bed when possible; this displaces the scapula laterally and stretches the rhomboid muscles, facilitating placement of the needle. The clinician should try to enter the interpleural space in a medial and posterior location. We choose a more cephalic entry point (superior to the T4 or T5 rib) if attempting to achieve denervation of the upper thoracic sympathetic chain and stellate ganglion. Alternatively, one should insert the needle more distally if sympathetic block of the splanchnic nerves is desired.

For blocks of the upper thoracic sympathetic chain, one should insert an epidural or special interpleural needle about 4 to 6 cm lateral to the thoracic spine and perpendicular to all planes. The needle is positioned sufficiently medial to the scapula to avoid subsequent trauma from the scapula if catheter insertion is anticipated. The clinician should seek contact with the rib, then direct the needle incrementally cephalad off the rib until the interpleural space is found using a loss-of-resistance technique with saline solution. The bevel of needle faces medically and cephalad, and a catheter can be inserted 10 to 15 cm if desired.

Side Effects and Complications

Pneumothorax represents a significant potential risk any time a needle is inserted into the interpleural space. This risk can be kept to a minimum with careful control and advancement of the needle and not leaving the stylet out of the needle once placed in the interpleural space.

A significant theoretical risk of prolonged catheter insertion in the pleural space is infection. Even though most infections are treatable with antibiotics, the risk of development of a potentially serious empyema cannot be excluded.

THORACIC SYMPATHETIC BLOCK

Anatomic Considerations

The thoracic sympathetic chain lies close to somatic nerves as they emanate from the intervertebral foramen. Their posterior orientation on the vertebral bodies is constant throughout the thoracic space. Ten pair of ganglia can be found as the chain courses through the thoracic cavity. The pleura is directly anterior to the ganglia, separated in most places by only the thin endothoracic fascia (Fig. 23C–7).

Indications

Few indications exist for thoracic sympathetic block. Thoracic epidural block can provide similar results without the high risk of pneumothorax. Some oncologic processes can produce a relatively specific sympathetic pain of the thoracic viscera, which can be alleviated by a neurolytic injected onto the thoracic sympathetic chain. This avoids potential complications of a neurolytic intraspinal block.

Technique

The clinician should position the patient prone and outline the spinous processes. One should use image intensification whenever possible. A skin wheal is raised 4 to 5 cm lateral to the spinous process. One should direct the needle to the lamina, then walk it laterally. A skin marker is placed 1 cm above the skin, and the loss-of-resistance technique is used as the needle passes from the lamina. One should never advance the needle in a lateral direction because this invariably results in a pneumothorax. If lamina is still contacted with the needle in a perpendicular plane, a skin wheal is raised 2 cm lateral to the original, and the previous steps are repeated. After a needle passes from the lamina, it engages the costotransverse ligament and, immediately on piercing the ligament, one encounters a loss of resistance. A dose of 1.5 to 2 ml of solution should anesthetize the chain at this point, although posterior diffusion to the corresponding somatic nerve can occur.

Complications

The risk of pneumothorax must be considered the main reason this block is not performed more often. The risk after neurolysis also includes the likelihood of diffusion of medicine to the nearby somatic nerves, producing neuralgic pain. The needle can also be inadvertently placed into the intraspinal space or adjacent to the intervertebral foramen, with resultant injection of medicine onto the spinal cord.

CELIAC PLEXUS AND SPLANCHNIC NERVE BLOCK

Anatomic Considerations

Sympathetic innervation of the abdominal viscera originates in the anterolateral horn of the spinal cord. Preganglionic axons from T5 to T12 leave the spinal cord with the ventral spinal routes to join the white communicating rami en route to the sympathetic chain. In contradistinction to other preganglionic sympathetic nerves, these axons do not synapse in the sympathetic chain; rather, they pass through the chain to synapse at distal sites, including the celiac, aortic renal, and superior mesenteric ganglia. Postganglionic nerves accompany blood vessels to their respective visceral structures (Fig. 23C–8).

Preganglionic nerves from T5 to T9 and occasionally T4 to T10 travel caudally from the sympathetic chain along the lateral and anterolateral aspects of the vertebral bodies. At the level of T9 and T10, the axons coalesce to form the greater splanchnic nerve, course through the diaphragm, and end as numerous terminal endings in the celiac plexus.

The celiac plexus lies anterior to the aorta and epigastrium (Fig. 23C–9). It is also located just anterior to the crus of the diaphragm and becomes an important consideration in selection of the approach for blockade. The plexus extends for several centimeters in front of the aorta and laterally

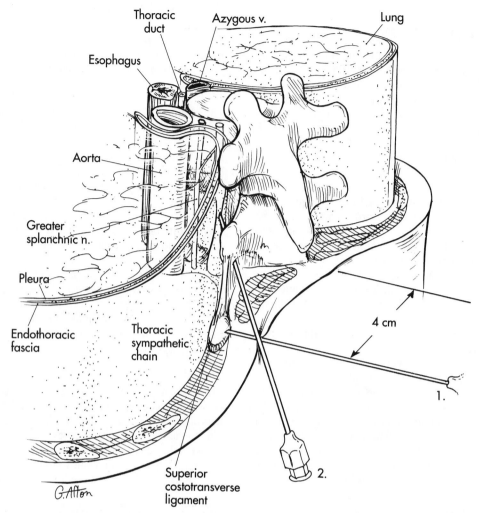

Thoracic duct

Azygous v.

Lung

Esophagus

Aorta

Greater splanchnic n.

Pleura

Endothoracic fascia

Thoracic sympathetic chain

4 cm

1.

2.

Superior costotransverse ligament

G. Afton

FIG. 23C–7 Midthoracic sympathetic block.

around the aorta (see Fig. 23C–9). Fibers within the plexus arise from preganglionic splanchnic nerves, parasympathetic preganglionic nerves from the vagus, some sensory nerves from the phrenic and vagus nerves, and sympathetic postganglionic fibers. Afferent fibers concerned with nociception pass diffusely through the celiac plexus and represent the main target of celiac blockade.

These fibers coalesce to form a dense, intertwining network of autonomic nerves. Three pairs of ganglia exist within the plexus: (1) the celiac ganglia, (2) the superior mesenteric ganglia, and (3) the aortic renal ganglia.

Indications

Any pain originating from visceral structures and innervated by the celiac plexus can be effectively alleviated by blockade of the plexus. These structures include the pancreas, liver, gallbladder, omentum, mesentery, and alimentary tract from the stomach to the transverse portion of the large colon (see Fig. 23C–1). The particular disease state determines the effectiveness of a celiac plexus block in producing sustained pain relief beyond the duration of the local anesthetic solution. The pain syndrome invoiced should dictate whether a local anesthetic block, neurolytic injection, catheter placement, or steroid injection should be anticipated.

The best indication for neurolytic celiac plexus block is upper abdominal malignancy, in particular, pancreatic cancer. An additional benefit to patients may be the effect of celiac plexus block on gastric motility. Complete sympathetic denervation of the gastrointestinal tract allows unopposed parasympathetic activity and increased peristalsis.

An alternative to neurolysis for patients who have had multiple abdominal surgeries and continue to complain of pain involves the addition of a corticosteroid preparation to the local anesthetic solution. Best results can be expected in patients who have an inflammatory component involving the celiac plexus.

The cause of abdominal pain cannot always be clearly elucidated at initial evaluation, especially in patients who have undergone multiple abdominal operations. In these patients, it can be difficult to differentiate abdominal wall pain from underlying visceral pain. Either a local anesthetic celiac plexus block or an intercostal nerve block should be considered a pain-specific block and differentiates visceral from somatic pain, respectively.

Lateral Technique

Before blockade, the clinician should obtain informed consent and insert an IV catheter. The patient is positioned with a

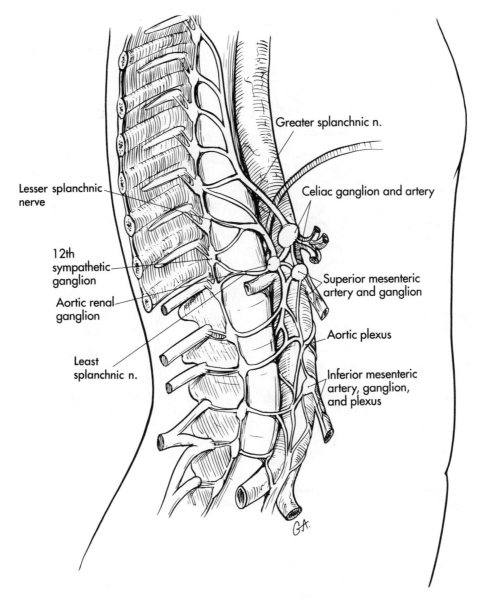

FIG. 23C–8 Splanchnic nerves: greater, lesser, and least. Formation of the respective abdominal plexuses is shown.

pillow under the lower abdomen to minimize the lumbar lordosis and allow easier palpation of the spinous processes.

Landmarks drawn with an indelible skin marker greatly facilitate needle placement, even for operators experienced with the procedure (Fig. 23C–10). This may be done before preparing and draping the patient or with a sterile marker after preparation. Landmarks to be drawn include the spinous processes of T12 and L1 and the inferior border of the 12th rib. The T12 spinous process must be correctly identified and marked by following the 12th rib medially and counting cephalad from the L5 spinous process.

The site for needle entry is marked 7 to 8 cm lateral from the spinous process. One should use either 20- or 22-gauge needles, 12- to 18-cm long; the exact length depends on body habitus. The insertion point should be immediately inferior to the border of the 12th rib. Entry site should not exceed 8 cm from the midline to avoid the risk of placing the

needle through renal parenchymal tissue. It is also extremely important that both needles not be immediately placed beneath the T11 rib, because a pneumothorax can result.

The ultimate directional positioning of the needle toward the midline depends on whether the splanchnic nerves or celiac plexuses are to be blocked (Fig. 23C–11). Classically, needles have been directed to the L1 spinous process for block of the celiac plexus. Splanchnic nerves are blocked by positioning the needles more cephalad toward the 11th or 12th thoracic spinous process.

Anatomically, the crus of the diaphragm determines whether the block performed represents a true celiac plexus block or a splanchnic nerve block. If the tip of the needle lies posterior to the crus, the nerves blocked belong to the splanchnic nerves. When needles are advanced anteriorly, they pass transcrurally and the solution injected blocks nerves to the celiac plexus.

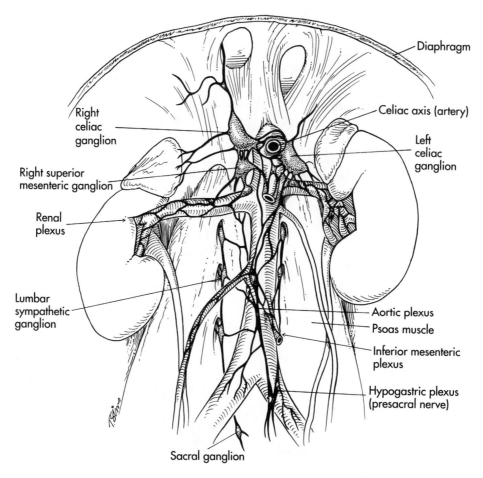

FIG. 23C–9   Anterior view of the celiac plexus. The relationship to nearby structures is shown. Note the dense, diffuse intertwining network of nerves that form the plexus.

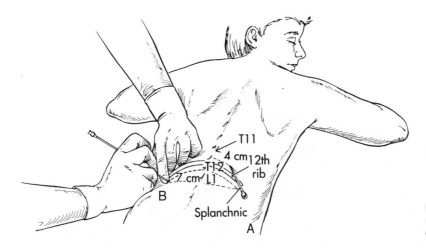

FIG. 23C–10   Surface landmarks for splanchnic nerve block (A) or celiac plexus block (B). The diagram drawn resembles a flat isosceles triangle.

Infiltration with local anesthetics of deep muscular structures and periosteum lessens the need for sedation. One should avoid heavy sedation, especially when a diagnostic block is being performed. With advancement of the needle, two bony landmarks, the 12th rib and the transverse process of L1, can be mistaken for the vertebral body. If any question remains after bone is encountered, the clinician should remove the needle and redirect it cephalad.

Once the vertebral body has been reached, one should place a skin marker on the needle 2 to 3 cm from the skin and then walk the needle laterally until it just slips from the lateral surface of the vertebral body (Fig. 23C–12). To make accurate small adjustments in the needle placement, one should first withdraw it to superficial, subcutaneous structures.

Once the lateral aspect of the vertebral body has passed, a "pop" is often felt when the needle passes through the psoas

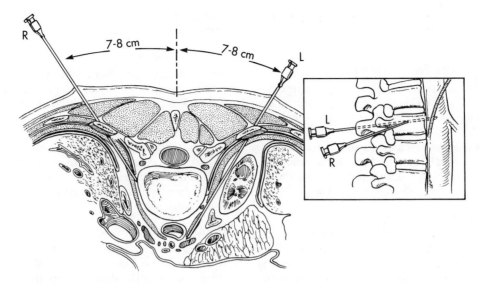

FIG. 23C–11 Retrocrural and transcrural needle placement for celiac plexus block. *Inset,* The left needle *(L)* is retrocrural and results in solution to spread and block the splanchnic nerves. The right needle *(R)* is transcrural and blocks the celiac plexus directly.

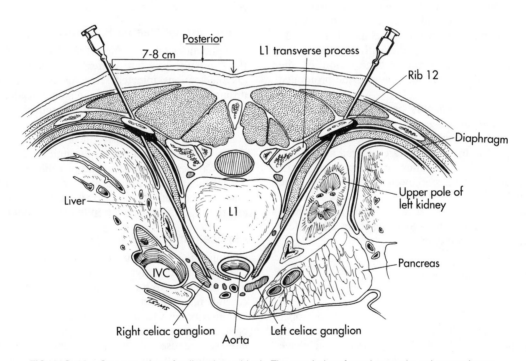

FIG. 23C–12 Cross section of celiac plexus block. The proximity of renal parenchymal necessitates placing needles no farther than 7 to 8 cm from midline.

fascia. At this point, the needles approach the great vessels and should be advanced slowly. The aorta is encountered from the left, and the inferior vena cava from the right. Pancreatic or other intra-abdominal masses often distort these structures laterally and posteriorly along the vertebral column. One can easily check for optimal location of the needle by feeling for arterial pulsations.

After proper needle placement, a careful aspiration of both needles is performed before injection.

Initially, inject 2 to 3 ml of a local anesthetic solution containing epinephrine to further test for either intravascular or

intraspinal placement. If results for intravascular or intraspinal placement are negative, one may inject 15 ml bupivacaine 0.5% with epinephrine 1:200,000 through each needle.

Image Intensification

Image intensification techniques can aid the performance of celiac plexus blocks and include x-rays, fluoroscopy, and CT.[33–35] Because many pain clinics do not have these facilities on site, these blocks must be performed in the radiology department. This is rarely necessary when diagnostic blocks are performed or when local anesthetic injections are the sole agents used. The potential seriousness and permanency of complications with neurolytic solutions make image intensification preferable.

Alternative Approach: Single-Needle

A single-needle approach using the left side has been reported with good results.[36,37] This technique for needle placement is similar to that previously described for bilateral placement. Final location of the needle has been reported both posterior to the aorta and anterior to it by a transaortic approach.

Adequate volume must be used because only one needle is used, and the celiac plexus is a diffuse network. One should consider 20 ml and, possibly, 30 ml whenever feasible.

Anterior Approach

An anterior approach to the celiac plexus has been employed with the needle inserted through the abdominal wall at the T12 level. A thin 22-gauge needle is used, because bowel is often perforated. The needle tip location is anterior to the aorta at the exact position of the celiac plexus.

Catheter Placement

Patients with nonmalignant abdominal pain often fare poorly after neurolytic blockade of the celiac plexus, yet many derive temporary benefit from local anesthetic blockade. Because this pain is sympathetically mediated and reflexively perpetuated, continuous denervation of the plexus by local anesthetic infusion may provide prolonged analgesia.

The technique for placement is similar to that described previously.[38] Instead of 22-gauge needles, the clinician should use a 6- or 8-inch catheter system placed bilaterally. Once they are placed, the catheters are secured at the skin with either a 2-cm silk skin suture or benzoin and Steri-Strips. One should place a sterile, clear dressing over the catheters, which are connected to local anesthetic solutions of bupivacaine 0.1%, given at 6 to 8 ml/hour. These catheters can be maintained for 4 to 7 days if placed sterilely and if the sites are checked daily.

NEUROLYTIC BLOCK

Indications

Patients with pancreatic cancer or other isolated upper abdominal malignancies are most commonly chosen for a neurolytic celiac plexus block. Specific indications have been discussed in the preceding section. The technique is similar to that previous described, with image intensification employed whenever possible.

In selecting patients for a neurolytic celiac plexus block, one should try to differentiate somatic pain from visceral pain. Diagnosis of pancreatic cancer does not always underlie the mechanism of pain. Pain from retroperitoneal extension into somatic structures or distant metastases is not effectively blocked with a celiac plexus block. If both visceral and somatic causes are present, the celiac plexus block may serve only to unmask the somatic component of pain.

Agents

Debate continues regarding which agent should be employed.[39] No comparative studies have been performed examining the effectiveness of the two most commonly used compounds: alcohol and phenol.

Complications

The main side effect from celiac plexus block is backache, which usually results from the passage of needles through the back muscles. This result can be minimized by gentle positioning of the needles, minimal repositioning, and adequate local infiltration. Although self-limiting, back pain can be a significant complaint and can require use of a nonsteroidal anti-inflammatory drug, muscle relaxant, or heating pad. Celiac catheter placement and subsequent maintenance can be distressing enough to require the on-going treatments listed previously.

Hypotension

Hypotension can be expected from a well-placed celiac block and occurs secondary to vasodilatation of the large splanchnic bed. The difference in the hypotensive response between a local anesthetic and a neurolytic occurs after compensatory mechanisms have adjusted for splanchnic vasodilatation. Orthostatic hypotension can persist after a neurolytic block despite compensation.

Inappropriate Needle Placement

Complications of celiac plexus block can be subdivided into those resulting from either (1) needle placement or (2) medications injected. Needles can inadvertently pass through a dural cuff, resulting in spinal headache. Repeated puncture of an intervertebral disk produces back pain that can be slow to resolve. Puncture of the great vessels, most commonly the aorta, can result in a retroperitoneal hemorrhage. Placement of a needle through the L1 somatic nerve root produces a paresthesia and possibly a painful neuropathy. A final, potentially serious complication from needle placement occurs if the 12th rib is not correctly identified and the needles are inadvertently inserted under the 11th rib.

Medication Complications

Complications from medications can result from the local anesthetic or neurolytic agent. Local anesthetic complications secondary to intravascular injection can easily occur if careful, repeated aspirations are not performed. The aorta and inferior vena cava can be punctured and may not be recognized with the longer needles necessary to perform these blocks. The use of epinephrine-containing solutions and incremental dosing may avoid this potential problem. Inadvertent injection of a local anesthetic solution into a dural cuff of the intraspinal canal can result in a total spinal block. The clinician should always keep resuscitative equipment readily available to handle such emergencies. Accidental injection of either alcohol or phenol into the intraspinal space can be catastrophic. Another catostrophic result has been the development of anterior spinal artery syndrome following neurolytic celiac plexus block. The mechanism is unclear, but may result from intra-arterial injection.

A more common complication of neurolytic blockade occurs when the drug diffuses laterally and posteriorly into the psoas muscle. The effect can be greatly reduced with the use of image intensifiers. When it does happen, the effect is most often limited to the L1 nerve root.

One potentially devastating complication after neurolytic celiac plexus block is aortic wall dissection.

LUMBAR SYMPATHETIC BLOCK

Anatomic Considerations

The lumbar sympathetic chain lies at the anterolateral border of the vertebral bodies. Unlike the more cephalad portions, the lumbar chain reveals many inconstant findings. The chain rarely appears in the same size or shape, or in the same location, within a given individual. The ganglia are also variable, with four sets being more common than five, a result of fusion of the T12 and L1 ganglia.[10] Their position also varies; they can be segmentally located or closely grouped between the second and fourth lumbar vertebrae. The size of the ganglion also varies from 3 to 5 mm wide and 10 and 15 mm in length.

The anatomic positioning of the lumbar sympathetic chain at the anterolateral border of the vertebral border differs from more cephalad portions of the chain and allows it to be removed from somatic nerves (Fig. 23C–13). The aorta is positioned anteriorly and slightly medial to the chain on the left side. The inferior vena cava is more closely approximated to the chain on the right in an anterior plane. Many other small lumbar arteries and veins are positioned near the sympathetic chain. The psoas muscle is situated posteriorly and lateral to the sympathetic chain.

Indications

Lumbar sympathetic blockade has been used extensively in the treatment of reflex sympathetic dystrophy and causalgia. Blockade of the sympathetic nerves can also be performed with a spinal, epidural, or peripheral nerve block, but relief of pain after a lumbar sympathetic block most

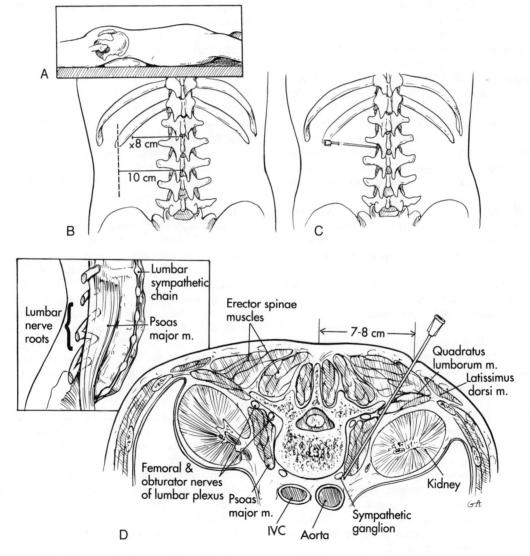

FIG. 23C–13 Lateral approach to lumbar sympathetic nerve block. *A,* The patient should be positioned with a pillow beneath the anterior iliac spines. *B,* Spine landmarks include the 12th rib, the posterior iliac crest, and the cephalad tip of the L2 spinous process. *C,* Insertion of the needle is 7 to 8 cm from the midline, perpendicular to the spinal canal at L2. *D,* Cross-sectional view of final needle placement. IVC, inferior vena cava.

clearly delineates the painful mechanism as sympathetically mediated.

Patients with acute herpes zoster and, possibly, postherpetic neuralgia can benefit from lumbar sympathetic blockade. Acute radiation neuritis and some chronic postradiation neuralgias can be partially relieved by sympathetic blocks. Finally, patients with chronic, ill-defined pelvic pain can derive benefit from sympathetic blockade, which can be helpful when pain presents a diagnostic dilemma.

Technique

Two techniques are described: (1) a lateral approach first described by Reid[40] and (2) a classic prone position initially reported by Mandl.[41] The clinician should obtain informed consent before the block, and place an IV line.

Lateral Approach

The patient is positioned prone with one or two pillows placed under the lower abdomen across the anterior iliac crest. One should mark and outline the spinous processes of L2, L3, and L4. This step is further checked by marking the inferior border of T12 and the posterior iliac crest. The midpoint between these two lines, 7 cm from the midline, places the mark at the L2-3 region. This mark should be adjusted to be perpendicular to the caudal aspect of the L2 vertebra.

The optimal distance from midline for needle insertion is reportedly anywhere from 4 to 10 cm.[7,31] Any of these distances has been used successfully by different operators.

Classically, two or three needles have been individually placed at the L2, L3, and L4 levels. Contrast material injected with subsequent x-ray or image intensification has repeatedly demonstrated good longitudinal spread of solution along the anterolateral border of the vertebral bodies with a single-needle technique. The use of multiple-needle techniques can be reserved for situations in which a temperature increase does not occur despite adequate placement or in which pain relief is not achieved despite good location in patients with know sympathetic pain.

Once a skin wheal is raised, deeper infiltration of the local anesthetic solution should be performed along the anticipated tract for subsequent needle placement.

A 22-gauge, 12- to 18-cm needle is advanced slowly until it comes in contact with the vertebral body. The angle of the needle with respect to the skin can be as shallow as 45 degrees in thin individuals or somewhat steeper in more obese patients.

If one bypasses the transverse process, one should recognize that the bone felt is vertebral body. The clinician should not confuse the transverse process for vertebral body whenever shallow bone is encountered.

Once the vertebral body has been appropriately identified, a rubber skin marker is placed on the needle 2 to 3 cm from the skin. One should remove the needle toward the skin, and redirect it at a slightly steeper angle. The length of the needles necessitates small-angle changes at the skin to prevent large changes at the distal end. With correct repositioning, the needle passes just lateral to the vertebral body and rests at the anterolateral border.

Before injection, one should perform careful aspiration in two planes. The aorta on the left and the inferior vena cava on the right both lie reasonably close to the sympathetic chain.

Most preservative-free local anesthetics at commercially prepared concentrations block the sympathetic chain. If a single-needle technique is used, one should inject 15 ml of volume to ensure proper cephalad and caudal spread of solution. Initial injection with 2-chloroprocaine yields a faster onset of block, as manifested by a recorded temperature rise of the distal extremity.

Classic "Paramedian" Approach

The clinician should place the patient prone, and outline the spinous processes of L2, L3, and L4. Skin wheals are raised 4 to 5 cm lateral to the midline. One should use shorter 8- to 12-cm, 20-gauge needles and insert them at a 70- to 80-degree angle toward the midline. The needle is advanced until it makes contact with the transverse process; at a depth of 4 to 6 cm, a skin marker is placed 3 to 5 cm from the skin. One should reposition the needle inferiorly and medially to slip off the transverse process and pass to the vertebral body, approximately 2 cm deep to the transverse process. The clinician should further reposition the needle to slip off the vertebral body and advance it to the previously positioned skin marker. The needle should now lie anterior to the psoas fascia at the anterolateral border of the vertebral body. One should repeat the process with the other two needles and inject the solution as previously described.

Neurolytic Block

Neurolysis of the lumbar sympathetic chain is easily performed and is one of the most useful neurolytic procedures.[42] It can be indicated for recalcitrant reflex sympathetic dystrophy, causalgia, peripheral vascular disease, pelvic malignancies, and deafferentation pain syndromes. Neurolysis should be considered only after local anesthetic blocks of the lumbar sympathetic chain have documented efficacy but have failed to produce long-lasting relief.

Needle placement for neurolysis does not differ from that of a local anesthetic lumbar sympathetic block. Image intensification, in particular, fluoroscopy, greatly facilitates placement, allows real-time visualization of drug diffusion, and helps prevent possible complications by ill-placed needles or neurolytic solution. When a single-needle technique is used, fluoroscopy can document adequate cephalad spread to the upper limits of L2 and caudal diffusion of drug to L4.

Significant longitudinal spread of drug along the sympathetic chain is required for adequate neurolysis. One needle is positioned at the inferior aspect of L2, and the second needle is positioned at the inferior aspect of L3. Needle placement is checked before injecting contrast material in both the anteroposterior and the lateral planes.

One should monitor distal skin temperatures during neurolysis for further documentation of block. If any questions remain after the placement of needles, the clinician should inject a local anesthetic solution before neurolysis and evaluate the efficacy by a temperature rise and relief of symptoms.

The spread of contrast is characteristic and reproducible. The dye confines itself to the anterolateral border of the vertebral body in a tight, linear fashion.

Phenol is the agent of choice for neurolysis.

RADIOFREQUENCY DENERVATION

An alternative to chemical neurolysis of the lumbar sympathetic chain involves thermal destruction using RF technique. A study from 1991 demonstrated no advantage of RF over chemical neurolysis; however, recent modifications in RF, including larger (15-mm) active tips, may increase the efficacy of this technique.[43]

Catheter Placement

Specially designed catheters are easily placed on the lumbar sympathetic chain for short-term infusions of local anesthetic solutions.

The technique for catheter placement is best performed with the lateral approach as previously described. The length of infusion necessary varies with each clinical situation. The most common long-term management problem with a catheter system is posterior dislodgment into the psoas muscle, manifested by decreased sensation and weakness of the quadriceps muscles.

Bupivacaine has been the agent of choice for infusions. Initial doses and infusion settings are 0.1% at 6 ml/hr.

A catheter system and infusion of local anesthetics can provide continuous denervation of the sympathetic nervous system.

Complications

The most common side effect after a lumbar sympathetic block is backache, which results from the placement of the needles through the paravertebral muscles of the back.

Intravascular injections of larger volumes of local anesthetics can produce serious systemic toxic reactions. Inadvertent subarachnoid injections occur rarely if the needle is mistakenly repositioned from bone into a dural cuff. Not uncommonly, the needle passes through the intervertebral disk. The sensation of passing through Swiss cheese is easily noted, necessitating removal of the needle and repositioning. Renal trauma or puncture of a ureter can occur if proper technique is not followed. Blockade of the genitofemoral nerve or lumbar plexus within the psoas muscle can occur if the needle is placed too far laterally or posteriorly. If a local anesthetic solution is used, a resulting numbness or weakness can occur in the groin, anterior thigh, or quadriceps.

Lateral spread of neurolytic solution from the lumbar sympathetic chain can result in genitofemoral neuralgia and, less often, lumbar plexus involvement.[44–46]

INTRAVENOUS REGIONAL SYMPATHETIC BLOCK

Mechanism of Action

Guanethidine monosulfate selectively inhibits the sympathetic nervous system while leaving the parasympathetic system intact. The site of action is postganglionic neuron at the neuroeffector junction. Guanethidine is actively transported into the postganglionic neuron by the norepinephrine pump. It displaces norepinephrine from presynaptic vesicles and inhibits reuptake of norepinephrine. A brief release of norepinephrine is followed by depletion, although the relative degree of each varies among patients.

With sympathetic stimulation, guanethidine and norepinephrine are both released from storage vesicles. It is believed that guanethidine does not act as a false neurotransmitter, because the sympatholytic effect does not depend on the degree of norepinephrine depletion. Rather, the mode of action is hypothesized to result from inhibition of neuronal transmission at the outer membranes of the postganglionic sympathetic axon.

Technique

The extremity is prepared for a Bier block. After inflating the tourniquet, the clinician should inject 20 mg guanethidine with lidocaine 0.5% for the upper extremities of 40 ml guanethidine for the lower extremities. Lidocaine is used to decrease the burning that is otherwise seen with the injection of guanethidine. Heparin, 500 to 1000 units, has been advocated by some to prevent stasis. One should keep the tourniquet inflated for 20 to 30 minutes to "fix" the guanethidine and prevent its release into the systemic circulation.

Reserpine is administered in a similar fashion to that for guanethidine, except 1 or 1.5 mg reserpine is substituted for upper and lower extremities, respectively.[47]

Drugs Used

The most widely studied drug for IV regional sympathetic block has been guanethidine. Unfortunately, guanethidine is not available in the Untied States. Bretylium has been advocated as an alternative to guanethidine.

Alpha$_2$-agonists have been demonstrated in the periphery and appear to have an important role in controlling blood flow to nutritive tissue at the precapillary shunt site.[48] Abnormal shunting of blood from nutritive tissue, as seen in reflex sympathetic dystrophy patients, may result via an α_2 mechanism.

Complications

Guanethidine should not be administered to patients taking monoamine oxidase inhibitors or those with a known or suspected pheochromocytoma.

Reported complications of IV regional sympathetic guanethidine include orthostatic hypotension, local piloerection, pain on injection, and edema of the extremity. With release of guanethidine into the systemic circulation, potential complications of bradycardia, diarrhea, edema, nausea, and bleeding can occur.

SUPERIOR HYPOGASTRIC PLEXUS BLOCK

Both pelvic pain associated with cancer[49,50] and chronic benign conditions[51,52] may be alleviated by blockade of the superior hypogastric plexus. Analgesia to the organs in the pelvis is possible because the afferent fibers innervating these structures travel in the sympathetic nerves, trunks, ganglia, and rami. Thus, a sympathectomy for visceral pain has the same effect as a peripheral neurectomy or dorsal rhizotomy for somatic pain.[53] Moreover, because visceral pain may be an important component of pelvic pain associated with cancer,[49,50,54] significant pain control may be achieved with percutaneous neurolytic blocks of the superior hypogastric plexus.

The superior hypogastric plexus is in the retroperitoneum, bilaterally extending from the lower third of the fifth lumbar vertebral body to the upper third of the first sacral vertebral body (Fig. 23C–14).

Techniques

Patients are placed in the prone position with a pillow under the pelvis to flatten the lumbar lordosis. The L4-5 intervertebral space is then found and marked. Antisepsis with

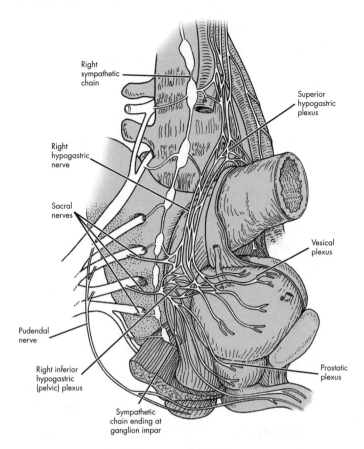

FIG. 23C–14 Oblique view of the pelvic in the male illustrating the location of the superior hypogastric plexus. *(Adapted from Bonica J: The management of pain. Philadelphia, Lea & Febiger, 1990.)*

an iodine solution and placement of sterile sheets in the lumbosacral area is performed. Sedation is provided with combinations of opioids and benzodiazepines. Skin wheals are raised 5 to 7 cm bilaterally to the midline at the level of the L4-5 interspace with 1% lidocaine.

Two 15-cm, 22-gauge Chiba needles are then inserted through the skin wheals with the bevel directed medially. Both needles are inserted 45 degrees mesiad and 30 degrees caudad so that the needle tips lie anterolateral to the L5-S1 intervertebral space (Fig. 23C–15). Although the transverse process of L5 is often encountered, slight change in the angle of insertion or use of insertion points 1 cm more lateral or medial to the original point of entry allows needle advancement. When the vertebral body of L5 is encountered, retrieval of the needle to superficial planes and reinsertion with slight concavity of the shaft help correct placement.

Careful aspiration to determine intravascular placement should always be done. Biplanar fluoroscopy and 2 to 3 ml of water-soluble contrast medium is used to verify accurate placement of the needles and to rule out intravascular injection. Accurate placement of the needles is determined by the collection of contrast medium just anterior to the L5-S1 intervertebral space. A diagnostic block with 8 ml of 0.25% bupivacaine injected through each needle may be performed. If the patient reports a 50% reduction in the pain intensity, a neurolytic block should be done.

For neurolysis, 8 ml of 10% phenol is used on each side. Although a suspension may be formed when the phenol is mixed with the sterile water, it is clinically effective if it is

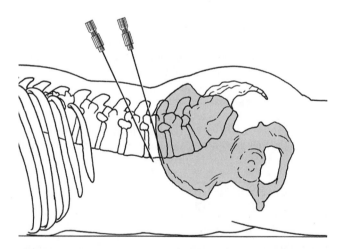

FIG. 23C–15 Cross-lateral view of a patient lying in the prone position, illustrating correct placement of needles for performance of a superior hypogastric plexus block. *(Adapted from Plancarte R, Velasquez R, Patt R: Neurolytic blocks of the sympathetic axis. In Patt R, editor: Cancer pain, Philadelphia, JB Lippincott, 1992.)*

prepared immediately after adequate needle placement has been confirmed via fluoroscopy.[49,50,54]

Following the block, patients are taken to the postanesthesia care unit (PACU), where vital signs are evaluated on arrival and again 30 to 60 minutes later. Patients are then discharged home and are re-evaluated by telephone 24 and 48 hours later.

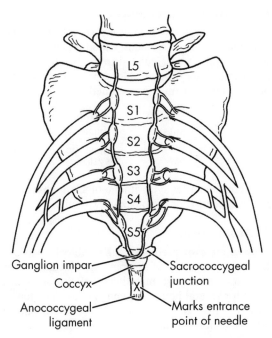

FIG. 23C–16 Simplified anatomy of the ganglion impar. *(Redrawn from Plancarte R, Velasquez R, Patt R: Neurolytic blocks of the sympathetic axis. In Patt R, editor:* Cancer pain, *Philadelphia, JB Lippincott, 1992.)*

Complications

The three studies[49,50,54] available for scrutiny have not reported complications associated with this procedure.

GANGLION IMPAR BLOCK

Anatomy

The ganglion impar is the most caudal ganglion of the sympathetic trunk. Thus, it marks the end of the two sympathetic chains (Fig. 23C–16). Commonly, it is a single ganglion produced by fusion of the ganglia from both sides. Because of this, it is usually located in the midline; however, it may also be lateral to the midline.

Indications

Visceral pain or sympathetically maintained pain in the perineal area associated with malignancies of the pelvic area may be effectively treated with neurolysis of the ganglion impar. Patients with a clinical picture of vague, burning, and localized perineal pain that is often associated with urgency may benefit from this block.

Technique

The patient is placed in the lateral decubitus position with hips flexed toward the abdomen. The right lateral decubitus is used if the operator is right-handed. Local anesthesia is injected at the level of anococcygeal ligament, which is situated midway between the anus and the tip of the coccyx (Fig. 23C–17). A 22-gauge spinal needle that has been previously bent according to the curvature of the coccyx is then introduced, while efforts are made to maintain the tip of the needle in the midline and outside the posterior rectal wall. Inserting the index finger in the rectum facilitates placement

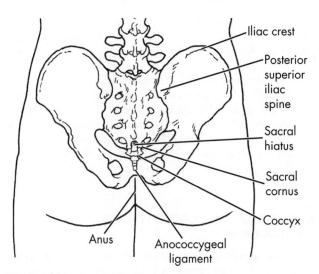

FIG. 23C–17 Surface anatomy of the lower back indicating the position of the anococcygeal ligament. *(Redrawn from Plancarte R, Velasquez R, Patt R: Neurolytic blocks of the sympathetic axis. In Patt R, editor:* Cancer pain, *Philadelphia, JB Lippincott, 1992.)*

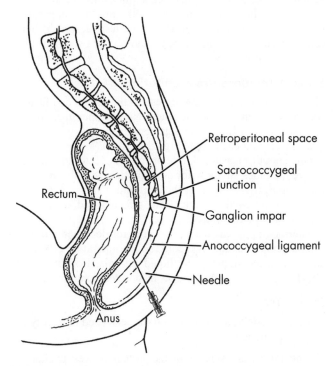

FIG. 23C–18 Later view of the sacrococcygeal area illustrating the ideal needle tip position for ganglion impar neurolysis. *(Redrawn from Plancarte R, Velasquez R, Patt R: Neurolytic blocks of the sympathetic axis. In Patt R, editor:* Cancer pain, *Philadelphia, JB Lippincott, 1992.)*

of the needle's tip at the level of the sacrococcygeal junction (Fig. 23C–18). Two ml of water-soluble contrast medium and biplanar fluoroscopy is used to verify adequate needle placement. Neurolysis is then performed with 4 to 6 ml of 6% to 10% phenol dissolved in sterile distilled water. For this purpose, we dissolve 1 g of phenol crystals in 10 to 15 ml of the solvent to obtain a 6% to 10% solution.

Two alternative approaches have been described for this block. In the trans-sacrococcygeal approach, a 22-gauge,

3.5-inch needle is placed directly in the retroperitoneal space, in the midline at the level of the sacrococcygeal junction.[55] An advantage of this approach is that the physician does not have to insert a finger in the rectum, which may be extremely painful in some patients, thus increasing the patient's tolerance. In the second alternative approach, the patient is placed in the lithotomy position. The resulting curvature of the coccyx is decreased, allowing access to the ganglion impar with a straight 22-gauge spinal needle and facilitating needle positioning. However, placement of the finger in the rectum and fluoroscopy guidance are still required.

EVALUATION OF COMPLETENESS OF BLOCKADE

Whenever possible, the clinician should monitor the effectiveness of a sympathetic block. Except for blocks involving visceral structures, one should evaluate all sympathetic blocks for completeness.

Many tests have been reported to monitor sympathetic activity. Unfortunately, many lack applicability for the practicing clinician secondary to their intricate apparatus involved, cost, and time for setup. The tests described here can be performed at the bedside, and one or two should be used to monitor all blocks.

Surface Temperature Monitoring

Skin temperature recording represents the easiest and fastest way to test sympathetic blockade. New temperature monitors have two or three channels combined with very sensitive sensors and easily read digital displays.

One should measure skin temperatures 15 to 20 minutes before the block to allow for equilibration with the ambient surroundings. Wrapping of the extremities subjects them to less environmental change. Both affected and unaffected sides should be monitored.

Thermography has been advocated for documentation of sympathetic blockade. It records skin temperature either by an infrared technique or by liquid crystals. Both methods effectively demonstrate changes in skin temperature.

Sweat Test

Three methods of sweat testing have been used clinically to test sympathetic blockade:

1. The ninhydrin test relies on the protein in sweat to change color to yellow.[56] A blocked extremity cannot sweat and shows no color change.
2. The cobalt blue test involves filter papers that are saturated with cobalt blue and then dried and stored in a desiccator. When needed, the papers are removed from the desiccator and placed on a clean, dry surface; the blocked and unblocked extremity is pressed onto the respective paper. The presence of sweat changes the paper from blue to pink. An extremity that has been sympathetically denervated shows no color.
3. The starch-iodine test also relies on color change. Its major drawback concerns the lengthy clean-up involved after the starch-iodine application.

Blood Flow Measurements

The most common blood flow measurements has been the Doppler indirect measurement. Blood pressures obtained by a Doppler probe are calculated in the brachial and dorsalis pedis arteries after standard blood pressure cuffs have been applied. An index is then determined:

$$\frac{ankle}{brachial} = \frac{systolic \quad \dfrac{systolic}{diastolic}}{diastolic \quad \dfrac{diastolic}{systolic}}$$

This is repeated after sympathetic block, with a decrease in pressure expected for the blocked extremity.

Pain Assessment

The assessment of preblock and postblock pain also provides some indication of sympathetic blockade. Pain relief can be reported almost immediately after a block or can be delayed for several hours in some patients. The long-lasting neurolytic effect of phenol is often delayed, but its local anesthetic action is usually more immediate.

References

1. Galen C: *Opus de usu partium corporis humani.* Paris, Apud Simonem Colinateum, 1528.
2. Estienne C: *De dissectione partium corporis humani libri tres.* Paris, Apud Simonem Colinateum, 1528.
3. Winslow JB: *Exposition anatomique de la structure du corps humain.* Paris, Guillaume Desperes et Jean Desessartz, 1732.
4. Whytt R: *An essay on the vital and other involuntary motions of animals.* Edinburgh, Hamilton, Balfour and Neill, 1751.
5. Whytt R: *Observations on the nature, causes and cure of those disorders which have commonly been called nervous, hypochondriac, or hysteric; to which are prefixed some remarks on the sympathy of the nerves.* Edinburgh, T Becket, 1765.
6. Langley JN, Dickinson WL: On the local paralysis of the peripheral ganglia and on the connection of different classes of nerve fibers with them. *Proc R Soc* 46:423, 1889.
7. Bonica JJ: *The management of pain.* Philadelphia, Lea & Febiger, 1953.
8. Bonica JJ: Autonomic innervation of the viscera in relation to nerve block. *Anesthesiology* 29:793, 1968.
9. White JC, Sweet W: *Pain: Its mechanisms and neurosurgical treatment.* Springfield, Ill, Charles C Thomas, 1955.
10. Bonica JJ: *Sympathetic nerve blocks for pain diagnosis and therapy.* New York, Breon Laboratories, 1984.
11. Brunn F, Mandl F: Die paravertebral injektion zur bekampfung visceraler schmerzen. *Wien Klin Aschsch* 37:511, 1924.
12. Kappis M: Weitere erfahrungen mit der sympathektomie. *Klin Wehr* 2:1441, 1923.
13. Von Gaza W: Die resektion der paravertebralen nerven und die isolirte durchsneidung des ramus communicans. *Arch F Klin Chir* 133:479, 1924.
14. Leriche R: *La chirurgie de la douleur.* Paris, Masson et Cie, 1949.
15. Appenzeller O: *The autonomic nervous system: An introduction to basic and clinical concepts.* New York, Elsevier Biomedical Press, 1982.
16. Harriman DGF, Sumner DW, Ellis FR: Malignant hyperpyrexia myopathy. *Q J Med* 42:639, 1973.
17. Monro PAG: *Sympathectomy.* London, Oxford University Press, 1959.
18. Randall WC, Cox JW, Alexander WF: Direct examination of the sympathetic outflows in man. *J Appl Physiol* 7:688, 1955.
19. Faden AI, Petras JM: An interspinal sympathetic preganglionic pathway: Anatomic evidence in the dog. *Brain Res* 144:358, 1978.
20. Kuntz A: *The autonomic nervous system.* Philadelphia, Lea & Febiger, 1953.

21. Kuntz A: Components of splanchnic and intermesenteric nerves. *J Comp Neurol* 105:251, 1956.
22. Becket RF, Grunt JA: The cervical sympathetic ganglia. *Anat Rec* 127:1, 1956.
23. Grant RT, Holling HE: Further observations on vascular responses of human limb to body warming: Evidence for sympathetic vasodilator nerves in human subjects. *Clin Sci* 3:273, 1952.
24. Jamieson RW, Smith DB, Anson BJ: The cervical sympathetic ganglia: An anatomical study of 100 cervicothoracic dissections. *Q Bull Northwest Univ Med School* 26:219, 1952.
25. Hoffman HH: An analysis of the sympathetic trunk and rami in the cervical and upper thoracic regions in man. *Ann Surg* 145:94, 1957.
26. Mitchell GAG: *Anatomy of the autonomic nervous system.* Edinburgh, E & S Livingstone, 1953.
27. Hogan QH, Erickson SJ, Haddox JD et al: The spread of solutions during stellate ganglion block. *Reg Anesth* 17:78, 1992.
28. Malmqvist ELA, Bengtsson M, Sorensen J: Efficacy of stellate ganglion block: A clinical study with bupivacaine. *Reg Anesth* 17:340, 1992.
29. Carron H, Litwiller R: Stellate ganglion block. *Anesth Analg* 54:567, 1975.
30. Moore DC: *Regional block,* ed 4. Springfield Ill, Charles C Thomas, 1975.
31. Bridenbaugh PO, Cousins MJ: *Neural blockade in clinical anesthesia and management of pain.* Philadelphia, JB Lippincott, 1988.
32. Czop CL: Sympathetic denervation to the upper extremity in CRPS: Stellate ganglion block vs interpleural block. *Anesthesiology* 87:A754, 1997.
33. Jackson SH, Jacobs JB, Epstein RA: A radiographic approach to celiac plexus block. *Anesthesiology* 31:373, 1969.
34. Jacobs JB, Jackson SH, Doppman JL: A radiographic approach to celiac ganglion block. *Radiology* 92:1372, 1969.
35. Moore DC, Bush WH, Burnett LL: Celiac plexus block: A roentgenographic, anatomic study of technique and spread of solution in patients and corpses. *Anesth Analg* 60:369, 1981.
36. Filshie J, Golding S, Robbie DS et al: Unilateral computerized tomography guided celiac plexus block: A technique for pain relief. *Anaesthesia* 38:498, 1983.
37. Hankemeier U: Neurolytic celiac plexus block for cancer-related upper abdominal pain using the unilateral puncture technique and lateral position. *Pain* 4:S135, 1987.
38. Gorbitz C, Leavens ME: Alcohol block of the celiac plexus for control of upper abdominal pain caused by cancer and pancreatitis. Technical note. *J Neurosurg* 34:575, 1971.
39. Racz G: *Techniques of neurolysis.* Boston, Kluwer Academic Publishers, 1989.
40. Reid W, Watt JK, Gray TG: Phenol injection of the sympathetic chain. *Br J Surg* 57:45, 1970.
41. Mandl F: *Die paravertebral injection.* Vienna, Springer Verlag, 1926.
42. Boas RA, Hatangdi VS, Richards EG: Lumbar sympathectomy: A percutaneous chemical technique. *Adv Pain Res Ther* 1:685, 1976.
43. Haynesworth RF, Noe CE: Percutaneous lumbar sympathectomy: A comparison of radiofrequency denervation versus phenol neurolysis. *Anesthesiology* 74:459, 1991.
44. Cousins MJ, Reeve TS, Glynn CJ et al: Neurolytic lumbar sympathetic blockade: Duration of denervation and relief of rest pain. *Anaesth Intensive Care* 7:121, 1979.
45. Dam WH: Therapeutic blockades. *Acta Chir Scand* 343(suppl):89, 1965.
46. Raskin NH, Levinson S, Hoffman PM et al: Postsympathectomy neuralgia: Amelioration with diphenylhydantoin and carbamazepine. *Am J Surg* 128:75, 1974.
47. Bengon HT, Chomka CM, Brenner EA: Treatment of reflex sympathetic dystrophy with regional intravenous reserpine. *Anesth Analg* 59:500, 1980.
48. Li Z, Koman LA, Smith BP et al: Alpha adrenoceptors in the rabbit ear thermoregulatory microcirculation. *Microvasc Surg* 55:115, 1998.
49. Plancarte R, Amescua C, Patt RB et al: Superior hypogastric plexus block for pelvic cancer pain. *Anesthesiology* 73:236, 1990.
50. De Leon-Casasola OA, Kent E, Lema MJ: Neurolytic superior hypogastric plexus block for chronic pelvic pain associated with cancer. *Pain* 54:145, 1993.
51. Freier A: Pelvic neurectomy in gynecology. *Obstet Gynecol* 25:48, 1965.
52. Lee RB, Stone K, Magelssen D et al: Presacral neurectomy for chronic pelvic pain. *Obstet Gynecol* 68:517, 1986.
53. Loeser JD, Sweet WH, Tew JM et al: Neurosurgical operations involving peripheral nerves. In Bonica JJ et al, editors: *The management of pain.* Philadelphia, Lea & Febiger, 1990.
54. Wang JK: Intrathecal morphine for intractable pain secondary to cancer of pelvic organs. *Pain* 21:99, 1985.
55. Wemm K, Saberski L: Modified approach to block the ganglion impar (ganglion of Walther)[letter]. *Reg Anesth* 20:544, 1995.
56. Dhuner KG, Edshage S, Wilhelm A: Ninhydrin test: Objective method for testing local anesthetic drugs. *Acta Anaesthesiol Scand* 4:189, 1960.

CHAPTER **23**

Interventional Techniques

P. PRITHVI RAJ

Infusion techniques with catheters located in the epidural and subarachnoid spaces and on the peripheral nerves are now commonly used for patients with acute and chronic pain. For patients with acute pain, continuous infusion has been beneficial for trauma, the postoperative period, and acute medical diseases. For patients with chronic pain, the technique has been useful for rehabilitation of low back pain, peripheral neuropathy, and cancer pain. If a sensory, motor, or sympathetic blockade is needed for a period considerably longer than that provided by long-acting local anesthetics, continuous regional anesthesia is indicated. The goal is to provide prolonged pain relief to a segregated portion of the body using the smallest doses of the drugs infused, thus minimizing the side effects. Infusion technique is also indicated for facilitation of early mobilization, increased distal limb vascularity, and improved nutrition. This section describes the technique, efficacy, and side effects of continuous infusion. Figure 23D–1 shows the closed circuit of this infusion technique, which decreases the incidence of infection.

EPIDURAL INFUSION

Continuous epidural infusion (CEI) offers therapeutic advantages over intermittent boluses. Its primary advantage is continuous analgesia compared with intermittent dosing. Although single boluses of opioids, such as epidural morphine, may provide 12 hours of pain relief, a wide variability has been reported in the duration of effective analgesia ranging from 4 to 24 hours.[1,2] Continuous infusions provide for easier titration, especially when shorter-acting opioids such as fentanyl and sufentanil are used. Epidurally administered fentanyl has an onset of action within 4 to 5 minutes and a peak effect within 20 minutes.[3–5] This rapid onset of relief facilitates adjustment in dosage because the patient quickly appreciates the subjective pain relief.

For the intermittent bolus technique to be successful, longer-acting agents such as morphine must be administered to provide a reasonable duration of analgesia. These opioids are associated with a higher risk of delayed-onset respiratory depression.[2]

Catheter Location

Segmental limitation of epidural analgesia mandates placing the epidural catheter at sites adjacent to dermatomes covering the field of pain. This reduces dose requirements while increasing the specificity of spinal analgesia.[6,7] Suggested interspaces where catheters may be located for epidural infusion of analgesic solutions are as follows:

- Thoracic surgery, T2 to T8
- Upper abdominal surgery, T4 to L1
- Lower abdominal surgery, T10 to L3
- Upper extremity surgery, C2 to C8
- Lower extremity surgery, T12 to L3

Figure 23D–2 shows the insertion of a thoracic epidural catheter and the spread of contrast solution in the thoracic epidural space.

Analgesic Agents

Continuous epidural analgesia is commonly provided with a local anesthetic, an opioid, or an opioid and local anesthetic combination.

Local Anesthetic

Local anesthetic agents are best used to provide analgesia and anesthesia for patients undergoing surgery and to maintain postoperative pain relief. Lidocaine and bupivacaine are both effective to achieve and maintain adequate analgesia.[5,8] In general, lidocaine use is limited to the bolus form to establish or rescue a block, whereas bupivacaine can be used as an infusion. Development of tachyphylaxis is a problem inherent with bolus administration of a local anesthetic through the epidural catheter.

Local anesthetic agents alone can accumulate in the systemic circulation.[5,9] This accumulation is more pronounced with the short-acting amides such as lidocaine. The decrease in systemic effects with longer-acting agents has been attributed to more nonspecific binding of the longer-acting agents in the fat of the epidural space compared with the shorter-acting amides.

A constant-rate infusion of 0.25% or more of bupivacaine has been associated with hypotension, muscle weakness,

Infusion technique

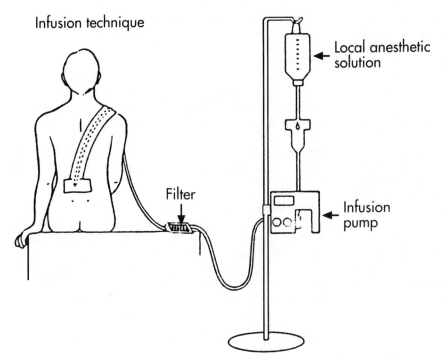

FIG. 23D–1 Closed circuit of continuous infusion technique. *(From Raj PP:* Pain medicine: a comprehensive review. *St. Louis, Mosby, 1995.)*

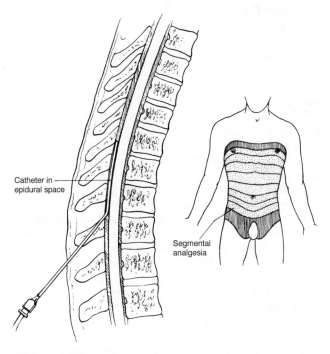

FIG. 23D–2 Insertion of thoracic epidural catheter and contrast solution spread in the thoracic epidural space. *(From Raj PP, Denson DD: Neurolytic agents. In Raj PP, editor:* Clinical practice of regional anesthesia. *New York, Churchill Livingstone, 1991.)*

sensory block, and possible accumulation of toxic levels of bupivacaine.[5] Higher plasma levels of the agent may occur in elderly and frail populations. Using lower concentrations can attenuate side effects. A low-dose, constant-rate infusion of epidurally administered bupivacaine (0.03% to 0.06%) close to the dermatomal level desired for pain relief can decrease the incidence of side effects. Although the low dose

of bupivacaine is effective, it provides a level of analgesia that is less profound than the combination of bupivacaine with low concentrations of epidurally administered morphine or the use of opioids alone.[5,10,11]

Opiate and Local Anesthetic Combinations

Extremely dilute concentrations of local anesthetics are capable of significantly decreasing high-frequency firing (somatic pain) of both afferent nerves and wide dynamic range (WDR) neurons, whereas opiate drugs work most efficiently on low-frequency WDR firing (visceral pain). The analgesia produced by this combination of epidural local anesthetics and opiates can be profound. In general, patients receiving epidural injections of local anesthetics plus narcotics have more rapid onset of analgesia, more profound and long-lasting pain relief, and less motor blockade than with a drug alone.

Bupivacaine, in concentrations of 0.035% to 0.125% (or ropivacaine in concentration of 0.02% to 0.1%), has been combined most often with morphine, fentanyl, or meperidine. Morphine and bupivacaine use has resulted in effective analgesia in the management of patients after thoracic, abdominal, and general surgery.[5,11–13] However, fentanyl combined with bupivacaine had a lower incidence of side effects than the morphine-bupivacaine combination.

Limitations of Continuous Epidural Analgesia

Epidural infusion analgesia cannot independently control pain occurring at multiple sites; normally it can provide analgesia for five to seven continuous dermatomal regions such as L4 to S5 or T2 to T8. Patients with multiple injuries may require other forms of pain control.

The site of the epidural catheter influences the adequacy of the pain relief and the maintenance of normal vital function. Placing the catheter within the dermatomal distribution of pain achieves the best results with the least amount of drug. For example, pain from a thoracotomy is best treated with a thoracic epidural infusion, and pain in the lower extremity calls for a lumbar epidural infusion.

Patient-Controlled Epidural Analgesia

Patient-controlled epidural analgesia (PCEA) is offered to patients recovering from intra-abdominal, major orthopedic, or thoracic surgery and for chronic pain states such as those resulting from cancer. The technique has several potential advantages. Patients can titrate analgesic doses in amounts proportional to the level of pain intensity. Because of large interindividual variations of pain relief,[14] this can optimize spinal opioid analgesia. Most of the published work describing PCEA comes from Europe.[14,15] Chrubasik and Wiemers[15] compared three different epidural opioids using the PCEA technique. These studies showed that the self-administered morphine dose required for effective analgesia was much smaller than the amount used with continuous epidural opioid and intravenous (IV) patient-controlled analgesia (PCA) techniques.[16–18]

Technique with Morphine[19]

Catheters are placed using the standard techniques. Patients are given a loading dose of 2 to 3 mg of preservative-free morphine, and a basal infusion of 0.4 mg/hr (0.02% solution) is started. Patients are allowed to self-administer 0.2 mg morphine every 10 to 15 minutes with a maximum dose of 1 to 2 mg/hour. The loading dose is only administered after a local anesthetic test dose (2 to 3 ml of lidocaine 2%) has demonstrated that the catheter is not in the subarachnoid space. The optimal size of the loading dose and the timing of administration have yet to be determined; however, because of morphine's latency to peak effect, the loading dose must be given as early as possible.

Breakthrough pain is common in these patients during the first 6 to 8 hours and is treated with epidural morphine boluses of 0.5 to 1 mg. If two doses are inadequate to provide analgesia, the catheter must be retested with local anesthetic to confirm epidural placement and to rule out dislodgment. The loading dose can be augmented with fentanyl 50 to 100 mg administered epidurally. This drug speeds the onset of the analgesia, possibly because of dural action and epidural intense neuroaxial action.

Alternative Choice of Analgesic Agents

Lipophilic Opioids

Fentanyl, sufentanil, and hydromorphone can be used with a PCEA infusion technique; however, the amount of drug needed to provide effective analgesia appears to be much greater than equivalent doses of morphine. Administration of lipophilic opioids by continuous infusions or PCEA has been questioned by several authors.[20,21] Estok and coworkers[21] showed that IV fentanyl administered by PCA or PCEA provided equivalent analgesia. Epidurally administered lipophilic opioids may have special use in the following circumstances:

- When the drug is administered via thoracic epidural catheters
- When there is a need to speed the onset of epidural opioid analgesia

- When the drug must be given in a large volume of dilute solution or combined with local anesthetic

Efficacy

Cohen and colleagues[22,23] compared combinations of fentanyl-bupivacaine and buprenorphine-bupivacaine for PCEA. The average hourly doses of opioid were minimized, presumably because of the effective analgesia provided by concurrently administered bupivacaine, so that 24-hour serum concentrations were low. Lipophilic agents may be useful for breakthrough pain, especially in the first few hours postoperatively.

Local Anesthetics

PCEA with local anesthetics has been reported to be safe and effective during labor. The technique was first described in 1988 by Gambling and coworkers,[24] who compared bupivacaine (0.125%) delivered as PCEA with continuous infusion. They found that PCEA was better than CEI of bupivacaine because patients in the PCEA group required significantly less bupivacaine to provide similar analgesia. The technique was believed to be safe, reliable, and not associated with excessive sensory blockade (Table 23D–1).

Efficacy of Continuous Epidural Analgesia for Labor Pain

Until recently, local anesthetics for continuous labor analgesia were usually injected intermittently into the epidural space by bolus injections. However, increased knowledge of the risks of this method, combined with the development of reliable and inexpensive infusion pumps, has produced widespread interest in the use of truly CEI techniques for the relief of labor pain. Several investigators have demonstrated that the continuous infusion of local anesthetic produces more reliable pain relief with similar or lower blood levels of local anesthetics than is achieved by giving intermittent boluses of these drugs.[29,30] Most importantly, the possibility of disastrous complications secondary to the administration of a large dose of local anesthetics is avoided.

If an epidural catheter enters an epidural vein during continuous infusion, the analgesia merely ceases, without producing central nervous system or cardiovascular toxicity.[31] If the catheter enters the subarachnoid space, the level of sensory and motor blockade slowly increases without the sudden onset of complete subarachnoid blockade, which may occur when using bolus techniques.[32] The infusion technique is safe and simple, but continuous monitoring of the patient for improper catheter placement or pump malfunction is essential. It is highly recommended that a different type or model of pump than that used for magnesium or oxytocin infusions be employed in the parturient to minimize the danger of adjusting the wrong pump.[33]

Local Anesthetic Agents

The choice of drug for continuous infusion remains controversial. Solutions of lidocaine, bupivacaine, and chloroprocaine have all been successfully used to produce labor analgesia.[34,35] Considerable controversy also exists regarding the concentration and volume required as a loading dose before the inception of the continuous infusion. Recent studies suggest that the common practice of initiating epi-

TABLE 23D–1 Patient-Controlled Epidural Analgesia Techniques

Author	Analgesic Drug	Additional Drug	Continuous Infusion (ml/hr)	Patient-Controlled Analgesia Dose	Lockout (min)	Comment
Gambling et al, 1988[25]	Bupivacaine	1:400,000	—	4	20	Greater satisfaction (1990) of 0.125% epinephrine with PCEA than continuous infusion
Gambling et al, 1988[24]	Bupivacaine 0.125%	—	4	4	20	PCEA group used less local than CI group
Lysak et al, 1990[26]	Bupivacaine 0.125%	Fentanyl 1 mg/ml	6	4	10	Fewer top-ups needed compared with CI group
Viscomi and Eisenach, 1989[27]	Bupivacaine 0.125%	Fentanyl 1 mg/ml	4	4	10	Fewer top-ups needed compared with CI
Naulty et al, 1990[28]	Bupivacaine	Sufentanil	5	2	6	No advantage over CI

CI, continuous infusion; PCEA, patient-controlled epidural analgesia.

dural local anesthetic blockade with a dose of 10 to 12 ml of concentrated local anesthetic (e.g., 0.5% bupivacaine) may be no more effective in producing analgesia than a slightly larger volume (e.g., 15 to 20 ml) of a lower concentration of local anesthetic (e.g., 0.125% bupivacaine), except that the higher concentration in some cases provides a slightly faster onset.[36] Furthermore, the volume of local anesthetic required for continuous infusion also may be less than that currently recommended.

Epidural Local Anesthetic-Opiate Combinations

A few studies have attempted to quantify the advantages and disadvantages of the use of these narcotic and local anesthetic combinations in labor. The major advantage appears to be a reduction in motor blockade, inasmuch as very low doses of local anesthetics are required. However, these studies contain too few patients to draw meaningful conclusions regarding the effects of decreased motor blockade on outcome.

Disadvantages of this technique consist of potential adverse maternal and fetal effects from epidural narcotics. These are essentially the risks from narcotics in general; the most serious is maternal and fetal respiratory depression. Large numbers of mothers and neonates exposed to epidural narcotics must be further evaluated to determine whether advantages of this technique outweigh risks. It must be understood, however, that parturients in the United States routinely receive much larger parenteral doses of these same narcotics in labor without excessive concern on the part of obstetricians and neonatologists. The benefits of combining epidural local anesthetics, particularly bupivacaine, and opiates appear to outweigh the potential risks.

It appears that complete analgesia for labor using epidural and subarachnoid opiates alone, with a minimum of side effects, remains an unfulfilled goal. However, the combination of extremely small doses of local anesthetics and opiate drugs seems to provide excellent analgesia with minimal side effects.

This concept of combined opiates and local anesthetics corresponds to that of modern "balanced" general anesthesia, in which small amounts of several drugs are used to provide excellent anesthesia with a minimum of the side effects seen with large doses of any single drug. Balanced regional anesthesia holds great promise for the future, especially with the discovery of new drugs that produce spinal analgesia through a variety of mechanisms. These drugs include catecholamines, clonidine, γ-aminobutyric acid (GABA) agonists, substance P antagonists, prostaglandin synthetase inhibitors, and many other drugs capable of altering neural transmission in such a way that analgesia results. Obviously, labor analgesia is one area in which these combinations will be explored extensively.

CONTINUOUS SUBARACHNOID INFUSION

Acute Pain

Continuous spinal anesthesia may be an option in patients in whom regional anesthesia is desirable and in whom epidural anesthesia proves to be inadequate. In patients with severe kyphoscoliosis or otherwise altered spinal anatomy in whom continuous spinal anesthesia with hyperbaric local anesthetics has resulted in an inadequate or patchy block, the addition of isobaric local anesthetic may provide adequate anesthesia.[37]

Chronic and Cancer Pain

Intraspinal infusion of narcotics has commonly been used for the management of intractable cancer pain.[38,39] These infusions have been maintained with implanted pumps connected to intrathecal catheters. Figure 23D–3 shows one of the types of programmable intrathecal infusion pumps in common use today. The treatment of patients with severe, chronic noncancer pain in the lower body has been a difficult problem. Included among the possible causes of this pain are arachnoiditis, epidural scarring, vertebral body compression fracture, reflex sympathetic dystrophy, phantom limb pain, and post-thoracotomy pain. Intraspinal infusions are increasingly used with minimal complications and limited instances of drug tolerance in these noncancer patients.[40–44] For these infusions, programmable infusion pumps have infusion rates that can be changed and tailored to the patient's needs at any time with an external programmer. These pumps have been extensively tested and found to be reliable and cost effective.[44]

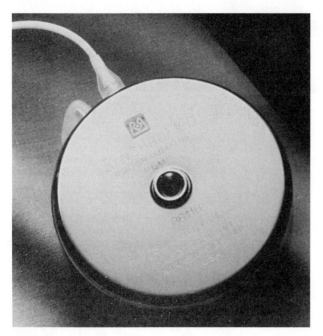

FIG. 23D–3 One type of programmable intrathecal infusion pump commonly used today.

Analgesic Agents

Morphine has been the usual agent for these infusions. In resistant cases for temporary or prolonged intraspinal infusions, the addition of dilute bupivacaine to the morphine infusion has resulted in improved pain relief.[45,46]

Efficacy

The Nitescu study[46] notes that spinal morphine dose requirements increase over time. All patients need to be started at the lowest dose possible to avoid early toxicity, overdosing, or overtreating. Most patients need greater doses over time to maintain adequate pain relief. Each patient reaches pain relief at a different level, as evidenced by the effective therapeutic range of morphine extending from 6.275 to 57 mg per 24 hours among the patients in this study group.[46] Most patients respond fairly well with a continuous infusion at the onset of therapy. When they become active as their pain decreases, they become aware that the pain is more intense at certain times of the day. As a result, individual dose patterns must be established. Such individualization can be efficient only with an externally programmable infusion system.

The medication is well tolerated in most cases and is without significant side effects, but increasingly larger doses may be necessary over time. The medications may allow a return to a more normal lifestyle, including improved ability to perform activities of daily living and resumption of vocational activities in many cases. The best results are found among well-motivated patients with realistic goals and a clear understanding of spinal morphine therapy who have demonstrated appropriate responses during a screening trial. Meticulous attention to detail in the care and maintenance of the system and a willingness of the clinician to devote ample time to the patient should maximize the effectiveness of this modality.

CONTINUOUS (PERIPHERAL NERVOUS SYSTEM) INFUSION

Peripheral continuous techniques are usually carried out exactly like a single injection technique. Various catheter-needle systems are available for use in providing continuous blockade. Early on, catheters were inserted through needles. Although the catheter was protected during insertion, the hole made by the needle in the sheath was often larger than the catheter, resulting in leakage of local anesthetic after the removal of the needle. The use of thin-bore needles with catheters over the needle has improved the success of continuous techniques. When the sheath has been penetrated, identified by either paresthesia or the use of a nerve stimulator, the catheter is advanced slightly as the needle is withdrawn. Sometimes it is best to first inject a test dose of local anesthetic through the needle to expand the perivascular space. If the catheter is to be used for several days or if movement is a problem, a second smaller catheter, similar to a nylon epidural catheter, can be advanced through the first catheter further into the perivascular compartment.

Continuous Brachial Plexus Infusion

Indications

For 10 decades, prolonged brachial plexus blocks have been performed perioperatively for trauma and postoperative pain; prolonged sympathetic blocks have also been performed for vascularly comprised patients. Catheters have been placed on the brachial plexus after surgery, providing postoperative pain relief for up to 48 hours. With the experience obtained in acute perioperative patients, prolonged brachial plexus analgesia has now been tried for difficult intractable patients such as those with Complex Regional Pain Syndrome (CRPS) I and II and phantom pain.

Site

The brachial plexus is an ideal location for a continuous regional technique because of its well-defined perivascular compartment and the close approximation of the large number of nerves supplying the upper extremity. All techniques of brachial plexus blockade have been described as continuous techniques, but some are easier to achieve than others are.

An *axillary approach* is easy to perform, and the technique is familiar to many. Unfortunately, movement of the upper extremity, either passive or active, can dislodge the catheter. Hair and moisture in the axilla also can make maintaining a sterile environment difficult at best.

The *interscalene technique* can be difficult to place because the approach is 90 degrees to the skin, making it difficult to thread the catheter.

A *subclavian perivascular approach* allows threading of the catheter, and the catheter position is not affected by head or neck movements.

The *infraclavicular approach* to the brachial plexus allows easy threading of the catheter and is not affected by patient movement.[47]

All four approaches to the brachial plexus have been used to insert a catheter for continuous infusion. The technique most often performed is at the axillary site, possibly because of the anesthesiologist's familiarity with inserting an intra-arterial catheter. This was the impetus to attempt this technique initially. It has remained popular ever since. The interscalene approach has been used by some clinicians. Technically, it is simple to do; however, the catheters do not stay at the site for more than 48 hours. The infraclavicular approach has been preferred by another group of clinicians who perform this block routinely. It has the advantage of maintaining the catheter in the same position for long durations, sometimes as long as 3 weeks.

Drugs and Technique

Although lidocaine and mepivacaine have been used for continuous infusion, the most commonly chosen local anesthetic is bupivacaine. In a typical case, after the catheter is placed on the brachial plexus, a bolus of 20 to 30 ml of 0.5% bupivacaine or a 1:1 mixture of 2% lidocaine and 0.5% bupivacaine is administered. Monitoring is mandatory for at least 45 minutes, during which time the onset of block is tested. If adequate block is present, then up to 10 ml/hr of either 0.25% or 0.125% bupivacaine is administered via an infusion pump. Steady state is reached in five half-lives (~18 hours). The infusion should be started within 2 hours, before the bolus effect wears off. Before 18 hours is reached, however, the bolus block is expected to wear off (usually after 6 hours). The infusion of 0.25% bupivacaine is not effective to maintain analgesia for another 12 hours. If there is intolerable pain at 6 hours, it is imperative to provide another bolus of 20 ml of 0.5% bupivacaine. Monitoring is required for 45 minutes, as with the initial bolus.

Efficacy

For periods up to 48 hours, continuous brachial plexus analgesia is reliably efficacious. After this period, the efficacy drops precipitously for A-delta fiber blocking. Sympathetic blocking can still be maintained reliably for as long as 2 to 3 weeks with 0.125% or 0.25% bupivacaine if catheters are well anchored.

The best site for catheter insertion seems to be the infraclavicular region. The second best site is at the axilla. The interscalene site is too superficial for reliable anchoring over prolonged periods.

Continuous Lower Extremity Peripheral Nerve Infusion

Lumbosacral Plexus Catheterization

Placement of a lumbosacral catheter with an epidural needle has been reported by Vaghadia and coauthors.[48] Successful blockade of the lumbar and sacral plexuses was achieved for unilateral lower extremity surgery. The catheter is placed between the quadratus lumborum and psoas muscles between the transverse processes of L4 and L5. The technique is not difficult and seems highly successful. The main disadvantage is the volume of local anesthetic needed, which is 40 to 70 ml.

Sciatic Nerve Catheterization

Many of the nerves innervating the lower extremity can be blocked. Blockade of the sciatic nerve has been described by Smith and others.[49] Continuous regional anesthesia can be obtained anywhere along the course of the nerve. A 16-gauge IV infusion needle and catheter or a Tuohy needle with an epidural catheter can be used. The catheter is usually advanced 4 to 6 cm into the perivascular space. The lateral approach described by Guardini and colleagues[50] can be very useful for obtaining a continuous block. The catheter is placed along the nerve just posterior to the quadratus femoris muscle in the subgluteal space.

Femoral Nerve Catheterization

Continuous techniques for the femoral nerve have been used for various surgeries. In 1992, Edwards and Wright[51] reported significantly lower postoperative pain scores and reduced opioid requirements in patients undergoing total knee replacement with continuous infusion of 0.125% bupivacaine at 6 ml/hr within the femoral sheath compared with analgesia from conventional intramuscular injections of opioids.

The drugs administered for lower extremity infusions follow the same principles as for brachial plexus infusions. The concentration of drug infusion depends on the need to block A-alpha, A-delta, or C-fibers, and the rate of infusion is usually 10 to 15 ml/hr. Complications include peripheral neuropathy, motor weakness, dysesthesias, and decubitus ulcers secondary to sensory loss.

Efficacy

Technically, lower extremity infusion is difficult and unreliable. At best, this technique is an alternative to lumbar epidural infusion when it cannot be performed. Postoperative knee pain and CRPS I and II may be best indications for these procedures.

CONTINUOUS SYMPATHETIC INFUSION

Some clinicians are routinely performing continuous sympathetic infusion,[52] such as continuous stellate ganglion and continuous lumbar sympathetic infusions. The stellate ganglion infusion is often unreliable because of catheter dislodgment. The continuous celiac and lumbar sympathetic infusions are successful even in outpatients with no significant problems. These techniques are most useful for treatment of visceral pain secondary to cancer and CRPS I and sympathetically maintained pain.[53]

Drugs

The drugs administered for sympathetic infusions follow the same principles as those for brachial plexus infusion. The drug choice has been bupivacaine (0.125% to 0.25%), usually without a narcotic. Morphine, fentanyl, and sufentanil have been mixed with the local anesthetic to prolong the analgesia. A solution of 6 ml to 20 ml is continuously infused.

Efficacy

Stellate ganglion infusion is unreliable because of catheter dislodgment. Lumbar sympathetic infusion is reliable even though the lumbar plexus is eventually blocked by the diffusion of the local anesthetic solution into the psoas muscle. Hypotension and nausea are rare complications of bilateral celiac plexus infusion. Not enough data are available to state that continuous sympathetic infusion is a safe, reliable, and efficacious technique at present.

SUMMARY

Continuous regional infusion by a local anesthetic or an opiate or a combination of both is now commonly performed in clinical practice. Infusions are performed centrally as well as peripherally. These techniques are indicated when prolonged analgesia is required for moderate to severe acute, chronic, and cancer pain. If done with due care and appropriate monitoring, the techniques are safe, reliable, and unique. Further research is required to compare them with other analgesic techniques.

References

1. Akerman B, Arwestrom E, Post C: Local anesthetics potentiate spinal morphine antinociception. *Anesth Analg* 67:943, 1988.
2. Bromage PR, Camporesi E, Chestnut D: Epidural narcotics for postoperative analgesia. *Anesth Analg* 59:473, 1950.
3. Cousins MJ, Mather LE: Intrathecal and epidural administration of opioids. *Anesthesiology* 61:276, 1984.
4. Rutter DV, Skewes DG, Morgan M: Extradural opioids for postoperative analgesia: A double-blind comparison of pethidine, fentanyl and morphine. *Br J Anaesth* 53:915, 1981.
5. Scott NB, Mogensen T, Bigler D et al: Continuous thoracic extradural 0.5% bupivacaine with or without morphine: Effect on quality of blockade, lung function and the surgical stress response. *Br J Anaesth* 62:253, 1989.
6. Lubenow TR, Durrani Z, Ivankovich AD: Evaluation of continuous epidural fentanyl/butorphanol infusion for postoperative pain. *Anesthesiology* 69:381, 1958.
7. Rosseel PM, van den Broek WG, Boer EC et al: Epidural sufentanil for intra- and postoperative analgesia in thoracic surgery: A comparative study with intravenous sufentanil. *Acta Anaesthesiol Scand* 32:193, 1988.
8. Raj PP, Denson D, Finnason P: Prolonged epidural analgesia: Intermittent or continuous? In Meyer J, Nolte H, editors: *Die kontinuerlick peridural anesthesia.* Seventh international symposium uber die regional anesthesia, January 7, 1982, Miden, Germany. Stuttgart, Germany, George Themaverlag, 1983.
9. Tucker GT, Cooper S, Littlewood D et al: Observed and predicted accumulation of local anesthetic agents during continuous extradural analgesia. *Br J Anaesth* 49:237, 1977.
10. Gregory MA, Brock-Utne JG, Bux S et al: Morphine concentration in brain and spinal cord after subarachnoid morphine injection in baboons. *Anesth Analg* 64:929, 1985.
11. Rawal N, Sjöstrand U, Dahlström B: Postoperative pain relief by epidural morphine: A comparative study with intramuscular narcotic and intercostal nerve block. *Anesth Analg* 60:726, 1981.
12. Magora F, Olshwang D, Eimerl D et al: Observations on extradural morphine analgesia in various pain conditions. *Br J Anaesth* 52:247, 1980.
13. Rutberg H, Hakanson E, Anderberg B et al: Effects of extradural administration of morphine, or bupivacaine, on the endocrine response to upper abdominal surgery. *Br J Anaesth* 56:233, 1984.
14. Sjöstrom S, Hartvig D, Tamsen A: Patient-controlled analgesia with extradural morphine or pethidine. *Br J Anaesth* 60:358, 1988.
15. Chrubasik J, Wiemers K: Continuous-plus-on demand epidural infusion of morphine for postoperative pain relief by means of a small, externally worn infusion device. *Anesthesiology* 62:263, 1985.
16. Downing JE, Stedman PM, Busch EH: Continuous low volume infusion of epidural morphine for postoperative pain. *Reg Anesth* 13(suppl):84, 1988.
17. Planner RS, Cowie RW, Babarczy AS et al: Continuous epidural morphine analgesia after radical operations upon the pelvis. *Surg Gynecol Obstet* 166:229, 1988.
18. Rauck R, Raj PP, Knarr DC et al: Comparison of the efficacy of epidural morphine given by intermittent injection of continuous infusion for the management of postoperative pain. *Reg Anesth* 19:316, 1994.
19. Marlowe S, Engstrom R, White PF: Epidural patient-controlled analgesia (PCA): An alternative to continuous epidural infusions. *Pain* 37:97, 1989.
20. Loper KA, Ready LB, Sandler AN: Epidural and intravenous fentanyl infusions are clinically equivalent after knee surgery. *Anesthesiology* 71:A1149, 1989.
21. Estok PM: Use of PCA to compare IV to epidural administration of fentanyl in the postoperative patient. *Anesthesiology* 67:A230, 1989.
22. Cohen S, Amar D, Pantuck CB: Continuous epidural-PCA postcesarean section: buprenorphine-bupivacaine 0.03% vs. fentanyl-bupivacaine 0.03%. *Anesthesiology* 73:A975, 1990.
23. Cohen S, Amar D, Pantuck CB: Continuous epidural-PCA caesarean section: Buprenorphine-bupivacaine 0.015 with epinephrine vs. fentanyl-bupivacaine 0.015 with and without epinephrine. *Anesthesiology* 73:A91A, 1990.
24. Gambling DR, Yu P, Cole C et al: A comparative study of patient controlled epidural analgesia (PCES) and continuous infusion epidural analgesia (CIEA) during labour. *Can J Anaesth* 35:249, 1988.
25. Gambling DR, McMorland GH, Yu P et al: Comparison of patient controlled epidural analgesia and conventional intermittent "top-up" injections during labor. *Anesth Analg* 70:256, 1990.
26. Lysak SZ, Eisenach JC, Dobson CE 2nd: Patient-controlled epidural analgesia during labor: A comparison of three solutions with a continuous infusion control. *Anesthesiology* 72:44, 1990.
27. Viscomi C, Eisenach JC: Patient-controlled epidural analgesia during labor. *Obstet Gynecol* 77:348, 1991.
28. Naulty JS: Epidural PCA vs. continuous infusion of sufentanil-bupivacaine for analgesia during labor and delivery. *Anesthesiology* 73:A963, 1990.
29. Rosenblatt R: Continuous epidural infusions for obstetric analgesia. *Reg Anesth* 8:10, 1983.
30. Hicks JA, Jenkins JG, Newton MC et al: Continuous epidural infusion of 0.075% bupivacaine for pain relief in labour: A comparison with intermittent top-ups of 0.5% bupivacaine. *Anesthesia* 43:289, 1988.
31. Dathis F: Epidural analgesia with a bupivacaine-fentanyl mixture in obstetrics: comparison of repeated injections and continuous infusion. *Can J Anaesth* 35:116, 1988.
32. Li DF, Rees GA, Rosen M: Continuous extradural infusion of 0.0625% or 0.125% bupivacaine for pain relief in primigravid labour. *Br J Anaesth* 57:264, 1985.
33. Sapsford DJ, Howard C: Epidural infusions—Shortage of infusion device [letter]. *Anaesthesia* 43:332, 1988.
34. Abboud TK, Afrasiabi A, Sarkis F et al: Continuous infusion epidural analgesia in parturients receiving bupivacaine, chloroprocaine, or lidocaine—Maternal, fetal, and neonatal effects. *Anesth Analg* 63:421, 1984.
35. Chestnut DH, Bates JN, Choi WW: Continuous infusion epidural analgesia with lidocaine: Efficacy and influence during the second stage of labor. *Obstet Gynecol* 69:323, 1987.
36. MacLeaod DM: The loading dose for continuous infusion epidural analgesia: A technique to reduce the incidence of hypotension. *Anaesthesia* 42:377, 1987.
37. Moran DH, Johnson MD: Continuous spinal anesthesia with combined hypobaric and isobaric bupivacaine in a patient with scoliosis. *Anesth Analg* 70:445, 1990.
38. Penn RD, Paice JA, Gottschalk W et al: Cancer pain relief using chronic morphine infusion: Early experience with a programmable implanted drug pump. *J Neurosurg* 61:302, 1984.
39. Coombs DW, Saunders RL, Lachance D et al: Intrathecal morphine tolerance: Use of intrathecal clonidine, DADLE, and intraventricular morphine. *Anesthesiology* 62:358, 1985.
40. Auld AW, Maki-Jokela A, Murdoch DM: Intraspinal narcotic analgesia in the treatment of chronic pain. *Spine* 10:777, 1985.
41. Carl P, Crawford ME, Ravlo O et al: Longterm treatment with epidural opioids: A retrospective study comprising 150 patients treated with morphine chloride and buprenorphine. *Anaesthesia* 41:32, 1986.
42. Glynn C, Dawson D, Sanders R: A double-blind comparison between epidural morphine and epidural clonidine in patients with chronic non-cancer pain. *Pain* 34:123, 1988.
43. Murphy TM, Hinds S, Cherry D: Intraspinal narcotics: Nonmalignant pain. *Acta Anaesthesiol Scand Suppl* 85:75, 1987.
44. Penn RD, Paice JA: Chronic intrathecal morphine for intractable pain. *J Neurosurg* 67:182, 1987.

45. Coombs DW, Pageau MG, Saunders RL et al: Intraspinal narcotic tolerance: Preliminary experience with continuous bupivacaine HCL infusion via implanted infusion device. *Int J Artif Organs* 5:379, 1982.

46. Nitescu P, Appelgren L, Linder LE et al: Epidural versus intrathecal morphine-bupivacaine: Assessment of consecutive treatments in advanced cancer pain. *J Pain Symptom Manage* 5:18, 1990.

47. Kanoff RB: Intraspinal delivery of opiates by an implantable, programmable pump in patients with chronic intractable pain of nonmalignant origin. *J Am Osteopath Assoc* 94:487, 1994.

48. Vaghadia H, Kapnoudhis P, Jenkins LC et al: Continuous lumbosacral block using a Tuohy needle and catheter technique. *Can J Anaesth* 39:75, 1992.

49. Smith BE, Fischer HB, Scott PV: Continuous sciatic nerve block. *Anesthesia* 39:155, 1984.

50. Gaurdini R, Waldron BA, Wallace WA: Sciatic nerve block: A new lateral approach. *Acta Anaesthesiol Scand* 29:515, 1985.

51. Edwards ND, Wright EM: Continuous low-dose 3-in-1 nerve blockade for postoperative pain relief after total knee replacement. *Anesth Analg* 75:265, 1992.

52. Rauck R: Sympathetic nerve blocks: Head & neck and trunk. In Raj PP, editor: *Practical management of pain,* ed 2. St. Louis, Mosby, 1992.

53. Racz GB et al: Sympathetic nerve block: Pelvic. In Raj PP, editor: *Practical management of pain,* ed 2. St. Louis, Mosby, 1992.

CHAPTER **23**

Interventional Techniques

HEMMO A. BOSSCHER

Chronic back pain, radiculopathy, and its associated disabilities represent a significant health problem. Back pain is considered a major cause of absence from work and long-term disability. Most patients suffering acute back pain recover spontaneously in several weeks.[1] However, a significant fraction of these have recurrence of symptoms within a year.[2] Many patients who have a relapse or whose back pain does not subside in time are eventually referred to a pain clinic if surgery is not indicated. By this time the patient may have undergone a variety of treatments with limited success. It is likely that at some point during therapeutic intervention, the patient will receive spinal steroid injections. Injections of substances into the epidural or subarachnoid space to treat back pain has been practiced for almost 100 years, and injection of epidural steroids is currently the foundation of many pain practices. Controversies over efficacy and safety have led to the decline of its use in some countries.[3,4]

BACK PAIN AND RADICULOPATHY

Anatomy

Pain is the most important and often the only symptom of most spinal disorders. In an early stage of the disease process, pain develops because of stimulation of pain sensitive structures. These structures include bones, joints, disks, nerves, muscles, and soft tissues. They may be affected by an inflammatory, infectious, neoplastic, or traumatic disease or a congenital or developmental mechanical defect. One might distinguish between a ventral and dorsal compartment, which are divided by a virtual frontal plane through the dorsal wall of the intervertebral foramen.[5,6] The dorsal compartment contains facet joints, the dorsal part of the dura, and intrinsic back muscles and ligaments. The ventral compartment consists of the vertebral bodies, disks, anterior and posterior ligaments, ventral dura, nerve roots, and prevertebral muscles. The innervation of these structures is complex[7] (Fig. 23E–1).

The ventral compartment is supplied by interconnected neural networks; one is in the anterior ligament (via the sympathetic chain), and one is in the posterior longitudinal ligament (via the sinuvertebral nerve). Both plexuses are connected via the rami communicantes from which the sinuvertebral arises. The dorsal compartment is supplied by the dorsal rami, of which the medial branch innervates the facet joints. The lateral branch innervates the paraspinal musculature and the adjacent skin. There are neural connections between the two compartments as well. These interconnections, multisegmental innervation, and involvement of the autonomic nervous system explain the lack of specificity of pain in relation to the underlying pathologic condition. Furthermore, the underlying pathologic condition is rarely limited to one anatomic structure. Thus, injection of corticosteroid in the epidural space for treatment of back pain yields results that often depend on unknown pathologic conditions and that are highly unpredictable. It is likely that epidural steroids are not highly valuable in the treatment of disorders of the dorsal compartment. Pain-sensitive structures in the ventral compartment include the posterior longitudinal ligament, the disk, the nerve root, and the dorsal root ganglion. It is generally thought that back pain that originates from pathologic conditions of the longitudinal

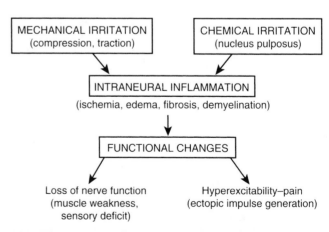

FIG. 23E–1 Mechanical or chemical stimulation initiates a sequence of events responsible for the generation of back pain and radiculopathy. *(Redrawn from Racz GB, Heavner JE, Raj PP: Epidural neuroplasty. Semin Anesth 16:302, 1997.)*

ligament and disk is referred and is nociceptive pain. Under normal conditions, stimulation of these structures does not cause pain. However, in the context of nerve injury, such as that mediated by inflammation or ischemia, these fibers may become easily excitable or even show spontaneous activity.[8,9] In contrast, pain radiating into an extremity that originates from a pathologic condition of the nerve root is thought to be neuropathic. Because the nerve root and dorsal root ganglia are innervated by sympathetic nerve fibers, neuropathic pain associated with an irritated nerve root may have a sympathetically mediated component, which may be associated with mechanical allodynia and hyperalgesia.[10] These processes may explain back pain that results from movements of the spine with flexion and extension[11] or radicular pain that results from minor stretch of the nerve root, such as with the straight leg raise test.[12] The pathologic process that causes nerve injury is the target of steroids placed in the epidural space. Thus, the effectiveness of epidurally injected steroids may differ entirely for back pain and radiculopathy and depends strongly on the underlying disease process.

Pathology

Mixter and Barr[13] initially introduced the idea that disk degeneration, disk rupture with herniation, and subsequent nerve impingement causes the syndrome of sciatica. Back pain was explained by posterior (central) disk herniation or protrusion, with activation of nociceptors in the annulus fibrosis, posterior longitudinal, and dorsal root ganglia.[14-17] However, some patients with large herniations have no radicular symptoms,[18] and in contrast, some patients with no evidence of disk herniation have severe radiculopathy. Mechanical irritation of a normal nerve root results in a neurologic deficit but not in pain. When the nerve root is swollen and hyperemic, mechanical stimulation results in pain in the distribution of the nerve root.

The process of disk degeneration has been associated with alterations of the chemical and cellular balance of the disk. Incision of the annulus has been shown to lead to disk degeneration. In a reparative response, vascular proliferation with production of several angiogenic factors may lead to the activation of latent enzymes that cause the breakdown of proteoglycans and collagens.[19] Independent of its cause, release of enzymes and products of enzymatic action may lead to a response similar to the inflammatory response seen in osteoarthritis, which in turn may lead to chemical nerve injury.[20,21] Indeed, histopathologic findings of inflammation of the nerve root may be demonstrated in samples obtained during surgery on the spine.[22]

McCarron and colleagues[23] used homogenized autologous nucleus pulposi material and injected it into the lumbar space of four dogs. The result of this study demonstrated well-developed fibrosis of the dura and the epidural fat and inflammatory changes of the spinal cord, dura, and nerve roots. The relative seclusion of the avascular nucleus pulposi to the immune system might explain how extrusion of disk components might induce an autoimmune response that results in inflammation.

Both a humoral and a cellular immune response have been suggested as well.[18,21] However, several substances found in the degenerated disk may cause responses associated with inflammation in the absence of an immune response or significant cellular infiltration. Substances such as lactic acid, hydrogen ions, histamine, nitric oxide, prostaglandins, and interleukins may be released by direct activation of certain biochemical pathways.[18] Phospholipase A_2 (PLA_2) activity was measured in disk material obtained from patients with a radiculopathy, caused by a herniated or protruded disk, who underwent laminectomy and discectomy. PLA_2 activity was found to be 20 to 10,000 times higher in the diseased disk than in normal tissue.[24] Phospholipase is responsible for the breakdown of phospholipids in the cell membrane, with the production of prostaglandins and leukotrienes.[25,26]

Release of these substances and other biochemical mediators in the process of inflammation or by leakage from an injured disk may induce a peripheral sensitization by decreasing the nociceptive threshold and the recruitment of new nociceptors resulting in back pain and radiculopathy.[8,9]

Although the theory of inflammation in the pathogenesis of back pain and radiculopathy may be attractive, not all investigations support the concept.[18] Gronblad and colleagues[27] compared the PLA_2 content in prolapsed degenerative disks to normal disks obtained from organ donors. These investigators were unable to demonstrate a lower activity in normal disks. Furthermore, using immunohistologic techniques, several investigators were unable to show an inflammatory response of the periradicular tissues.[24,28,29]

The periradicular tissues associated with a herniated disk in cadavers demonstrated congestion, venous thrombosis, and severe perineural fibrosis but no inflammatory cells. The role of inflammation may be important in early stages of disk herniation. First, it would explain the gradual, spontaneous resolution of symptoms seen in many patients with acute back injury and the more favorable response to epidural steroids in patients with (sub)acute back pain and radiculopathy. Second, this inflammatory process may result in permanent changes that can lead to a chronic pain syndrome.

Vascular Abnormalities, Fibrosis, and Mechanical Tension

Disk degeneration and protrusion in the context of an already narrowed intervertebral foramen by osteophytes, facet hypertrophy, or other abnormalities of the bony structures may cause pressure on the epidural venous plexus causing venous obstruction.[30] Venous dilation can indeed be observed with magnetic resonance imaging (MRI) or epiduroscopy.[31] Venous obstruction may lead to decreased perfusion pressure of the nerve root. Unlike peripheral nerves, blood supply to the nerve root is limited. Nutrition of the nerve root is primarily via direct cerebrospinal fluid (CSF) transport, which may be compromised by the disk herniation and scar tissue formation.[32] Olmarker[33] studied the effects of nerve root compression on basic physiologic events such as blood flow, nutrition, and nerve conduction in animals. Pressures equal to the mean arterial blood pressure decrease arterial blood flow, but venular blood flow may cease at pressures as low as 5 mm Hg. Pressures of 50 mm Hg and changes in the permeability of endoneural capillaries lead to intraneural edema. Edema leads to fibrosis and further compromise of nutrition of the nerve root.

Fibrosis develops intraneurally but also outside the nerve root as a result of ischemia, inflammation, or trauma (e.g., surgery). Indeed, fibrosis seems a consistent finding in epidurograms and can often be seen during epiduroscopy.[2,31] Fibrosis in the narrow intervertebral foramen and the epidural space leads to further venous congestion. Venous congestion in turn may lead to further edema and swelling of the nerve root. Eventually, the nerve root is fixed in the foramen.[12,15,16,30,34] Lack of a perineurium[35] and poorly developed connective tissue makes the nerve root more susceptible to mechanical deformation.[36] Movement of 1 to 5 mm at the intervertebral foramen with straight leg raising has been documented.[12] These movements may cause mechanical tension on a nerve root and pain if it is fixed in the intervertebral foramen by adhesions.[12,15,30,37,38] The degree of swelling of the nerve root, as measured by MRI, has been correlated to pain generation with straight leg raising.[38]

Back Pain

Typical back pain can be reproduced by pressure on the posterior longitudinal ligament and posterior disk during surgery under local anesthetic.[15] However, the mechanism of this type of pain is not well explained. Degenerative disk disease may lead to central protrusion or extrusion of disk material with mechanical activation of nociceptors in the disk, ligaments, and dura. Primary ligament pain can be caused by instability of the spine causing stress on the anterior and posterior longitudinal ligaments.[11] Degenerative disease may lead to an annular tear. This may lead to continuous leakage of nucleus pulposi material, which has been associated with chronic inflammation.[21] The sinuvertebral nerve contains mostly sympathetic fibers; therefore, a sympathetically maintained pain component cannot be ruled out.[11] Finally, persistent pain may be the result of altered central modulation of pain signals. This can occur at the spinal or supraspinal level and makes the condition difficult to treat.

EPIDURAL CORTICOSTEROID INJECTION

Mechanism of Action

The adrenal cortex synthesizes corticosteroids (e.g., glucocorticoids, mineralocorticoids, and androgens). In humans, cortisol is the primary glucocorticoid and aldosterone is the main mineralocorticoid. However, physiologic production and circulating rates of these agents varies considerably, and each adrenal corticosteroid differs in relative glucocorticoid and mineralocorticoid activities. Cortisol production is roughly 10 mg/day, and relative potencies of representative corticosteroids vary considerably[39] (Table 23E–1).

The usual dose for methylprednisolone ranges from 80 to 120 mg.[40] The dose of triamcinolone ranges from 40 to 80 mg.[41,42] Beta-methasone is not as commonly used. Fewer complications have been reported with this drug. The usual dose is 1 ml (5.7 mg). Steroids can be mixed with either saline or local anesthetic.[43,44] The advantage of local anesthetic may be the presence of a sensory block, confirming the epidural administration of the steroid. An injection of 6 to 10 ml has been recommended in lumbar epidural injection, because this amount may be adequate to reach the target issues.[45]

Changes in nerve conduction and nerve fiber degeneration, after epidural application of autologous nucleus pulposus material in pigs, were significantly reduced by intravenous administration of methylprednisolone 30 mg/kg.[46] PLA_2 induces injury to membranes and edema by generating membrane perturbants, unsaturated fatty acids, and lysoderivatives. PLA_2 is the enzyme responsible for the liberation of arachidonic fatty acids from cell membranes leading to the production of eicosanoids.[47] Steroids interfere

---

TABLE 23E–1   Current Formulations of Steroid Preparations Commonly Used for Epidural Injection*

Formulation	Formulation 1	Formulation 2	Formulation 3
Depo-Medrol Multidose Vials			
Methylprednisolone	20	40	80
Polyethylene glycol 3350	29.5	29.1	28.2
Polysorbate 80	1.97	1.94	1.88
Monobasic sodium phosphate	6.9	6.8	6.59
Dibasic sodium phosphate USP	1.44	1.42	1.37
Benzyl alcohol (NaCl to adjust tonicity)	9.3	9.16	8.88
Depo-Medrol Single-Dose Vials†			
Methylprednisolone acetate	40	80	
Polyethylene glycol 3350	29	28	
Myristyl-Ō-picolinium chloride NaCl to adjust tonicity	0.195	0.189	
Aristocort Intralesional‡			
Triamcinolone diacetate	25		
Polyethylene glycol 3350	30		
Polysorbate 80	2		
Benzyl alcohol	9		
NaCl		8.5	

*All amounts in mg/ml.
†Upjohn, Kalamazoo, Michigan.
‡Fujisawa USA, Deerfield, Illinois.
NaCl, sodium chloride.

with the PLA_2 cascade and, therefore, reduce arachidonic acid metabolites, products that include prostaglandins, and leukotrienes that sensitize small neurons and enhance pain generation. Altered permeability in response to these inflammatory mediators result in intraneural edema and venous congestion, eventually resulting in abnormal conduction and generation of pain. Corticosteroids suppress the autoimmune response triggered by glycoproteins from the nucleus pulposus[48] and inhibit cytokine production by leukocytes.[49] Beta-methasone decreases secretion of several leukotrienes, tumor necrosis factor, and prostaglandin PGE_2 in intervertebral disk tissue.[50]

These mechanisms may explain the effect of corticosteroids in early stages of back pain and/or sciatica, when inflammation is the predominant pathologic process. Because inflammation plays a role in enhanced nociceptive activity in the posterior longitudinal ligament and disk, steroids may actually be effective in the treatment of back pain without radiculopathy.

Corticosteroids have a direct inhibiting action on fibrous tissue forming adhesions. Long-term pain relief may be mediated by the inhibiting effects of corticosteroids on fibrosis and adhesion formation in and around the nerve root in the intervertebral foramina. This mode of action may be particularly important when used in conjunction with other techniques, such as topical application of corticosteroids during surgery or as part of a decompressive neuroplasty.[2,51] One would expect these techniques to be more successful when used for radicular pain.

Corticosteroids exert a membrane stabilizing effect on injured nerve segments, reducing ectopic discharge from the affected nerve root.[10] In experimental neurinomas, corticosteroids prevent the development of ectopic neural discharge; in chronic neurinomas, they suppress on-going discharge.[52] This stabilizing effect is probably achieved through stimulation of a membrane-bound corticosteroid receptor, resulting in hyperpolarization of the membrane.[53]

Corticosteroids reduce conduction in nociceptive C-fibers in an animal model. It has been shown that onset of this effect was instantaneous and for the duration of the steroid application.[54] This suggests a direct membrane action rather than an intracellular receptor effect or an anti-inflammatory effect. It would also explain the effect primarily on thin unmyelinated C-fibers and not on thick myelinated A-fibers. Local anesthetic properties of corticosteroids may produce immediate pain relief that is occasionally seen in a patient after epidural steroid injections (ESIs). This mode of action may also be effective in the relief of pain originating from the dorsal compartment, including pain from facet arthropathy and myofascial pain. The C-fiber plays an important role in sympathetically mediated pain by a reduction in efferent and/or afferent activity from sympathetic fibers.

Central mechanisms in the processing of pain may be a target for corticosteroids as well. Corticosteroids have been shown to reduce the sensitization of dorsal horn neurons by persistent activation of nociceptors in the affected nerve root, possibly through their affect on spinal prostaglandin production.[55]

Corticosteroids may also exert a direct central nervous system affect by interfering with neurotransmitter production and metabolism in the brainstem and the spinal cord.[56]

Euphoric effects of corticosteroids are well known[49] and can add to the favorable response of ESIs.

Drug Deposition

There are several ways of administering corticosteroids to the affected area. The simplest method is systemic administration by either oral or parenteral route. Success has been reported with the intramuscular administration of dexamethasone.[57] However, these results have not been confirmed in several randomized controlled studies.[58]

Winnie and colleagues[59] compared intrathecal administration with epidural administration. Methylprednisolone, in a dose of 80 mg in 2 ml given either intrathecally or epidurally, was highly effective, with nearly identical success rates of 80% to 100%. Subsequent studies have found epidural steroids to be slightly more effective.[60,61] Although intrathecal administration in the subarachnoid space is probably safe, this treatment modality is currently inadvisable because of the controversy of possible serious side effects.[62,63]

Technique

Several approaches to the epidural space are used. The lumbar, cervical, or caudal epidural routes are the most commonly used. No study has supported one particular technique. Recently, new techniques have been introduced, including the caudal approach using a Racz catheter or epiduroscopy and the transforaminal approach to the epidural space.[2,64–67]

Only a brief description of the lumbar epidural technique is described here.[40] The patient may be in the sitting or lateral decubitus position. The patient's back is prepped aseptically with povidone-iodine solution and then draped. The appropriate interspace is selected, and the skin infiltrated with a local anesthetic. An introducer and then the epidural needle are inserted. Some prefer to use the 17-gauge Tuohy or Weiss needle; other people use a smaller (20-gauge) needle. A well-lubricated glass syringe is attached to the needle. The epidural needle is inserted slowly through the supraspinous and interspinous ligaments and ligamentum flavum until the epidural space is reached. Either intermittent or continuous pressure on the plunger of the syringe is applied while the needle is advanced slowly. Sudden loss of resistance to pressure on the plunger signifies that the tip of the needle has reached the epidural space. Aspiration is performed to ensure that the dura has not been punctured unintentionally. Methylprednisolone, 80 mg in 6 to 8 ml saline, is injected. This is followed by 2 to 3 ml saline to flush the needle of any remaining steroid. Some anesthesiologists use 2 to 3 ml (50 to 75 mg) triamcinolone. If a local anesthetic is used as a diluent, a test dose of 2 to 3 ml should be injected first. After a test dose is found negative for CSF and blood, the rest of the dose is injected in fractional (4 to 5 ml) increments. Whether saline or local anesthetic is used, a repeat aspiration should be done before final injection of the steroid solution.

Fluoroscopy has been advocated by several investigators.[2,68–70] Several factors may make blind needle placement inadvisable. Identification of the level of the pathologic condition, using surface anatomy, is notoriously unreliable. Correct placement of the needle occurs in 30% to 75% of patients.[71,72] Adhesions, particularly after decompressive surgery,[73] may make the spread to the affected nerve root difficult to impossible.[2] In a recent study on patients with "failed back surgery syndrome," disposition of epidural steroids at the site of the pathologic condition occurred in only 25% of the patients, despite accurate needle placement.[69]

Placement of a catheter using fluoroscopy, through the sacral canal or through an intervertebral foramen into the ventral epidural space, has been advocated. In a prospective study, 49% of patients had pain relief at 1-year follow-up.[2]

Transforaminal injection of epidural steroids has the theoretical advantage of direct placement at the site of the pathologic condition. However, damage to the nerve root is a potential complication. Lutz and colleagues[66] reported a successful outcome in 75% of 69 patients. No complications were reported. Several other studies support this technique, but the safety of this procedure has not yet been established.[65,67]

Lumbar Epidural Steroid Injection

Efficacy

Lumbar epidural steroid injections (LESIs) have gained widespread acceptance as a conservative treatment for low back pain with or without radiculopathy. The number of injections performed annually in Britain has been estimated at approximately 30,000.[74] Although currently no information is available, the number of LESIs performed in the United States may exceed 300,000 yearly. According to the report of the Quebec Task Force on Spinal Disorders, interventions practiced commonly, but without scientific evidence, constituted the third strongest type of evidence possible for treatment efficacy.[75,76] However, LESI remain controversial. The Agency for Health Care Policy and Research rate the quality of evidence of LESI as "C," which means that there is no good evidence, particularly clinical trials, for efficacy.[75,77] Even if one considers the currently available data to support the use of LESI, many questions remain unanswered. Who are the appropriate candidates for LESI? What is the ideal volume and content of the injectate? How many injections should a patient receive in a specific time?[75]

The studies currently available can be divided in three groups. The first group is represented by the older studies.[44,78–81] These are usually small, often lack a control group, and may have major design flaws. This group is important because these studies have made LESI accepted in clinical practice and have set the standard. The second group of studies contains the more recent randomized controlled trials.[4,82–85] However, these studies, reviewed by many prominent investigators, have yielded varied results. The third group consists of systematic reviews of the second group.[4,43,86,87] Several techniques are used to make groups comparable.

Early Studies

In the United States, the results from early studies[44,78–81,88] have led to the current standard of practice and can be summarized as follows:

1. LESI are indicated for patients with back pain with radicular pain. Efficacy is reported between 25% and 89%

with an average of 60%. Efficacy in less specific cases, such as spinal stenosis, spondylosis, and spondylolisthesis, is not clearly defined.[44,59,79–81,87]
2. LESI seems to be more effective in early stages (less than 3 months) of back pain with or without radiculopathy.[79–81]
3. Repeated LESI are more effective. However, there is no clinical benefit beyond three injections.[80,88]
4. Onset of pain relief occurs in most patients after the second day.[89]
5. No significant difference can be demonstrated between the caudal versus lumbar approach to the epidural space.[44]
6. Corticosteroids are more effective than either local anesthetic or saline injections. Dilution with either local anesthetic or saline demonstrate comparable results.[44]
7. The volume of the injection depends on the site of the injection. In general, larger volumes do not offer an advantage.[90]

Randomized Controlled Trials

Dilke and coworkers[84] conducted a double-blind, randomized trial on 100 patients with degenerative disk disease and unilateral sciatica with neurologic deficit. Patients received either 80 mg of methylprednisolone in 10 ml saline or 1 ml of normal saline injected in the interspinous ligament. Those patients from these comparable groups who received epidural steroids manifested improvement judged by decreased use of analgesics. Significantly more patients had clear pain relief at timed post-treatment assessments, required fewer surgical referrals, and had a significant reduction in time to return to work. There was no difference with respect to neurologic deficit and straight leg raise test.

In contrast to these positive findings, Snoek and colleagues performed a double-blind randomized study on 51 highly selected patients with lumbar root compression syndrome. All patients had symptoms, neurologic deficit, and myelographic findings consistent with herniated lumbar disk. The control group received 2 ml of normal saline, and the treatment group received 80 mg of methylprednisolone in 2 ml of normal saline in the epidural space at the level of the lesion. Although both groups showed improvements, they were not statistically different.[85]

Differences in results of the studies by Dilke and Snoek may be attributed to the different injection volumes used and timing of post-treatment assessment. Although Snoek evaluated patients between 24 and 48 hours after the injection, Dilke did his post-treatment assessment after 6 days. Green and colleagues[89] found that 37% of responders to epidural steroids do so within 2 days; 59% experienced relief between 4 and 6 days. The control group in the study by Snoek was more similar to the treatment group than in Dilke's study.

Cuckler[82] studied 73 patients with lumbar radicular pain syndromes in a prospective, randomized, double-blinded fashion. The authors found some short-term improvement in approximately 60% of the patients but could not demonstrate a significant difference between the two groups. However, patients were evaluated after 24 hours, and long-term assessment was done mainly by telephone. All injections were given at the L3-4 level irrespective of pathologic condition, and the important second ESI was given in both treatment and control groups for ethical reasons.

More recently, Carette and colleagues[83] conducted a blinded, placebo-controlled trial in 158 patients with sciatica resulting from herniated nucleus pulposus. In this carefully conducted study, the authors were able to show significant improvement in sensory deficit, finger-to-floor distance, and leg pain in the treatment group at 3 weeks and 6 weeks, but not at 3 months. Differences in other measures, such as straight leg raise test, motor deficit, and several pain and disability scores, did not reach statistical significance. At 12 months, the probability of surgery in the treatment and the control groups was similar, approximately 25%. The authors concluded that the treatment may result in short-term improvement but offers no significant functional benefit, nor does it reduce the need for surgery. However, because of the variety of signs and symptoms in these patients and the number of outcome measures, one might question the statistical power of this investigation.[75]

Systematic Reviews

Recently, several more systematic reviews have addressed the efficacy of LESI. Koes and colleagues[4] reviewed 15 trials, subject to certain conditions of design, in which a detailed analysis of the methodologic quality of each study was evaluated. In the five highest ranked studies, two studies had a favorable outcome; in the next six studies, four had positive outcomes. Overall, the authors concluded that the efficacy of ESIs had not been established and that benefits, if any, seem to be of short duration only.

This review was criticized by McQuay and Moore.[86] They stated that the study by Koes and colleagues was merely an in-depth examination of the methodologic quality of the trials rather than a meta-analysis of their results. In contrast, efficacy was investigated by a meta-analysis of all 11 randomized studies, involving a total of 907 patients. Data analysis used O-E differences (number of responders in the experimental group minus the numbers of responders in the control group), and odds ratios were calculated. Thus, patients in one trial were never compared with patients in another. They found little evidence of significant heterogeneity. Short-term effects of ESIs increased the odds ratio of pain relief to 2.6, and for long-term pain relief the odds ratio was 1.8. The investigators concluded that epidural administration of corticosteroids is effective in the management of lumbosacral radicular pain.[86,87]

McQuay and Moore elaborated on the work of Watts and colleagues.[87] They concluded from these studies that epidural steroid injections indeed work. To answer the question of how well this treatment works, these investigators reanalyzed the same data, and added the study by Carette and colleagues,[83] in which they used the number needed to treat (NNT) as a measure of clinical benefit. They found that short-term pain relief of 75% or more occurred in one out of seven patients. Long-term pain relief of 50% or more occurred in 1 out of 13 patients. They concluded that, given the data available, results should be interpreted in the clinical context: "In the case of chronic painful disease, intervention may be attractive even if the success rate is far lower than would be acceptable in acute postoperative pain."[86]

Several studies have shown decay in the overall success rate over time.[59,86,92–94] In a carefully conducted study by White and colleagues,[72] there was a drop in success rate from 82% on the first day to 7% at 6 months. Only 4 out of 300 patients were pain free after 2 years.[72] A more sustained response to LESI, approximately 30% of patients with significant pain relief after 6 months, was found by several other investigators.[82,84,89]

Several factors have been shown to affect the outcome of LESI. The nerve root is the main target of LESI. However, the underlying pathologic processes causing nerve root irritation may vary. Use of LESI in patients with spinal stenosis, spondylosis, intervertebral narrowing by osteophytes, or spondylolisthesis is questionable. Because proper correlation of the clinical syndrome with the underlying pathologic process is not always reliable,[95] selection of the appropriate candidates for LESI may be difficult.

In a randomized controlled trial, Fukusaki and colleagues[96] investigated the effect of LESI on 53 patients with degenerative spinal canal stenosis. The selection criteria included symptoms of unilateral or bilateral pseudoclaudication and intolerable leg pain on a walking distance of less than 20 m. The investigators were unable to show a beneficial effect of LESI in these patients.

The use of LESI in patients with prior surgery on the spine is highly controversial. One older study reports a high success rate (76%) after three caudal injections of 125 mg hydrocortisone acetate and 30 ml of 1% procaine.[81]

More recently Devulder and colleagues[97] used a randomized single-blinded design to compare steroid (methylprednisolone) with a local anesthetic (bupivacaine) with hyaluronidase and a local anesthetic via the transforaminal approach. After 6 months, 27% of all patients obtained more that 50% pain relief. There was no difference in efficacy between the two groups.

Cervical Epidural Steroid Injections

Information on cervical ESIs is limited and may reflect a lack of experience with this technique. Studies support the use of epidural steroids in patients with neck pain and/or radiculopathy. However, no randomized controlled studies exist to establish the role of cervical ESIs. Electromyographic results, in the pursuit of documenting radicular symptoms, did not correlate well with the likelihood of response to ESIs.

Indications

The principal indication for epidural corticosteroid injection is nerve root irritation. This irritation can be due to mechanical pressure, inflammation, ischemia, or a combination of these three processes. Nerve root irritation expresses itself as radicular pain and may be associated with neurologic deficits in the distribution of the nerve root. Classically, the patient has sharp, shooting pain that radiates into the leg and below the knee. Patients with upper extremity radiculopathy may not have the distinct symptoms of shooting pains below the elbow. Often, there is an increase in pain with coughing, sneezing, or straining. Onset of symptoms is often associated with lifting or twisting injury to the spine. Repetitious strain on the spine can also be contributory as can overall poor health, fatigue, and anxiety.[98]

The most significant finding in physical examination is the straight leg raise test.[38,42,88] In one study all patients with nerve root swelling, confirmed by computed tomography (CT), had a positive straight leg raise test at 50 degrees or less.[38] The femoral nerve tension test and tension tests of the major nerves of the upper extremity are less specific. Presence of neurologic deficit correlates well with nerve root irritation.[88,92,99]

Laboratory studies are less helpful. Eighty-five percent of patients with low back pain cannot be given a definitive diagnosis because of poor correlation between symptoms, pathologic processes, and imaging results.[95] Indeed poor correlation between radiographic findings and symptoms is a consistent finding in several studies.[91,93,100]

Selection of the appropriate candidate for ESI is not always easy. The patient population presenting with back pain and/or radiculopathy is not a homogeneous group. First, there is a wide range of pathologic processes that may be the cause of patients' symptoms. Classically, radicular pain is associated with degeneration and herniation of an intervertebral disk. However, stenosis of the central or foraminal canal by osteophytes, compression fractures, or tumor infiltration may cause a typical radiculopathy as well. Second, patients' dependent factors directly related to the pain (nature, onset, duration, previous treatments including surgery) or indirectly related factors (sleep deprivation, stress) play a roll in the success of ESI. Factors related to socioeconomic status (age, education, marital status, employment, litigation, and compensation) and psychologic issues are also important.[101]

Factors that make outcome less favorable were identified by Abram and Hopwood[101]: patients who were unemployed, received compensation, had a long duration of symptoms, and had nonradicular pain complaints.

Jamison and colleagues[102] found the following factors to be the best predictors of poor outcome after ESI: number of previous treatments, amount of medication taken for pain, presence of pain independent of activity, and nonradicular nature of back pain.

Sandrock and coworkers[103] found the most important factors to be accuracy of diagnosis, duration of symptoms, history of previous surgery, age of patient, and proper location of the needle.

As Rowlingson[98] states: "It is clearly a challenge to select those patients, who meet criteria for ESIs and still have enough flexibility in their attitude and behavior to respond positively to a marked reduction in pain by regaining a productive physical and emotional approach to life."

In summary, based on the previous considerations and the literature currently available, the following criteria can be used to select patients for ESIs:

1. Evidence of root involvement[40,74,94,98,104,105]
2. The objective to produce short-term pain relief alongside rehabilitation[74]
3. Absence of contraindications: infection, coagulopathy, history of untoward reaction to steroids, and poorly controlled diabetes
4. Absence of a favorable response to 4 weeks of conservative treatment[74]

Patients should belong to one of the following groups[55,98,105]:

1. Patients with radicular pain and a corresponding sensory change

2. Patients with clinically significant herniation of a disk, diagnosed by characteristic physical or laboratory findings with symptoms
3. Motivated patients with postural back pain, with radicular-like features
4. Patients with cancer, in whom tumor infiltration of the nerve root may cause radicular pain
5. Patients with acute back pain and radicular symptoms, superimposed on chronic back pain

Safety

Few complications of ESI have been reported in the literature, which now encompasses more than 6000 cases. More complications are related to the invasive nature of the procedure than to the procedure itself. Symptoms may include nausea, mild headache, dizziness, vasovagal reactions, or other transient benign phenomena.[106] Only four minor complications of this nature and no major complications were reported in a large series of 5334 ESIs. All of these procedures were performed under fluoroscopy with epidurography.[70]

A potentially serious complication is direct damage to the nerve root. Two patients with numbness in a dermatome have been reported in a series of 58 injections[107]; neurologic deficit was transient in one patient and persistent in the other. Intrinsic spinal cord damage after cervical ESIs has been reported but seems exceedingly rare.[108]

The most common technical complication of ESIs is unintentional puncture of the dura. The incidence ranges somewhere between 1% to 5%. The potential danger of an inadvertent corticosteroid injection into the subarachnoid space after accidental dural puncture exists but is probably clinically insignificant.[59,62,63]

Injection of corticosteroids in the epidural space is generally considered to be a safe procedure, but subarachnoid injections and epidural injections have been associated with rare but serious complications including adhesive arachnoiditis,[109] meningitis,[110] and transient[111] and permanent paralysis.[104,106] Durocutaneous fistulae have been reported,[106] which may be related to poor wound healing commonly associated with the use of corticosteroids.

Recent case reports have documented the development of epidural lipomatosis after the administration of multiple ESIs. Thecal sac compression is a potential complication. Fortunately, the lipomas disappeared after discontinuation of the injections as demonstrated by sequential MRI studies.[112]

Neurotoxicity

Several studies have examined the effect of epidural or subarachnoid deposteroid injections on neural tissues and meninges.

Sehgal and coworkers[113] injected methylprednisolone in the subarachnoid space of human and found a transient increase in CSF protein and pleocytosis that persisted for weeks. However, a similar response can be seen with injections of normal saline.[114]

Single-shot epidural injection with triamcinolone (Aristocort) in a cat model showed minor inflammatory changes after 30 days and near complete resolution after 120 days. The investigators conclude that there was no evidence of tissue damage when compared with matched controls.[115]

Methylprednisolone (Depo-Medrol) contains polyethylene glycol, an agent known to cause damage to connective tissue, nerves, and muscle fibers.[62] However, it was shown that the 3% concentration of polyethylene glycol used in clinical practice was not neurotoxic[58] and did not have fibroblast activity.[116]

Recently, Latham and colleagues[117] investigated the intrathecal injection of various volumes and doses of betamethasone (Celestone Chronodose) in 20 sheep. The authors concluded that small amounts (1 ml) of betamethasone are safe, but larger doses form a potential hazard of arachnoiditis.

Arachnoiditis

Arachnoiditis has been associated with spinal corticosteroid injections in several studies.[62,105] However, arachnoiditis as a result of spinal corticosteroid injections should be differentiated from arachnoiditis resulting from spinal surgery,[118] use of contrast agents,[119] or underlying disease for which the patient is treated. Indeed, chronic arachnoiditis may be the result of fibrosis and adhesions associated with degenerative disk disease and chronic nerve root compression.[120]

The cause of arachnoiditis has been attributed to the additives of the corticosteroid containing solutions. Triamcinolone and methylprednisolone contain the preservatives glycol and benzyl alcohol. Neurotoxicity at a concentration of 3% polyethylene glycol, the concentration used in clinical practice, was not shown to be significant.[121] However, fibrosis and adhesions leading to arachnoiditis is not equivalent to neurotoxicity. Signs of inflammation and fibrosis observed in the investigation by Latham and colleagues may be due to the vehicle benzyl alcohol, a preservative used in many corticosteroid preparations.

Wilkinson[122] reviewed the literature on the safety of subarachnoid steroid injections and concluded that most of the evidence of neurologic injury after intrathecal injections is circumstantial. If such a relationship exists, then arachnoiditis is more likely with higher dose corticosteroids or multiple injections.[63] In eight series of subarachnoid steroid injections involving 358 patients, no complications of arachnoiditis were reported.[123]

Based on extrapolation of the concerns with subarachnoid injections, use of ESIs has been questioned as well, for example, through the mechanism of accidental dural puncture.[62] The association between ESIs and arachnoiditis is a very weak one. Case reports of arachnoiditis following an ESI are exceedingly rare.[124,125]

Aseptic Meningitis

Few reports have documented aseptic meningitis following subarachnoid steroid injections,[105,112] and even fewer have been reported after ESIs.[126] The syndrome is characterized by fever, nausea, headaches, and neurologic signs including burning paining in the lower extremities, convulsions, and confusion after spinal steroid injections. CSF studies may reveal pleocytosis, roughly proportional to the steroid dose given,[113] elevated protein, and low glucose. Cultures are negative for bacteria, fungi, and mycobacteria. Changes in cell count or protein content of CSF are not obligatory following subarachnoid steroid injections, and pleocytosis may occur after the subarachnoid injection of normal saline alone.[127]

Symptoms and CSF abnormalities are of short duration, and no long-term complications have been reported.[104,105]

Epidural Abscess and Bacterial Meningitis

Bacterial meningitis seems unlikely in the absence of dural puncture. The few cases that are reported are unusual infections (i.e., tuberculosis and torula) and/or are not well documented.[110,127,128]

Epidural abscess after ESI has been reported but is rare.[129,130] Diabetes seems to predispose patients to this complication.[110,127,128] *Staphylococcus aureus* is most often implicated, presumably through contamination with skin flora.[129]

In a recent, large multicenter study, epidural abscess, as a complication of epidural catheter placement, was more common than once thought.[130] Corticosteroids may be associated with an increased risk of epidural abscess as was recently suggested in a report by Lowell[131] and co-workers in which 3 of 31 patients who received epidural methylprednisolone during lumbar microdiscectomy developed an epidural abscess.

Systemic Effects

Epidurally injected corticosteroids in conventional doses have been reported to cause iatrogenic Cushing's syndrome and adrenal suppression.[132–134]

Acute suppression of adrenocorticotropic hormone and plasma cortisol level can occur in the absence of cushingoid features. The duration of suppression varies from approximately 2 to 4 weeks, depending on dose and age.[133,135]

Cushingoid lesions, including moon facies, abnormal fat depositions, and skin lesions, can last for several months. Cortisol levels are elevated for more than 2 weeks after the injection of methylprednisolone into the epidural space.[44]

The exact mechanism by which epidural steroids suppress the neuroendocrine axis remains unclear. Slow release from the epidural space is most likely, because intra-articular injected triamcinolone can be found in the systemic circulation for up to 3 months.[135] A central mechanism, through absorption into CSF, is less likely because dura acts as a barrier to deposteroids.[114]

Because corticosteroid increases blood glucose concentration by an increase in glycogenolysis and neoglycogenesis, epidural corticosteroids may make control of blood sugar levels in diabetic patients more difficult.

References

1. Nachemson A: Advances in low back pain. *Clin Orthop* 200:266, 1985.
2. Racz GB, Heavner JE, Raj PP: Epidural neuroplasty. *Semin Anesth* 16:302, 1997.
3. Bogduk N: *Epidural use of steroids in the management of back pain and sciatica of spinal origin.* Canberra, Australia, Australian National Health and Medical Research Council, 1994.
4. Koes BW, Rob JPM, Scholten M et al: Epidural steroid injections for low back pain and sciatica: An updated systematic review of randomized clinical trials. *Pain Dig* 9:241, 1999.
5. Bogduk N: The innervation of the lumbar spine. *Spine* 8:286, 1983.
6. Steindler A, Luck JV: Differential diagnosis of pain low in the back: Allocation of the source of pain by the procaine hydrochloride method. *JAMA* 110:106, 1938.
7. Groen GJ, Baljet B, Drukker J: Nerves and nerve plexus of the human vertebral column. *Am J Anat* 188:282, 1990.
8. Cavanaugh JM: Neural mechanisms of lumbar pain. *Spine* 20:1804, 1995.

9. Woolf CJ, Safieh-Garabedian B, Ma QP: Nerve growth factor contributes to the generation of inflammatory sensory hypersensitivity. *Neuroscience* 62:327, 1994.

10. Devor M, Govrin-Lippmann R, Raber P: Corticosteroids suppress ectopic neural discharge originating in experimental neuromas. *Pain* 22:127, 1985.

11. Stolker RJ, Vervest AC, Groen GJ: The management of chronic spinal pain by blockades: A review. *Pain* 58:1, 1994.

12. Goddard MD, Reid JD: Movements induced by straight leg raising in the lumbo-sacral roots, nerves and plexus and the intra pelvic section of the sciatic nerve. *J Neurol Neurosurg Psych* 28:12, 1965.

13. Mixter WJ, Barr JS: Rupture of the intervertebral disc with involvement of the spinal cord. *N Eng J Med* 211:210, 1934.

14. Kelly M: Pain due to pressure on nerves: Spinal tumors and the intervertebral disc. *Neurology* 6:32, 1956.

15. Kuslich SD, Ulstrom CL, Michael CJ: The tissue origin of low back pain and sciatica: A report of pain response to tissue stimulation during operations on the lumbar spine using local anesthesia. *Orthop Clin North Am* 22:181, 1991.

16. Murphey F: Sources and patterns of pain in disc disease. *Clin Neurosurg* 15:343, 1968.

17. Smythe MJ, Wright V: Sciatica and the intervertebral disc: An experimental study. *J Bone Joint Surg* 40A:1401, 1958.

18. Goupille P, Jayson MI, Valat JP: The role of inflammation in disc herniation-associated radiculopathy. *Sem Arthritis Rheum* 28:60, 1988.

19. McLaughlin B, Weiss JB: Endothelial-cell-stimulating angiogenesis factor (ESAF) activates progelatinase A (72 kDa type IV collagenase), prostromelysin 1 and procollagenase and reactivates their complexes with tissue inhibitors of metalloproteinases: A role for ESAF in non-inflammatory angiogenesis. *Biochem J* 317:739, 1996.

20. Pankovich AM, Korngold L: A comparison of the antigenic properties of nucleus pulposus and cartilage protein polysaccharide complexes. *J Immunol* 99:431, 1967.

21. Saal JS: The role of inflammation in lumbar pain. *Phys Med Rehab* 4:191, 1990.

22. Lindahl O, Rexed D: Histological changes in the spinal nerve roots of operated cases of sciatica. *Acta Orthop Scand* 20:215, 1951.

23. McCarron RF, Wimpee MW, Hudkins PG et al: The inflammatory effect of nucleus pulposus: A possible element in the pathogenesis of low-back pain. *Spine* 12:760, 1987.

24. Saal JS, Franson RC, Dobrow R et al: High levels of inflammatory phospholipase A2 activity in lumbar disc herniations. *Spine* 15:674, 1990.

25. O'Donnel JL, O'Donnel AL: Prostaglandin E2 content in herniated lumbar disc disease. *Spine* 21:1653, 1996.

26. Willburger RE, Wittenburger RH: Prostaglandin release from lumbar disc and facet joint tissue. *Spine* 19:2068, 1994.

27. Gronblad M, Virri J, Ronkko S et al: A controlled biochemical and immunohistochemical study of human synovial-type (group II) phospholipase A2 and inflammatory cells in macroscopically normal, degenerated, and herniated human lumbar disc tissues. *Spine* 21:2531, 1996.

28. Gronblad M, Virri J, Tolonen J: A controlled immunohistochemical study of inflammatory cells in disc herniation tissue. *Spine* 19:2744, 1994.

29. Habtemariam A, Gronblad M, Virri J: Immunocytochemical localisation of immunoglobulins in disc herniations. *Spine* 21:1856, 1996.

30. Hoyland JA, Freemont AJ, Jayson MIV: Intervertebral foramen venous obstruction. A cause of periradicular fibrosis? *Spine* 14:558, 1989.

31. Heavner J: Personal communication, 1998.

32. Olmarker K, Rydevik B: Pathophysiology of sciatica. *Orthop Clin North Am* 22:223, 1991.

33. Olmarker K, Rydevik B, Holm S: Edema formation in spinal nerve roots induced by experimental, graded compression. *Spine* 14:569, 1989.

34. Jayson MIV: Presidential address: When does acute back pain become chronic? *Spine* 22:1053, 1997.

35. Sunderland S, Bradley KC: Stress-strain phenomena in human spinal nerve roots. *Brain* 84:120, 1961.

36. Sharpless SK (Goldstein M, editor): *Susceptibility of spinal roots to compression block. The research status of spinal manipulative therapy.* Washington, DC, NIH Workshop, February 2–4, 1975. NINCDS Monograph No 15, 1975.

37. Breig A: Biomechanical considerations in the straight-leg-raising test. Cadaveric and clinical studies of the effect of medial hip rotation. *Spine* 4:242, 1979.

38. Takata K, Inoue S, Takahashi K: Swelling of the cauda equina in patients who have herniation of lumbar disc: A possible pathogenesis of sciatica. *J Bone Joint Surg* 70:361, 1988.

39. Esteban NV, Loughlin T, Yergey AL: Daily cortisol production rate in man determined by stable isotope dilution/mass spectrometry. *J Clin Endocrinol Metab* 72:39, 1971.

40. Benzon HT: Epidural steroids. In Raj PP, editor: *Pain medicine: A comprehensive review.* St. Louis, Mosby, 1996.

41. Arnhoff FN, Triplett HB, Pokorney B: Follow-up status on patients treated with nerve blocks for low-back pain. *Anesthesiology* 46:170, 1977.

42. Yates DW: A comparison of the types of epidural injections commonly used in the treatment of low back pain and sciatica. *Rheumatol Rehab* 17:181, 1978.

43. Merry A, Schug SA, Rodgers A: Epidural steroid injections for sciatica and back pain a meta-analysis of controlled clinical trials. *Reg Anesth* 21(suppl 2):64, 1996.

44. Swerdlow M, Sayle-Creer W: A study of extradural medication in the relief of the lumbosciatic syndrome. *Anaesthesia* 25:341, 1970.

45. Harley C: Extradural corticosteroid infiltration: A follow-up study of 50 cases. *Ann Phys Med* 9:22, 1967.

46. Olmarker K, Rydevik B, Nordborg C: Autologous nucleus pulposus induces neurophysiologic and histologic changes in porcine cauda equina nerve roots. *Spine* 18:1425, 1993.

47. Famaey JP: Phospholipases, eicosanoid production and inflammation. *Clin Rheumatol* 1:84, 1982.

48. Marshall LL, Trethewie ER, Curtain CC: Chemical radiculitis: A clinical, physiological and immunological study. *Clin Orthop* 129:61, 1977.

49. Haynes RC: Adrenocorticotropic hormone: Adrenocortical steroids and their synthetic analogs; inhibitors of the synthesis and actions of adrenocortical hormones. In Hardman JG, Limbird LE, editors: *Goodman and Gilman's the pharmacological basis of therapeutics,* ed 9. Philadelphia, McGraw-Hill, 1996.

50. Takahashi H, Suguro T, Okazima Y: Inflammatory cytokines in the herniated tissue of the lumbar spine. *Spine* 21:218, 1996.

51. Haughton VM, Nguyen CM, Ho KC: The etiology of focal spinal arachnoiditis: An experimental study. *Spine* 18:1193, 1993.

52. Pateromichelakis S, Rood JP: Prostaglandin E2 increases mechanically evoked potentials in the peripheral nerve. *Experientia* 37:282, 1981.

53. Shao-Ying H, Yi-Zhang C: Membrane receptor-mediated electrophysiological effects of glucocorticoid on mammalian neurons. *Endocrinology* 124:687, 1989.

54. Johanson A, Hao J, Sjolund B: Local corticosteroid application blocks transmission in normal nociceptive C-fibres. *Acta Anesthesiol Scand* 34:335 1990.

55. Abram SE, Marsala M, Yaksh TL: Analgesic and neurotoxic effects of intrathecal corticosteroids in rats. *Anesthesiology* 81:1198, 1994.

56. Fuxe K, Harfstrand A, Agnati LF et al: Immunocytochemical studies on the localisation of glucocorticoid receptor immunoreactive nerve cells in the lower brain stem and spinal cord of the male rat using monoclonal antibody against rat liver glucocorticoid receptor. *Neurosci Lett* 60:1, 1985.

57. Green NP: Dexamethasone in the management of symptoms due to herniated lumbar disc. *J Neurol Neurosurg Psychiatry* 38:1211, 1975.

58. Kepes ER, Duncalf D: Treatment of backache with spinal injections of local anesthesia, spinal and systemic steroids: A review. *Pain* 22:33, 1985.

59. Winnie AP, Hartman JT, Meyers HL Jr et al: Pain clinic II: Intradural and extradural corticosteroids for sciatica. *Anesth Analg* 51:990, 1972.

60. Abram SE: Subarachnoid corticosteroid injection following inadequate response to epidural steroids for sciatica. *Anesth Analg* 57:313, 1978.

61. Hartman JT, Palumbo F, Hill BJ et al: Intradural and extradural corticosteroid injections for sciatic pain. *Orthop Rev* 3:21, 1974.

62. Nelson DA: Intraspinal therapy using methylprednisolone acetate: Twenty-three years of clinical controversy. *Spine* 18:278, 1993.

63. Wilkinson HA: Intrathecal Depo-Medrol: A literature review. *Clin J Pain* 8:49, 1992.

64. Barendse G, van Kleef J, Sluijter M: Technique of transforaminal epidural steroid injection. *Pain Dig* 9:254, 1999.

65. Kraemer J, Ludwig J, Bickert U: Lumbar epidural perineural injection: A new technique. *Eur Spine J* 6:357, 1997.

66. Lutz GE, Vad VB, Wisneski RJ: Fluoroscopic transforaminal lumbar epidural steroids: An outcome study. *Arch Phys Med Rehabil* 79:1362, 1998.

67. Viton JM, Rubino T, Peretti-Viton P: Short-term evaluation of peri-radicular corticosteroid injections in the treatment of lumbar radiculopathy associated with disc disease. *Rev Rheum Engl Ed* 65:195, 1998.

68. el-Khoury G, Ehara S, Weinstein JN: Epidural steroid injection: A procedure ideally performed with fluoroscopy control. *Radiology* 168:554, 1988.

69. Fredman B, Nun MB, Zohar E: Epidural steroids for treating "failed back surgery syndrome": Is fluoroscopy really necessary? *Anesth Analg* 88:367, 1999.

70. Johnson BA, Schellhas KP, Pollei SR: Epidurography and therapeutic epidural injections: Technical considerations and experience with 5334 cases. *Am J Neuroradiol* 20:697, 1999.

71. Steward HD, Quinell RC, Dann N: Epidurography in the management of sciatica. *Br J Rheumatol* 26:424, 1987.

72. White AH, Derby R, Wynne G: Epidural injections for the diagnosis and treatment of low-back pain. *Spine* 5:78, 1980.

73. Greenwood J, McGuire TH, Kimbell F: Study of the causes of failure in herniated intervertebral disc operation: Analysis of 67 reoperated cases. *J Neurosurg* 9:5, 1952.

74. Nash TP: Current guidelines in the use of epidural steroids in the United Kingdom. *Pain Dig* 9:231, 1999.

75. Hopwood MB, Manning DC: Lumbar epidural steroid injections: Is a clinical trial necessary or appropriate? *Reg Anesth Pain Med* 24:5, 1999.

76. Spitzer WO, Leblanc FE, DuPuis M: Report of the Quebec Task Force on Spinal Disorders. *Spine* 12:S9, 1987.

77. Acute low back pain problems in adults: Clinical practice guidelines #14. AHCPR publication no 95-0642. December 1994.

78. Beliveau P: A comparison between epidural anesthesia with and without corticosteroids in the treatment of sciatica. *Rheumatol Phys Med* 11:40, 1971.

79. Berman AT, Garbarino JL Jr, Fisher SM et al: The effects of epidural injection of local anesthetics and corticosteroids on patients with lumbosciatic pain. *Clin Orthop* 188:144, 1984.

80. Warr AC, Wilkinson JA, Burn JM et al: Chronic lumbosciatic syndrome treated by epidural injections and manipulation. *Practitioner* 209:53, 1972.

81. Goebert HW Jr: Painful radiculopathy treated with epidural injections of procaine and hydrocortisone acetate: Results in 113 patients. *Anesth Analg* 40:130, 1961.

82. Cuckler JM: The treatment of epidural steroids in the treatment of radicular pain. *Anesthesia* 25:346, 1970.

83. Carette S, Leclaire R, Marcoux S et al: Epidural corticosteroid injections for sciatica due to herniated nucleus pulposus. *N Engl J Med* 336:1634, 1997.

84. Dilke TFW, Burry HC, Grahame R: Extradural corticosteroid injection in the management of lumbar nerve root compression. *BMJ* 2:635, 1973.

85. Snoek W, Weber H, Jorgensen B: Double blind evaluation of epidural methylprednisolone for herniated lumbar disc. *Acta Orthop Scand* 48:635, 1977.

86. McQuay HJ, Moore RA: *An evidence-based resource for pain relief.* Oxford, UK, Oxford University Press, 1998.

87. Watts RW, Silagy CA: A meta-analysis on the efficacy of epidural corticosteroids in the treatment of sciatica. *Anaesth Intensive Care* 23:564, 1995.

88. Hickey RJ: Outpatient epidural steroid injections and lumbosacral radiculopathy. *N Z Med J* 100:594, 1987.

89. Green PW, Burke AJ, Weiss CA et al: The role of epidural cortisone injection in the treatment of discogenic low back pain. *Clin Orthop* 153:121, 1980.

90. Heyse-Moore GH: A rational approach to the use of epidural medication in the treatment of sciatic pain. *Acta Orthop Scand* 49:366, 1978.

91. Wiesel SW, Tsourmas N, Feffer HI: A study of computer assisted tomography. 1. The incidence of positive CAT scans in an asymptomatic group of patients. *Spine* 9:549, 1984.

92. Warfield CA, Biber MP, Crews DA: Epidural steroid injections as a treatment for cervical radiculitis. *Clin J Pain* 4:201, 1988.

93. Thornbury JR, Fryback DG, Turski PA et al: Disk-caused nerve compression in patients with acute low back pain: diagnosis: Diagnosis with MR, CT myelography, and plain CT. *Radiology* 186:731, 1993.

94. Breivik H, Hesla PE, Molnar I et al: Treatment of chronic low back pain and sciatica: Comparison of caudal epidural injections of bupivacaine and methylprednisolone with bupivacaine followed by saline. In Bonica J, editor: *Advances in pain research and therapy,* vol 1. New York, Raven Press, 1976.

95. Deyo RA: Fads in the treatment of low back pain. *N Engl J Med* 325:1039, 1991.

96. Fukusaki M, Kobayashi I, Hara T et al: Symptoms of spinal stenosis do not improve after epidural steroid injection. *Clin J Pain* 14:148, 1998.

97. Devulder J, Deene P, De Laat M: Nerve root sleeve injections in patients with failed back surgery syndrome: A comparison of three solutions. *Clin J Pain* 15:132, 1999.

98. Rowlingson JC: Epidural steroids: Do they have a role in pain management? *APS J* 3:20, 1994.

99. Rowlingson JC, Kirschenbaum LP: Epidural analgesic techniques in the management of cervical pain. *Anesth Analg* 65:938, 1986.

100. Hitselberger WE, Witten RM: Abnormal myelograms in asymptomatic patients. *J Neurosurg* 28:204, 1968.

101. Abram SE, Hopwood MB: Factors associated with failure of lumbar epidural steroids. *Reg Anesth* 18:238, 1993.

102. Jamison RN, VadeBocouer T, Ferrante FM: Low back pain patients unresponsive to an epidural steroid injection: Identifying predictive factors. *Clin J Pain* 7:311, 1991.

103. Sandrock NJG, Warfield CA: Epidural and facet injections. In Warfield CA, editor: *Principles and practice of pain management.* New York, McGraw-Hill, 1993.

104. Abram SE: Treatment of lumbosacral radiculopathy with epidural steroids. *Anesthesiology* 91:1937, 1999.

105. Raj, PP: Epidural steroid injections. *Pain Dig* 9:235, 1999.

106. Haddox JD: Lumbar and cervical epidural steroid therapy. *Anesth Clin North Am* 10:179. 1992.

107. Purkins EI: Cervical epidural steroids. *Pain Clin* 1:3, 1986.

108. Hodges SD, Castleberg RL, Miller T: Cervical epidural steroid injection with intrinsic spinal cord damage: Two case reports. *Spine* 23:2137, 1998.

109. Ryan MD, Taylor TK: Management of lumbar nerve-root pain by intrathecal and epidural injections of depot methylprednisolone acetate. *Med J Aust* 2:532, 1981.

110. Shealy CN: Dangers of spinal injections without proper diagnosis. *JAMA* 197:156, 1966.

111. McLain RF, Fry M, Hecht ST: Transient paralysis associated with epidural steroid injection. *J Spinal Disord* 10:441, 1997.

112. Sandberg DI, Lavyne MH: Symptomatic spinal epidural lipomatosis after local epidural corticosteroid injections: Case report. *Neurosurgery* 45:162, 1999.

113. Sehgal AD, Tweed DC, Gardner WJ et al: Laboratory studies after intrathecal corticosteroids. *Arch Neurol* 9:64, 1963.

114. Bedford THB: The effect of injected solutions on the cell count of the cerebrospinal fluid. *Br J Pharmacol* 3:80, 1948.

115. Delaney TJ, Rowlingson JC, Carron H et al: Epidural steroid effects on nerves and meninges. *Anesth Analg* 59:610, 1980.

116. Cicala RS, Turner R, Moran E et al: Methylprednisolone acetate does not cause inflammatory changes in the epidural space. *Anesthesiology* 72:556, 1990.

117. Latham JM, Fraser RD, Moore RJ et al: The pathological effects of intrathecal betamethasone. *Spine* 22:1558, 1997.

118. Matsui H, Tsuji H, Kanamori M: Laminectomy-induced arachno-radiculitis: A postoperative serial MRI study. *Neuroradiology* 37:660, 1995.

119. Dullerud R, Morland TJ: Adhesive arachnoiditis after lumbar radiculopathy with Dimer-X and Depo-Medrol. *Radiology* 119:153, 1976.

120. Burton CV: Lumbosacral arachnoiditis. *Spine* 3:24, 1978.

121. Benzon HT, Gissen AJ, Strichartz GR et al: The effect of polyethylene glycol on mammalian nerve impulses. *Anesth Analg* 66:553, 1987.

122. Wilkinson HA: Intrathecal Depo-Medrol: A literature review. *Clin J Pain* 8(1):49, 1992.

123. Abram SE, O'Connor TC: Complications associated with epidural steroid injections. *Reg Anesth* 21:149, 1996.
124. Rovira E, Garcia-Escrig M, Catala J: Chronic adhesive arachnoiditis following epidural paramethasone. *Rev Neurol* 25:2067, 1997.
125. Sekel R: Epidural Depo-Medrol revisited. *Med J Austr* 3:688, 1982.
126. Morris JT, Konkol KA, Lonfield RN: Chemical meningitis following epidural methylprednisolone injection. *Infect Med* 11:439, 1994.
127. Dougherty JH Jr, Fraser RA: Complications following intraspinal injections of steroids: Report of two cases. *J Neurosurg* 48:1023, 1978.
128. Roberts M, Sheppard GL, McCormick RC: Tuberculous meningitis after intrathecally administered methylprednisolone acetate. *JAMA* 200:894, 1967.
129. Chan S-T, Leung S: Spinal epidural abscess following steroid injection for sciatica. *Spine* 14:106, 1989.
130. Wang LP, Hauerberg J, Schmidt JF: Incidence of spinal epidural abscess after epidural analgesia: a national 1-year survey. *Anesthesiology* 91:1928, 1999.
131. Lowell TD, Errico TJ, Eskenazi MS: Use of epidural steroids after discectomy may predispose to infection. *Spine* 25:516, 2000.
132. Edmonds LC, Vance ML, Hughes JM: Morbidity from paraspinal depo-corticosteroid injections for analgesia: Cushing's syndrome and adrenal suppression. *Anesth Analg* 72:820, 1991.
133. Kay J, Findling JW, Raff H: Epidural triamcinolone suppresses the pituitary-adrenal axis in human subjects. *Anesth Analg* 79:501, 1994.
134. Knight CL, Burnell JC: Systemic side-effects of extra-dural steroids. *Anaesthesia* 35:593, 1980.
135. Cook DM, Meikle AW, Bowman R: Systemic absorption of triamcinolone after a single intraarticular injection suppresses the pituitary-adrenal axis [abstract]. *Clin Res* 36:21A, 1988.

CHAPTER 23

Interventional Techniques

M O N I C A   N E U M A N N,   P.   P R I T H V I   R A J,
L L O Y D   J O S E P H   F I T Z G E R A L D,   A N D
M A H M O O D   A H M A D

THE FACET SYNDROMES

The facet joints of the spine may be otherwise known as the apophyseal joints. The Greek word *apophysis* means an "off-shoot," and the anatomic definition of the word is a natural outgrowth or process on a vertebra or other bone.[1] The degenerative changes and associated muscle spasm that develop when a facet joint is involved in a sprain from a forceful or violent twisting motion were termed the "facet syndrome" by Ghormley in 1933.[2] The intra-articular facet joints at all levels are subject to trauma.

Anatomy

The apophyseal articulations are formed by the superior articular facet of one vertebra and the inferior articular facet of the adjacent vertebra above (Fig. 23F–1). The articular surfaces of the facets are covered by hyaline cartilage. The joints are lined by synovium and, where the surfaces of the facets are not in contact, tabs of synovial tissue project into the joint from the joint margins.[3] The fibrous joint capsule forms superior and inferior joint recesses that may contain synovial villi.[4] The inferior and posterior portions of the recesses are larger, allowing a wide range of motion. Medially and anteriorly, the capsule blends with the ligamentum flavum and is adjacent to the neural foramen and the nerve root.

The joint capsule is richly innervated.[3,5–7] Each dorsal ramus sends branches to the facet joint at its own level and to the level below (Fig. 23F–2). Consequently, each posterior ramus innervates two facet joints, and each facet joint has innervation from two levels.

The articular facets in the cervical spine extend laterally from the junction of the lamina and pedicles and are oriented in the coronal plane to permit flexion, extension, and lateral bending. In the thoracic spine, the facets extend superiorly and inferiorly from the junctions of the lamina and pedicles, and the apophyseal joints are oriented approximately 20 degrees off the coronal plane. The superior facets

in the lumbar spine are concave posteriorly, and the inferior facets are convex anteriorly. The lumbar facet joints are oriented approximately 45 degrees off the sagittal plane; however, because of the curvature of the joints, the posterior portion of the joint is much closer to the sagittal plane.

Cervical Facet Syndrome

A cervical facet syndrome may result from the sudden stop of a vehicle, athletic or occupational injuries, sleeping with a twisted neck, or a sudden jerk of the neck resulting in over-riding of the superior on the inferior articular facet. Degenerative changes may cause intense muscle spasm on the ipsilateral side. Pain on palpation of the transverse process and decreased range of motion at the involved level are present. Rotating motion and hyperextension may exacerbate the pain, which is described as dull and aching, most often radiating to the occipital region, shoulder, arm, and cervicoscapular area. The head may be held to one side, and the patient cannot touch the ear to the shoulder of the affected side.[8]

The diagnosis is made through history, physical examination, and x-ray evaluation. Treatment includes conservative measures such as local heat, traction, nonsteroidal anti-inflammatory drugs (NSAIDs), local myofascial trigger point injections, and local injection in the paravertebral muscles. Manual manipulation may be required to reduce the subluxation. Arthrography with local anesthetic and steroid injection under fluoroscopy may prove beneficial, with up to 12 months of pain relief.[9] Because of the possibility of subarachnoid and epidural injection, it is recommended that the cervical facet joint injections be undertaken with fluoroscopic control.

Thoracic Facet Syndrome

The thoracic facet joint syndrome is similar to that of the cervical facet syndrome, resulting from a sudden twisting motion, twisting while lifting overhead, or an unguarded rotating motion of the thoracic spine. The resultant pain may

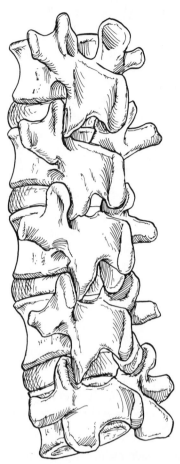

FIG. 23F–1 The lumbar facet joints are best visualized with 30- to 45-degree obliquity. The inferior articular facet from the vertebra above and the superior articular facet from the vertebra below articulate to form the facet joint.

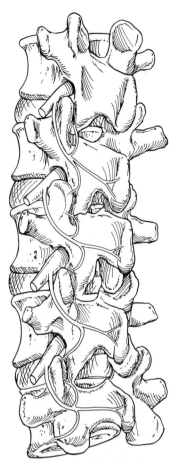

FIG. 23F–2 Each articular facet is innervated by branches from the posterior ramus at the same level above, resulting in a dual nerve supply.

be mild, dull, and aching, with radiation encircling that chest, or it may be sharp, pleuritic-type pain that can affect functional vital capacity or become overwhelming to the patient. There is usually decreased motion in the portion of the spine involved.

Diagnosis is made through history, physical examination, and plain x-ray films. Computed tomography (CT) may provide a more precise diagnosis of the area of involvement, but radiographic findings may not correlate with the clinical picture.

Treatment consists of local heat, NSAIDs, or local muscle (myofascial) injections. Intercostal nerve blocks may help with the splinting and guarding in the affected areas, especially if functional vital capacity is decreased.[8] Hydrotherapy involving swimming and prescribed exercises in warm water (95°F) may alleviate the syndrome. If the articular facet involved is identified, the joint may be injected in an indirect fashion with a paravertebral somatic nerve block using an adequate volume of local anesthetic and steroid solution, usually 3 to 5 cc.

Lumbar Facet Syndrome

The lumbar facet joints present the most often encountered problems involving any of the facet joints of the spine. Low back pain with or without radiation is the primary present-

ing complaint. The lumbar facet syndrome should be one of the differential diagnoses of low back pain once other etiologic factors, such as degenerative disk disease, disk herniation, and trauma, have been evaluated.

The pain of an aggravated lumbar facet is described as a dull ache that radiates into the low back, buttocks, hip, or posterior or lateral thigh down to the knee. Hamstring pain and muscle spasm, decreased straight leg raising, and depressed deep tendon reflexes may be present.[5] The pain only occasionally radiates below the knee, and, when it does, it is usually associated with prolonged pathologic changes of the involved facet. The pain then may present as sciatica.

On examination, the patient complains of tenderness to the deep palpation over the facet joint, sharp, aching pain on extension of the lumbar spine, and pain with simultaneous rotation and flexion of the lumbar spine. Often, there is muscle spasm of the ipsilateral paraspinous muscles.

The diagnosis is made based on history and physical examination and possibly by changes noted on radiographic or CT scan examination.

Treatment consists of local heat, NSAIDs, electroacupuncture therapy, local myofascial trigger point injections to the paraspinous muscles, and, more precisely, injection of a single joint or a multiple lumbar articular facet joint.

Facet Arthrography with Blockade

The normal facet joint has an S-shaped contour in the oblique projection. Small superior and larger inferior recesses are present. The articular cartilage is seen as a thin lucency between the contrast and cortex of the adjacent facets. The capacity of the joint is between 1 to 2 ml.[10] The joint usually ruptures along the medial or lateral aspect of the inferior recess with injection of local anesthetic and steroid solution.[11,12]

Indications

The major indications for facet joint injection include (1) focal tenderness over a facet joint, (2) chronic low back pain with or without radiation but with a normal radiographic evaluation, (3) back pain with evidence of disk disease and facet arthritis, and (4) postlaminectomy syndrome without arachnoiditis or recurrent disk disease.[11,13]

The findings on conventional radiographs correlate poorly with the clinical symptoms.[11,14] There may be better correlation between symptoms and findings on CT scans.[15,16] Facet arthrography with injection of local anesthetic and an anti-inflammatory agent is a diagnostic procedure that that is often therapeutic, with relief of symptoms lasting much longer than expected from the pharmacologic effects of the injected agents.[5,9,11,14]

Contraindications

The only absolute contraindication to facet joint block is infection in the overlying soft tissues. A relative contraindication is allergy to injected agents. Facet joint block can be accomplished, however, without injection of contrast, and the newer nonionic contrast agents also decrease the risk in allergic individuals.

Complications

Complications following facet blocks are rare but include infection, allergic reaction, and transient radicular pain. Theoretically, the subarachnoid space can be entered during a facet block. It is important to aspirate before any injection to ensure that there is no return of cerebrospinal fluid (CSF). Placement of the needle under fluoroscopic visualization and proper technique are safeguards to prevent this possibility.

Technique of Injection

Although the lumbar facet joint injection may be attempted by a blind technique, it is not recommended. A blind technique should be considered only for the lumbar joints, not the cervical or thoracic.

Radiographic localization of the facet joints for needle insertion with arthrography for documentation of the intra-articular position of the tip of the needle eliminates any question as to whether the response to the injection was related to technique. Although arthrography and injection of the cervical facets using fluoroscopy have been described,[9] most referrals for facet injection are for low back pain. The discussion of technique, therefore, deals with the lumbar facets.

Patients with facet syndrome usually have localized to one side. The localization of the level is made difficult, however, (1) because of the frequency of multiple-level disease and the dual nerve supply of each facet joint and (2) because similar symptoms can result from disease at different levels.[13-15] It may be necessary to inject two or three levels to determine the cause of the symptoms. Facet joints can be entered only from a posterior approach in the lumbar and thoracic regions. However, cervical facets from levels 2 to 5 are preferentially approached in the supine position.

Efficacy

Most patients experience little or no pain during injection of the facet joints. If the injected facet is the cause of the pain, often dramatic relief of pain immediately follows the injection. The patient is asked to sit, climb off the table, and walk while still in the radiographic procedure room. The patient is questioned concerning any immediate change in symptoms and is instructed to keep track of any change in pain over the next 24 hours as well as during the following weeks.

The immediate response to the injection, as well as long-term relief of pain, is significant. The test is considered positive if (1) complete relief of low back pain and sciatica follows intra-articular facet block, (2) the pain does not return during the 24 hours afterward, and (3) the patient's normal activities do not exacerbate the pain.[12-14]

Initial relief of pain has been reported in 54% to 65% of patients undergoing facet block. Between 20% and 30% of these patients experienced continued relief of pain for more than 6 months.[6,11,14] Patient selection and technique are important factors in achieving satisfactory results.

Radiofrequency

Cervical Facets

Patients with cervical facet disease tend to complain of pain in the neck, shoulder girdle, ear, or head. Clinical experience has suggested that tender points exist anterior, over, and posterior to the trapezius muscle.[17] Anatomically, the medial branch wraps around posteriorly, sending two branches along the waist of the body.

Technique

The patient is positioned supine for C2-3 to C5-6 lesions and prone for levels below C6. A 5-cm cannula with a 5-mm active tip is used. The camera is rotated in the oblique view, 30 degrees from horizontal, so that the vertebral foramen are well visualized. The camera axis is then oriented 10 degrees caudocranially. The posterior border of the facets is palpated and marked on the skin. The examiner identifies the craniocaudad level of approach by holding a clamp over the lateral neck and the cannula inserts in this plane at the premarked posterior border of the facet. The cannula is advanced with a slight anterior angle, and the bone is typically encountered in 1.5 to 2.5 cm. Cannula progress is followed in the 30-degree oblique view, with care taken not to advance in the direction of the foramen.

Once the cannula reaches the bone, an anteroposterior (AP) view is taken to confirm placement at the waist of the body. Sensory stimulation at 50 Hz up to 1.0 V is employed, and the examiner looks for stimulation in the region of the neck and the shoulder. Motor stimulation at 2 Hz up to 2.0 V should reveal the absence of upper extremity motor fasciculations. The area is treated with 0.5 cc of 2% lidocaine, and a lesion is created at 80 degrees for 20 seconds. Possible complications include neuritis and segmental nerve injury.

The posterior primary ramus of C2 goes on to become the greater occipital nerve and must not be lesioned. To denervate the branches of the C2 posterior primary ramus, the examiner places the radiofrequency cannula on the C2 arch at a point cranial to the C2-3 facet joint and level with the C3 foramen. Stimulation is performed at this point to identify the C2 communicating branch, and an AP view is taken to confirm placement on the lateral pillar. Lesions below the C5-6 level are made from a posterior approach, with the camera angled slightly cephalad, and lateral oblique. The cannula is placed so that its tip is lying on the superior, medial, and anterior border of the transverse process. Possible complications include mild to severe neuritis, patchy numbness, and, occasionally, vertigo when the C2-3 level is injected.

Thoracic Facets

The anatomy of the thoracic facet median branch differs from that of the lumbar region. Specifically, from T5-8, the median branch can be found more superior than the inflection point of the transverse process. Candidates for the procedure are identified with low-volume diagnostic median branch blocks.

Technique

The patient is placed in a prone position, and the camera is rotated cephalad or caudad, as needed, to line up the intervertebral disks. The C-arm is them rotated 10 to 15 degrees oblique so that the most medial aspect of the superior articulating process is visualized. A 10-cm cannula with a 10-mm curved, blunt active tip is advanced in tunnel view toward the "eye of the Scottie dog" until bone is struck. The bevel of the cannula is then turned cephalad, and then the cannula is advanced another 2 mm, laying the body of the cannula in the groove between the rib and the transverse process. A lateral view should confirm that the anterior most aspect of the tip is located dorsal to the posterior foraminal line.

Sensory stimulation up to 1.0 V should produce paravertebral tingling. Motor stimulation at 2 Hz usually produces paravertebral muscle contraction at less than 1.0 V. Then, 1 cc of 2% lidocaine is injected; after a 30-second delay, a lesion is created for 60 seconds at 80 degrees. Potential complications include pneumothorax and thoracic neuritis.

Lumbar Facets

Many authors agree that lumbar facet disease is a common cause of diffuse low back pain. Lumbar facet pain can be referred to the buttocks, hips, and thighs. Anatomically, the median branch at the lumbar level travels across the medial most border of the transverse process, innervating the facet at its own level and below.

Technique

The patient is placed in a prone position on the procedure table. The camera is rotated to 10 to 50 degrees oblique, so that the medial-most aspect of the transverse process is visualized. A 20-gauge curved, blunt cannula with a 10-mm active tip is inserted in a tunnel view and advanced toward the target until it strikes bone. The bevel of the cannula is then turned cephalad; the cannula is advanced another 2 mm, laying the body of the cannula in the groove. Approaching is to be laid alongside the course of the medial branch.

A lateral view should confirm that the tip of the electrode is dorsal to the posterior foraminal line. Sensory stimulation at 1.0 V causes a paresthesia to the back or hips when the cannula is in good position. Motor stimulation at 2 Hz ideally causes paraspinal muscle contraction and at 2.0 V does not cause lower extremity fasciculations. Then, 1 cc of 2% lidocaine is injected; after a 30-second delay, a lesion is created at 80 degrees for 60 seconds. In a small percentage of these patients, a postprocedure neuritis develops that can last as long as 6 weeks.

CRYONEUROLYSIS AND RADIOFREQUENCY LESIONING

Neurodestructive techniques may be helpful in the management of certain painful conditions. This section does not provide a detailed description of each procedure, but rather provides an overview of both cryoneurolysis and radiofrequency lesioning.

Selection of Patients

Before neurodestruction is initiated, it is important to diagnose accurately the pain generator. The peripheral nerve in question must always be examined in conjunction with the central nervous system. Combining physical examination with appropriate diagnostic data improves the chances of success.

When making neurodestructive lesions, the physician must avoid unnecessary procedures. Both cryoneurolysis and radiofrequency are best used when a single nerve or site is involved. They are not suitable for diffuse processes in multiple sites. In certain conditions, one technique may be superior to the other. For example, for trigeminal neuralgia the cryoneurolysis results are poorer than those obtained by radiofrequency lesioning.[18,19] Many physicians believe that it is inappropriate to use radiofrequency lesioning on large peripheral nerves because the risk of neuroma formation is greater than that with cryoneurolysis. Technical considerations may also determine which technique should be used.

After initial clinical impressions and usually after the failure of more conservative measures, diagnostic microinjections (typically 0.2 to 0.5 ml) of local anesthetic are performed at the peripheral nerve or nerves. A favorable response to diagnostic injections does not always predict a successful result with radiofrequency or cryoneurolysis. Failure of palliation of symptoms by neurodestruction after successful diagnostic block may occur in up to 30% of cases.[20] There are several reasons for this:

1. Placebo response, which is at least 30%.
2. Poor needle placement leading to a nonspecific diagnostic block
3. Excessive volumes of local anesthetic causing a diffuse neural blockade without specificity. For example, the

stellate ganglion may be blocked with volumes as small as 1.5 ml, although volumes of 8 to 10 ml are widely used.[21,22]

4. Systemic volumes of absorbed local anesthetic. The analgesic effects of local anesthetics in certain neuropathic conditions are well known. Certain blocks, for example, intercostal and lumbar sympathetic blocks, are known to lead to significant local anesthetic plasma levels.

5. Technical problems that prevent generation of the lesion.

Contraindications

Among the contraindications are the following:

1. Undiagnosed condition
2. Coagulopathy
3. Infection
4. Patient who is unwilling or unable to cooperate
5. Psychopathologic condition, including anxiety, that makes toleration of the procedure unlikely

Cryoneurolysis

Cryoneurolysis is a technique in which the application of low temperatures produced by cryosurgical equipment achieves anesthesia or analgesia by blocking peripheral nerves or destroying nerve endings. It is best reserved for situations in which analgesia is required for weeks to months.[23]

Physical Principles and Equipment

Expansion of gas enclosed in the cryoprobe results in the Joule-Thompson or Kelvin effects; that is, gas under pressure escaping through a small orifice expands and cools (Fig. 23F–3). The probes are made of stainless steel insulated with a coating of polytetrafluoroethylene (Teflon) and are coaxial in design. Thermocouples and stimulators with variable voltages and frequencies are built into the exposed tip surface, and, by using a console with a variable flow control, it is possible to achieve a wide range of subzero temperatures.

The ice ball encompasses the end of the probe and is about 3.5 mm in diameter for a 1.3-mm tipped probe. The variables involved in ice ball size include probe size, freeze time, tip temperature, tissue thermal conductivity, tissue permeability to water, and presence or absence of vascular structure (i.e., a heat sink). When thermal equilibrium between the probe and tissues is achieved, there is no further increase in the size of the ice ball; however, repetition of the freeze-thaw cycle increases the size of the cryolesion.[24]

When the probe is used percutaneously, it is difficult to ensure close proximity to the nerve, and large ice balls have a greater chance of producing the desired lesion. For myelinated fibers a direct lesion 3 mm in diameter with a freeze time of 1 minute produces a conduction block.[25] When the nerve is frozen amid other tissues, the duration of exposure should be approximately 90 to 120 seconds. Rapid defrosting aids removal of the probe from tissues.

Lesion Characteristics

Freezing involves removal of pure water from solution and its isolation into biologically inert ice crystals. The extent of the lesion depends primarily on the rates of freezing and thawing.[26] When cooling is slow, ice crystal nucleation occurs in the extracellular fluid. When freezing is rapid, crystal nuclei develop uniformly throughout the tissue. The central zone close to the probe tip cools rapidly compared with the peripheral zone, which is influenced by heat generated by the surrounding tissues. Therefore, intracellular ice is formed at the periphery.[27,28] Tissue destruction is more complete at the center of a cryolesion. It is also likely that the areas at the edge of the cryolesion undergo ischemic necrosis.

Application of cold to peripheral nerves induces a reversible block of conduction similar to that produced by local anesthesia. The extent and duration of the effect depend on the temperature attained in the tissue and the duration of exposure. Large myelinated fibers are initially affected with relative sparing of smaller sensory nerves.

A prolonged conduction block occurs when the nerve is frozen at temperatures between −5°C and −20°C.[29,30] This causes axonal disintegration and breakdown of myelin sheaths. Wallerian degeneration occurs with the perineurium and epineurium remaining intact. The absence of external damage to the nerve and the minimal inflammatory reaction following freezing ensure that regeneration is accurate and complete. Recovery depends on the rate of axonal regeneration and the distance of the cryolesion from the end organ. All elements of the nerve are involved. The rate of axonal regrowth is 1 to 3 mm/day. Histologic sectioning of nerve suggests that regeneration is still occurring in functionally intact nerves.

Technique

The cryolesion is attempted only after successful temporary reduction of symptoms by a diagnostic block. After a small skin wheal is raised with local anesthetic, a 1.3-mm or 2-mm probe is passed via a 16-gauge or 12 gauge catheter, respectively, depending on the nerve size. Larger probes counteract arterial warmth where heat sinks are expected. Localization is facilitated with stimulation between 50 and 100 Hz at less than 0.5 V for sensory nerves or at 2 to 5 Hz for motor nerve. Two or three 2-minute cycles are usually sufficient. During the freezing, care is taken to prevent frostbite if the probe comes in direct contact with the skin. Continuous irrigation with 0.9% saline solution at room temperature reduces the possibility of skin injury.

Common Procedures

Head and Neck

Supraorbital Nerve. Irritation of the nerve occurs primarily at the supraorbital notch. Supraorbital neuralgia may be secondary to blunt trauma, entrapment neuropathy, acute herpetic infection, Paget's disease, or neoplasm.

Cryoneurolysis can be accomplished via an open operative technique or percutaneously. The importance of cosmesis should be considered in avoiding thermal damage to the sensitive skin around the eye. Entry of the catheter and probe should be below or above the eyebrow line to avoid damage to the brow follicles. Potential risks include nerve trauma after insertion of the probe, hematoma, infection, and skin necrosis.

Infraorbital Nerve. The infraorbital nerve is a terminal branch of the second division of the trigeminal nerve as it

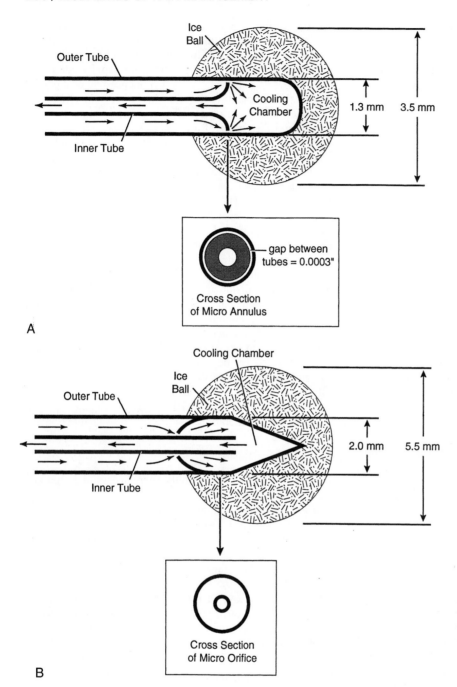

FIG. 23F–3 *A* and *B,* Two typical cryoprobe designs. High-pressure gas flows through the outer tube and expands after passing through the orifice. The gas is vented through the center tube. *(From Saberski LR: Cryoneurolysis in clinical practice. In Waldman SD, Winnie AP, editors:* Interventional pain management. *Philadelphia, WB Saunders, 1996.)*

exits through the infraorbital foramen. It is in the same vertical plane as the pupil when the eye is in a forward gaze. It is a sensory nerve to the lower eyelid, cheek, lateral aspect of the nose, upper lip, and part of the temple.

Infraorbital neuralgia is typically characterized by maxillary pain worsened by smiling or laughing. Patients sometimes experience referred pain in the teeth.

Cryoneurolysis can be accomplished via an open operative technique or percutaneously. It can also be accomplished by an intraoral approach to minimize cosmetic damage. The same introducer and probe are inserted through the superior buccal-labial fold. The probe is then advanced until it lies over the infraorbital foramen.

Mandibular Nerve. After emerging from the foramen ovale, the mandibular nerve runs through the infratemporal fossa posterior to the posterior border of the pterygoid plate. It provides motor supply to lateral pterygoid, masseter, and temporalis muscles and sensory supply to the skin and buccal mucosa of the cheek and gingiva. The auriculotemporal and lingual nerves constitute a posterior division.

Neuropathy of the mandibular nerve may result from muscular hypertrophy of the pterygoids caused by chronic bruxism and loss of vertical dimension of the oral cavity with loss of posterior dentition.

An insulated needle is introduced through the mandibular notch and advanced through the infratemporal fossa until it encounters the lateral pterygoid plate. It is then walked back off the lateral pterygoid plate, maintaining the same depth, until paresthesia or stimulation with a nerve stimulator is achieved. The depth of the needle is noted, and then it is removed. The cryoprobe is advanced to the same depth using stimulation to localize the nerve.

Mental Nerve. The mental nerve emerges from the mental foramen. The foramen becomes progressively cephalad with advancing age.

Irritative peripheral neuropathy occurs principally at the mental foramen. The pain of mental neuralgia is typically manifested in the chin, lower lip, and gum line. The nerve may also become entrapped in surgical scars.

Closed extraoral or intraoral cryoneurolysis can be preformed. Intraorally, the probe is advanced through the gingivobuccal reflection at the level of the premolar tooth and makes contact with the mandible. Care must be taken not to enter the foramen because of the risk of nerve injury.

Greater Occipital Nerve. The greater occipital nerve is a branch of the cervical plexus located halfway between the mastoid process and the greater occipital protuberance at the crest of the occipital bone and lies adjacent to the occipital artery.

Cryoneurolysis is performed for relief of occipital neuralgia and relief of occipital muscle tension headaches. The procedure is often performed bilaterally.

Spinal Accessory Nerve. The spinal part of the 11th cranial nerve emerges from the posterior border of the sternocleidomastoid muscle at the junction of the lower and middle thirds to cross the neck and supply the trapezius muscle.

Cryoneurolysis is used for severe tonic or clonic spasms of the trapezius muscle, spasmodic torticollis, and certain whiplash injuries.

The nerve is identified by motor stimulation and can be frozen either at its exit from the sternocleidomastoid or close to its entry into the trapezius.

Spine

Although it is possible to cryodenervate cervical, thoracic, and lumbar facet joints, denervation is best performed with radiofrequency probes because of the smaller probe size and better maneuverability. Radiofrequency is also preferred for sacral nerve root pain. Coccygodynia is amenable to cryoanalgesia at the sacral hiatus.

Abdomen/Pelvis

Iliohypogastric Nerve. The iliohypogastric nerve arises from the T11 and T12 nerve roots and passes anteriorly to the rectus sheath. Neuropathy results in an upper quadrant pain, which may mimic that of cholecystitis or pancreatitis or may be caused by the surgical treatment of upper abdominal pathology.

Ilioinguinal Nerve. The ilioinguinal nerve arises from the T12 and L1 nerve roots. It is often injured at lateral rectus sheath, approximately 5 cm from the midline, 10 cm inferior to the umbilicus. At this point, the nerve perforates the superior crus of the superficial inguinal ring. The nerve may be injured during inguinal herniorrhaphy, by compression resulting from bladder retraction during abdominal surgery, or, rarely, by tight-fitting garments.

Genitofemoral Nerve. The genitofemoral nerve arises from the L1 and L2 nerve roots. The genital branch of the nerve passes under the inguinal ligament and over the symphysis pubis immediately lateral to the pubic tubercle. This sensory nerve then travels to the labia or scrotum. It can be injured as the result of surgical trauma during abdominal surgery and inguinal herniorrhaphy.

The clinical presentation of genitofemoral neuralgia and ilioinguinal pathologic conditions consists of dull, aching pain in the lower quadrants of the abdomen. Pain worsens with Valsalva's maneuver, cough, bowel movement, and lifting. Patients often experience increased pain intensity and frequency with menstruation and sexual intercourse. Irritation of either nerve can result in referred pain to the testicle or vulva, interior thigh, or upper lumbar region.

The abdominal wall nerves can be localized percutaneously or with laparoscopic guidance. In the latter procedure, lower than usual intra-abdominal insufflation pressures are used with minimal sedation to permit active feedback from the patient during nerve localization. The internal inguinal ring can be identified, nerve entrapment isolated, and the nerve released. A cryoprobe can be inserted percutaneously and the nerve lesion made under direct vision.

Upper Extremity

Suprascapular Nerve. The supraclavicular nerve passes through the suprascapular notch and provides innervation to the supraspinatus, infraspinatus, and shoulder joint. Clinically, the patient complains of a poorly localized upper shoulder pain. Tenderness is elicited by palpation of the suprascapular notch. Fluoroscopic guidance is helpful in locating the superior scapular border during cryoneurolysis.

Radial Nerve. Cryoneurolysis can be preformed at the elbow and wrist. The radial nerve passes over the anterior aspect of the lateral epicondyle. Probe entry is 2 cm lateral to the biceps tendon on the intercondylar line. Localization is facilitated by stimulation. At the wrist, branches of the radial nerve are located in the anatomic "snuff box" close to the exterior pollicis longus and extensor pollicis brevis tendons.

Ulnar Nerve. Cryoneurolysis can be achieved at the elbow 2 to 3 cm proximal to the ulnar groove in the medial epicondyle. Similarly, at the wrist the nerve lies medial to the ulnar artery and beneath the flexor carpi ulnaris. The nerve is approached from the ulnar side of the tendon to block the cutaneous branches.

Median Nerve. The median nerve lies medial to the brachial artery along the intercondylar line at the elbow. At the wrist, the nerve is approached 2 cm proximal to the distal wrist crease beneath the palmaris tendon. If the tendon is absent, the point of entry is 1 cm to the flexor carpi radialis tendon.

Digital Nerves. The volar and dorsal digital nerves can be frozen at each side by insertion of the cryoprobe at the dorsolateral aspect of the base of the involved finger. Cryoneurolysis of the common volar digital nerve can also be done in the web space.

Lower Extremity

Lateral Femoral Cutaneous Nerve. The lateral femoral cutaneous nerve passes under the inguinal ligament near the anterior superior iliac spine. It is amenable to cryoneurolysis for the treatment of meralgia paresthesia. The procedure can be performed after surgical exposure or percutaneously, medial to the anterior superior iliac spine.

Superior Gluteal Nerve. The superior gluteal nerve is a branch of the sciatic nerve. After exiting the sciatic notch, it passes caudal to the inferior border of the gluteus minimus and penetrates the gluteus medius. It is injured as a result of shearing between the gluteal muscles with forced external rotation of the leg extension of the hip. The neuralgia presents as pain in the lower back; dull pain in the buttock; vague pain in the popliteal fossa; and occasionally pain extending to the foot, mimicking radiculopathy. Patients describe a "giving way" of the leg and sit with the weight on the contralateral buttock.

Saphenous Nerve. Neuralgia caused by irritation of the infrapatellar branch of the saphenous nerve is seen weeks to years after blunt injury to the tibial plateau, varicose vein surgery, or knee replacement. The nerve is vulnerable as it passes superficially to the tibial collateral ligament, piercing the sartorius tendon and fascia lata, inferior to the medial tibial condyle. The clinical presentation consists of dull pain in the knee joint and aching below the knee. Patients have trouble localizing the pain and tend to walk in a way that minimizes flexion of the knee.

Cryotherapy may be performed posteromedially to the patella at the level of the knee or more distally superior to the medial malleolus.

Peroneal Nerves. Neuralgia caused by irritation of the deep peroneal and superficial peroneal nerves can be seen weeks to years after injury to the knee, ankle, and foot. These superficial sensory nerves pass through strong ligamentous structures and are vulnerable to stretch injury with innervation of the ankle, compression injury resulting from edema, and sharp trauma caused by bone fragmentation.

The course of the superficial peroneal nerve is superficial and medial to the lateral malleolus and superficial to the inferior extensor retinaculum, terminating in the fourth and fifth toes. The clinical presentation consists of dull ankle pain aggravated by passive inversion of the ankle.

The deep peroneal nerve runs beneath the tendon of the extensor hallucis brevis, superficial to the dorsal interosseous muscle, in between the first and second metatarsal heads, terminating in the first and second toes. Patients with diabetes and women seem most vulnerable to this injury, but it is also seen occasionally after blunt injury to the dorsum of the foot. The clinical presentation consists of dull pain in the great toe that is often worse after prolonged standing. There may also be pain in the ball of the foot that is poorly localized and occasionally burning.

Cryotherapy of these nerves is best performed as far distally as possible. Lesions of the common peroneal nerve may cause significant motor weakness.

Interdigital Nerve. Entrapment neuropathy at the metatarsal head presents as Morton's neuroma. Cryoanalgesia is performed at the apex of the metatarsal bones.

Radiofrequency Lesioning

The first attempts to use direct current (DC) electricity experimentally were made in the 1870s, and it was introduced into clinical practice in the 1940s. The DC generators produced irregular unpredictable lesions. The current gene-

rators represent several important advantages over earlier DC generators:

1. The mechanism of lesion generation is different. With DC generators, the lesions were generated by dielectric mechanisms. With radiofrequency, the lesions are generated by ionic means. These lesions are more predictable.
2. The tissue temperature and thus the extent of the lesion are more controllable. Modern generators have automatic temperature controls that prevent overheating and boiling of tissue. Active electrode design has improved. Most electrodes have low thermal coefficients, which lead to faster warming of the electrode and thus more accurate depiction of the tissue temperature.
3. Electrical stimulation can be used to locate the nerve and also to prevent unwanted nerve damage.
4. Tissue resistance (impedance) can be measured. Low tissue impedance may affect the size and characteristics of the lesion generated.

Physical Principles and Equipment

The circuit consists of an active electrode, which delivers the current; a method for measuring tissue temperature; a radiofrequency generator; and a passive electrode with large surface area. Current in the region of the active electrode generates heat. The heat generated is a function of the amount of current per unit area (current density) that flows in the region of the electrode. The active electrode does not generate heat but is heated as a result of local tissue warming. The current flows from the active to the passive electrode. However, because of the much greater surface area of the passive electrode, the current density is much less. Therefore, heating and tissue damage do not usually occur at the passive electrode.

Heating of the active electrode is an important safety feature of this system, because tissue damage is related to the temperature generated. The newer electrodes have a low thermal coefficient, meaning that the electrode absorbs heat well and heats rapidly, leading to a faster response and improved safety of the system. Excessive heating causes more diffuse and permanent tissue damage. It is possible to boil tissues, and these tissues may then adhere to the electrode and be avulsed when the electrode is removed. The thermocouple lends itself better to miniaturization than the thermistor and is, therefore, more widely used.

Most electrodes are available in a number of sizes and lengths. Both reusable and disposable needles are used. Most have varying lengths of the exposed tip, and the electrode must be selected for the desired purpose.

Lesion Characteristics

It is critical to control lesion size. The size and consistency of the lesion are governed by four major factors:

1. Temperature generated. At higher temperatures, the local tissue reaction is greater.
2. Rate of thermal equilibrium. If there is more rapid equilibrium between tissues, the lesion is more uniform. Conversely, if there is slow and incomplete equilibrium, the lesion is erratic. Usually thermal equilibrium is complete by 60 seconds.

TISSUE TEMPERATURE VS. DISTANCE FROM ELECTRODE

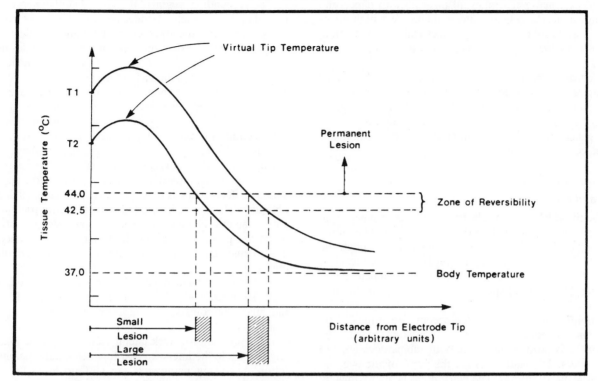

FIG. 23F–4 Tissue injury after radiofrequency lesioning. Note the shape of the lesion and also the large area of reversibility. *(From Cosman ER, Nashold BS, Ovelman-Levitt J: Theoretical aspects of radiofrequency lesions in the dorsal root entry zone. Neurosurgery 15:945, 1984.)*

3. Electrode size and configuration. Larger electrodes generate larger lesions. Larger electrodes generate bigger lesions but at the expense of more tissue trauma on insertion, unwanted neural destruction, and larger reversible zones (Fig. 23F–4).
4. Local tissue characteristics. Lesions in tissues in contact with tissues of low electrical resistance such as blood and CSF may be reduced or irregular in size and shape. Blood may also act as a heat sink, removing heat from the area and thereby limiting local tissue temperature rise and lesion size.

The size of the lesion does not correlate well with either the time or the power used, because the temperature generated depends on tissue characteristics. The lesion generated is usually an inverted cone. In vitro evidence suggests that the lesion radius is maximal at the part of the exposed electrode farthest from the tip.[31] The actual tip may not even be incorporated in the lesion, and this has important clinical implications. Nerves in contact with the tip may only be partially blocked, and an electrode placed tangential to the nerve generates a more effective lesion. The effect on tissues depends on the temperature generated. Above 45°C, irreversible tissue injury occurs. Between 42° and 45°C, temporary neural blockade occurs. In general, the larger the lesion, the larger the zone of reversibility (see Fig. 23F–4).

The histologic appearance of lesions generated by radio frequency is one of local tissue burn. Nerve architecture is destroyed. After the lesion is created, wallerian degeneration becomes apparent. The perineurium may also be destroyed. Therefore, with radiofrequency lesioning, unlike cryoneurolysis, neuroma formation is possible. Clinically, it appears that there is relative selectivity for small unmyelinated fibers at lower temperatures. Therefore, by limiting the temperature, it may be possible to damage pain fibers selectively. This selectivity has not been borne out in in vitro experiments. There is no evidence of selectivity for white or gray matter.[32,33]

Technique

Minimal sedation is used so that the patient can participate fully and accurately report the stimuli. All of the equipment, in particular the cables and thermocouple or thermistor, are checked before beginning the procedure. The lesion parameters, especially the maximal temperature, are preset. The radiofrequency probe must be of the appropriate size for the length for the needle. In particular, the correct exposed tip length, needle diameter, and the length are critical in improving the efficacy of the procedure and reducing the risk of inadvertent tissue injury. Fluoroscopy is mandatory.

The most common reason for failure to generate a lesion is a poor electrical connection, usually related to cable damage. Occasionally, the insulation on the active electrode is disrupted, with a subsequent reduction of current density and poor lesion generation. This may also lead to lesions farther up along the shaft in other tissues traversed by the needle. Poor connection may also occur at the passive electrode, leading to poor conduction or even local tissue burning. The newer machines all measure impedance and can help isolate the source of the problem. Very high impedance (>2000 ohms) suggests electrical disconnection, whereas very low impedance (<200 ohms) implies a short circuit.

Inadequate temperature generation may occur if the temperature selected is too low. Lesions tend to be smaller when lower temperatures are used (see Fig. 23F–4). Poor needle placement accounts for many technical failures. Newer lesion generators incorporate an electrical nerve stimulator to help locate the nerve.

Common Procedures

Head and Neck

Trigeminal Rhizotomy. The trigeminal nerve synapses in the gasserian ganglion before dividing into the ophthalmic, maxillary, and mandibular nerves, which pass through the foramen ovale. The gasserian ganglion is best reached through the foramen ovale, which is 7 mm in diameter and 7 mm long. The classical approach is an anterior one through the foramen ovale.

Positioning and adequate fluoroscopy are critical. The patient is positioned with the head hyperextended. The fluoroscope is positioned to give both submentovertex and lateral views. The landmarks are the pupil of the eye and external auditory meatus. The entry point is approximately 1 cm lateral to the angle of the mouth, and it should be superimposed on the foramen ovale on fluoroscopy.

The tract is anesthetized with local anesthetic solution, and generous sedation is given to the patient. The needle is advanced down the beam of the fluoroscope, aiming for the intersection of a line drawn from the external auditory meatus and a perpendicular line drawn from the pupil of the eye. Care is taken not to penetrate the buccal mucosa. When the base of the skull or lateral pterygoid plate is reached, the needle is walked into the foramen ovale and advanced. The needle is then followed on the lateral view and is advanced until it is superimposed on the clivus. CSF should flow at that stage. The active electrode is then inserted and stimulation commenced.

Paresthesia after stimulation at 50 Hz should be evident in the affected division at less than 1 V (ideally, <0.5 V). Depending on the division required, the needle might have to be repositioned for maximal paresthesia. There should be little spread of paresthesia to other divisions. Motor stimulation at 2 Hz should be minimal. Ideally, the threshold for motor stimulation should be at least twice the sensory stimulation threshold. The probe position should be checked in both submentovertex and lateral positions before the lesion is created. Sequential low-temperature burns are used, starting at 60°C for 1 minute. Sensory loss is checked between lesions, especially loss of corneal sensation. Two additional 1-minute lesions are then made at 63° and 65°C.

Spine

Cervical Facet Denervation. Chronic cervical pain is one of most difficult syndromes to treat. Cervical zygapophyseal denervation, ganglionotomy, and partial rhizotomy have been used widely for persistent cervical pain without radiculopathy and with a response to diagnostic local anesthetic block.

The facet joints are innervated by the primary ramus of the corresponding segmental nerve and the nerve more cephalad. This branch separates nerve immediately from the nerve as it exits the intervertebral foramen. It then loops around the waist of the transverse process and passes posteriorly. Lower cervical facets C6 to T1 are similar in anatomy to lumbar facets, and the technique is similar.

Two approaches can be used for upper cervical facets (C2 to C6). In the traditional approach, the patient is in a prone position and the anteroposterior view is used. The needle is advanced until it makes contact with the transverse process at or near the waist. This approach has the disadvantage of having a small area of contact. Alternatively, the patient can be in a supine position with the head rotated to the opposite side. The fluoroscope is positioned approximately 10 degrees obliquely. The needle is inserted in the posterior triangle and passed anteriorly under intermittent fluoroscopy until the transverse process is reached. In this approach the needle is more tangential to the nerve and better results should be obtained.[34]

A 22-gauge, 5-cm needle with a 4-mm exposed tip is used. Stimulation should be performed at 50 and 2 Hz. Few radicular symptoms should be reported, and no motor stimulation should be seen.

It is important to check lateral views to exclude inadvertent entry into the intervertebral foramen before making the lesion. Lesioning parameters are 60°C to 80°C for 60 to 90 seconds.

Thoracic Facet Denervation. Denervation is indicated for thoracic facet joint syndrome. The thoracic facet is innervated by the medial branch of the dorsal ramus of the corresponding segmental nerve and by the nerve from the more cephalad ramus, in a manner similar to the innervation of the lumbar facet joint. The nerve passes over the junction of the superior articular process and the transverse process.

Stimulation should be at 50 Hz and less than 1 V. Motor stimulation should not be seen when 2 Hz is used at 2 V. Lesions are usually created at 80°C for 90 seconds.

Lumbar Facet Denervation. Denervation is indicated for persistent facet-mediated low back pain with good response to diagnostic blocks. The lumbar facet is innervated by the medial branch of the posterior ramus of the corresponding nerve root cephalad to it. The nerve loops over the junction of the transverse process and superior articular process. On a 10-degree oblique view under fluoroscopy, this loop resembles the eye of a Scottie dog.

The skin directly over the target area is marked. A skin wheal is raised with local anesthetic. Care is taken to avoid inadvertent block of the target nerve when infiltrating more superficial tissues. The needle is inserted parallel to the fluoroscopy beam and advanced with intermittent fluoroscopy until the target area is reached. The radiofrequency probe is then inserted and stimulation commenced at 50 and 2 Hz. Minimal radicular paresthesia and no motor fasciculation should be seen. Reproduction of the pain should be obtained at less than 1 V. The needle may have to be repositioned for this purpose.

Before creating the lesion, it is important to check a lateral view and impedance. If the impedance is too low, there may be a short circuit or the needle may be positioned in an area of low impedance such as a blood vessel or CSF. In either case, the lesion would be unpredictable. Lesions are generated at 80ºC for 90 seconds. The chances of success can be improved by positioning the needle tangentially to the nerve.

Reported side effects include major nerve injury, inadvertent dural puncture, hemorrhage, and infection.

Dorsal Root Ganglionotomy. Dorsal root ganglionotomy is a procedure reserved for patients with radicular unresponsive to less interventional techniques. Usually, both diskal and posterior elemental causes are ruled before embarking on this form of therapy.

Cervical Ganglion Rhizotomy. The C2 ganglion lies on the arch of the second cervical vertebra. The patient is in a supine position. Using a lateral projection, the needle is inserted between the first and second cervical vertebrae. The target is the upper two thirds of the second cervical arch. The needle is then advanced under an anteroposterior view (through the mouth) until it appears to lie approximately halfway across the C1 to C2 facet joint. The other cervical ganglia are approached laterally or obliquely with the patient supine. The needle should lie in the posterior intervertebral foramen and not project beyond the midpoint of the corresponding facet joint.

Thoracic Ganglion Rhizotomy. In the thoracic spine, the approach is complicated by the presence of the ribs and close proximity of the pleura. Here the oblique approach is associated with increased risk of pneumothorax. In the upper thoracic spine it is difficult to obtain good needle position by the oblique approach because the needle tends to lie too far anteriorly or laterally. The recommended posterior approach involves drilling through the lamina using a K wire and inserting the probe through this and into the intervertebral foramen.

Lumbar Ganglion Rhizotomy. Before rhizotomy, diagnostic nerve sleeve blocks are performed to isolate the source of the pain. Using fluoroscopy, the needle is inserted in an oblique manner, aiming slightly cephalad under the transverse process. The position is checked frequently with anteroposterior and lateral projections. The needle should lie in the posterosuperior part of the intervertebral foramen, and the tip should not project beyond the midpoint of the corresponding facet joint; otherwise, it is possible to puncture the dura.

Lumbar Disk and Ramus Communicans. Lesions of the lumbar disk and ramus communicans are indicated for persistent pain of disk origin. The disk level is usually confirmed by discography before the procedure. The innervation of the disk is complex, involving many different nerves. From posterior to anterior, the disk is innervated by segmental nerve rami, communicating rami, and the sympathetic chain. Full disk denervation involves lesioning all these nerves bilaterally. Interest has focused on the L2 dorsal root ganglion as a possible common entry point for the sinuvertebral nerves, which may make disk denervation ore feasible.[35]

Two procedures are commonly performed. The offending disk can be directly lesioned, or, alternatively, the ramus communicans may be lesioned.

Percutaneous Sympathectomy

Stellate Ganglionotomy

Stellate ganglionotomy is most commonly performed for long-term control of sympathetically maintained pain of the upper extremity and face. Less commonly, it may be per-

formed for intractable angina, Prinzmetal's angina, and hyperhidrosis.

The stellate ganglion is formed by the fusion of the lowest cervical and first thoracic ganglia. It lies over the transverse process of the C7 vertebra, being separated from it by the longus colli muscle. The traditional anterior approach is most commonly used. The transverse process of C7 is identified. A 5-cm, 22-gauge needle with a 4-mm exposed tip is passed medial to the neurovascular bundle until the junction of the vertebral body and the transverse process is reached. The needle is then withdrawn at least 2 mm to avoid making a lesion in the longus colli. Real-time fluoroscopy with a contrast medium is important to rule out intravascular needle placement.

Stimulation at 50 and 2 Hz is performed to avoid inadvertent lesioning of a sensory or motor nerve. The recurrent laryngeal nerve is vulnerable, and phonation should be checked during motor stimulation and before lesioning. No change in phonation should be observed at 2 V and 2 Hz. High-frequency stimulation may generate diffuse pain in the ipsilateral face and upper extremity. Changes in regional blood flow should be apparent after the procedure.

Three lesions are made along the junction of the vertebral body and transverse process. Lesioning at 80ºC for 30 to 60 seconds is recommended. Using plethysmography or temperature can monitor the efficacy. Adverse events include pneumothorax, recurrent laryngeal nerve palsy, vascular injury, and inadvertent somatic nerve injury.

Thoracic Sympathectomy

Percutaneous thoracic sympathectomy is occasionally performed for intractable angina, Raynaud's phenomenon, causalgia, and hyperhidrosis. The proximity of the pleura makes pneumothorax common. The advent of laparoscopic surgery has reduced the number of these procedures performed. Needle placement guided by CT allows improved efficacy and reduced complications.

Lumbar Sympathectomy

Lumbar sympathectomy is indicated for sympathetically maintained pain and ischemia of the lower extremity. The sympathetic chain lies on the anterolateral aspect of the lumbar vertebra and anterior to the psoas sheath. The kidney and ureter lie laterally and the great vessels and the viscera anteriorly. Communicating rami pass between the posterior rami and the sympathetic chain. The needle used is a 15-cm, 18-gauge needle with a 5-mm exposed tip. The patient is in a prone position. Using fluoroscopy, the L3 vertebra is identified. The tip of the transverse process is encountered. The needle is then walked off the transverse process superiorly and advanced under fluoroscopic guidance until the vertebral body is reached. The needle is then repositioned to pass along the body and to lie posterior to the anterior border of the vertebral body. Needle position is confirmed on a lateral projection. Contrast material is injected to confirm placement anterior to the psoas sheath. A further needle may be positioned at either L2 or L4 to improve the efficacy of the procedure.

Stimulation at 50 Hz may reproduce diffuse pain in the lower extremities. There should be no radicular pain with stimulation at 50 Hz and 1 V and no motor stimulation at 2 Hz. After the initial lesion, the needle may be advanced to reach the anterior border of the vertebral body. Multiple lesions at 90°C for up to 3 minutes are used.

References

1. *Webster's new collegiate dictionary,* ed 9. Springfield, Mass, Merriam-Webster, 1985.
2. Ghormley RK: Low back pain: With special reference to the articular facets, with presentation of an operative procedure. *JAMA* 101:1773, 1933.
3. Hadley LA: Anatomic-roentgenographic studies of the posterior spinal articulations. *AJR* 86:270, 1961.
4. Lewin T, Moffett B, Viidik A: The morphology of the lumbar synovial intervertebral joints. *Acta Morphol Neurol Scand* 4:299, 1961.
5. Mooney V, Robertson J: The facet syndrome. *Clin Orthop* 115:149, 1976.
6. Pederson HE, Blunck CFJ, Gardiner E: The anatomy of lumbosacral posterior rami and meningeal branches of spinal nerves (sinu-vertebral nerves). *J Bone Joint Surg Am* 38A:377, 1956.
7. Nade S, Bell E, Wyke BD: The innervation of the lumbar spinal joints and its significance. *J Bone Surg* 62:255, 1980.
8. Bonica JJ: *The management of pain.* Philadelphia, Lea & Febiger, 1953.
9. Dory MA: Arthrography of the cervical facet joints. Radiology 148:379, 1983.
10. Glover JR: Arthrography of the joints of the lumbar vertebral arches. *Orthop Clin North Am* 8:37, 1977.
11. Destouet JM, Gilula LA, Murphy WA et al: Lumbar facet joint injection: Indication, technique, clinical correlation, and preliminary results. *Radiology* 145:321, 1982.
12. Dory MA: Arthrography of the lumbar facet joints. *Radiology* 140:23, 1981.
13. Ghelman B, Goldman AB: Lumbar facet injection. In Goldman AB, editor: *Procedures in skeletal radiology.* Orlando, Fla, Grune & Stratton, 1984.
14. Carrera GF: Lumbar facet joint injection in low back pain and sciatica: Preliminary results. *Radiology* 137:665, 1980.
15. Carrera GF, Williams AL, Haughton VM: Computed tomography in sciatica. *Radiology* 137:433, 1980.
16. Risius B, 1: Modic MT, Hardy RW Jr et al: Sector computed tomographic spine scanning in the diagnosis of lumbar root entrapment. *Radiology* 143:109, 1982.
17. Sluijter ME: *Radiofrequency lesions in the treatment of cervical pain syndromes.* Burlington, Mass, Radionics, 1990.
18. Zakrzewska JM: Cryotherapy for trigeminal neuralgia: A 10 year audit. *Br J Oral Maxillofac Surg* 29:1, 1991.
19. Zakrzewska JM, Thomas DG: Patient's assessment of outcome after three surgical procedures for the management of trigeminal neuralgia. *Acta Neurochir* 122:225, 1993.
20. North RB, Kidd DH, Zahurak M et al: Specificity of diagnostic nerve blocks: A prospective, randomized study of sciatica due to lumbosacral spine disease. *Pain* 65:77, 1996.
21. Hogan QH, Erickson SJ, Abram SE: Computerized tomography-guided stellate ganglion blockade. *Anesthesiology* 77:596, 1992.
22. Hogan QH, Erickson SJ, Haddox JD et al: The spread of solutions during stellate ganglion block. *Reg Anesth* 17:78, 1992.
23. Saberski LR: Cryoneurolysis in clinical practice. In Waldman SD, Winnie AP, editors: *Interventional pain management,* ed 1. Philadelphia, WB Saunders, 1996.
24. Gill W, Da Costa J, Fraser J: The control and predictability of a cryolesion. *Cryobiology* 6:347, 1970.
25. Douglas WW, Malcolm JL: The effects of localized cooling on conduction in cat nerves. *J Physiol (Lond)* 130:53, 1955.
26. Mazur P: Physical and chemical factors underlying cell injury in cryosurgical freezing. In Ranh RW, editor: *Cryosurgery.* Springfield, Ill, Charles C Thomas, 1968.
27. Whittaker DK: Ice crystals formed in tissues during cryosurgery. I. Light microscopy. *Cryobiology* 11:192, 1974.
28. Whittaker DK: Ice crystals formed in tissues during cryosurgery. II. Electron microscopy. *Cryobiology* 11:202, 1974.
29. Denny-Brown D: The pathology of injury to nerve induced by cold. *J Neuropathol Exp Neurol* 4:305, 1945.
30. Carter DC, Lee PW, Gill W et al: The effect of cryosurgery on peripheral nerve function. *J R Coll Surg Edinb* 17:25, 1972.
31. Bogduk N, Macintosh J, Marsland A: Technical limitations to the efficacy of radiofrequency neurotomy for spinal pain. *Neurosurgery* 20:529, 1987.
32. Cosman ER, Nashold BS, Ovelman-Levitt J: Theoretical aspects of radiofrequency lesions in the dorsal root entry zone. *Neurosurgery* 15:945, 1984.
33. Smith HP, McWhorter JM, Challa VR: Radiofrequency neurolysis in a clinical model: Neuropathological correlation. *J Neurosurg* 55:246, 1981.
34. Sluyter ME: Radiofrequency lesions in the treatment of cervical syndromes. In *Procedure Technique Series.* Burlington, Mass, Radionics, 1990.
35. Nakamura SI, Takahashi K, Takahashi Y et al: The afferent pathways of discogenic low-back pain: Evaluation of L2 spinal nerve infiltration. *J Bone Joint Surg Br* 78:606, 1996.

CHAPTER **23**

Interventional Techniques

JOHN C. OAKLEY, PETER S. STAATS, AND SAMUEL HASSENBUSCH

IMPLANTABLE INFUSION PUMPS

In the search for a more convenient, more effective, and safer method for delivering intraspinal opioids, an adaptation was made of a constant flow pump manufactured by the Strato-Infusaid Corporation (now Arrow, Inc.) for the administration of intravascular, and occasionally intrathecal, chemotherapeutic agents. This device is a hollow titanium cylinder separated into two chambers by metal bellows, as illustrated in Figure 23G–1. In one chamber, a two-phase (gas-liquid) charging fluid (Freon) is permanently sealed between the bellows and the outside wall of the cylinder. The other chamber is the drug reservoir, which is percutaneously filled with the infusate via a self-sealing septum.

Filling the drug reservoir compresses the charging fluid and returns it to a liquid state. As the body temperature warms the charging fluid, it becomes a vapor and exerts a continuous pressure on the drug reservoir. This pressure forces the infusate from the reservoir through an outlet filter and flow-restricting capillary tube assembly. The infusate then enters the silicone rubber delivery tube exiting the pump. The result is a continuous delivery of medication at a constant flow rate if temperature and pressure remain unchanged. An inconvenience of this device is that it is necessary to change the concentration of the drug in the reservoir to alter the prescription of medication. An advantage of this type of delivery system is its long lifetime, which is limited only by the number of punctures the refill septum can tolerate.

Largely because of the clinical demand for a drug delivery system with which the prescription of intraspinal medication could be changed without draining and refilling the reservoir, the Medtronic Corporation in 1988 introduced an externally programmable, fully implantable pump. It was initially released for cancer-related pain of all types in 1991, after 7 years of clinical trials. This device is an implantable, programmable, battery-powered pump that stores and delivers medication according to instructions delivered by an external programmer (Fig. 23G–2).

SELECTION OF PATENTS

In general, intraspinal pain therapy using implantable drug administration systems has been reserved for patients whose condition is considered chronic.

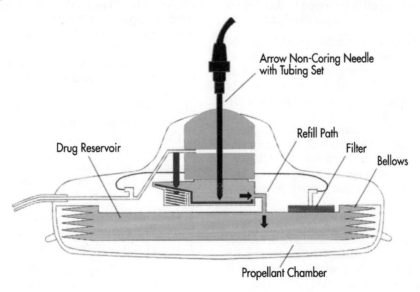

FIG. 23G–1 Infusaid-Arrow pump. *(Courtesy of Arrow International, Inc.)*

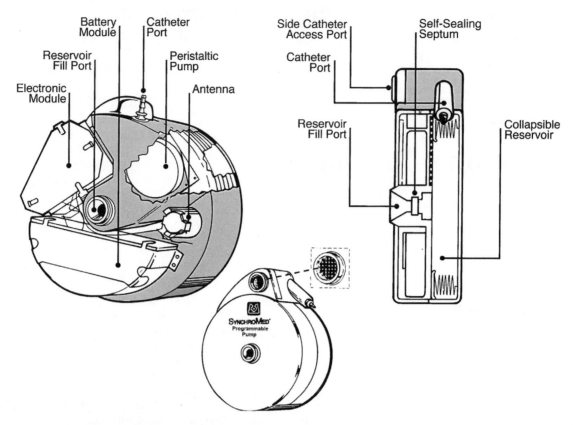

FIG. 23G–2 The SynchroMed Infusion System (Medtronic, Inc., Minneapolis, Minn) allows a precise amount of drug into the space around the spinal cord. The programmable delivery device is implanted under the skin near the patient's abdomen. A liquid form of the drug baclofen is placed in a reservoir inside the pump and is delivered through a small-diameter catheter into the space around the spinal cord where it is needed. The pump is available in sizes of 18 ml and 10 ml. *(Courtesy of Medtronic, Inc., Minneapolis, Minn.)*

With regard to cancer-related pain, although the disease is progressive, if the pain is expected to last beyond 3 months, it can be thought of as chronic. The indication for use of implantable drug administration systems then includes the treatment of chronic pain of both cancer-related and noncancer-related varieties.

Classifying patients with regard to pain type further refines selection. There are two nonspecific categories of pain:

1. *Nociceptive pain* is mediated at receptors widely distributed in cutaneous tissue, bone, muscle, connective tissue, vessels, and viscera. These nociceptors are classified as thermal, chemical, and mechanical. The pain is usually described as sharp, dull, aching, and/or throbbing. In general, nociceptive pain is opioid-responsive.
2. *Neuropathic pain* is elicited by damage to the peripheral or central nervous system and is described as burning, tingling, shooting, electric-like, or lightning-like. Although the pain responds to opioid analgesics in high concentrations, it is less responsive than nociceptive pain at the usual clinical levels.[1–3]

Beyond the requirements for an adequate history and physical examination to assess pain type and medical risk factors, there are general inclusion and exclusion criteria for the use of implantable devices that may help improve outcomes if rigorously applied. These are shown in Table 23G–1.

Psychologic assessment is an important part of the selection process. It is performed to identify any psychologic problems that, if left untreated, might prevent a successful outcome of therapy.[4]

Screening

Patients selected as candidates for intraspinal opioid administration should not have benefited from optimal medical management. The implanting physician must be certain that more conservative interventions have been adequately tried and that a trial of systemic opioid therapy has been undertaken. Before an implanted pump is used, it is important to perform an appropriate trial to assure the patient and the physician that they will do well with long-term administration of intrathecal opiates.

There is no proven method of screening for the safety and efficacy of intraspinal opioids, but the response to the acute administration of such medication is thought to predict the long-term efficacy of the treatment. The goals for any screening trial are primarily two:

1. Does the patient have side effects with the administered drug that would contraindicate the therapy?
2. Does the patient demonstrate pain relief?

Just as there are no proven methods of screening, there is no proven length of screening trial.[5]

TABLE 23G–1 Exclusion and Inclusion Criteria for Intraspinal Opioids

Exclusion Criteria
Absolute exclusion
    Aplastic anemia
    Systemic infection
    Known allergies to the materials in the implant
    Known allergies to the intended medication(s)
    Active intravenous drug abuse
    Psychosis or dementia
Relative exclusion
    Emaciated patient
    Ongoing anticoagulation therapy
    Child before fusion of the epiphyses
    Occult infection possible
    Recovering drug addict
    Opioid nonresponsivity (other drugs may be considered)
    Lack of social or family support
    Socioeconomic problems
    Lack of access to medical care

Inclusion Criteria
Pain type and generator appropriate
    Demonstrated opioid responsivity
    No untreated psychopathologic condition that might
        predispose to an unsuccessful outcome
    Successful completion of a screening trial

Single intrathecal bolus dosing, epidural infusion, and intrathecal infusion are the predominant screening methods employed.[1] Bolus intrathecal doses are administered by lumbar puncture, and the patient is monitored for side effects and pain relief. This technique may maximize reports of nausea and may provoke a higher incidence of urinary retention. Reported pain relief can persist for up to 24 hours but tends to peak in the first few hours. In a retrospective review of a number of centers with 429 physicians conducted by Paice and coworkers,[1] 33.7% used this method.

Although this approach can be helpful in determining whether pain relief exists and whether intractable side effects develop, many practitioners feel that it does not control for the placebo effect. Few clinicians feel that a blinded placebo trial is helpful. In the study of Paice and colleagues, 18.3% still used such a trial. The placebo response occurs in 0% to 100% of patients, and there are no data indicating that a patient will not do well with an implanted morphine pump.[6,7] In fact, data have indicated that the words patients say to themselves about their pain drastically affects their tolerance endurance and threshold for pain.[8] Thus, it is not appropriate to deny a patient implantable therapy on the basis of a positive placebo response.[9]

Screening Technique

There are two widely used and accepted approaches to the screening technique. The percutaneous approach is often used by one of us (P.S.S.). In this technique a paramedian approach is used to enter the intrathecal space. Under fluoroscopic guidance the catheter is threaded to the level of the substantia gelatinosa at which pain transmission is modulated. Dye is the often injected to confirm appropriate catheter placement and document free flow of cerebrospinal fluid (CSF). After a tract of local anesthetic is applied, the stylet of a Tuohy needle is placed beside the first needle and threaded laterally. A second 17-gauge Tuohy needle is advanced over the stylet. At this point the first Tuohy needle is withdrawn and the catheter is threaded down the second Tuohy needle. After the patient has completed the trial, this catheter cannot be internalized and must be removed and discarded. This approach has the advantages that it does not create incisional pain that can confuse the trial and that the device can easily be removed if the trial is unsuccessful. On the other hand, instrumenting the spine twice is necessary if the patient does well and then undergoes implantation.

The surgical approach, employed successfully by one of us (J.O.), avoids instrumenting the spine twice when the patient has a successful trial. With this technique, the patient is taken to the operating room and placed prone on a fluoroscopic operating table, and the back is prepared in sterile fashion. The area is squared off with sterile towels, and a "chest-breast" drape with a large fenestrated opening is applied. This wide exposure enables placement of the catheter and tunneling to the side. A 1- to 2-inch incision is made, and a paraspinous intrathecal puncture is performed with the needle appropriate to the intrathecal catheter used. The catheter is then introduced under fluoroscopic control to the desired spinal level, most often T10, but may be more focally located according to the pathologic condition or drug used. A second catheter, the extension catheter, which is designed to be disposable, is tunneled using a malleable cardiac pacemaker tunneling trocar to the flank opposite the surgeon from the back skin incision. This catheter is then connected to the intrathecal catheter with a suitable connector, tied with 2-0 silk, and then anchored to the lumbar fascia with 2-0 silk in a figure-of-eight fashion. The wound is closed with an interrupted inverted layer of 3-0 absorbable suture and Steri-Strips are applied to the skin edge. Alternatively, staples may be used. An antiseptic bandage is placed around the percutaneously exiting catheter. A Biopatch (Johnson & Johnson) impregnated with chlorhexidine gluconate (Hibiclens) is used in the author's (J.O.) clinic. Some external extension catheters require fitting a Luer-Lok connector on the externalized end to facilitate mating with the infusion catheter coming from the pump. The back wound is dressed, and the patient is now ready to begin receiving medication using an external infusion pump as a screening trial.

An important concern is the patient's current opioid use and how to manage it at the time of screening. Eliminating opioids before screening may cause unwarranted discomfort to the patient and may add to the expense of the trial.[5] A complete conversion from systemic opioid to intraspinal opioid may result in an abstinence syndrome. Therefore, a clinical protocol during the screening trial is necessary to prevent withdrawal effects.

IMPLANTATION

Pump Preparation

When the decision to proceed to a permanent implant is made, the surgical aspects are similar. Variation arises in the pump preparation sequence. It is efficient in terms of time and ultimately cost to have an implant assistant perform pump preparation while the implant surgery is being performed. With proper timing, both procedures can be performed to allow the pump to be ready for implantation as the surgical preparation is completed.

Surgical Implantation Technique

Implantation may take place with the patient under general or local anesthesia with monitoring. Local anesthesia is often preferred in an outpatient setting because it lends itself to rapid recovery after the procedure. When general anesthesia is chosen, the use of muscle relaxants is often deferred until after the catheter is threaded into the intrathecal space. The steps are as follows:

1. Before the implantation, the clinician should spend time with the patient to decide on the side and location of the pump. About the only area amenable to the implantation of these generally large devices is the right or left lower quadrant of the abdomen. The anatomic constraints tend to be the iliac crest, the symphysis pubis, the ilioinguinal ligament, and the costal margin. These structures should not touch the pump when the patient is in the seated position. The task is easier with more obese patients and can be very difficult with cachectic cancer patients.

2. One should position the patient in the lateral decubitus position on the operating table with the side of implantation upward. At this stage, C-arm fluoroscopy may be necessary if a new intrathecal catheter is to be placed.

3. The instrument is positioned to permit an anteroposterior view, allowing easy lumbar puncture and identification of the catheter tip level.

4. The clinician should implant the catheter through a paramedian approach after making a 5- to 8-cm incision in the skin down to the lumbar fascia.

5. One should document a good flow of spinal fluid and clamp the catheter to the drape to prevent CSF loss.

6. The incision is packed with an antibiotic-soaked sponge.

7. If the existing catheter is to be used as the permanent delivery catheter, as in the screening technique of the first author (P.S.S.), one should place the patient on the operating table in the decubitus position, with the implantation side upward and the exiting screening extension catheter downward. Preparation and draping for implantation then proceed as usual.

8. One should reopen the previous back incision and disconnect the disposable extension catheter from the permanent intrathecal catheter. The circulating nurse should pull it out from under the patient.

9. The clinician should clamp the intrathecal catheter to prevent CSF loss. The rest of the implantation proceeds in the usual manner.

10. Turning attention to the lower quadrant of the abdomen, a 10-cm incision is made down to the underlying subcutaneous fat layer. A subcutaneous pocket is fashioned that is large enough to admit the particular pump being used. Generally, if all four fingers can be admitted to the metacarpal phalangeal joints in the pocket, it is large enough.

11. One should undermine the upper side of the incision roughly the width of the pump or about 2.5 cm to allow closure without tension. The eccentric location of the pocket allows the pump to be placed in such a fashion that the refill port is clear of the incisional scar and easier to locate. An ideal pocket is one that allows placement of the pump without struggle but is tight enough to aid in preventing pump rotation. The depth of the pocket below the skin is critical for programmable pumps. A depth greater then 2.5 cm may not allow reliable telemetry.

12. In fashioning the pocket, one should maintain meticulous hemostasis to avoid postoperative hematoma formation. At this point, the pocket is packed with an antibiotic-soaked sponge.

13. Next, one should tunnel the catheter connecting the intrathecal catheter to the pump, the extension catheter, from the pump pocket to the back incision using a malleable tunneling device. The author (J.O.) uses a cardiac pacemaker tunneling tool. Shunt tunneling tools may also be used, and the tunneling system provided with the programmable pump works well. Because most constant flow rate pumps come with the extension catheter connected to the pump at the factory, the catheter must be attached to the programmable pump.

14. A connection is made between the extension catheter and the intrathecal catheter using a male-to-male tubing connector. This connector may be made of titanium or plastic material.

15. This construct is covered with some type of anchoring device, which is secured to the connector with 2-0 nonabsorbable braided tie, and the construct is anchored to the underlying muscle fascia in a figure-of-eight fashion. One should not skip the anchoring; without it, the intrathecal catheter will migrate, usually coiling under the skin.

16. The extension catheter is connected to the previously prepared programmable pump and secured to the pump with a 2-0 braided tie. Pumps with a previously attached catheter must be placed into the pocket at the time of catheter tunneling.

17. The programmable pump is placed into the subcutaneous pocket. The Synchromed pump in its polyester pouch may be placed without need for further suturing. Pumps without this pouch may have anchoring loops manufactured around the pump circumference. The use of these structures is problematic. A nonabsorbable stitch is placed into a tissue that does not necrose rapidly, as do fat and muscle. At least two stitches should be used to prevent rotation; three may be necessary to prevent flipping. A dermal or fascial stitch is usually required, and there is a risk that the anchor will be painful. If this technique is used, one should place the stitches into the pocket first, then through the pump suture loops. One should place the pump into the pocket and tie the sutures. If the pocket is carefully fashioned, even a pump lacking a Dacron pouch may be placed without suturing, especially in thin patients.

18. The clinician should carefully close the incisions. An interrupted, inverted layer of 2-0 absorbable suture in the abdomen and 3-0 absorbable suture in the back is sufficient. Then the skin edges are apposed with Steri-Strips. If tension is a problem, surgical staples should be used to reinforce the closure.

OUTCOMES

Although most patients with chronic noncancer-related and cancer-related pain are adequately managed with oral analgesic medications, electrostimulation, or behavioral techniques, studies indicate that only about half of the patients so treated with back pain or neuropathic pain achieve good reduction of pain, and a full 21% are unresponsive to opioid therapy.[10,11] Long-term results are even less satisfactory, with only 16.7% reporting adequate relief.[12]

COMPLICATIONS

Any technique involving a surgical procedure, a prosthetic device, and the infusion of medication has complications. With implantable drug administration systems, complications may be divided into three categories: surgical complications, device-related complications, and drug-related complications.

Surgical Complications

In the perioperative period, bleeding with subsequent development of a pocket hematoma is perhaps the most troublesome and preventable problem. Meticulous attention to hemostasis during pump pocket formation prevents this problem. Prevention is aided by placing an abdominal binder, such as a 6-inch Ace wrap, around the abdomen and lightly compressing the fresh pump pocket for 24 to 48 hours. This compression dressing helps to avoid accumulation of blood or fluid in the pocket.

The possibility of epidural and intrathecal hemorrhage with the obvious risk of neurologic injury is often mentioned. This complication, unfortunately, is likely to be unnoticeable at the time of catheter implantation. Preoperatively, care should be taken to discontinue nonsteroidal anti-inflammatory drugs and reverse any anticoagulation. Signs of a developing hematoma are usually a sudden increase in focal back pain associated with tenderness, progressing numbness or weakness in the lower extremities, and loss of bowel or bladder control resulting in either retention or incontinence. This clinical presentation warrants immediate imaging studies with magnetic resonance imaging (MRI) or computed tomography (CT)-myelography and emergent neurosurgical intervention if there is neurologic deterioration.

With implantable devices, one of the most feared complications is that of wound infection. Prophylactic antibiotics have been controversial, but a consensus seems to have developed for using some preoperative antibiosis. One method is to use a cephalosporin intravenously 1 hour before surgery without subsequent antibiosis. Some clinics use daily prophylaxis while an externalized screening electrode trial is performed. Intraoperatively, antibiotic irrigation may be used. Attention on the part of surgical personnel to handling all parts with care and avoiding unnecessary contact with any, even prepared, skin may cut down on contamination.

With catheter placement, the spinal cord is at risk. Catheters that are spring wound or have stiffening wires internally must not be forced through the spinal canal because the tip may be buried in an intramedullary position. Penetration of the spinal cord often results in the production of dysesthesias or a burning, stinging pain below the lesion that is nondermatomal and may not result in noticeable neurologic signs immediately. Intramedullary infusion of drug may result in progressive signs of a spinal cord lesion, and this should be immediately evaluated with MRI or CT myelography and dealt with appropriately by the neurosurgeon.

CSF leaks are a natural consequence of placing catheters in the subarachnoid space. The opening created in the dura mater by the introducing needle is larger than the entering catheter, predisposing to some potential leakage. The dura mater has a moderate amount of elasticity, which probably explains why the incidence of leaks is not higher. If the particular technique used seems to result in a relatively high incidence of spinal headache or CSF collection under the skin, a blood patch injecting 10 to 20 ml of autologous venous blood one level above the catheter entry point or at the entry point under fluoroscopic control (to avoid shearing the intrathecal catheter) may treat this problem effectively.

Device-Related Complications

The most frequently reported complications with implantable pump systems involve some failure in the catheter system. Pump complications are rare. Early reports contained many catheter-related complications.[13,14] With the development of more thick-walled and reinforced catheters, new anchoring techniques, and paraspinous approaches to placement, this problem seems to have decreased.[15]

Infusate-Related Complications

Errors related to the infusate may occur if meticulous attention is not paid to the type of system used, the drug used, the drug concentration used, the dead space present in the system, and the prescription entered with the programmable systems. Errors that occur may result in a life-threatening overdose. Some mechanism for verification of these parameters should be in place at the initial filling and at each refill procedure. When more than one drug is placed in the pump, the potential errors in dosing are compounded and a skilled operator and careful calculation are required.

References

1. Paice JA, Penn RD, Shott S: Intraspinal morphine for chronic pain: A retrospective multicenter study. *J Pain Symptom Manage* 11:71, 1996.
2. Hassenbusch SJ, Stanton-Hicks M, Covington EC: Long-term intraspinal infusions of opioids in the treatment of neuropathic pain. *J Pain Symptom Manage* 10:527, 1995.
3. Portenoy RK, Foley KM: Chronic use of opioid analgesics in non-malignant pain: Report of 38 cases. *Pain* 25:171, 1986.
4. Olson K: *An approach to psychological assessment of chronic pain patients.* Minneapolis, Minn, NCS Assessments, 1992.
5. Turner JA, Loeser JD: The importance of placebo effects in pain treatment and research. *JAMA* 271:1609, 1994.
6. Tyler DB: The influence of a placebo and medication on motion sickness. *Am J Physiol* 146:458, 1946.
7. Liberman R: An experimental study of the placebo response under three different situations of pain. *J Psychiatr Res* 2:233, 1964.
8. Staats PS, Staats AW, Hekmat H: Placebo suggestion and pain: Negative as well as positive. *J Pain Symptom Manage* 15:235, 1998.
9. Staats PS: Implications of the placebo response for interventional pain specialists. *J Inter Neuromod* 5(2):69, 2002.
10. Winkelmuller M, Winkelmuller W: Long-term effects of continuous intrathecal opioid treatment in chronic pain of nonmalignant etiology. *J Neurosurg* 85:458, 1996.
11. Zenz M, Strumpf M, Tryba M: Long-term oral opioid therapy in patients with chronic nonmalignant pain. *J Pain Symptom Manage* 7:69, 1992.
12. Schulzech S, Gleim M, Maier C: Morphintabletten bei chronischen nicht-tumorbedingten schmerzen. Welche faktoren beeinflussen erfolg oder misserfolg einer langzeittherapie. *Anaesthesist* 42:545, 1993.
13. Coffey JR, Cahill D, Steers W et al: Intrathecal baclofen for intractable spasticity of spinal origin: Results of a long-term multicenter study. *J Neurosurg* 78:226, 1993.
14. Penn RD, York MM, Paice JA: Catheter systems for intrathecal drug delivery. *J Neurosurg* 83:215, 1995.
15. Krames ES: Intrathecal infusion therapies for intractable pain: Patient management guidelines. *J Pain Symptom Manage* 8:36, 1993.

1. In a patient whose headaches are positional and are associated with diplopia, vertigo, tinnitus, nystagmus, hearing loss, photophobia, nausea, and vomiting, the headache can be termed

   A. Cervicogenic headache
   B. Migraine headache
   C. Episodic cluster headache
   D. Postdural puncture headache

2. The most common indication for gasserian ganglion block is

   A. Glossopharyngeal neuralgia
   B. Atypical facial pain
   C. Trigeminal neuralgia
   D. Migraine headache

3. A lateral approach first described by Reid should be done in the following manner except

   A. Place the patient prone.
   B. Mark the inferior part of T12 and the posterior iliac crest.
   C. Take the midpoint between the two lines and mark the point of entry 7 cm from midline to lie at the L2-3 region.
   D. Perform the procedure blindly.

4. The catheter location for continuous infusion for postoperative pain relief for lower abdominal surgery should be

   A. T2 to T8
   B. T4 to L1
   C. T10 to L3
   D. T12 to L3

5. Cushingoid lesions including moon facies can last for several months after the following procedure

   A. Lumbar sympathetic block
   B. Trigeminal gangliolysis
   C. Epidural steroid injection
   D. Facet medial branch block

ANSWERS

1. D
2. C
3. D
4. C
5. C

CHAPTER 24

Surgical Techniques

SAMUEL HASSENBUSCH

The surgical techniques for management of chronic pain can be conceptually divided into those that affect various anatomic sites and those that are possibly reversible. The procedures in this chapter are presented in an anatomic progression from anterior intracranial targets to spinal procedures to techniques that affect peripheral nerves (Fig. 24–1). Each anatomic compartment also addresses the irreversible ablative techniques, generally using radiofrequency methods or neurolytic solutions, as well as the augmentative procedures, such as electrical stimulation and selective drug infusion.

This examination does not distinguish the procedures used predominantly for cancer from those used mainly for noncancer-related pain, although these indications are discussed as needed. As survival times become longer with aggressive cancer treatment, more pain syndromes have resulted from the actual treatment or even have been coincidental and not related to the cancer or its treatment. For this reason, the selection of a procedure should be based on the nature of the pain (e.g., nociceptive vs. neuropathic). Notable exceptions are some of these procedures, especially ablative techniques at intracranial sites, that might provide a limited time of pain relief. In that situation, the expected survival time of a patient with extensive cancer pain should be considered.

Although numerous techniques are described in this chapter, their role is at the bottom of a long treatment continuum. These invasive procedures should be used only after appropriate consideration and application of the following:

1. Systemic treatments, such as various medications or physical therapy
2. Direct operations, such as spinal stabilization or surgical decompression
3. Thorough psychologic evaluation and treatment as appropriate
4. Chemotherapy or radiotherapy (for cancer patients)

THALAMOTOMY

Lesions in the thalamus are generally considered effective and useful for intermittent shooting and hyperpathic or allodynic pain. In contrast, thalamotomy may not be effective for the burning or dysesthetic components of deafferentation or central pain.[1] Although thalamotomy is usually reserved for noncancer pain, it can be effective for cancer pain.[1,2]

One of the most effective sites within the thalamus appears to be the inferior posteromedial thalamus, which contains the intralaminar, centromedian, and parafascicularis nucleus, all of which might be part of the putative paleospinothalamic tract.[3] Other thalamic targets have included the basal thalamus, medial thalamus, and dorsomedian thalamus.

HYPOPHYSECTOMY

For lesions in the pituitary gland, percutaneous stereotactic lesions are generally favored using alcohol instillation, radiofrequency thermal therapy, cryotherapy, or the interstitial placement of radioactive seeds.[4–7] Most recently, focused radiotherapy using the Gamma Knife has been used as an essentially noninvasive modality for creating similar lesions.

The analgesic mechanism of action for hypophysectomy remains unclear, with evidence both in favor of and against theories that involve hormonal, hypothalamic, and neurotransmitter release mechanisms. Actions on the limbic system and effects on the psychologic aspects of the suffering are most unlikely, however.

Hypophysectomy generally is recommended in the treatment of pain from bone metastases from breast or prostate carcinoma regardless of whether the individual tumor is hormonally responsive or unresponsive.[8–12] The instillation of alcohol into the pituitary gland via stereotaxic methods is perhaps the best described technique.

CINGULOTOMY

Although cingulotomy has most commonly been applied to patients with affective disorders, there are numerous reports of its use for control of severe pain.[13–19] The mechanism of pain relief is unclear, although it presumably derives from interruption of the limbic system. This procedure appears most effective for either diffuse (massively widespread) cancer or cancer with tumors in multiple areas of the body.[20,21]

PULVINOTOMY

Lesions in the pulvinar of the thalamus for pain relief have been reported since 1966.[22] Electrophysiologic study has suggested that the pulvinar is a way station for afferent stimuli, including nociceptive transmission with outflow to the temporal lobe and from there to the posterior sensory cortex.[23,24] This procedure is indicated mainly in the treatment of intractable cancer pain with qualities and areas of involvement similar to those indicated for cingulotomy or hypothalamotomy.[25] Based on previous reports, pulvinotomy might be indicated for cancer patients with expected

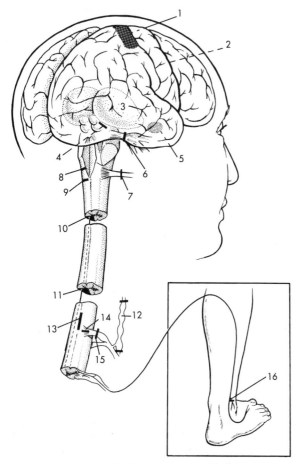

FIG. 24–1 Schematic illustration of the various sites for ablative neurosurgical operations to relieve pain. *1,* Postcentral gyrectomy; *2,* Prefrontal lobotomy (leucotomy); *3,* Thalamotomy; *4,* Mesencephalotomy; *5,* Hypophysectomy; *6,* Trigeminal rhizotomy; *7,* Glossopharyngeal rhizotomy; *8,* Medullary tractotomy; *9,* Trigeminal tractotomy; *10,* C1-2 anterolateral cordotomy; *11,* Thoracic cordotomy; *12,* Sympathectomy; *13,* Commissural myelotomy; *14,* Lissauer tractotomy; *15,* Dorsal rhinotomy; *16,* Peripheral neurectomy. *(From MacCarty CS: Neurosurgical procedures for the control of pain. Staff Meet Mayo Clin 31:208, 1956).*

survival times as long as 18 months. Although lesions have been created in one hemisphere, contralateral to the site of pain, bilateral lesions appears to be more effective.[25–27]

COMBINED PROCEDURES

Combinations of the aforementioned intracranial procedures have also been examined, for example, cingulotomy combined with anterior capsulotomy (lesions in both the cingulate gyrus and the anterior limb of the internal capsule). In the treatment of severe cancer-related pain, this combination appears to provide better relief for pain, including neuropathic pain, than cingulotomy alone.[28] The combination is more commonly used, however, in the treatment of various psychiatric conditions, such as intractable obsessive-compulsive disorder. Various combinations of targets for thalamotomy have also included the pulvinar as an additional target with improved pain relief over a single site in the talamus.[29] With continued clinical experience, a research

basis, ideally, will be developed to provide for rational combinations of these procedures and better long-term efficacy

HYPOTHALAMOTOMY

Hypothalamic lesions, although first reported for psycho-affective disorders, have also been used in the treatment of chronic pain in a limited number of patients.[30,31] Indications are similar to those for cingulotomy in terms of cancer pain from multiple sites, especially when there is an emotional or visceral component.[32] Cancer pain appears to respond better than noncancer pain.[32,33]

Although the exact mechanism of action remains unclear, beta-endorphin concentrations in ventricular cerebrospinal fluid are elevated by electrical stimulation of the hypothalamotomy target before the actual ablation.[33]

PONTINE AND MIDBRAIN SPINOTHALAMIC TRACTOTOMY

Stereotactic pontine spinothalamic tractotomy for cancer pain has been described in limited reports.[34,35] In theory, the pontine target is logical, because the sensory and autonomic fibers (respiration, micturition) are more widely separated than in the spinal cord, whereas the neospinothalamic and paleospinothalamic fibers are closer together than in the midbrain. Pain relief lasting until death has been noted in approximately 75% of cancer patients, with pain involving the upper extremity, trunk, hip, sacrum, and even all four limbs.

Since its introduction by Spiegel and Wycis in 1947, stereotactic spinothalamic tractotomy at the midbrain level (stereotactic mesencephalotomy) has remained a useful and relatively commonly performed operation to relieve cancer pain involving the face, head, neck, and upper extremity or trunk.[36–44] Significant pain relief has been noted by 65% to 75% of patients in both short-term and long-term (2- to 4-year) follow-ups, especially in the treatment of head and neck cancers.

Radiosurgical techniques have also been used to create a mesencephalotomy lesion, although experience is limited. As with the use of radiosurgery for thalamotomy, the radiosurgery for mesencephalotomy eliminates risks of hemorrhage or infection but does not allow physiologic confirmation of proper electrode placement.

INTRAVENTRICULAR INFUSION OF OPIOID

At the intracranial level, one of the most useful augmentative techniques is the intraventricular infusion of opioid. The intraventricular delivery of opioids can be accomplished by an implanted infusion pump-ventricular catheter system or by a subcutaneous Ommaya reservoir-type device with bolus injections. There appears to be a much longer duration of action with intraventricular delivery compared with the intraspinal delivery of morphine.[45]

There are two main indications for the intraventricular delivery of morphine: (1) patients with head and neck cancer pain and (2) patients with an initial good response to intraspinal infusions of opioids and subsequent development of apparent tolerance but with limited (1 to 3 months)

remaining survival time. Most studies indicate that the safety and side effects of intraventricular injections are similar to those for intraspinal infusions.

DEEP BRAIN STIMULATION

Deep brain stimulation for pain relief received its biggest support with the 1969 report that brain stimulation in the rat could produce sufficient analgesia to allow a laparotomy without chemical anesthetics.[46,47] Subsequent clinical studies have reported the benefits of deep brain stimulation in more than 1000 patients.[36–38,46,48–63]

The two principle stimulation sites have been the periaqueductal/periventricular gray region of the midbrain and caudal thalamus, and the ventroposteromedial/ventro-posterolateral (VPM/VPL) thalamic somatosensory relay nuclei. Despite the clinical efficacy, however, the mechanisms, pathways, and neurotransmitters involved in stimulation-produced analgesia remain an area of active investigation. For periaqueductal/periventricular gray stimulation, both endogenous opioid-dependent and nonopioid-dependent mechanisms have been found. VPM/VPL stimulation may activate the medullary nucleus raphe magnus, which inhibits deafferentation-facilitated activity in the spinal trigeminal system.

The periaqueductal/periventricular gray stimulation has been thought to be most effective for nociceptive and cancer pain, whereas stimulation of targets in the VPM/VPL/internal capsule has been used most often for deafferentation pain.

For noncancer pain, deep brain stimulation of either the periaqueductal gray region or thalamic sensory nuclei is effective in the short term in 61% to 80% of patients and has an overall success rate of 50% to 63%.[64–67]

The best results for deafferentation pain (67% to 73% success) have been obtained in patients with peripheral nerve disorders (neuropathy, trauma) and partial spinal cord injuries (postcordotomy dysesthesias). Generally, poor results have been obtained in patients with thalamic syndrome, anesthesia dolorosa (especially facial), and complete spinal cord injuries (0% to 42% success).

In the application of cancer pain, deep brain stimulation can be used for pain not well treated by ablative procedures, including pain from diffuse bone metastases, midline or bilateral pain (especially of the lower body), brachial or lumbosacral plexopathy, and recurrent pain from head and neck cancer.[68]

TRIGEMINAL NEURALGIA

Patients with cranial neuralgias form the largest group with surgically treatable painful disorders of the head and neck. Surgical referral is warranted after a patient has been unable to obtain satisfactory relief or has experienced significant side effects from anticonvulsant or antispasmodic medications.

Percutaneous Techniques

Percutaneous operations are recommended for:

1. Patients older than age 60 or 65 years

2. Patients whose medical conditions increase the risks of general anesthesia and open intracranial surgery
3. Younger patients who decline open surgery

Percutaneous surgical treatments for trigeminal neuralgia include:

- Radiofrequency
- Thermal rhizotomy
- Glycerol rhizolysis
- Balloon-catheter compression

Stereotactic or open trigeminal tractotomy for the treatment of typical trigeminal neuralgia is currently only of historical interest.[69,70]

Thermocoagulation of the gasserian ganglion or trigeminal root remains the most widely practiced percutaneous procedure for the treatment of medically refractory trigeminal neuralgia (Fig. 24–2).

An aggressive lesion can lead to better long-term pain relief but perhaps with dense anesthesia, although a more conservative lesion is less likely to cause motor weakness, unwanted sensory loss in a nonaffected division, or diplopia from excessive heating of cranial nerves III, IV, or VI in the cavernous sinus. Especially in patients with first division (V1) trigeminal neuralgia, the risk of corneal anesthesia and subsequent keratitis is lower with an incomplete lesion.

Radiosurgery Techniques

Trigeminal neuralgia was one of the earliest diseases treated by radiosurgery by Lars Leksell.[71] More recently, a multicenter study using this modality was undertaken for patients with facial pain.[72] Of 50 patients with a mean follow-up of 9.2 months, 50% were pain free and another 34% experienced pain reductions of at least 50%. The mean latency for relief is generally 14 days but can range from as early as 1 day to as long as 4 months. Failure of pain relief was seen in 16% of patients, and in 6% of the patients altered facial sensation occurred after the procedure.

Open Surgical Techniques
Microvascular Decompression

Microvascular decompression of the trigeminal nerve has been claimed to be the only nondestructive and potentially curative operation for trigeminal neuralgia. A successful microvascular decompression carries virtually no risk of anesthesia dolorosa, dysesthesia, motor weakness, cerebellar hemorrhage, cranial nerve injuries, or infection. Other serious complications have been reported, albeit rarely.[73] Microvascular decompression is a demanding microsurgical procedure that is performed through a limited, deep exposure.

Subtemporal Sensory Rhizotomy

Subtemporal sensory rhizotomy, sparing the motor root and V1, was the standard operation performed for trigeminal neuralgia during the first half of the 20th century. Immediate postoperative pain relief was reported in 95% to 99% of patients, with a long-term recurrence rate of 5% to 20%. However, middle fossa rhizotomy has been accompanied by a 26% overall incidence of unpleasant paresthesias, an 8% incidence of anesthesia dolorosa, and a 4.8% incidence of

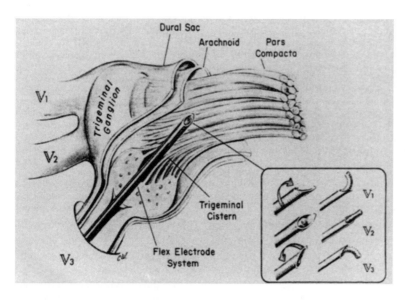

FIG. 24–2 Anatomic relationships of the foremen ovale, trigeminal divisions, ganglion, and root applied to percutaneous radiofrequency rhizotomy using a flexible electrode system. *(From Van Louveren H, Tew JM Jr, Keller JT, et al: A 10-year experience in the treatment of trigeminal neuralgia: Comparison of percutaneous stereotaxic rhizotomy and posterior fossa exploration. J Neurosurg 57:757, 1982).*

keratitis (0.2% to 15%). The high rate of immediate and delayed morbidity has led to the demise of subtemporal retrogasserian rhizotomy as a primary procedure for trigeminal neuralgia.

Selective Trigeminal Rhizotomy

Selective trigeminal rhizotomy via the posterior fossa approach for trigeminal neuralgia is recommended only after thorough exploration of the root entry zone has failed to reveal an arterial or venous source of neural compression. Conservative partial V2-3 section, internal neurolysis, and sparing of the motor root help minimize postoperative dysesthesias, painful anesthesia, and masticatory muscle weakness.

Electrical Stimulation Techniques

Trigeminal anesthesia dolorosa after retrogasserian rhizotomy for trigeminal neuralgia or other conditions is relieved in fewer than 25% of patients by further ablative surgery at the brainstem or thalamic level. Unfortunately, thalamic or periaqueductal/periventricular gray deep brain stimulation provides long-term pain relief in only 25% of patients as well. In post-traumatic or postsurgical patients with injury of the trigeminal divisions or branches distal to the ganglion, electrical stimulation of the gasserian ganglion has been tried with modest success. Temporary percutaneous trigeminal ganglion stimulation has been used as a screening procedure.[74]

Trigeminal Tractotomy (Nucleus Caudalis)

Lesions in the descending trigeminal tract and the adjacent nucleus caudalis may affect pain and temperature but not touch sensation.[69] It appears that the nucleus caudalis is a relay station for pain and temperature transmission from cranial nerves V, VII, IX, and X. Anatomically, the nucleus lies on the surface of the medulla, posterior to the dorsal spinocerebellar tract, lateral to the fasciculus cuneatus, and inferior to the restiform body.[75]

There are two main indications for trigeminal tractotomy: (1) head and neck cancer and (2) intractable trigeminal

distribution pain. Unfortunately, these types of pain often involve more diffuse areas of the head and neck, and mesencephalotomy is more appropriate in this situation.[76] Destruction of the trigeminal nucleus caudalis at the medulla and C1 levels is actually a modification of the spinal dorsal root entry zone (DREZ) lesion.[77]

As an alternative to the open method, a percutaneous technique has been reported with needle penetration at the C1 foramen magnum area under stereotaxic guidance.[78,79] Electrical stimulation (50 Hz) helps to confirm correct localization:

1. With ventral placement, stimulation is felt in contralateral body areas via the spinothalamic tract.
2. With dorsal placement, stimulation is felt in ipsilateral areas via the fasciculus cuneatus.
3. With correct placement, stimulation is perceived in the face.

With either technique (often combined with other nerve and/or root sections in the same area), generally 75% to 85% of patients with head and neck cancer report good pain relief, although the tractotomy often is combined with other nerve or root sections in the same area. Pain relief is often short lived, with pain recurrence after 1 or more years, although the overall recurrence rate might be as low as 22%.[75,80]

GLOSSOPHARYNGEAL NEURALGIA

Glossopharyngeal neuralgia affects only 1.0% to 1.3% as many individuals as trigeminal neuralgia does; the lancinating pain is similar in character but is located in the throat of the base of tongue or deep in the ear. Paroxysms of pain are triggered by eating or swallowing. All such patients should undergo a thorough clinical evaluation by an otolaryngologist before neurosurgical intervention. Invasive carcinomas of the skull base or posterior pharynx can produce a pain syndrome identical to idiopathic glossopharyngeal neuralgia. In some patients with essential glossopharyngeal neuralgia, bradycardia, and syncope either accompany the painful attacks or occur in the absence of pain.

Before referral for surgery, patients usually have tried the medication most effective for trigeminal neuralgia. Unfortunately, the drugs are effective in fewer than 50% of patients with glossopharyngeal neuralgia.

Percutaneous Techniques

Surgical treatment consists of (1) percutaneous cranial nerve IX radiofrequency rhizotomy in the jugular foramen or (2) open microsurgical section of the cranial nerve IX and upper vagal rootlets in the posterior fossa. Patient preparation, anesthetic monitoring, and the use of fluoroscopy in the operating or radiology department are as described for radiofrequency rhizotomy for trigeminal neuralgia.

Open Surgical Techniques

Open intradural section of the glossopharyngeal nerve and the first one to three rootlets of the vagus nerve is the most effective treatment for glossopharyngeal neuralgia not associated with malignancy.[81–83] Microvascular decompression of cranial nerves IX and X does not yield better short-term results than root section and may have a higher recurrence rate.[82] Special intraoperative considerations include cardiovascular instability during manipulation of the cranial nerve IX and nerve roots IX. Application of small lidocaine-soaked cottonoid pledgets to the rootlets can blunt this response.

GENICULATE NEURALGIA

Open Surgical Techniques

The otalgic type of geniculate neuralgia described by Hunt consists of pain centered within the ear and sometimes radiating to deep facial structures. The pain can be paroxysmal and neuralgic in character, but more often it is felt as a deep aching that lasts for hours. Attacks may occur in clusters and are rarely evoked or worsened by tactile stimuli in or around the ear. In eight cases of true geniculate neuralgia reviewed by White and Sweet, all patients were relived of pain by one or more operations that coupled intracranial section of the nervus intermedius with sectioning of cranial nerves VII, VIII, IX, or X or the medullary trigeminal descending tract.[75]

The surgical exposure of the nervus intermedius is similar to that of cranial nerves IX and X, only carried more rostrally. It lies between the superior vestibular nerve (VIII) and facial nerve (VII) within the superior portion of the internal auditory meatus and may consist of single or multiple fibers. Nervus intermedius section is technically more difficult than either trigeminal or glossopharyngeal procedures.

OCCIPITAL NEURALGIA

Recurrent, episodic neuralgic pain in the distribution of the greater occipital nerve (C2) or the lesser occipital nerve (C3) may occur as a result of spondylitic root entrapment after cervical trauma or, more often, as a nonspecific manifestation of cervical myofascial pain. In virtually all cases the pain is relieved by local anesthetic blocks, a series of which may induce a long-lasting remission. In occipital nerves or C2 and C3 roots may be considered. A thorough neurologic examination, including imaging studies of the posterior fossa and foramen magnum region, is recommended to ensure that the pain is not caused by a mass lesion or Arnold-Chiari malformation.

Percutaneous Techniques

Although long-term results after this operation are not clear, at least one study has reported excellent or good pain relief in 65% to 75% of patients at follow-up periods of 24 months.[84,85] In patients who underwent a second procedure on the same or opposite side, only 50% and 67%, respectively, were relieved of their pain. The presence or absence of antecedent trauma, cervical spondylosis, or disk disease did not affect the outcome.

Open Surgical Techniques

Avulsion of the greater occipital nerve has relieved occipital neuralgia in as many as 83% of patients during short-term follow-up. The nerve is surgically exposed below the subcutaneous tissue as it pierces the trapezius muscle. Although avulsion of both the distal and proximal nerve segments have been described, the latter carries a greater risk of hemorrhage from damage to the occipital artery as well as a potential risk of spinal cord injury.

CORDOTOMY

Percutaneous C1-2 radiofrequency cordotomy by the lateral approach is among the most useful procedures for patients with unilateral cancer pain below the C5 dermatome level.[86–89] Complete or satisfactory pain relief has been reported in 59% to 96% of patients with cancer pain. Half of the patients who failed to obtain relief or who experienced early pain recurrence after a single procedure did find relief after another percutaneous cordotomy. Bilateral staged cordotomies have yielded satisfactory pain relief in 70% to 90% of patients at the time of hospital discharge. The percutaneous C1-2 cordotomy is performed by the lateral approach with the use of local anesthesia with fluoroscopic monitoring.

MIDLINE MYELOTOMY

Midline myelotomy is a procedure to section the midline fibers posterior to the central canal of the spinal cord. It has been reported using various techniques, including mechanical ablation, radiofrequency techniques, and carbon dioxide laser.[90] Although the usual site of the lesion is at the lower thoracic spinal cord level, lesions at C1 also have been reported.[91] It is thought that myelotomy interrupts the putative paleospinothalamic tract, and, thus, analgesia to hyperpathia and background pain is usually obtained without sensory loss but with preserved ability to localize and discriminate between sharp and dull stimuli.[92]

DORSAL ROOT ENTRY ZONE LESIONS

The DREZ procedure, introduced by Nashold in 1976, is beneficial for noncancer pain, especially central pain, from an injury or other damage to the central nervous system (Fig. 24–3).[93] Creation of lesions at the entry zone disrupts much of the dorsal horn of the spinal cord, in addition to the

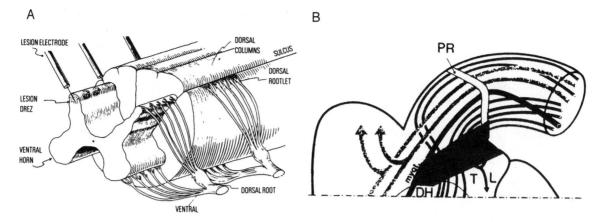

FIG. 24–3 *A,* Schematic representation of the dorsal root entry zone (DREZ) operation. A continuous series of coagulations is made through dorsal intermediate sulcus into Lissauer's tract, the substantia gelatinosa, and the superficial layers of the dorsal horn at spinal cord levels corresponding to the patient's painful zone. *B,* Organization of the dorsal root and site of Sindou's DREZ-otomy incision *(large black arrow).* The lemniscal fibers turn dorsally and are spared. DH, dorsal horn; LT, Lissauer's tract; PR, pial ring. *(A from Nashold BS Jr, Ostdahl RH: Dorsal root entry zone lesions for pain relief. J Neurosurg 51:59, 1979; B from Sindou M, Jeanmonod D: Microsurgical DREZ-otomy for the treatment of spasticity and pain in the lower limbs. Neurosurgery 24:655, 1989).*

actual Lissauer tract, at the level where the pain impulses are entering. Applications include brachial plexus avulsion pain, spinal cord injury pain, phantom limb or stump pain, or postherpetic pain.[94]

DORSAL RHIZOTOMY

The use of open dorsal rhizotomy for treatment of nociceptive pain of nonmalignant origin has been questioned over the past 2 decades. Although White and Sweet reported relief of pain in 66% of patients 2 months to 20 years postoperatively, Loeser[95] reported only a 21% long-term success rate in a similar group of patients. The addition of ganglionectomy to rhizotomy has relieved pain in only 46.6% of the patients in combined series.

SPINAL NERVE DENERVATION

More proximal radiofrequency thermocoagulation of the primary spinal nerve trunk and ganglion has also been described. This latter procedure must not be confused with facet denervation. Percutaneous spinal rhizotomy can result in a motor and sensory deficit if performed at a functioning root level. As described by Uematsu and coworkers,[96] the procedure relieves nociceptive pain and spasticity in the affected limbs of patients with preexisting neurologic deficits because of multiple sclerosis or spinal injury.

SYMPATHECTOMY

The constant, burning pain of complex regional pain syndrome (CRPS)—also known as reflex sympathetic dystrophy and causalgia—that occurs after injury to peripheral nerves in the limbs has been relieved by cervicothoracic (upper extremity) or lumbar (lower extremity) sympathectomy in up to 100% of patients in several series.

Sympathectomy has also been of value in the treatment of painful vasospastic disorders of the extremities (e.g., Raynaud's phenomenon).[97] Less certain is whether sympathectomy improves limb salvage and reduces pain in patients with atherosclerotic or vasculitic arterial occlusive disease. Before referral for surgery, patients with CRPS should undergo a diagnostic and therapeutic series of sympathetic blocks using local anesthetic agents as well as placebo injections. Only patients who respond unequivocally to the active agent and not to placebo should be considered for surgical sympathectomy. Patients who experience a recurrence of pain after initial long-term relief from one or more blocks are also good candidates for surgery.

Open surgical exposures for sympathetic denervation of the upper limb include the (1) supraclavicular extrapleural (anterior cervical), (2) anterior transthoracic (transpleural), (3) axillary transthoracic (transpleural), and (4) posterior extrapleural paramedian (Smithwick) or midline (Cloward) approaches.

Lumbar sympathectomy is indicated for the treatment of CRPS type II (causalgia) involving the lower extremity and for selected classes of ischemic peripheral vascular disease with rest pain and vasospasm.

References

1. Tasker RR: Thalamotomy. *Neurosurg Clin North Am* 1:841, 1990.
2. Sano K: Neurosurgical treatments of pain—A general survey. *Acta Neurochir Suppl* 38:86, 1987.
3. Sweet WH: Central mechanisms of chronic pain (neuralgias and certain other neurogenic pain). *Res Publ Assoc Res Nerv Ment Dis* 58:287, 1980.
4. Gros C: Place of hypophysectomy in the neurosurgical treatment of pain. *Adv Neurosurg* 3:264, 1975.
5. Silverberg GD: Hypophysectomy in the treatment of disseminated prostate carcinoma. *Cancer* 39:1727, 1977.
6. Tindall GT, Payne NS, Nixon DW: Transsphenoidal hypophysectomy for disseminated carcinoma of the prostate gland: Results in 53 patients. *J Neurosurg* 50:275, 1979.

7. Tindall GT, Ambrose SS, Christy JH et al: Hypophysectomy in the treatment of disseminated carcinoma of the breast and prostate gland. *South Med J* 69:579, 1976.

8. Miles J: Chemical hypophysectomy. *Adv Pain Res Ther* 2:373, 1979.

9. Katz J, Levin AB: Treatment of diffuse metastatic pain by instillation of alcohol into the sella turcica. *Anesthesiology* 46:115, 1977.

10. Levin AB, Ramirez LF, Katz J: The use of stereotaxic chemical hypophysectomy in the treatment of the thalamic pain syndrome. *J Neurosurg* 59:1002, 1983.

11. Perrault M: L'hypophysectomie totale dans le traitement du cancer sein: Premier cas Francais. Avenir de la method. *Therapie* 7:290, 1952.

12. Williams NE, Miles JB, Lipton S et al: Pain relief and pituitary function following injection of alcohol into the pituitary fossa. *Ann R Coll Surg Engl* 62:203, 1980.

13. Faillance LA: Cognitive deficits from bilateral cingulotomy for intractable pain in man. *Dis Nerv Sys* 32:171, 1981.

14. Foltz EL, White LE: Pain "relief" by frontal cingulotomy. *J Neurosurg* 19:89, 1962.

15. Hurt RW, Ballantine HT Jr: Stereotactic anterior cingulate lesions for persistent pain: A report on 68 cases. *Clin Neurosurg* 21:334, 1974.

16. Mempel E, Dietrich RZ: Favorable effect of cingulotomy on gastric crisis pain. *Neurol Neurochir Pol* 11:611, 1977.

17. Ortiz A: The role of the limbic lobe in central pain mechanisms: An hypothesis relating to the gate control theory of pain. In Laitinen LV, Livingston KE, editors: *Surgical approaches in psychiatry.* Baltimore, University Park Press, 1972.

18. Sharma T: Abolition of opiate hunger in humans following bilateral anterior cingulotomy. *Tex Med* 70:49, 1974.

19. Sharma T: Absence of cognitive deficits from bilateral cingulotomy for intractable pain in humans. *Tex Med* 69:79, 1973.

20. Hassenbusch SJ, Pillay PK: Cingulotomy for treatment of cancer-related pain. In Arbit E, editor: *Advances in surgical management of cancer-related pain.* Mount Kisco, NY, Futura Publishing, 1993.

21. Pillay PK, Hassenbusch SJ: Cingulotomy for cancer pain: Two year experience. *Stereotact Funct Neurosurg* 59:33, 1992.

22. Kudo T, Yoshii N, Shimizu S et al: Effects of stereotactic thalamotomy to intractable pain and numbness. *Keio J Med* 15:191, 1966.

23. Kudo T, Yoshii N, Shimizu S et al: Stereotactic thalamotomy for pain relief. *Tohoku J Exp Med* 96:219, 1968.

24. Laitinen LV: Anterior pulvinotomy in the treatment of intractable pain. In Sweet WH, Obrador S, Martin-Rodriguez JG, editors: *Neurosurgical treatment in psychiatry, pain, and epilepsy.* Baltimore, University Park Press, 1977.

25. Yoshii N, Mizokami T, Ushikubo Y et al: Comparative study between size of lesioned area and operative effects after pulvinotomy. *Appl Neurophysiol* 45:492, 1982.

26. Yoshii N, Fukuda S: Effects of unilateral and bilateral invasion of thalamic pulvinar for pain relief. *Tohoku J Exp Med* 127:81, 1979.

27. Sweet WH: Central mechanisms of chronic pain (neuralgias and certain other neurogenic pain). *Res Publ Assoc Res Nerv Ment Dis* 58:287, 1980.

28. Hassenbusch SJ, Pillay PK: Ablative intracranial neurosurgery for cancer pain: Three-year experience and modification of techniques [abstract]. *J Neurosurg* 76:396A, 1992.

29. Mayanagi Y, Bouchard G: Evaluation of stereotactic thalamotomies for pain relief with reference to pulvinar intervention. *Appl Neurophysiol* 39:154, 1976.

30. Fairman D: Hypothalamotomy as a new perspective for alleviation of intractable pain and regression of metastatic malignant tumors. In Fusek V, editor: *Present limits of neurosurgery.* Prague, Avicenum Czechoslovakian Medical Press, 1971.

31. Sano K: Sedative neurosurgery with reference to posteromedial hypothalamotomy. *Neurol Medicochir* 4:112, 1962.

32. Amano K, Kitamura K, Sano K et al: Relief of intractable pain from neurosurgical point of view with reference to present limits and clinical indications—A review of 100 consecutive cases. *Neurol Med Chir (Tokyo)* 16:141, 1976.

33. Mayanagi Y, Sano K, Suzuki I et al: Stimulation and coagulation of the posteromedial hypothalamus for intractable pain, with reference to beta-endorphins. *Appl Neurophysiol* 45:136, 1982.

34. Barbera J, Barcia-Salorio JL, Broseta J: Stereotaxic pontine spinothalamic tractotomy. *Surg Neurol* 11:111, 1979.

35. Hitchcock ER: Stereotaxic pontine spinothalamic tractotomy. *J Neurosurg* 39:746, 1973.

36. Frank F, Tognetti F, Gaist G et al: Stereotaxic rostral mesencephalotomy in treatment of malignant faciothoracobrachial pain syndromes: A survey of 14 treated patients. *J Neurosurg* 56:807, 1982.

37. Frank F, Tognetti F, Gaist G et al: Rostral stereotactic mesencephalotomy in treatment of cancer pain: A survey of 40 treated patients. *Acta Neurochir* 33(suppl):437, 1984.

38. Gildenberg PL: Stereotactic treatment of head and neck pain. *Res Clin Stud Headache* 5:102, 1978.

39. Amano K, Kawamura H, Tanikawa T et al: Long-term follow-up study of rostral mesencephalic reticulotomy for pain relief—Report of 34 cases. *Appl Neurophysiol* 49:105, 1986.

40. Amano K, Iseki H, Notani M et al: Rostral mesencephalic reticulotomy for pain relief: Report of 15 cases. *Acta Neurochir* 30(suppl):391, 1980.

41. Nashold BS: Stereotactic mesencephalotomy. *Prog Neurol Surg* 8:35, 1977.

42. Nashold BS, Wilson WP, Slaughter DG: Sensations evoked by stimulation of the midbrain in man. *J Neurosurg* 30:14, 1969.

43. Tasker RR: Neurological concepts of pain management in head and neck cancer. *Can J Otolaryngol* 4:480, 1975.

44. Wycis HT, Spiegel EA: Long-range results in the treatment of intractable pain by stereotactic midbrain surgery. *J Neurosurg* 19:101, 1962.

45. Branenor GA: Long term intrathecal administration of morphine: A comparison of bolus injection via reservoir with continuous infusion by implanted pump. *Neurosurgery* 21:484, 1987.

46. Levy RM, Lamb S, Adams JE: Treatment of chronic pain by deep brain stimulation: Long term follow-up and review of the literature. *Neurosurgery* 21:885, 1987.

47. Reynolds DV: Surgery in the rat during electrical analgesia induced by focal brain stimulation. *Science* 164:444, 1969.

48. Tasker RR: Thalamic stereotaxic procedures. In Schaltenbrand G, Walker AE, editors: *Stereotaxy of the human brain.* Stuttgart, Germany, George Thieme Verlag, 1982.

49. Boivie J, Meyerson BA: A correlative anatomical and clinical study of pain suppression by deep brain stimulation. *Pain* 13:114, 1982.

50. Demierre B, Siegfried J: Le syndrome douloureux thalamique. *Neurochirurgie* 31:281, 1985.

51. Dieckmann G, Krainick JU, Thoden U: Stereotaxic induction stimulation for pain. In Schaltenbrand G, Walker AE, editors: *Stereotaxy of the human brain: Anatomical, physiological and clinical applications.* New York, Thieme-Stratton, 1982.

52. Gildenberg PL: The use of pacemakers in functional neurological disorders. In Marino R, editor: *Functional neurosurgery.* New York, Raven Press, 1979.

53. Hosobuchi Y: Chronic brain stimulation for the treatment of intractable pain. *Res Clin Stud Headache* 5:122, 1978.

54. Hosobuchi Y: The current status of analgesic brain stimulation. *Acta Neurochir* 30(suppl):219, 1980.

55. Hosobuchi Y: Combined electrical stimulation of the periaqueductal gray matter and sensory thalamus. *Appl Neurophysiol* 46:112, 1983.

56. Hosobuchi Y: Subcortical electrical stimulation for control of intractable pain in humans: Report of 122 cases (1970-1984). *J Neurosurg* 64:543, 1986.

57. Hosobuchi Y, Adams JE, Rutkin B: Chronic thalamic stimulation for the control of facial anesthesia dolorosa. *Arch Neurol* 29:158, 1973.

58. Plotkin R: Results in 60 cases of deep brain stimulation for chronic intractable pain. *Appl Neurophysiol* 45:173, 1982.

59. Richardson DE, Akil H: Pain reduction by electrical brain stimulation in man: Part 1. Acute administration in periaqueductal and periventricular sites. *J Neurosurg* 47:178, 1977.

60. Richardson DE, Akil H: Pain reduction by electrical brain stimulation in man: Part 2. Chronic self-administration in the periventricular gray matter. *J Neurosurg* 47:184, 1977.

61. Roldan P, Broseta J, Barcia-Salorio JL: Chronic VPM stimulation for anesthesia dolorosa following trigeminal surgery. *Appl Neurophysiol* 45:112, 1982.

62. Turnbull IM, Shulman R, Woodhurst WB: Thalamic stimulation for neuropathic pain. *J Neurosurg* 52:486, 1980.

63. Young RF, Kroening R, Fulton W et al: Electrical stimulation of the brain in treatment of chronic pain: Experience over 5 years. *J Neurosurg* 62:389, 1985.

64. Gybels J, Kupers R: Deep brain stimulation in the treatment of chronic pain in man: Where and why? *Neurophysiol Clin* 20:389, 1990.

65. Kumar K, Wyant GM, Nath R: Deep brain stimulation for control of intractable pain in humans, present and future: A ten-year follow-up. *Neurosurgery* 26:774, 1990.

66. Young RF: Brain stimulation. *Neurosurg Clin North Am* 1:865, 1990.

67. Young RF, Tronnier V, Rinaldi PC: Chronic stimulation of the Kölliker-Fuse nucleus region of intractable pain in humans. *J Neurosurg* 76:979, 1992.

68. Young RF: Electrical stimulation of the brain for the treatment of intractable cancer pain. In Arbit E, editor: *Management of cancer-related pain.* Mount Kisco, NY, Futura Publishing, 1993.

69. Sjoqvist O: Studies on pain conduction in the trigeminal nerve. *Acta Psych Neurol* 18(suppl):93, 1938.

70. Hosobuchi Y, Rutkin B: Descending trigeminal tractotomy: Neurophysiological approach. *Acta Psych Neurol* 25:115, 1971.

71. Leksell L: Stereotaxic radiosurgery in trigeminal neuralgia. *Acta Chir Scand* 137:311, 1971.

72. Konziolka D: Stereotactic radiosurgery for trigeminal neuralgia: A multi-institutional study using the gamma unit. *J Neurosurg* 84:940, 1996.

73. Hanakita J, Kondo A: Serious complications of microvascular decompression operations for trigeminal neuralgia and hemifacial spasm. *Neurosurgery* 22:348, 1988.

74. Meyerson BA, Hakanson S: Suppression of pain in trigeminal neuropathy by electric stimulation of the gasserian ganglion. *Neurosurgery* 18:59, 1986.

75. White JC, Sweet WH, editors: *Pain and the neurosurgeon: A forty-year experience.* Springfield, Ill, Charles C Thomas, 1969.

76. Spiegel EA, Wycis HT: Mesencephalotomy in the treatment of "intractable" facial pain. *Arch Neurol* 69:1, 1953.

77. Bernard EJ Jr, Nashold BS Jr, Caputi F et al: Nucleus caudalis DREZ lesions for facial pain. *Br J Neurosurg* 1:81, 1987.

78. Nashold BS Jr, Crue BL Jr: Stereotaxic mesencephalotomy and trigeminal tractotomy. In Youmans JR, editor: *Neurological surgery,* ed 2. Philadelphia, WB Saunders, 1982.

79. Schvarcz JR: Spinal cord stereotactic techniques re trigeminal nucleotomy and extralemniscal myelotomy. *Appl Neurophysiol* 41:99, 1978.

80. Schvarcz JR: Stereotactic trigeminal tractotomy. *Confinia Neurol* 37:73, 1975.

81. Dandy WE: Glossopharyngeal neuralgia (tic douloureux): Its diagnosis and treatment. *Arch Surg* 15:198, 1927.

82. Laha RK, Jannetta PJ: Glossopharyngeal neuralgia. *J Neurosurg* 47:316, 1977.

83. Rushton JG, Stevens JC, Miller RH: Glossopharyngeal (vagoglossopharyngeal) neuralgia: A study of 217 cases. *Arch Neurol* 38:201, 1981.

84. Murphy JP: Occipital neurectomy in the treatment of headache: Results in 30 cases. *Md State Med J* 18:62, 1969.

85. Blume HG: *Radiofrequency denaturation for the treatment of occipital pain.* Burlington, Vt, Radionics, 1975.

86. Levin AB, Cosman ER: Thermocouple-monitored cordotomy electrode. Technical note. *J Neurosurg* 53:266, 1980.

87. Rosomoff HL, Brown CJ, Sheptak P: Percutaneous radiofrequency cervical cordotomy: Technique. *J Neurosurg* 23:639, 1965.

88. Taren JA, Davis R, Crosby FC: Target physiologic corroboration in stereotaxic cervical cordotomy. *J Neurosurg* 30:569, 1969.

89. Tasker RR: Percutaneous cordotomy: The lateral high cervical technique. In Schmidek HH, Sweet WH, editors: *Operative neurosurgical techniques, indications, methods, and results,* ed 2. Orlando, Fla, Grune & Stratton, 1988.

90. Fink RA: Neurosurgical treatment of nonmalignant intractable rectal pain: Microsurgical commissural myelotomy with the carbon dioxide laser. *Neurosurgery* 14:64, 1984.

91. Gildenberg PL, Hirshberg RM: Limited myelotomy for the treatment of intractable cancer pain. *J Neurol Neurosurg Psychiatry* 47:94, 1984.

92. Schvarcz JR: Stereotactic extralemniscal myelotomy. *J Neurol Neurosurg Psychiatry* 39:53, 1976.

93. Nashold BS Jr: Introduction to Second International Symposium on Dorsal Root Entry Zone (DREZ) Lesions. *Appl Neurophysiol* 51:76, 1988.

94. Iskandar BJ, Nashold BS: Spinal and trigeminal DREZ lesions. In Gildenberg PL, Tasker RR, editors: *Textbook of stereotactic and functional neurosurgery.* New York, McGraw-Hill, 1998.

95. Loeser JD: Dorsal rhizotomy for the relief of chronic pain. *J Neurosurg* 36:745, 1972.

96. Uematsu S, Udvarhelyi GB, Benson DW et al: Percutaneous radiofrequency rhizotomy. *Surg Neurol* 2:319, 1974.

97. Smithwick RH: The rationale and technic of sympathectomy for the relief of vascular spasm of the extremities. *N Engl J Med* 222:699, 1940.

Questions • Surgical Techniques

1. Thalamotomy may be effective for

   A. Intermittent shooting pain
   B. Burning pain
   C. Dysesthetic pain
   D. Lower motor neuron lesion pain

2. The intraventricular infusion of opioids is accomplished by an implanted infusion pump with a ventricular catheter system. Compared with intraspinal delivery of morphine the duration of action of intraspinal morphine is

   A. Shorter
   B. Longer
   C. Unpredictable
   D. Similar

3. For nociceptive and cancer pain the most effective site for deep brain stimulation is the

   A. Thalamus
   B. Internal capsule
   C. Periaqueductal gray region
   D. Frontal cortex

4. Microvascular decompression for trigeminal neuralgia has been widely performed because it carries minimal risk of all of the following except

   A. Anesthesia dolorosa
   B. Motor weakness
   C. Cerebellar hemorrhage
   D. Trigeminal tract injury

5. Recurrent episodic neurologic pain in the greater or lesser occipital nerve may occur as a result of root entrapment. During radiographic workup, all of the following lesions should be eliminated before occipital nerve blocks except

   A. Posterior fossa lesion
   B. Foramen magnum lesion
   C. Arnold-Chiari malformation
   D. C2-3 facet arthropathy

ANSWERS

1. A

2. B

3. C

4. D

5. D

CHAPTER 25

Psychologic Techniques

GEORGE F. BLACKALL
AND KEVIN E. WILSON

Pain, like all human experiences, is subjective and idiopathic. The shift in understanding illness from a biomedical model to a more complex biopsychosocial model[1] and the introduction of the gate-control theory of pain[2] have expanded the treatment of the pain patient to include the entire experience of pain, specifically nociception, pain, and the resulting suffering and distress. Consideration is also given to the context within which the pain is occurring (family, friends, work). A multidisciplinary approach to treating pain that includes the medical, psychologic, and physical therapy aspects of pain has proved to be more effective than no treatment or single-modality treatment.[3–6]

OPERANT INTERVENTIONS

Fordyce[7,8] introduced the concept that pain patients respond to reinforcement from the environment. The presence of positive reinforcers increases the likelihood that a certain behavior will be maintained or repeated. The goal of operant therapy is to alter *maladaptive* pain behaviors (i.e., avoidance, reduced activity levels, verbal pain behaviors, excessive use of medications) by reducing reinforcement for these behaviors and providing reinforcement for *well* behaviors (increased activity levels, reduction of pain medications, decreased verbal pain behaviors).

A common clinical dilemma is how to validate a patient's pain experience without reinforcing undesirable pain behaviors. It is important for the treating physician to convey a sense of understanding to the pain patient. Failure to convey an understanding of the impact of the pain experience may inadvertently lead a person to "raise the stakes" in the form of increasing pain behaviors. Restating the patient's complaints is a simple and effective way to demonstrate understanding.

Patients consistently express a sense of relief when they feel a physician finally understands their struggle and does not think the pain is "all in their head." This is not the same as reinforcing undesirable pain behaviors. For example, the pain patient who takes more narcotic medications than prescribed, calls the pain clinic in a panic, and then receives a refill early is receiving positive reinforcement for undesirable behavior.

Negative reinforcement refers to the removal of unpleasant or noxious stimuli. Expectations of pain and a perceived lack of self-efficacy can result in movement limitations and impaired functioning.[9] The absence of pain then serves to reinforce the avoidant behavior, thereby eliminating a feedback loop.[10] As long as the behavior is avoided, the person does not know whether it still causes pain.

Behavior therapy or operant conditioning programs have been demonstrated to reduce health care use,[11] decrease physical and psychologic disability,[12] and improve pain and decrease functional impairment.[13] Basic indications for the use of operant conditioning with pain patients have been presented by Sanders[10] as follows:

1. Overt pain behavior is chronic (3 months or longer).
2. Overt pain behavior occurs as a function of the environment, time of day, or persons present.
3. Overt pain behavior is acknowledged by others.
4. Overt pain behavior is sometimes followed by positive or negative reinforcers.
5. Overt pain behavior is in excess of known physical findings.
6. The patient exhibits significant concern about increased pain with increased physical activity or return to work.

The presence of these conditions does not imply any degree of psychopathology; rather, such conditions should be viewed as attempts to adapt to the pain experience.

The concept of receiving some reinforcement as a result of pain behaviors is referred to as *secondary gain*. Clinically, it is hazardous to make presumptions of secondary gain. In a busy pain clinic, it is unfair to patients to presume secondary gain is operating based on the limited information available to the health care provider. All behavior is determined by multiple factors, not just pain behavior. Viewing a person's behavior in terms of secondary gain may be too simplistic. It ignores the complexity of why we behave the way we do. The challenge that must be presented to the patient is one of maximizing adaptation and functioning despite the pain.

Operant interventions are specific and targeted. The patient sets goals and has a predefined reward for the attainment of each goal. The goals are increasingly difficult in an attempt to maximize functioning. Medical staff and family members are instructed to ignore pain behaviors and acknowledge adaptive behaviors.

It is critical to the success of behavioral interventions that the person be integrally involved in goal setting and determining rewards. Goals must be definable, realistic, and achievable to be effective.

COGNITIVE-BEHAVIORAL THERAPY

Cognitive-behavioral models of pain are driven by the theory that a person's beliefs about his or her pain can influence adjustment to the pain experience.[14] Jensen and Karoly[15] found that appraisals of pain control were positively associated with psychologic functioning in a diverse group of pain patients. Specifically, patients who tended to ignore the pain, who used coping self-statements, and who increased their activities had better psychologic functioning than those who did not engage in these behaviors. However, this correlation was maintained only with patients reporting relatively low levels of pain.

Another moderating factor in the relationship between pain beliefs and functioning is time. Jensen and coauthors[16] found that the belief that pain signaled on-going tissue damage was associated with physical dysfunction in patients with pain duration of less than 2.4 years. In addition, the authors reported that the beliefs that emotions affect pain, that others should be attentive during a pain episode, and that one is disabled by pain have also been positively associated with psychosocial dysfunction. Conversely, acceptance of pain has been demonstrated to be associated with lower reports of pain intensity, less anxiety related to pain, decreased avoidance and depression, decreased disability, and improved work status.[17]

Self-efficacy, or the belief that one can complete a desired course of action, is also believed to influence adjustment to chronic pain. *Catastrophizing* (viewing the pain as the worst thing in the world and believing it will never get better) is related to lower self-efficacy.

Turk and Rudy[18] provide five basic assumptions for the foundation of cognitive-behavioral interventions:

1. Individuals actively process information for internal and external stimuli. Accordingly, behavior is influenced by expectations of outcomes and perception of potential consequences of behavior.
2. Cognitions interact with emotions, physiologic sensations, and behavior. Altering one of these components, therefore, can alter other components.
3. The interaction between an individual and the environment is reciprocal. The person can influence the environment as readily as the environment can influence the person.
4. Effective interventions must address the cognitive, emotional, and behavioral aspects of the presenting problem.
5. Individuals must be active participants in treatment if they are to learn more adaptive ways to deal with their problems.

Cognitive-behavioral interventions are structured and time-limited. These interventions tend to include elements of relaxation training and the identification and alteration of maladaptive cognitions. The results of outcome studies of cognitive-behavioral techniques with chronic pain patients are mixed, although there appears to be enough support to suggest at least moderate effectiveness.

Cognitive processes have been associated with adjustment to chronic pain. The most positive include ignoring pain, using coping self-statements, and indicating acceptance of the pain; the most detrimental is catastrophizing. Cognitive-behavioral interventions should strike a balance between identifying and altering maladaptive cognitions, while reinforcing adaptive thoughts and behaviors.

GROUP THERAPY

Group therapy provides the advantage of exposing pain patients to others with similar problems, thereby creating the

opportunity to feel less isolated; it also tends to be less expensive than individual therapy. Group therapy has proved effective in reducing pain and in improving function.

The primary goals of group therapy with pain patients include targeting behavior change, providing patient education, and offering social support.[19] Group therapy should be structured and time-limited. Group size typically ranges from four to eight people, with therapy sessions lasting from 60 to 90 minutes. With pain patients, treatment tends to be for a predetermined number of sessions.

Patient selection is crucial to facilitating group functioning. Poor candidates include patients who are severely depressed, who are not willing to regularly attend group sessions, who are violent, or who have severe personality disorders.

FAMILY THERAPY

Consistent with the biopsychosocial model of illness, pain exists within the context of a person's life. A primary part of that context is the family. Because pain can alter the life of an individual, it too can alter the life of a family. The depression and irritability that can accompany pain can easily be directed toward family members. Family members may be unfamiliar with the behavioral manifestations of pain and may unknowingly reinforce pain behaviors.[8]

The application of family therapy models to chronic illness is an established form of intervention.[20,21] However, controlled studies on the effectiveness of family therapy for chronic pain patients is lacking. There is evidence that spouses can influence the level of pain behaviors expressed[22] and alter levels of disability.[23] Turk and colleagues[23] found decreased pain and disability in pain patients whose spouses were generally positive but tended to avoid paying attention to expressions of pain.

Patterson and Garwick[24] propose the Family Adjustment and Adaptation Response (FAAR) Model as a way of understanding the balancing act families are faced with in chronic illness. The authors suggest that families who successfully adapt to chronic illness are able to use their resources and coping behaviors to respond to the dynamic nature of the illness experience.

HYPNOSIS

Hypnosis is generally considered a process in which a hypnotist offers suggestions to a subject to experience alterations in sensation, perception, or cognition.[25] Although clinical reports describe patients as achieving total anesthesia via hypnosis,[26] the goal of hypnosis with chronic pain patients is the reduction, not the total elimination, of pain. Hypnosis is often used as part of a comprehensive psychotherapeutic intervention. In addition to using hypnotic induction and suggestion, it is often necessary to address other parts of the patient's psychologic functioning.

How hypnosis can be used to alter the pain experience is limited only by the imaginations of the patient and the hypnotist. Common techniques for achieving pain control include such suggestions as[27]:

1. Injection of a local anesthetic into the afflicted area

2. Achieving anesthesia in a nonpainful part of the body and then transferring it to the painful area (glove anesthesia)
3. Displacing the pain and converting it to something less painful
4. Amnesia
5. Directing attention away from the pain

BIOFEEDBACK AND RELAXATION

Biofeedback and relaxation are used together to provide the pain patient with a set of skills that have proved useful in pain reduction.

Biofeedback is a process that includes the use of electronic or electromechanical instruments to monitor physiologic processes and to "feed back" that information to the subject being monitored.[28] The primary goal is to develop psychophysiologic self-regulation. The physiologic processes often assessed include muscle tension, skin temperature, blood flow, and heart rate. Feedback to patients usually takes the form of computer-generated information (i.e., a graph of skin temperature) or auditory cues, such as a tone, when there is a change in the physiologic parameter being measured. The most frequent types of biofeedback used with chronic pain patients include electromyographic (EMG) biofeedback, thermal biofeedback, electrodermal activity (EDA), electroencephalogram (EEG), and cephalic blood volume pulse (BVP).

Relaxation is a term used to describe a decrease in sympathetic nervous system arousal, also referred to as the *relaxation response*.[29] The state of relaxation can be induced through various procedures, including progressive muscle relaxation, controlled breathing, and visual imagery.[30] Relaxation procedures are coupled with biofeedback in an effort to facilitate alterations in the physiologic process being monitored. Once a baseline value for the physiologic process is established (i.e., muscle tension), the patient is taught relaxation techniques and observes changes in the parameter being assessed.

Relaxation and biofeedback therapy have been effective in the treatment of pain patients. The exact physiologic and psychologic mechanisms of change in both biofeedback and relaxation are not known. Clinical observation suggests that noninvasive procedures that instill a sense of control, perhaps even hope, for the chronic pain patient may be a powerful mitigating factor in the pain experience. Further studies that address the specific treatment effects of biofeedback and relaxation are needed.

PAIN DEFINITIONS

Pain, as defined by the International Association for the Study of Pain, is "an unpleasant sensory and emotional experience associated with actual or potential tissue damage."[31] The definition empathizes pain as a complex multidimensional sensory-perceptual phenomenon that represents a unique subjective experience for each individual. Pain researchers have traditionally delineated categories of pain as (1) acute pain, (2) cancer-related pain, and (3) chronic nonmalignant pain subgroups.

Acute Pain

Acute pain is viewed as the reaction to a nociceptive trauma or disease onset, with the pain symptoms viewed as directly proportional to the disease, injury, or tissue damage. Furthermore, the symptoms follow a typical expected time course for the injury or condition, which may be days, weeks, or months.

Chronic Pain

When pain does not resolve during the acute phase and persists beyond expected recovery intervals or remains present because of the nature of the disease or injury, chronic pain disorders may develop. In cancer-related conditions, the pain may often present with an identifiable somatogenic cause and progression. The malignant condition, by its nature, may pose unique coping and adaptation demands and involve significant psychosocial adjustment issues that are not present in nonmalignant pain disorders.

Chronic Nonmalignant Pain

Chronic nonmalignant pain represents a complex group that has been the focus of many medical and mental health researchers. This category has usually been defined as a complex pain state in which the pain symptoms have persisted long after the original injury, trauma, or disease onset. The symptoms are viewed as exceeding the typical expected time course for healing of the acute injury, and the symptom intensity and duration are also viewed as in excess of what would be predicted by the medical condition alone. Some researchers have noted that the patient's pain symptoms move beyond the initial acute disease or injury to a point at which the pain symptoms become the disease.[32]

Chronic nonmalignant pain is also usually associated with a broad array of functional impairments, psychologic symptoms, disability, and a high rate of medical service use.

MULTIDISCIPLINARY TREATMENT AND BIOPSYCHOSOCIAL MODEL

While treating pain disorders during World War II, Bonica[33] reported the need for multidisciplinary treatment, which led to the development of the multidisciplinary pain clinic. Despite 50 years of progress and development of the multidisciplinary model, many pain patients continue to receive treatment under unidimensional biomedical models with emphasis on the correct diagnosis and treatment of the nociceptive pain generators using procedures such as nerve blocks, pharmacologic approaches, surgery, or cryolysis without consideration of coexisting psychosocial factors. Although this approach can be effective with a broad array of acute and chronic pan conditions, it has been less efficacious with complex chronic pain subgroups in which there are often, by definition, symptoms that are disproportionate to the original injury, tissue damage, or disease. Furthermore, physical symptoms alone are often poorly associated with predictive value in return to work or functional outcomes.[34,35]

Most pain clinics are now oriented toward a multidisciplinary and biopsychosocial model that recognizes the importance of biologic and medical factors, psychologic factors, and sociocultural factors in complex chronic pain.

The *gate-control theory* of pain[36,37] served as a model that incorporates the multidimensional nature of pain. This model and the development of the biopsychosocial approach[38] illustrated theoretical mechanisms whereby biopsychosocial factors interact to influence pain symptoms and behavior. Despite some changes, challenges, and subsequent refinements, gate-control theory continues to have widespread acceptance in pain management as a theory that can integrate the biopsychosocial factors and demonstrate how cortical factors affect the processing of nociceptive information.[39]

Briefly, the gate-control model[37] (Fig. 25–1) illustrates the roles of both ascending and descending neural pathways, which operate to create a gating or control mechanism for the transmission of nociceptive impulse. The gate mechanism, operating in the dorsal horn of the spinal cord, involves the substantia gelatinosa and the transmission cells. The gate has both peripheral and central mechanisms that influence the transmission of pain. Gate-control theory incorporates the influence of cognitive, emotional, and motivational factors that can operate both at the gate and at higher nervous system levels, which also modulate pain perception.

Newer psychologic pain models also developed after publication of the gate-control theory and took a focus that differed from that of the pure psychodynamic-intrapsychic models. Two major models emerged:

- The *operant (behavioral) model*—focuses on observable measures of pain behavior, including verbal reports, activities, facial expressions, and motor behaviors such as guarding
- The *cognitive-behavioral model*—focuses on cognitions (pain attitudes, beliefs, self-control), affective factors, and coping mechanisms

Both models continue to shape theoretical and treatment efforts and fall under the wider biopsychosocial pain model.

PAIN-PRONE AND PSYCHOGENIC PAIN ISSUES

Over the past 30 years since the gate-control theory was published, a huge volume of psychologic research has developed in pain assessment methods, pain-related disorders, and pain treatment methods. In clinical practice and in research, the role of psychologic and social factors has become more prominent with pain disorders that progress from an acute to a chronic stage. Researchers in pain psychology have examined both preexisting psychologic problems that might contribute to the development of chronic pain and the psychologic problems that develop as pain disorders become chronic.

Overall, although no single personality type or psychogenic profile has been supported in the literature or has a diagnosis-specific psychologic profile, it has become clear that multiple psychologic distress variables and disorders are present in high incidence among chronic pain populations.

PSYCHIATRIC NOMENCLATURE AND CHRONIC PAIN

Psychiatric and psychologic diagnoses related to chronic pain can be grouped into three main areas:

1. Preexisting conditions such as depression or personality disorders that were present before pain onset
2. Reactive conditions that occur as a result of chronic pain such as depression, anxiety, or adjustment problems
3. Conditions related to the pain, such as somatoform pain disorder or factitious disorder

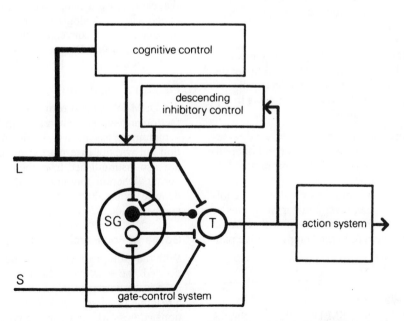

FIG. 25–1   The gate-control theory of pain: Mark II. The new model includes excitatory (*white circle*) and inhibitory (*black circle*) links from the substantia gelatinosa (SG) to the transmission (T) cells as well as descending inhibitory control from brainstem systems. The round knob at the end of the inhibitory link implies that its action may be presynaptic, postsynaptic, or both. All connections are excitatory, except the inhibitory link from SG to T cell. *(From Melzack R, Wall PD: The challenge of pain: Exciting discoveries in the new science of pain control. New York, Basic Books, 1982).*

The *Diagnostic and Statistical Manual for Mental Disorders, 4th edition* (DSM-IV),[40] published by the American Psychiatric Association, is a widely accepted diagnostic classification system used to diagnose all forms of mental disorders, including organic, substance abuse, developmental, personality, mood, and many other forms. Although this system is labeled as a classification of "mental disorders," implying a mind-body dualism, DSM-IV actually reflects a biopsychosocial multifactorial model. A basic familiarity with this system allows the pain practitioner to communicate with mental health disciplines on a common language and conceptual basis.

Axes

Full diagnosis of a disorder under DSM-IV requires assessment of five factors or axes[40]:

- Axis I contains clinical disorders (e.g., anxiety, depression, substance abuse) that are presenting problems. Individuals may have more than one of these conditions, requiring multiple Axis I listings.
- Axis II conditions meet specific criteria for personality disorders or mental retardation and also include maladaptive personality traits, features, or defense mechanisms. A subsequent section highlights the importance of this area in chronic pain populations.
- Axis III lists general medical conditions that are present and may relate to the mental disorder. The medical conditions are not seen as necessarily independent factors and may relate to the Axis I condition.
- Axis IV contains a listing of psychosocial and environmental stresses, problems that are thought to potentially relate to the Axis I clinical disorder or Axis II personality disorder. These psychosocial problems include issues such as loss of a job, death in the family, divorce, and relocation.
- Axis V reflects the clinician's assessment of the individual's overall level of functioning on the Global Assessment of Functioning (GAF) scale with a range of 1 to 100. Scores in a range of 50 or less reflect both serious clinical symptoms and severe impairments in multiple areas of life functioning.

Although all five axes are specified in comprehensive evaluations, it is also common for mental health practitioners to specify only the Axis I or II disorders that are prominent features of the clinical presentation.

For the pain specialist who is not a psychiatrist, psychologist, or mental health clinician, several major categories of DSM-IV diagnoses occur frequently along with chronic pain and should be considered in initial comprehensive pain evaluations.

Specific Disorders

Substance-Related Disorders

Substance-related disorders in DSM-IV include problems related to drug and alcohol abuse, medications, and also toxic exposure problems. Specific criteria for each disorder deal with issues of physical and psychologic abuse versus dependency, tolerance, and withdrawal.

Mood Disorders

Mood disorders under DSM-IV encompass an array of mood and depression disorders. Common major diagnoses in this category that the pain clinician will likely encounter are *major depressive disorder, dysthymic disorder,* and *bipolar disorder.*[40] *Adjustment disorder with depressed mood* is another common depression diagnostic category seen in individuals with chronic pain.

Anxiety Disorders

Anxiety disorders compose a significant subset of the psychologic disorders seen in groups with chronic pain. DSM-IV presents multiple categories of anxiety-based disorders, some of which occur frequently in chronic pain populations. Some of the disorders that may occur include *generalized anxiety disorders, panic disorder, post-traumatic stress disorder,* and *acute stress disorder.*

Somatoform Disorders

Somatoform disorders under DSM-IV[40] are defined as disorders that present primarily with physical symptoms that suggest but cannot be explained by a general medical condition. Furthermore, a diagnosis in this category requires that the physical symptoms must cause significant distress and functional impairments. Central to somatoform diagnoses is the concept that the physical symptoms are not under voluntary control, a criterion that distinguishes them from *factitious disorders* and *malingering,* in which voluntary control and intentional symptom production are present.

Additional forms of somatoform disorders encountered in the chronic pain setting include *conversion disorders* and *somatoform pain disorders.* Conversion disorders involve symptoms affecting voluntary sensory or motor functions that cannot be attributed to a medical condition but are associated with psychologic factors or stressors. Under DSM-IV, the diagnosis of conversion disorder is not limited to pain symptoms alone. Diagnostic criteria for somatoform pain disorders are listed in Box 25–1.

Factitious Disorders

All DSM-IV somatoform disorders are distinguished from factitious disorders, wherein an individual voluntarily feigns symptoms to assume a sick role and its accompanying attention but without external incentives. Somatoform disorders are also distinguished from the DSM-IV category of malingering, wherein the individual feigns symptoms but has definite external incentives, such as faking an injury for compensation.

Some Major Psychologic Risk Factors

With the multiple diagnostic issues of psychologic problems defined, the extent to which these psychologic conditions exist in chronic pain populations as an antecedent factor or a reactive problem to pain remains debatable. Further questions address whether chronic pain patients are in fact from (1) other groups in the general population, (2) other groups under significant psychologic stress, and (3) groups with general medical disorders but without persistent pain. Many psychologic risk factors or problems have been found to be

---

BOX 25–1 Pain Disorder as Characterized in DSM-IV

Diagnostic Criteria for Pain Disorder

A. Pain in one or more anatomical sites is the predominant focus of the clinical presentation and is of sufficient severity to warrant clinical attention.

B. The pain causes clinically significant distress or impairment in social, occupational, or other important areas of functioning.

C. Psychological factors are judged to have an important role in the onset, severity, exacerbation, or maintenance of the pain.

D. The symptom or deficit is not intentionally produced or freigned (as in Factitious Disorder or Malingering).

E. The pain is not better accounted for by a Mood, Anxiety, or Psychotic Disorder and does not meet criteria for Dyspareunia.

Code as follows:

307.80 Pain Disorder Associated with Psychological Factors: psychological factors are judged to have the major role in the onset, severity, exacerbation, or maintenance of the pain. (If a general medical condition is present, it does not have a major role in the onset, severity, exacerbation, or maintenance of the pain.) This type of Pain Disorder is not diagnosed if criteria are also met for Somatization Disorder.

Specify if:

Acute: duration of less than 6 months
Chronic: duration of 6 months or longer

307.89 Pain Disorder Associated with Both Psychological Factors and a General Medical Condition: both psychological factors and a general medical condition are judged to have important roles in the onset, severity, exacerbation, or maintenance of the pain. The associated general medical condition or anatomical site of the pain (see below) is coded on Axis III.

Specify if:

Acute: duration of less than 6 months
Chronic: duration of 6 months or longer
Note: The following is not considered to be a mental disorder and is included here to facilitate differential diagnosis.

Pain Disorder Associated with a General Medical Condition: a general medical condition has a major role in the onset, severity, exacerbation, or maintenance of the pain. (If psychological factors are present, they are not judged to have a major role in the onset, severity, exacerbation, or maintenance of the pain.) The diagnostic code for the pain is selected based on the associated general medical condition if one has been established (see Appendix G) or on the anatomical location of the pain if the underlying general medical condition is not yet cleary established —for example, low back (724.2), sciatic (724.3), pelvic (625.9), headache (784.0), facial (784.0), chest (786.50), joint (719.4), bone (733.90) abdominal (789.0), breast (611.71), renal (788.0), ear (388.70), eye (379.91), throat (784.1), tooth (525.9), and urinary (788.0).

From the American Psychiatric Association: *Diagnostic and Statistical Manual of Mental Disorders*, ed 4. Washington, DC, 1994, American Psychiatric Association.

---

prevalent in chronic pain populations. Four specific areas examined in the recent literature include:

- Abuse history
- Depression
- Personality disorders
- Coping

Physical, Sexual, and Emotional Abuse and Neglect

The negative effects of childhood abuse and neglect are well-recognized risk factors in the development of many Axis I and Axis II mental disorders of DSM-IV.[40] A recent Minnesota Multiphasic Personality Inventory (MMPI-2) study indicated that women with abuse histories scored significantly higher on multiple MMPI-2 scales than did those without a history of abuse, suggesting that they had higher levels of psychologic distress and symptoms.[41] Whether a history of childhood or adult abuse also creates an increased risk factor for chronic pain remains a research issue that has received increased attention.

Anderson and Hines[42] summarized the various forms of childhood abuse and neglect that potentially lead to an increased vulnerability to pain. These factors included physical abuse, sexual abuse, parental-caregiver alcohol or sub-

stance abuse, abandonment, and emotional neglect-abuse. These factors were viewed as traumatic psychologic experiences that interfered in the developmental attachment process of a child to their parent or caregiver. Other authors have also found significant correlations between a history of abuse, particularly physical and sexual abuse, and various types of chronic pain disorders.

Various theories have been offered to explain the possible mechanisms for the abuse and the interaction with chronic pain. Some authors have focused on the negative psychologic effects of abuse and neglect on the attachment process and psychologic development (e.g., Anderson and Hines[42]) in which abuse creates a hyperarousal state as a generator for chronic pain memory patterns. Other researchers have implicated links between psychologic trauma and the subsequent dysregulation-deficiency of endogenous opioid systems in post-traumatic stress disorder and chronic pain (e.g., Friedman[43]).

Depression

Depression symptoms are generally defined to include depressed mood; crying spells; low self-esteem; thoughts of death and suicide; disturbances of sleep, appetite, energy, and activity levels; anhedonia (inability to experience pleasure); concentration and short-term memory problems; and social withdrawal. Such symptoms are often seen in chronic pain populations and have led to questions about the incidence of clinical depression in chronic pain. One inherent problem is that symptoms of depression, especially somatic symptoms, can be the same symptoms associated with the disease or biomedical component of chronic pain. Given the high prevalence of major depressive disorder, a severe form of depression under DSM-IV, researchers have attempted to elucidate the underlying issues related to the pain-depression relationship. Another aspect of the pain-depression relationship is whether the depression was a preexisting condition or developed after the onset of pain. Considerable interest has been shown in the time course and mechanisms for depression that develop after the onset of pain.

Collectively, the pain-depression studies indicate the importance of assessing depression in chronic pain groups, including both preexisting depressive disorders and those that develop after acute pain onset. The cognitive factors that appear to mediate the development of depression are also an important issue for assessment and as a target of both preventive and treatment interventions. The need to address these areas is further underscored by the high rate (15%) of eventual suicide associated with major depression[40,44] and the demonstrated correlation between suicide and self-reported measures of depression (e.g., Beck Depression Inventory, Beck Hopelessness Scale).[45,46]

The chronic pain-depression relationship appears to be best explained by the diathesis-stress model adopted by several researchers.[47,48] This model proposes that the demand characteristics of living with chronic pain produce negative cognitive and behavioral changes, which then lead to depression. Chronic pain is a stressor that can lead to the preceding changes given sufficient intensity, duration, and effects of pain. Furthermore, in individuals who have biochemical, cognitive, or behavioral predispositions toward depression, the stress of chronic pain can result in a change from a nondiagnosed subclinical problem or trait to a full depressive episode meeting criteria for major depression or dysthymic disorder.

Personality Disorders

Personality disorders, as defined in DSM-IV,[40] are listed as a separate dimensional factor (Axis II) from clinical disorders (Axis I). Essential features of a personality disorder under DSM-IV are persistent and maladaptive patterns of inner experience and behaviors that fall outside normative cultural expectations and affect at least two of the following four areas: (1) cognition, (2) affect, (3) interpersonal function, and (4) impulse control.

By definition, personality disorders affect how an individual relates to others and often cause significant problems in interpersonal relationships. Because the personality disorders have developed into long-term stable dysfunctional patterns, they are usually apparent by adolescence and early adulthood. In individuals with chronic pain, the personality disorders generally precede the onset of acute to chronic pain progression. DSM-IV also specifically states that there must be a long-term pattern of maladaptive behaviors and problems that are not caused by an Axis I (clinical) disorder or an Axis II (medical) disorder.

DMS-IV lists 11 personality disorder subtypes (10 specific types and one mixed-nonspecific type).[40] These types are grouped into three clusters based on symptoms:

- Cluster A: paranoid, schizoid, and schizotypal disorders (characterized by odd or eccentric behaviors, cognitive disorganization)
- Cluster B: antisocial, borderline, histrionic, and narcissistic types (characterized by acting out; poor impulse control; behaviors that are overly dramatic, emotional, or erratic)
- Cluster C: avoidant, dependent, and obsessive-compulsive personality disorders (characterized by anxious, fearful, or compulsive behaviors)[40,44,49,50]

Prevalence information reveals Clusters B and C to be the groups most likely to be seen within the chronic pain setting. There has been greater inter-rater agreement on cluster group classification than on which of the specific 11 diagnostic subtypes applies.[50] Further complicating the diagnostic process are situations in which an individual presents with only a partial set of criteria, thus not warranting a specific personality disorder diagnosis yet still manifesting patterns of an overall personality disorder. Also, many individuals have specific personality traits that are characteristic of a DSM-IV personality disorder but do not receive a formal diagnosis, because all criteria are not applicable.

The personality disorders are important in the chronic pain setting because they affect how individuals react to life events, including pain, and they particularly affect the individual's pattern of relating to others, including spouses, family, employers, pain treatment staff, or rehabilitation staff.

Cognitive Factors and Coping Strategies

With the rapid development of cognitive-behavioral applications to pain treatment and conceptualizations, a large volume of research has developed that examines both pain beliefs and coping styles or strategies. Beyond the questions of how these factors relate to or predict chronic pain, this research has also examined the effects of interventions aimed at modifying maladaptive coping strategies and beliefs. *Pain beliefs* are subjective beliefs, attitudes, or expectations about pain and are distinguished in the coping literature from *coping strategies,* which are defined as the actual type of cognitive response an individual exhibits in response to pain. Turk and colleagues[51] outlined the application of the cognitive-behavioral model to chronic pain, and dozens of measures of pain belief and coping have been developed.[35,52,53]

Pain-coping studies have moved beyond coping assessment instruments to further investigation of the dynamic process of coping with chronic pain, mediating factors, and interventions to enhance adaptive coping. Numerous positive cognitive strategies or coping styles have been identified in individuals dealing with chronic pain, together with negative coping strategies that can intensify or exacerbate the pain experience.[51]

Rosensteil and Keefe,[54] for example, devised a Coping Strategies Questionnaire (CSQ) that has become a widely used measure across a spectrum of chronic pain conditions. The CSQ outlines six cognitive coping strategies (diverting attention, reinterpreting pain sensations, coping self-statements, ignoring pain, praying-hoping, and catastrophizing). In addition, the CSQ has two behavioral coping strategies (increasing activity level and increasing pain behavior) and two items measuring perception of self-efficacy in controlling or reducing pain. Although reviews of the CSQ have indicated some interpretation issues and factors structure issues, many studies with CSQ have indicated the increased functional disability and depression are associated with catastrophizing strategies for pain and beliefs of limited self-control over pain.[52,53,55]

References

1. Engel G: The clinical application of the biopsychosocial model. *Am J Psychiatry* 137:535, 1980.
2. Melzack R, Wall PD: Pain mechanisms: A new theory. *Science* 150:971, 1965.
3. Flor H, Fydrich T, Turk DC: Efficacy of multidisciplinary pain treatment centers: A meta-analytic review. *Pain* 49:221, 1992.
4. Maruta T, Malinchoc M, Offord KP et al: Status of patients with chronic pain 13 years after treatment in a pain management clinic. *Pain* 74:199, 1998.
5. Pfingsten M, Hildebrandt J, Leibing E et al: Effectiveness of a multimodal treatment program for chronic low-back pain. *Pain* 73:77, 1997.
6. Deardoff WW, Rubin HS, Scott DW: Comprehensive multidisciplinary treatment of chronic pain: A follow-up study of treated and non-treated groups. *Pain* 45:35, 1991.
7. Fordyce WE: An operant conditioning method for managing chronic pain. *Postgrad Med* 53:123, 1973.
8. Fordyce WE: *Behavioral methods for chronic pain and illness.* St. Louis, Mosby, 1976.
9. Council JR, Ahern DK, Follick MJ et al: Expectancies and functional impairment in chronic low back pain. *Pain* 33:323, 1988.
10. Sanders SH: Operant conditioning with chronic pain: Back to basics. In Gatchel RJ, Turk DC, editors: *Psychological approaches to pain management: A practitioner's handbook.* New York, Guilford Press, 1996.
11. Kerns RD, Turk DC, Rudy TE: Comparison of cognitive-behavioral and behavioral approaches to the out-patient treatment of chronic pain. *Clin J Pain* 1:195, 1986.
12. Turner JA, Clancy S: Comparison of operant-behavioral and cognitive-behavioral group treatment for chronic low back pain. *J Consult Clin Psychol* 56:261, 1988.
13. Nicholas MK, Wilson PH, Goyen J: Operant-behavioural and cognitive-behavioural treatment for chronic low back pain. *Behav Res Ther* 29:225, 1991.
14. Jensen MP, Turner JA, Romano JM et al: Coping with chronic pain: A critical review of the literature. *Pain* 47:249, 1991.
15. Jensen MP, Karoly P: Control beliefs, coping efforts and adjustment to chronic pain. *J Consult Psychol* 59:431, 1991.
16. Jensen MP, Turner JA, Romano JM et al: Relationship of pain-specific beliefs to chronic pain adjustment. *Pain* 57:301, 1994.
17. McCracken LM: Learning to live with the pain: Acceptance of pain predicts adjustment in persons with chronic pain. *Pain* 74:21, 1998.
18. Turk DC, Rudy TE: A cognitive-behavioral perspective on chronic pain: Beyond the scalpel and syringe. In Tollison CD, editor: *Handbook of chronic pain management.* Baltimore, Williams & Wilkins, 1988.
19. Keefe FJ, Beaupre PM, Gil KM: Group therapy for patients with chronic pain. In Gatchel RJ, Turk DC, editors: *Psychological approaches to pain management: A practitioner's handbook.* New York, Guilford Press, 1996.
20. Rolland JS: *Families, illness, and disability.* New York, Basic Books, 1994.
21. Minuchin S: *Families and family therapy.* Boston, Harvard University Press, 1974.
22. Kerns RD, Haythornthwaite J, Southwick S et al: The role of marital interaction in chronic pain and depressive symptom severity. *J Psychosom Res* 34:401, 1990.
23. Turk DC, Kerns RD, Rosenberg R: Effects of marital interaction on chronic pain and disability: Examining the down side of social support. *Rehabil Psychol* 37:259, 1992.
24. Patterson JM, Garwick AW: The impact of chronic illness on families: A family systems perspective. *Ann Behav Med* 16:131, 1994.
25. Kirsch I, Lynn SJ, Rhue JW: Introduction to clinical hypnosis. In Rhue JW, Lynn SJ, Kirsh I, editors: *Handbook of clinical hypnosis.* Washington, DC, American Psychological Association, 1997.
26. Gauld A: Reflections on mesmeric analgesia. *Br J Exp Clin Hypn* 5:17, 1988.
27. Hilgard ER, Hilgard JR: *Hypnosis in the relief of pain.* New York, Brunner/Mazel, 1994.
28. Schwartz MS: *Biofeedback.* New York, Guilford Press, 1995.
29. Benson H: *The relaxation response.* New York, Avon Books, 1976.
30. Smith JC: *Cognitive-behavioral relaxation training: A new system of strategies for treatment and assessment.* New York, Springer, 1990.
31. Lindblom U: Pain terms: A current list with definitions and usage. *Pain* 3(suppl):S215, 1986.
32. Sternback RA: *Pain patients: Traits and treatment.* New York, Academic Press, 1974.
33. Bonica JJ: Multidisciplinary/interdisciplinary pain programs. In Bonice JJ, editor: *The management of pain,* ed 2, vol 1. Malvern, Pa, Lea & Febiger, 1990.
34. Jamison RN: *Mastering chronic pain: A professional's guide to behavioral treatment.* Sarasota, Fla, Professional Resource Press, 1996.
35. Block AR: *Presurgical psychological screening in chronic pain syndromes: A guide for the behavioral health practitioner.* Mahwah, NJ, Lawrence Erlbaum Associates, 1996.
36. Melzack R, Wall PD: Pain mechanisms: A new theory. *Science* 150:971, 1965.
37. Melzack R, Wall PD: *The challenge of pain.* New York, Basic Books, 1983.
38. Loeser JD: Concepts of pain. In Stanton-Hicks M, Boas RA, editors: *Chronic low back pain.* New York, Raven Press, 1982.
39. Staats PS, Hekmat H, Staats AW: The psychological-behaviorism theory of pain. *Pain Forum* 5:194, 1996.
40. American Psychiatric Association: *Diagnostic and statistical manual of mental disorders,* ed 4. Washington, DC, American Psychiatric Association, 1994.
41. Griffith PL, Myers RW, Cusick GM et al: MMPI-2 profiles of women differing in sexual abuse history and sexual orientation. *J Clin Psychol* 53:791, 1997.
42. Anderson DJ, Hines R: Attachment and pain. In Grzesiak RC, Ciccone DS, editors: *Psychological vulnerability to chronic pain.* New York, Springer, 1994.
43. Friedman MJ: Biological diagnosis and treatment of PTSD. In Everly GS, Lating JM, editors: *Psychotraumatology: Key papers and core concepts in post-traumatic stress.* New York, Plenum Press, 1995.
44. Kaplan HI, Sadock BJ: *Pocket handbook of clinical psychiatry.* Baltimore, William & Wilkins, 1990.
45. Beck AT: *Depression: Causes and treatment.* Philadelphia, University of Pennsylvania Press, 1967.
46. Beck AT, Weissman A, Lester D et al: The measurement of pessimism: The hopelessness scale. *J Consult Clin Psychol* 42:861, 1974.
47. Banks SM, Kerns RD: Explaining high rates of depression in chronic pain: A diathesis-stress framework. *Psychol Bull* 119:95, 1996.
48. Maxwell TD, Gatchel RJ, Mayer TG: Cognitive predictors of depression in chronic low back pain: Toward an inclusive model. *J Behav Med* 21:131, 1998.
49. Scully JH: Personality disorders. In Scully JH, editor: *Psychiatry.* Media, Pa, Harwal Publishing, 1985.
50. Weisberg JN, Keefe FJ: Personality disorders in the chronic pain population: Basic concepts, empirical findings, and clinical implications. *Pain Forum* 6:1, 1997.
51. Turk DC, Meichenbaum D, Genest M: *Pain and behavioral medicine: A cognitive behavioral perspective.* New York, Guilford Press, 1983.
52. DeGood DE, Shutty MS: Assessment of pain beliefs, coping, and self-efficacy. In Turk DC, Malzack R, editors: *Handbook of pain assessment.* New York, Guilford Press, 1992.
53. Jensen MP, Turner JA, Romano JM: Correlates of improvement in multidisciplinary treatment of chronic pain. *J Consult Clin Psychol* 62:172, 1994.
54. Rosenstiel AK, Keefe FJ: The use of coping strategies in low back pain patients: Relationship to patient characteristics and current adjustment. *Pain* 17:33, 1983.
55. Block AR, Vanharanta H, Ohnmeiss DD et al: Discographic pain report: Influence of psychological factors. *Spine* 21:334, 1996.

1. Operant interventions are specific and targeted. These include all of the following except

   A. Patient sets goals and has a predefined award for attainment of goal
   B. Goals are increasingly more difficult in an attempt to maximize function
   C. Medical staff and family members are instructed to support the patient's pain behavior
   D. Medical staff and family members are asked to acknowledge adaptive behaviors by the patient

2. When a clinician offers suggestions to the patient to experience alteration in sensation, perception, or cognition, this technique is called

   A. Hypnosis
   B. Biofeedback
   C. Psychologic counseling
   D. Psychometric testing

3. Relaxation technique used in psychotherapy can be accomplished by all of the following except

   A. Progressive muscle relaxation
   B. Controlled breathing
   C. Visual imagery
   D. Measuring blood pressure

4. An electronic or electromechanical instrument is used to monitor physiologic processes and to provide feedback of this information to the patient in

   A. Hypnosis
   B. Biofeedback
   C. Relaxation technique
   D. Transcendental meditation

5. The psychiatric model that focuses on cognition (pain attitudes, beliefs, and self-control), affective factors, and coping mechanisms is termed

   A. Operant (behavioral) model
   B. Cognitive-behavioral model
   C. Medical model
   D. Psychosocial model

ANSWERS

1. C
2. A
3. D
4. B
5. B

CHAPTER 26

Physical Therapy Techniques

RICHARD M. LINCHITZ AND PAUL J. SORELL III

Physical therapy remains a major component of any successful pain management program and plays a key role in the overall rehabilitation of patients with both acute and chronic pain. Physical medicine and rehabilitation have traditionally been the medical specialty that oversees and prescribes the application of the physical modalities to treat disease and disorders, including the rehabilitation of patients with pain. All physicians, whether in primary care or in other medical and surgical specialties, and especially pain medicine specialists should understand the rationale for physical methods of controlling pain and the appropriate use of the methods in the rehabilitation of patients with both acute and chronic pain.

Physical therapy alone is sometimes all that is needed to return the pain patient to a more productive and rewarding life. However, especially for patients with chronic pain, physical therapy augments the other interventions provided by the pain rehabilitation team.

Modalities are both active and passive psychical agents and techniques used to produce a therapeutic response in tissue. For many modalities, the mechanism of action is well defined; for others, it is not. In clinical practice, it is more important that physicians know the indications, contradictions, and effects on the body of specific modalities than it is to understand the mechanism of action.

BOX 26–1 Outline of Therapeutic Modalities for Pain

- Therapeutic heat—hot packs, paraffin, heat lamps, hydrotherapy, fluidotherapy, ultrasound, phonophoresis, short-wave and microwave diathermy
- Therapeutic cold—cold packs, ice massage, cold water immersion, contrast bathing, vapocoolant spray
- Electrical stimulation—high-voltage pulsed galvanic stimulation, iontophoresis, functional neuromuscular electrical stimulation, transcutaneous electrical nerve stimulation (TENS)
- Passive physical therapeutic modalities—stretching, therapeutic exercise, massage and manipulation, mobilization, traction
- Behavioral approaches

Among the physical modalities are interventions such as:

1. Heat and cold (conduction, convection, radiation)
2. Water (whirlpool, aquatic/hydrotherapy)
3. Sound (ultrasound, phonophoresis)
4. Electricity (transcutaneous electrical nerve stimulation [TENS], iontophoresis)
5. Electromagnetic waves (infrared [IR], visible, and ultraviolet [UV] light; short waves; and microwaves)
6. Therapeutic exercise (Box 26–1)

Other physical modalities, such as traction, orthotics, assistive devices, acupuncture, biofeedback, and manual therapy are described in more extensive discussions provided by other sources.[1-3]

TEMPERATURE MODALITIES

Therapeutic Heat

Heat is one of the oldest physical modalities used to reduce and relieve pain. Although by themselves heat modalities may not lead to a cure, they are important additions to treatment. Heat is commonly used as an adjunct to other therapy in relieving painful conditions, even when the underlying disorder may not be treatable.

Heat therapy can be classified by depth of penetration (superficial vs. deep) and form of energy transfer. Superficial modalities include hot packs, heating pads, hot lamps, paraffin and whirlpool baths, and fluidotherapy. None of these agents can elevate temperature by more than a few degrees at depths of a few centimeters.[4] Deep heating agents, also known as diathermics, include ultrasound, short wave, and microwave. Energy transfer can be divided into several mechanisms as well:

1. Conduction
2. Convection
3. Conversion
4. Radiation

Physiologic Effects of Heat

Various mechanisms for the analgesic effect of heat have been proposed. First, localized heating produces a variety of hemodynamic effects. Vasodilation is believed to reduce the pain associated with ischemia via the resultant increased influx of oxygen and nutrients and the egress of carbon dioxide, metabolic waste products, and pain mediators.[5] Cell membrane permeability is also altered by heat.[6] Hence, heat is indicated in the treatment of chronic inflammatory conditions but contraindicated in acute inflammation because of the risk of increased bleeding and edema formation.[7,8]

Distant heating effects include the slowing of gastrointestinal peristalsis and peristalsis and decreased uterine contractions.[9] *Local* heating also increases the extensibility of collagen, which can help relieve joint stiffness.[10]

Indications

Among the indications for heat therapy are muscle spasm, myalgia, fibromyalgia, contracture, collagen vascular disease, and bursitis.

Contraindications

Heat should be avoided in the following instances[11]:

1. Tissues with inadequate vascular supply
2. Acute injury
3. Bleeding disorders
4. Regions of severely insensate tissue
5. Scar tissue

In addition, heat should be used with great caution for patients with impaired cognition or communication because of the inability to report pain.

Therapeutic Cold

Cryotherapy (therapeutic use of cold) has become the most useful modality in treating acute conditions but, like heat therapy, is also a useful tool in chronic pain management. All forms of cryotherapy are considered superficial cooling agents.

Indications

Cryotherapy is indicated in the management of spasticity, muscle spasm, and edema and in the reduction of local and systemic metabolic activity. Injuries such as sprains, strains, and contusions are treated initially with *r*est, *i*ce, *c*ompression, and *e*levation (RICE).

Physiologic Effects of Cold

Cold is often used because of its therapeutic value in decreasing metabolism, modulating the inflammatory response,[8] slowing nerve conduction velocity,[14,15] and decreasing muscle spindle activity resulting in decreased muscle spasm. Application of cold to the skin results in immediate cutaneous vasoconstriction through sympathetically medicated reflex mechanisms and by directly stimulating smooth muscle contraction.[16,17] Simultaneously, the firing rates of both group Ia and II muscle spindle fibers and group Ib Golgi tendon organ fibers are decreased.[18] Histamine release is also blocked by cold, which leads to decreased edema and hemorrhage.[10] The analgesic effect of cold most likely results from a combination of all these effects.

Contraindications

The use of any form of cryotherapy should be avoided in patients with angina, arterial insufficiency, Raynaud's phenomenon or disease, cold insensitivity, or allergy.[10,11] Patients who do not tolerate cold therapy well because of cold insensitivity tend to increase muscle guarding and co-contraction, which is directly counterproductive to the therapeutic goals.

Modalities

Some cold modalities include:

1. Cold packs
2. Ice massage
3. Cold water immersion
4. Contrast bathing
5. Vapocoolant spray

ELECTRICAL STIMULATION

Electricity has been used since ancient times to treat many types of medical problems. Electrical stimulation (ES) comes in many forms and can provide many beneficial effects. In patients who have lost voluntary control of a group of muscles for whatever reason, ES can actively stimulate these muscles to exercise them and prevent atrophy. Thanks to the work of Melzack and Wall[19] in 1965 and their discovery of the *gate theory of pain,* electroanalgesia is now widely applied in the form of what is commonly known as TENS.

Finally, improved electronics and neurosurgical techniques can now apply electrical signals directly to the dorsal column of the spine, providing yet another way of helping achieve pain relief for chronic pain. ES is often used in the control of pain as an adjunct to exercise and other applied modalities.

Physiologic Effects

Fast-twitch skeletal muscle fibers (type IIb) have been observed to transform into fibers with more *slow-twitch* type I characteristics.[19–24] The number of type IIa muscle fibers also increase in response to ES.[25] Both normally innervated and denervated muscles benefit from ES. If muscles are denervated, ES maintains nutrition by promoting blood flow, which decreases fibrotic changes and retards denervation atrophy. Innervated muscles benefit from ES via increased strengthening, prevention or reversal of disuse atrophy, maintenance or improvement of mobility, promotion of increased peripheral circulation, and provision of improved proprioceptive feedback.[10]

The effectiveness of ES depends on its (1) intensity (amplitude), (2) frequency, (3) waveform, and (4) duration.[26] Three basic types of waveforms exist:

- Direct current (DC)
- Alternating current (AC)
- Pulsed current

The pulsed waveforms are the most common waveforms applied for therapeutic purposes.[27] Both burst-modulated AC and asymmetric biphasic pulsed currents appear to induce the most forceful muscle contractions while providing the most comfort to patients.[28,29]

The electrodes through which ES is applied also play a significant role in its overall therapeutic effectiveness. The choice of an electrode type is based on the goal of the ES program and its ease of use for the patient. Electrodes are either *unipolar* (one active) or *bipolar* (two equally sized active). The active electrodes are placed over motor points.

Surface electrodes remain the most commonly used electrode type for most therapeutic interventions.

Indications and Contraindications

ES is effective in the management of both acute and chronic pain disorders. It can help reduce pain and edema while decreasing muscle spasm and alleviating inflammation through improved peripheral circulation. ES has also been used in the treatment of neuropathic pain conditions and assists in wound and fracture healing, prevention or reversal of osteoporosis as well as the pain sometimes associated with it, and prevention of deep venous thromboses.

ES should never be used in the presence of patients with pacemakers or in patients with thrombophlebitis and skin disorders. Patients with cardiac disease should also be monitored very carefully, because ES can rarely induce arrhythmias in patients who may be predisposed to them.

Modalities

Some modalities for ES include:

1. High-voltage pulsed galvanic stimulation
2. Iontophoresis
3. Functional neuromuscular ES
4. TENS

PASSIVE PHYSICAL THERAPEUTIC MODALITIES

Stretching

Stretching is a general term encompassing any therapeutic maneuver designed to lengthen pathologically shortened soft tissue structure leading to an increase in range-of-motion (ROM).[30] Adequate mobility and flexibility of all the soft tissue components surrounding a joint, including skin, fascia, muscle, and ligament, are necessary for proper pain-free motion.[30] The foremost goal to be sought when one is performing these techniques is an increase in soft tissue elasticity and plasticity, thereby decreasing contractures. Stretching can be either *passive* (when the patient is relaxed and the force is applied either manually or mechanically) or *active* (when the patient participates in the stretching maneuver).

Indications

Indications for stretching include:

1. Prolonged immobilization leading to adhesions and contractures
2. Restricted mobility
3. Connective tissue or neuromuscular diseases
4. Structural damage secondary to trauma
5. Congenital or acquired bony deformities

Contraindications

Stretching should be avoided in the following situations:

1. Restricted motion secondary to a bony block
2. After a recent fracture
3. Evidence of an acute inflammatory of infective process, either in or around a joint
4. Patients in whom contractures are the chief means of providing joint stability

Therapeutic Exercise

Therapeutic exercise is the cornerstone in achieving long-term benefits in the treatment of chronic pain. During the chronic phase of pain, the patient may have had a prolonged period of decreased activity, leading to weakened muscles and contracted joints, which contribute to increased pain.[31] Restoration of the body to its normal level of functioning is the long-term goal of therapeutic exercise. The short-term goals include[32]:

1. Strengthening the muscles
2. Improving flexibility of muscles and tendons
3. Increasing endurance
4. Reinstating the normal pattern of motion to the affected muscles and to the body in general

Systemically, exercise increases blood flow, cardiac output, and respiratory reserve. Locally, it has an effect on the muscle and joints being treated. Universally, exercise can strengthen weak muscles, mobilize stiff joints, build endurance and speed, and establish neuromuscular balance and coordination.[33]

Range-of-Motion Exercises

ROM refers to the amount or degrees of motion that can occur between two bones or the amount of motion from a neutral position when referring to the spine.

Passive Range-of-Motion Exercises

Passive movement is movement within an unrestricted range for a segment that is produced entirely by an external force; there is no voluntary muscle contraction.[30] These techniques help to manage chronic pain by increasing blood flow (and thereby nutrition), augmenting venous return and lymphatic drainage (thereby controlling edema), and preventing contracture formation secondary to immobility.[34,35]

Specific indications for passive ROM exercises include[30]:

1. Maintenance of joint and soft structure
2. Minimization of contracture formation
3. Decrease or inhibition of pain by mechanisms described previously
4. Assistance with healing following injury or surgery
5. Assistance in proprioceptive maintenance

These exercises do not prevent muscle atrophy or increase muscle strength or endurance.

Active Assisted Range-of-Motion Exercises

Active assisted movement is movement through a ROM by means of a muscular contraction supplemented by an external force either manually or mechanically.[30] The benefits seen with this type of exercise are identical to those of the passive type. These exercises usually serve as a transitional therapy.

Active Range-of-Motion Exercises

Active exercises entail voluntary muscle contraction by the patient to move the joint through the available ROM without assistance from the external force.[36] Physiologically, active ROM exercises facilitate greater circulation than that achieved with passive exercise, help to maintain soft tissue flexibility and elasticity, prevent muscle atrophy, improve coordination and kinesthetic responses, and avoid thrombus formation.[36]

Precautions and Contraindications

All forms of ROM exercises are contraindicated when motion to a segment (joint) is disruptive to the healing process; however, adhesions and contracture formation, sluggish circulation, and an extended recovery time can all result from complete immobilizations.[30] Active ROM is contraindicated in any patients with an unstable cardiac condition because the risk would outweigh any potential benefit.

Resistive Exercises

Once the goals of increased ROM and soft tissue elasticity have been reached, the next part of the therapeutic exercise program should begin.

Resistive exercise is any form of active exercise in which a dynamic or static muscular contraction is resisted by an outside force.[37] The external force may be applied manually or mechanically. The three basic types of resistive exercise are *isometric* (a static form of motion performed by contraction against an immovable object), *isotonic* (a dynamic form of motion preformed against a constant or variable load through the available ROM),[38] and *isokinetic* (a form of dynamic motion in which the velocity of muscle shortening or lengthening—and thus the velocity of the body part—is controlled by a rate-limiting device).[38]

Precautions and Contraindications

In general, precautions for resistive exercises include cardiovascular factors, overwork, fatigue, osteoporosis, and immediate muscle soreness associated with exercise.[30] A specific complication of isometric exercise is the potential for a large increase in blood pressure.[39] Relative contraindications include inflammation of the muscle or joint being exercised and pain.

Other Techniques of Therapeutic Exercise

A number of other techniques can be used either alone or in combination with most of the modalities described thus far.[36] These include:

1. Endurance activities
2. Desensitization
3. Breathing exercises
4. Relaxation
5. Proprioceptive neuromuscular facilitation
6. Coordination training

Manual Techniques

Throughout history, many different forms of massage and manipulation have been used to relieve pain.[40] Massage and manipulation together constitute a larger category known as manual medicine, manipulative therapy, or manual therapy.[40] All techniques whereby the hands are used to manipulate soft or bony tissue therapeutically are included under these titles. By far, most people who search for massage or manipulation, as a form of therapy, do so for the relief of muscle spasm, tension, or stiffness, all of which can cause pain. A multitude of theories have been proposed to explain how manual therapy may reduce pain[40]:

1. A change in pain threshold secondary to an increase in serum endorphins[41]
2. Relief of muscle spasm by multiple mechanisms[42]
3. Increased circulation by either local effects or sympathetic reflex[43]
4. Increased ROM[43]
5. Increased venous and lymphatic drainage, thereby decreasing local swelling and edema[43]

Massage

Massage is the scientific application of force by the hands to soft tissue, usually the skin, fascia, muscles, tendons, and ligaments, to produce a therapeutic effect. The effect can be mechanical or reflexive. All techniques grouped under the term *massage* are of the passive type, meaning the patient does not actively participate during the treatment. These techniques include:

1. Stroking or effleurage
2. Kneading and pétrissage
3. Friction massage
4. Percussion, tapotement, or clapping
5. Stroking and vibration

Myofascial Techniques

Myofascial techniques are soft tissue techniques often used by osteopathic physicians.[44] The difference between myofascial techniques and massage is that the former involves active or voluntary muscle contraction on the part of the patient along with passive massage. This active component adds additional physiologic mechanisms by which muscle spasm and pain may be treated. These proposed physiologic mechanisms include effects involving (1) the muscle spindle reflex, (2) the Golgi tendon organ reflex, (3) reciprocal inhibition, and (4) the crossed extensor reflex.[43]

Myofascial techniques have been postulated to aid in achieving the primary goal of homeostasis or the restoration and preservation of optimal bodily function. Myofascial techniques have been proposed to break the cycle thought to be at the core of chronic muscle pain.

Mobilization

As with passive ROM exercises, joint mobilization consists of passive oscillations that try to restore the normal ROM or decrease the restriction by rearranging and loosening the collagen fiber.[45] Mobilization techniques can be used to reduce muscle guarding, improve ROM, and decrease pain. These techniques are contraindicated if hypermobility, joint effusion, or acute inflammation is present.

Manipulation

Most modern textbooks of manual therapy define manipulation as a forceful thrust in which a joint is passively moved through its physiologic barrier. The "thrust" is of high velocity and low amplitude (HVLA). The difference between mobilization and manipulation is the application of this HVLA thrust to the joint.[40]

Manipulation is most commonly used by osteopathic physicians and chiropractors, with each profession adhering to its own specific techniques. HVLA is most commonly applied to the vertebral joints.

When performed precisely, manipulation usually relieves pain or other symptoms instantaneously.[33]

Contraindications include osteoporosis, acute inflammation, infection, tumor infiltration, fracture, any other cause of structural instability seen radiographically,[33] and vertebral-basilar insufficiency when applied to the cervical spine.

Traction

In the therapy of traction, the soft tissues of the body (cervical or lumbar spine) are stretched by pulling (traction) force. This force can be applied either manually or mechanically. Factors that determine the amount of separation (and thus pain reduction) include the position of the spine, the angle of pull, and the amount of force applied.[40] Traction, when applied properly, may prevent adhesion formation, subdue painful muscle spasm, relieve pain, maintain anatomic alignment, and prevent or correct a deformity.[33]

Contraindications to the use of traction include acute trauma, inflammation, hypermobility, increasing pain, and any spinal condition in which movement is to be avoided.[30]

BEHAVIORAL APPROACH TO EXERCISE

In chronic pain patients, factors other than an underlying pathologic process become important in the maintenance of chronic pain complaints and chronic pain behavior. The patient's pain complaints, gait, lack of activity, demands for medication, joblessness, and so forth may all be subtly (or not so subtly) reinforced by the patient's environment. In behavioral terms, the patient's behavior shifts from being purely *respondent* (i.e., in response to underlying tissue pathology) to *operant* (i.e., aimed at obtaining reinforcement from the environment). Reinforcement in the environment can take the form of monetary rewards, administration of pain medications, and especially attention from significant others and rest from responsibilities.

In an elegant and comprehensive classic, Fordyce[46] systematically outlined the principles of behavioral management of chronic pain patients, stating that:

> … changing behavior by contingency management is a precision enterprise. In general, the three potential behavior problems to be addressed include: (1) some desired behavior is not occurring often enough and needs to be increased (such as overall activity level); (2) a behavior is occurring too frequently and needs to be diminished or eliminated (e.g., bed rest, pain complaints, moaning); (3) some desired behaviors are entirely absent and need to be learned (e.g., methods of relaxation training, relaxed ways of movement, and so forth).

References

1. Foley KM, Payne RM: *Current therapy of pain.* Philadelphia, BC Decker, 1989.
2. Kaplan P, Tanner E: *Musculoskeletal pain and disability.* Norwalk, Conn, Appleton & Lange, 1989.
3. Leek JC, Gershwin ME, Fowler WM Jr: *Principles of physical medicine and rehabilitation in the musculoskeletal diseases.* Orlando, Fla, Grune & Stratton, 1986.
4. Lehmann JF, Silverman DR, Baum BA et al: Temperature distributions in human thigh, produced by infrared, hot pack and microwave application. *Arch Phys Med Rehabil* 47:291, 1966.
5. Guy AW, Lehmann JF, Stonebridge JB: Therapeutic applications of electromagnetic power. *Proc IEEE* 62:55, 1974.
6. Braddom RL, editor: *Physical medicine and rehabilitation.* Philadelphia, WB Saunders, 1996.
7. Guy AW, Lehmann JF, Stonebridge JB: Therapeutic applications of electromagnetic power. *Proc IEEE* 62:60, 1974.
8. Schmidt KL, Ott VR, Rocher G et al: Heat, cold and inflammation (review). *Z Rheumatol* 38:391, 1979.
9. Lehmann JF, deLateur BJ: Ultrasound, short-wave, microwave superficial heat, and cold in the treatment of pain. In Melzack R, Wall P, editors: *Textbook of pain,* ed 2. New York, Churchill Livingstone, 1989.
10. Hayes KW: *Manual for physical agents,* ed 4. East Norwalk, Conn, Appleton & Lange, 1993.
11. DeLisa A, Gans M: *Rehabilitation medicine principles and practice,* ed 2. Philadelphia, Lippincott-Raven, 1991.
12. Lehmann JF, deLateur BJ: Ultrasound, short-wave, microwave superficial heat, and cold in the treatment of pain. In Melzack R, Wall P, editors: *Textbook of pain,* ed 2. New York, Churchill Livingstone, 1989.
13. Michlovitz SL: *Thermal agents in rehabilitation.* Philadelphia, FA Davis, 1986.
14. Abramson DI, Chu LS, Tuck S Jr et al: Effect of tissue temperatures and blood flow on motor nerve conduction velocity. *JAMA* 198:1082, 1966.
15. Denys EH: AAEM minimonograph # 14: The influence of temperature in clinical neurophysiology. *Muscle Nerve* 14:795, 1991.
16. Guyton AC: Body temperature, temperature regulation, and fever. In Guyton AC, editor: *Textbook of medical physiology,* ed 8. Philadelphia, WB Saunders, 1991.
17. Perkins IF: Cooling as a stimulus to smooth muscles. *Am J Physiol* 163:14, 1950.
18. Eldred E, Lindsley DF, Buchwald JS: The effect of cooling on mammalian muscle spindles. *Exp Neurol* 2:144, 1960.
19. Melzack R, Wall PD: Pain mechanisms: A new theory. *Science* 150:971, 1965.
20. Heilmann C, Muller W, Pette D: Correlation between ultrastructural and functional changes in sarcoplasmic reticulum during chronic stimulation of fast muscle. *J Membr Biol* 59:143, 1981.
21. Mabuchi K, Szvetko D, Pinter K et al: Type IIB to IIA fiber transformation in intermittently stimulated rabbit muscles. *Am J Physiol* 242:373, 1982.
22. Eisenberg BR, Salmons S: The reorganization of subcellular structure in muscle undergoing fast-to-slow type transformation: A stereological study. *Cell Tissue Res* 220:449, 1981.
23. Brownson C, Isenberg H, Brown W et al: Changes in skeletal muscle gene transcription induced by chronic stimulation. *Muscle Nerve* 11:1183, 1988.
24. Lawrence JC Jr, Krsek JA, Salsgiver WJ et al: Phosphorylase kinase isozymes in normal and electrically stimulated skeletal muscles. *Am J Physiol* 250:84, 1986.
25. Greve JM, Muszkat R, Schmidt B et al: Functional electrical stimulation (FES): Muscle histochemical analysis. *Paraplegia* 31:764, 1993.
26. Shriven WJ: *Manual of electrotherapy.* Philadelphia, Lea & Febiger, 1975.
27. Lake DA: Neuromuscular electrical stimulation: An overview and its application in the treatment of sports injuries. *Sports Med* 13:320, 1992.
28. Kramer IF, Semple JE: Comparison of selected strengthening techniques for normal quadriceps. *Physiol Ther Can* 35:300, 1983.
29. Walsfley RP, Letts G, Booyf J: A comparison of torque generated by knee extension with a maximal voluntary muscle contraction: Vis-à-vis electrical stimulation. *J Orthop Sports Phys Ther* 6:10, 1984.
30. Kisner C, Colby LA: *Therapeutic exercise: Foundations and techniques,* ed 2. Philadelphia, FA Davis, 1990.
31. Grabois M: Treatment of pain syndromes through exercise. In Lowenthal DT, Bharadwaja K, Oaks WW, editors: *Therapeutics through exercise.* New York, Grune & Stratton, 1979.
32. Wells PE, Frampton V, Bowsher D: *Pain: Management by physical therapy,* ed 2. Oxford, Butterworth-Heinemann, Jordan Hill, 1994.
33. Lee HM, Yang FW, Eason AL et al: Physical therapy and rehabilitation medicine. In Bonica JJ, editor: *The management of pain,* ed 2, vol I. Philadelphia, Lea & Febiger, 1990.
34. Ebel A: Exercise in peripheral vascular disease. In Basmajian JV, editor: *Therapeutic exercise,* ed 3. Baltimore, Williams & Wilkins, 1978.

35. Swenson JR: Therapeutic exercise in hemiplegia. In Basmajian JV, editor: *Therapeutic exercise,* ed 4. Baltimore, Williams & Wilkins, 1984.

36. Fairchild VM, Salerno LM, Wedding SL et al: Physical therapy. In Raj PP, editor: *Practical management of pain.* Chicago, Year Book Medical Publishers, 1986.

37. Huddleston OL: *Therapeutic exercises: Kinesiotherapy.* Philadelphia, FA Davis, 1961.

38. Hislop HJ, Perrine JJ: The isokinetic concept of exercise. *Phys Ther* 47:114, 1967.

39. Donald KW, Lind AR, McNichol GW et al: Cardiovascular response to sustained (static) contractions. *Circ Res* 1(suppl) 10:15, 1967.

40. Haldeman S: Manipulation and massage for the relief of pain. In Melzack R, Wall P, editors: *Textbook of pain,* ed 2. New York, Churchill Livingstone, 1989.

41. Vernon HJ: Spinal manipulation and beta-endorphin: A controlled study of the effect of a spinal manipulation on plasma beta-endorphin levels in normal males. *J Manipulative Physiol Ther* 92:29, 115, 1986.

42. Grice AA: Muscle tonus changes following manipulation. *J Can Chiropract Assoc* 19:29, 1974.

43. DiGiovanna EL: Somatic dysfunction. In DiGiovanna EL, Schiowitz S, editors: *An osteopathic approach to diagnosis and treatment.* Philadelphia, Lippincott, 1991.

44. Murphy T: Myofascial techniques. In DiGiovanna EL, Schiowitz S, editors: *An osteopathic approach to diagnosis and treatment.* Philadelphia, Lippincott, 1991.

45. Saunders H: *Evaluation, treatment, and prevention of musculoskeletal disorders.* Eden Prairie, Minn, self-published, 1985.

46. Fordyce W: *Behavioral methods for chronic pain and illness.* St. Louis, Mosby, 1976.

Questions • Physical Therapy Techniques

1. Deep heating agents in temperature modalities of physical therapy includes all of the following except

   A. Ultrasound
   B. Short-wave diathermy
   C. Microwave
   D. Infrared

2. Cryotherapy has become the most useful modality in treating

   A. Chronic pain
   B. Cancer pain
   C. Acute pain
   D. Arthritic pain

3. The effectiveness of electrical stimulation depends on all of the following except

   A. Intensity
   B. Frequency
   C. Waveform
   D. Temperature

4. Modalities of electrical stimulation includes all of the following except

   A. High-voltage pulsed galvanic stimulation
   B. Iontophoresis
   C. Magnetic pulsing
   D. Transcutaneous electrical nerve stimulation

5. Therapeutic exercises prescribed by physical therapy include all except

   A. Endurance exercises
   B. Desensitization exercises
   C. Proprioceptive neuromuscular facilitation exercises
   D. Uncoordinated muscular activity exercises

ANSWERS

1. D
2. C
3. D
4. C
5. D

CHAPTER 27

Home Care

JUDITH A. PAICE, AND MICHAEL STANTON-HICKS

The population of patients being cared for in the home is greatly increasing. Many are referred to home care services for cardiovascular disease, cancer, human immunodeficiency virus (HIV) infection, and other chronic illnesses. Little is known about the experiences of patients admitted to home care with a diagnosis of chronic pain, yet there is little disagreement that home care services are necessary and beneficial for many individuals with chronic pain. Clear understanding of the purpose of home health care, the types of services available, the members of the team, and the costs associated with this care enables those considering home care services for their patients to make sound decisions about referral. Current experiences with parenteral, epidural, and intrathecal analgesic delivery in the home suggest that these techniques are safe and effective for selected populations of patients.

HISTORICAL PERSPECTIVES

The use of home care services has increased greatly in the past 3 decades.[1] This trend has been driven in large part by financial factors resulting in earlier discharge from the hospital and changes in reimbursement for care delivered in the home. However, home health care services are hardly new. Begun in the late 1700s, home nursing services originated in Boston to provide care to the poor.[2] Other home care services soon developed, designed primarily to meet the needs of the indigent. Hospital-based home care services were developed in the 1940s with an expansion of services beyond medical and nursing care to include nutritional support, social services, physical and occupational therapy, and custodial care.

Home care services were included from the onset in Medicare, yet initially benefits were provided only if patients were first hospitalized. This situation was eliminated in 1980, resulting in rapid growth of home care programs.[1,3]

Studies suggest that home care services have evolved to provide long-term care[3] rather than to replace hospital services. As families become smaller and more scattered, this long-term care may be a substitute for the care previously provided by large, extended families; neighbors; and friends.

GOALS OF HOME CARE

The primary goal of home care is to provide safe, effective, and efficient care in the home with the family as the basic unit of care. More specifically, home care includes the provision of services and equipment to restore and maintain health, function, and comfort.[4]

Most patients who receive home care services are older than 65 years and have limitations in one or more activities of daily living. Common diagnoses associated with home care include[5]:

1. Diseases of the circulatory system (26.6%)
2. Endocrine, nutritional, and metabolic diseases and immunity disorders (9.4%)
3. Diseases of the musculoskeletal system (8.2%)
4. Injuries (8.0%)
5. Diseases of the nervous system (7.8%)

All of these disorders are known to be associated with chronic pain.

Patients with chronic pain may be admitted to home care for a variety of services, including assistance with oral, parenteral, or spinal drug delivery. Pain is one of the most common problems that lead to home care in persons with cancer.[6] Other interventions related to pain measures that may be provided in the home include (1) comprehensive assessment of the pain, (2) adaptation of an analgesic regimen to fit the needs of the patient and the family in the home, (3) management of adverse effects of analgesics, (4) introduction of nonpharmacologic interventions to relieve pain, and (5) on-going assessment of the beliefs of the patient and family regarding opioids.[7]

General guidelines for accepting patients with chronic pain into home care are listed in Box 27–1.

TYPES OF HOME HEALTH SERVICES

Home health agencies include Medicare-certified home health agencies, Medicare-certified hospices, and non-Medicare-certified agencies.[1]

The Joint Commission on Accreditation of Healthcare Organizations (JCAHO) established a home care accreditation program in 1988. To be accredited, an agency must offer the following[4]:

1. Home medical equipment services
2. Home health services, including nursing; physical, speech, and occupational therapies; social work services; and nutritional support
3. Personal care services, such as custodial care
4. Pharmaceutical services
5. Respiratory care

1. The patient's home environment should be amenable to support the treatment program or protocol of care.
2. The patient must want and request therapy or services at home.
3. The patient and/or the caregiver must be knowledgeable about (a) the therapy, including names, dosages, side effects, and adverse reactions to drugs; (b) actions to prevent or minimize side effects; and (c) proper procurement, storage, handling, and disposal of drugs, as necessary.
4. The patient must have the financial means to pay for home care, treatments, therapies, and services.
5. The patient and/or the caregiver must understand the technology and operational aspects of the devices and equipment used, including their mechanisms, use of alarms and limits, troubleshooting, routine maintenance, and upkeep.
6. The diagnosis, prognosis, and course of the disease must be determined through a reasonable, logical, and thorough evaluation.
7. A physician or practitioner with expertise in pain control must be responsible and available for frequent reevaluation and monitoring of the patient's condition.
8. The patient's medical condition must be stable; if not, the patient is better off as an inpatient.
9. There must be access to communication between the patient, physician, home care providers or team, pharmacy, hospital, and health insurance payers.

Adapted from Rigor BM: Pain control in home care. In Spratt JS, Hawley RL, Hoye RE, editors: *Home health care: Principles and practices.* Delray Beach, Fla, GR/St. Lucie Press, 1997.

COMPONENTS OF THE HOME CARE TEAM

More than 500,000 people are employed by home care agencies.[1] Home care aides are the largest group of workers, followed by registered nurses and licensed practical nurses (LPNs). Other core members of the home care team include physical therapists, social workers, occupational therapists, and speech pathologists. Still other members may include psychologists, dietitians, respiratory therapists, and clergy.[2]

Home care would be impossible if not for the support of family and friends. A survey conducted in 1989 by the Bipartisan Commission on Comprehensive Health Care estimated that almost 75% of older persons receiving home care relied exclusively on family members or other uncompensated caregivers.[8]

Although the role of caregiver is potentially very rewarding, it can be associated with feelings of isolation, grief, fatigue, anxiety, resentment, depression, and guilt.[2,9] Home health care personnel must offer caregivers emotional support by encouraging discussion of feelings in an empathetic manner.

ASSESSMENT OF THE FAMILY AND HOME

The family is the unit of care in home care; therefore, assessment of both the home and the family is critical. Barriers to safe and effective pain control may be environmental or financial. Environmental barriers include lack of utilities, inadequate hygiene, and insufficient or unsafe storage areas for medications and supplies.[7] Financial barriers include inadequate coverage for durable medical equipment and pharmaceuticals.

Characteristics of the family to be assessed include[7]:

- Structure and composition of the family
- Patterns of authority in the household
- Family values
- Behavior and family activities
- Coping abilities
- Health and functional status of caregivers
- Stressors
- Support systems
- Knowledge of health practices

Among the specific areas of the family assessment that can reveal potential barriers to good pain control are (1) treatment-related concerns of the spouse or other family members, (2) family experience with cancer or with chronic pain, and (3) spiritual or sociocultural concerns regarding pain and its treatment.[10] The results of these assessments may lead to education of the patient, referral to social services, and possibly even removal from an unsafe home environment.

COST

Financial burden on patients and family caregivers is another significant source of stress on the family unit, and its effect has not been sufficiently studied.

Six types of care are reimbursed for patients who meet Medicare's eligibility criteria:

- Skilled nursing care
- Physical therapy
- Occupational therapy
- Speech therapy
- Medical social services
- Home health aide services

OUTCOMES AND QUALITY IMPROVEMENT

The successful home care program includes the following attributes: accessibility, amiability, acceptability, availability, adaptability, and accountability.[11] "Accountability" means that the home care agency must be accountable for the quality of care provided. Quality of care includes professional performances, efficient use of resources, reduced or minimal risk for patients and caregivers, and satisfaction of the patient and caregiver.[12] Chart audits regarding satisfaction with pain treatments give some evidence of the quality of care provided by a home care agency.[13] Both the JCAHO and the National League for Nursing's Community Health Accreditation Program (CHAP) have developed models for quality improvement (QI) measures in home health care settings.[14]

When selecting a home care agency, the referring physician or nurse should ask about QI monitoring regarding pain management as well as results of any recent audits of patients receiving care for chronic pain.

THERAPIES FOR PAIN CONTROL

Parenteral Infusion

Intravenous administration and subcutaneous administration of opioids have been used safely and effectively in the home. Bolus injections and continuous infusions, as well as patient-controlled analgesia (PCA) systems, have been used.[15–18] The intravenous route is often chosen when patients have existing vascular access, but the subcutaneous route can be used as an alternative. A retrospective study of home-based hospice patients reported a mean 4-hour subcutaneous morphine dose of 14.3 mg, with the mean duration of needle placement 4.62 days (range, 1 to 26 days).[16] The use of multiday (3 to 4 days) infusion pumps support the delivery of intravenous or subcutaneous opioids in the home by reducing costs without an increase in bacterial growth.[19]

Using spinal drug delivery system in the home has also been shown to be safe and effective.[20] The success of any of these therapies demands appropriate selection of patients and delivery method and ongoing communication between pain clinicians, home care personnel, and the patient and caregiver.

Epidural Infusion

The choice between an intrathecal and an epidural infusion system is based on many factors, including expected duration of use, nature of the pain, agents used, anatomic considerations, and cost. Either form of drug delivery has specific advantages and disadvantages. The management of patients undergoing intraspinal drug delivery requires considerable education of the patient and caregiver and technical support. Once implanted, these systems necessitate frequent reassessment in the home setting with constant clinical monitoring, dose adjustments, and immediate treatment of any side effects or complications.

Selection of Patients and Technique

On the basis of guidelines of the Agency for Health Care Policy and Research of the U.S. Public Health Service[21] and the American Pain Society,[22] patients are selected by the presence of continued pain that is refractory to adequate systemic opioid therapy.

Selection criteria include the following:

- Untoward or unacceptable side effects
- Refractory neuropathic or incident pain or both
- Failure of regional anesthetic techniques
- Successful inpatient trial of epidural analgesia
- No surgical or neuroablative considerations
- Availability of systems and home care nursing

Patients considered suitable for long-term epidural analgesia are those with incident pain such as that related to pathologic fractures or neuropathic pain, particularly that associated with nerve roots, plexus, or peripheral nerves. In certain circumstances, however, prolonged epidural infusions or intermittent administration of opiates for terminal cancer can be effectively used in the home care setting. In general, however, the cost effectiveness of epidural infusion limits its use to less than 6 months.[23] For longer duration, intrathecal infusion is more suitable and involves a much lower risk of infection.

Another factor most important in the successful use of an externalized epidural drug delivery system is a proficient caregiver that can monitor the patient's care to ensure that adequate aseptic technique is employed for maintenance of the system. Some useful applications of prolonged epidural infusion are facilitation of rehabilitation for patients with chronic pain after unsuccessful surgery, restoration of function after orthopedic surgery in patients with concomitant long-standing neuropathic pain, and relief of pain for patients with complex regional pain syndromes (reflex sympathetic dystrophy and causalgia).[24]

When a technique has been selected, the patient is admitted for a short inpatient stay to titrate the dose of local anesthetic, with or without an opiate or other adjuncts, thought to be appropriate for the particular circumstances. Systems that are expected to be used for several weeks or months generally require stabilization by tunneling, surgical placement and attachment to spinal tissues, or use of a subcutaneous port. For the utmost efficiency, epidural catheters require radiographic imaging for their placement to favor ipsilateral or bilateral infusion. The success of long-term epidural catheterization depends on strict attention to asepsis, the use of periprocedural broad-spectrum antibiotics for 72 hours, and, if surgical implantation is used, appropriate attention to tissue technique.

The use of "permanent" as opposed to "temporary" systems has been evaluated.[25] An algorithm for determining the use of an intrathecal versus epidural system has been proposed by Bedder and colleagues.[23] Certainly, the success of any "high-tech" system depends on such factors as:

- Intensity and character of the pain
- Physical status of the patient
- Immune system integrity
- Education of the patient
- Social structure of the home
- Knowledge of the system by the visiting nurse
- Frequency of home visits
- Strict attention to a maintenance protocol

The availability of nurses experienced in and having an understanding of as well as training in the maintenance of epidural infusions (as opposed to completely implanted intrathecal systems) is critical to the protracted maintenance of epidural infusion systems.

Awareness and recognition of complications such as infection of the epidural catheter site, paravertebral or intraspinal tissues, and migration of the catheter require a good understanding of the associated clinical signs and symptoms expressed by the patient. Now that implantable intrathecal infusion systems have become an accepted therapy for chronic intractable and malignant pain that is unmanageable by other means; the epidural route lends itself more to managing cancer pain for short duration or pain relief to facilitate rehabilitation.

Commencement of Therapy

After selection of the level at which the catheter tip is sited, radiographic visualization of the epidural space, with contrast if necessary, should both precede and follow catheter placement.[26–28] After tunneling and stabilization of the epidural catheter, it is common to commence an infusion of bupivacaine at a dose of 0.06 to 0.1 ml, infusing at a rate of 3 to 6 ml/hour. Clinical monitoring of these patients can be achieved only in an inpatient setting with dose titration occurring every 3 to 4 hours; the endpoint is "working" analgesia without motor or significant proprioceptive impairment. It should be obvious within 24 hours whether analgesia adequate for physical or occupational therapy can be realized with local anesthetic alone.

During the short (3- to 4-day) hospital admission, satisfactory parameters for both hospital and home use can be achieved effectively. Any changes in the subsequent treatment plan should be dictated by pain and function.

It is essential during the course of a patient's rehabilitation that immediate and frequent communication between the patient, home care nurse, and therapist is maintained between appointments.

Complications

The complications associated with long-term epidural catheters can be summarized as follows: (1) mechanical and technical problems; (2) medication-related side effects or toxicity; and (3) infection, most commonly subcutaneous at the catheter exit site and more rarely paravertebral or intraspinal. Adverse side effects rarely occur and then usually only because of a breakdown in the constant communication that should be maintained between the physician initiating the treatment and local home care nurse or therapist and patient.

Mechanical problems may be associated with the pump, the catheter, or its connections. Displacement of the catheter is not uncommon because most catheters are percutaneously inserted and, therefore, are attached to the skin and not to spinal structure.

The side effects of medication include toxicity or drug withdrawal or both. Opiate side effect may be evident. If any of these side effects occur in the home setting, they require immediate treatment and, if necessary, return to the implanting institution for another brief period of hospital admission to re-establish pain control with another analgesic agent.

Local anesthetic toxicity is unusual and is generally manifested during the initial period of titration. Subcutaneous infection at the catheter site can occur at any time and, if minor, may be successfully treated with a 7-day course of broad-spectrum antibiotic. The signs of epidural infection that require immediate diagnosis and radiographic imaging, when suspected, can also be treated by removal of the catheter and a 5- to 6-week course of antibiotics.

Nursing Care of the Catheter Site

It is usual to retain the catheter with a monofilament suture, but Steri-Strips may be used as an alternative. The exit site should be covered by an occlusive dressing that is vapor permeable. It is essential that the wound site remains dry, but the dressing should be changed as infrequently as possible.

Specific Home Care Aspects

It is essential to understand the social environment to which the patient is returning. Awareness of hygiene and identification of a specific site for storage of opiate-containing solutions are important, requiring education of the patient beforehand.

Implanted Delivery Systems

Implanted drug delivery systems include continuous-flow devices and programmable pumps. Both require skilled clinicians to assess the patient's pain, evaluate pump function, refill the device, and troubleshoot when relief is inadequate. The use of home care services varies widely by clinician. Some routinely consult home care for all refills, whereas others limit home care referrals to patients too disabled to return to the outpatient setting.[29]

Considering Home Care Before Implantation

The primary reason for using implanted delivery systems to relieve pain is to maintain ambulation and physical activity while reducing the potential for infection.[30,31] Unfortunately, many patients have progressive illnesses that accompany their pain and may require home care services with worsening of disease. Thus, the possibility of home care should be seriously entertained for every patient before pump implantation. Lack of available home care services equipped for and skilled in pump refills, particularly in less populated areas, may preclude consideration of this therapy.[29]

Selecting a Home Care Agency

The implanting team should select a home care agency with expertise in the care of patients with implanted pumps for pain. These agencies have the necessary equipment, including programmers and refill kits, as well as pharmacy services to obtain or compound preservative-free opioids and other agents. Because expertise develops with experience, a selected group of nurses should be specially trained to make these home visits. Training should include pain assessment, pump refills, programming, and troubleshooting system or drug complications.

Developing a Treatment Plan

Communication among patient, caregivers, the implanting team, and the home care team is also essential. All parties must first agree on the treatment plan. Patients and family members or caregivers should be queried regarding their goals for home therapy. There may be discordance between the what the patient wants and expects and what the professionals believe is required.[2] This requires a frank discussion of the meaning of pain and outlook for relief.[10] This discussion is essential for all persons with implantable drug therapy delivery systems to relieve pain, whether the pain is due to cancer or a nonmalignant process.

Communication

Communication is enhanced by having the home care nurse meet the patient, the caregivers, and the implanting team before the first home visit.[32] The home care nurse observes the refill procedure, which is particularly important for patients with difficult access, such as very obese patients. The home care nurse and implanting team should explain the roles of each health care professional to the patient and family.[2] Guidelines should be given regarding when to call the home care nurse or when to call the implanting team.

To provide seamless delivery of care across the hospital, outpatient clinic, and home care setting, computer bases must be integrated within these environments.

References

1. National Association of Home Care (NAHC): *Basic statistics about home care.* Washington, DC, NAHC, 2001.
2. Navarra T, Ferrer M: *An insider's guide to home health care.* Thorofare, NJ, Slack, 1997.
3. Welsh HG, Wennberg DE, Welsh WP: The use of Medicare home health care services. *N Engl J Med* 335:324, 1996.
4. Spratt JS, Hawley RL, Hoye RE, editors: *Home health care: Principles and practices.* Delray Beach, Fla, GR/St. Lucie Press, 1997.
5. Strahan GW: *National Center for Health Statistics: An overview of home health and hospice patients.* 1994 National Home and Hospice Care Survey, Advance Data, No. 274, Hyattsville, Md, Division of Health Care Statistics, April 24, 1996.
6. Yost LS: Cancer patients and home care: Extent to which required services are not received. *Cancer Pract* 3:83, 1995.
7. McNally JC: Home care. In Groenwald SL, Goodman M, Frogge MH et al, editors: *Cancer nursing: Principles and practice,* ed 4. Sudbury, Mass, Jones & Bartlett, 1997.
8. U.S. Bipartisan Commission on Comprehensive Health Care: The Pepper Commission final report: A call for action. S Prt 101–114. Washington, DC, Government Printing Office, 1990.
9. Ferrell BR, Dean GE: Ethical issues in pain management at home. *J Palliat Care* 10:67, 1994.
10. Rhiner M, Coluzzi PH: Family issues influencing management of cancer pain. In McGuire DB, Yarbro CH, Ferrell BR, editors: *Cancer pain management,* ed 2. Boston, Jones & Bartlett, 1995.
11. Rigor BM: Pain control in home care. In Spratt JS, Hawley RL, Hoye RE, editors: *Home health care: Principles and practices.* Delray Beach, Fla, GR/St. Lucie Press, 1997.
12. Davis ER: *Total quality management for home care.* Gaitherburg, Md, Aspen, 1994.
13. Joint Commission on Accreditation of Healthcare Organizations (JCAHO): *Using performance improvement tools in home care and hospice organizations.* Oakbrook Terrace, Ill, JCAHO, 1996.
14. Carefoot J: Total quality management implementation in home care agencies: Common questions and answers. *J Nurs Admin* 24:31, 1994.
15. Coyle N, Cherny NI, Portenoy RK: Subcutaneous opioid infusion at home. *Oncology* 8:21, 1994.
16. Crane RA: Intermittent subcutaneous infusion of opioids in hospice home care: An effective, economical, manageable option. *Am J Hosp Palliat Care* 11:8, 1994.
17. Murphy D: Home pain management: Continuous infusion of narcotics. *J Intravenous Nurs* 13:355, 1990.
18. Patt RB: PCA: Prescribing analgesia for home management of severe pain. *Geriatrics* 47:69, 1992.
19. Ohlsson LJ, Rydberg TS, Eden T et al: Microbiologic and economic evaluation of multiday infusion pumps for cancer pain. *Ann Pharmacother* 29:972, 1995.
20. Smith DE: Spinal opioids in the home and hospice setting. *J Pain Symptom Manage* 5:175, 1990.
21. Agency of Health Care Policy and Research (AHCPR): *Clinical guidelines: Cancer pain management.* Bethesda, Md, US Public Health Service, 1994.
22. American Pain Society: *Principles of analgesic use in the treatment of acute pain and cancer pain,* ed 4. Skokie, Ill, American Pain Society, 1999.
23. Bedder MD, Burchiel K, Larson A: Cost analysis of two implantable narcotic delivery systems. *J Pain Symptom Manage* 6:368, 1991.
24. Stanton-Hicks M, Janig W, Hassenbusch S et al: Reflex sympathetic dystrophy: Changing concepts and taxonomy. *Pain* 63:127, 1995.
25. Ali N, Hanna N, Hoffman J: Percutaneous epidural catheterization for intractable pain in the terminal cancer patients. *Gynecol Oncol* 32:22, 1989.
26. Patt R, Jain S: Long-term management of a patient with perineal pain secondary to rectal cancer. *J Pain Symptom Manage* 5:127, 1990.
27. Asari H, Inoue K, Shibata T et al: Sequential effect of morphine injected into the epidural space in man. *Anesthesiology* 54:75, 1981.
28. Hunt R, Massolino J: Spinal bupivacaine for the pain of cancer. *Med J Aust* 150:350, 1989.
29. Gianino JM, York MM, Paice JA: *Intrathecal drug therapy for spasticity and pain.* New York, Springer, 1996.
30. Krames ES, Olson K: Clinical realities and economic considerations: Patient selection in intrathecal therapy. *J Pain Symptom Manage* 14:S3, 1997.
31. Penn RD, Paice JA: Chronic intrathecal morphine for intractable pain. *J Neurosurg* 67:182, 1987.
32. Paice JA, Williams AR: Intraspinal drugs for pain. In McQuire DB, Yarbro CH, Ferrell BR, editors: *Cancer pain management,* ed 2. Boston, Jones & Bartlett, 1995.

Questions • Home Care

1. Most patients who receive home care services are

    A. Younger than 30 years
    B. Younger than 55 years
    C. Older than 65 years
    D. Older than 75 years

2. Common diagnosis associated with home care include

    A. Disease of the circulatory system
    B. Endocrine, nutritional, and metabolic diseases
    C. Psychiatric diseases
    D. Injuries

3. Quality of care in a home care program includes all of the following except

    A. Adequate professional performance
    B. Efficient use of resources
    C. Reduced or minimal risk to the patient or the caregiver
    D. High cost to patient and family

4. When using implanted delivery systems in patients, the following criteria must be met. Skilled clinicians are available to provide all but one of the following.

    A. Assess the patient's pain
    B. Evaluate pump function
    C. Troubleshoot the pump when relief is inadequate
    D. Prescribe systemic medications

5. Parenteral infusions of opioids have been used safely and effectively in the home. These include all except one of the following

    A. Intravenous administration of opioids
    B. Subcutaneous infusion of opioids
    C. Patient-controlled analgesic systems
    D. Peritoneal infusion of analgesics

ANSWERS

1. C
2. C
3. D
4. D
5. D

CHAPTER 28

Alternative Medicine

WINSTON C. V. PARRIS

Pain and illness continue to be the scourge of mankind even with tremendous strides that have been made in the cure and relief of several diseases. Over the past 10 to 20 years, great progress has been made in the management of pain derived from disease, trauma, or idiopathic origin. However, pain continues to be a problem in the very young, the very old, cancer patients, diabetic patients, patients after stroke, and almost all patients whose disorder produces unrelenting pain.

Since the advent of the pain medicine specialty, significant developments have contributed to modest success in resolving chronic pain,[1] although much remains to be done in optimizing pain control. While physicians await these advances, patients become disappointed and at times disgusted with the inadequacy of their pain management. This disillusionment has led many people to seek nontraditional, unconventional, and at times dangerous remedies to control pain. Naturally, a few unscrupulous "practitioners" take advantage of this situation, but it is heartening to note that a number of these nontraditional remedies are effective in controlling, if not eliminating, chronic pain syndromes in selected patients. The whole arena is known as alternative or complementary medicine.[2] This chapter explores the role of alternative medicine in chronic pain management and examines how these methods can contribute to traditional or conventional pain medicine.

PREVALENCE OF ALTERNATIVE MEDICINE

Many patients use alternative medicine as their main therapeutic option, and a majority of patients use alternative medicine along with conventional medicine, occasionally with the assent of a traditional physician. There is some regional bias, in that alternative medicine, including herbal medicine,[3] is used more commonly in the Western states and, to a lesser extent, in the South than in the northern and eastern regions of the United States.

DEFINITION

In this chapter, alternative medicine may be defined as unconventional or unorthodox medical interventions not routinely taught at American medical schools or not generally available in American hospitals.[4]

Alternative medicine covers a wide scope of healing philosophies, methodologic approaches, and clinical therapies (Box 28–1). In addition to the fact that they are not taught in medical schools, most alternative medical practices are not reimbursed by medical insurance companies. This situation is changing slowly; for example, acupuncture services are now recognized as effective and are also reimbursed by several medical insurers.

Alternative medicine has been labeled "holistic medicine," and although there are some common areas, the comparison is not an accurate one. The term *holistic* generally implies that the health care practitioner considers the whole person, including physical, mental, emotional, and spiritual aspects. In today's health conscious society, many therapies are labeled as "preventive," implying that the practitioner is involved primarily in educating the patient about the disease, its symptoms, its complications, and its treatment but, even more important, is committed to instructing the patient regarding the techniques and methods of preventing disease.

CLASSIFICATION

To a large extent, alternative medicine has not been evaluated or scrutinized according to accepted scientific principles or methods. Consequently, the architects of individual alternative modalities have been more concerned with acceptance and positive results rather than an open and unconditional evaluation of their efficacy. As a result, no consistent organization existed before the creation of the Office of Alternative Medicine,[5] and there were no attempts at classifying modalities used for alternative medicine. Under the aegis of the National Institutes of Health (NIH), a task force was created to address classification issues. The result is seven categories of complementary or alternative medicine practices, including:

1. Alternative systems of practice
2. Bioelectromagnetic applications
3. Diet, nutrition, and lifestyle changes
4. Herbal medicine
5. Manual healing methods
6. Mind-body interventions
7. Pharmacologic and biologic treatments

The task force also reported on corresponding issues, such as research methodology, research and training needs, the peer review process, and information dissemination activities.[6]

OFFICE OF ALTERNATIVE MEDICINE

Since its inception, the Office of Alternative Medicine has served a number of important functions that have helped to legitimize some modalities of alternative medicine. Most notably, it has served as an institution that compiles data and serves as a granting agency for sponsoring some of those research projects.

BOX 28–1   Classification of Alternative Medicine Practices

Alternative Systems of Medical Practice
  Acupuncture
  Anthroposophically extended medicine
  Ayurveda
  Community-based health care practices
  Environmental medicine
  Homeopathic medicine
  Latin American rural practices
  Native American practices
  Natural products
  Naturopathic medicine
  Past life therapy
  Shamanism
  Tibetan medicine
  Traditional Asian (Oriental) medicine

Bioelectromagnetic Applications
  Blue light treatment and artificial lighting
  Electroacupuncture
  Electromagnetic fields
  Electrostimulation and neuromagnetic stimulation
    devices
  Magnetic resonance spectroscopy

Diet, Nutrition, Lifestyle Changes
  Changes in lifestyle
  Diet
  Gerson therapy
  Macrobiotics
  Megavitamins
  Nutritional supplements

Herbal Medicine
  Echinacea (purple coneflower)
  Ginger rhizome
  Ginkgo biloba extract
  Ginseng root
  Wild chrysanthemun flower
  Witch hazel
  Yellowdock

Manual Healing
  Acupressure
  Alexander technique
  Aromatherapy
  Biofield therapeutics
  Chiropractic medicine
  Feldenkrais method
  Massage therapy
  Osteopathy
  Reflexology
  Rolfing
  Therapeutic Touch
  Trager method
  Zone therapy

Mind/Body Control
  Art therapy
  Biofeedback
  Counseling
  Dance therapy
  Guided imagery
  Humor therapy
  Hypnotherapy
  Meditation
  Music therapy
  Prayer therapies
  Psychotherapy
  Relaxation techniques
  Support groups
  Yoga

Pharmacologic and Biologic Treatments
  Antioxidizing agents
  Cell treatment
  Chelation therapy
  Metabolic therapy
  Oxidizing agent (ozone, hydrogen peroxide)

Data from Astin JA: Why patients use alternative medicine: Results of a national study. JAMA 279(11):1548–1553, 1998.

Other functions can be outlined as follows[7]:

1. To provide and evaluate a research database
2. To serve as a clearinghouse of alternative medicine data
3. To organize media relations
4. To facilitate sponsored research
5. To create and fund alternative medicine specialty research centers
6. To facilitate an international and professional liaison program that participates in and promotes cooperative efforts in research and education
7. To organize intramural research training

SCOPE

In an attempt to determine prevalence, costs, and patterns of use of alternative medicine in the United States, Eisenberg and colleagues[8] demonstrated that alternative modalities are used not only for chronic pain but also for cancer, arthritis, AIDS, gastrointestinal problems, chronic renal failure, and eating disorders. Among the commonly used therapies were:

- Relaxation techniques
- Chiropractic manipulation
- Massage
- Imagery
- Spiritual healing
- Promotional weight loss programs
- Lifestyle diets (e.g., macrobiotics, herbal medicine, megavitamin therapy)
- Self-help groups
- Energy healing
- Biofeedback
- Hypnosis
- Magnetic therapy
- Low-power laser therapy
- Homeopathy
- Acupuncture

- Folk remedies
- Exercise
- Prayer

More than 60% of the patients who use unconventional therapy did so without medical supervision and without active consultation with a provider of either conventional or unconventional therapy. The medical conditions for which most patients sought alternative therapy included back pain, allergies, arthritis, insomnia, sprains, strains, headaches, high blood pressure, digestive problems, anxiety, and depression. Except for allergies and depression, all of the other medical conditions are associated with some form of chronic pain.

A satisfying observation is that most of the users of alternative therapy do not replace conventional therapy but use those alternative therapy modalities as adjuncts to conventional therapy. For example, few patients use alternative therapy modalities for the treatment of high blood pressure or digestive problems, which suggests that patients have been satisfied with the validity and efficacy of traditional therapy for these ailments. However, many patients do not use alternative medicine for the treatment of chronic back pain, headaches, arthritis, strains, or sprains.

As part of the medical evaluation of chronic pain patients, an attempt should be made to determine whether the patient is receiving alternative therapy and the frequency, amount (units), or intensity with which that particular modality is used.

ALTERNATIVE THERAPY MODALITIES

Although it is impossible to describe all of the modalities used in alternative medicine, a few have been arbitrarily selected and are discussed here.

Music Therapy

Schorr[9] demonstrated in a study of 30 women with chronic pain secondary to rheumatoid arthritis that chronic pain might be effectively controlled using music as a unitary-transformative intervention. Hanser[10] also described the effective use of music as a distraction during lumbar punctures. Unfortunately, this study was a series of anecdotal reports and not a scientifically conducted investigation. Nevertheless, it is reasonable to propose that in some patients with well-defined pathologic conditions music therapy may be effective by itself and can be a useful adjunct to conventional modalities in pain management.

Intercessionary Prayer and Spiritual Healing

Several claims have been made regarding the effectiveness of intercessionary prayer, spiritual healing, divine intercessions, and meditation in controlling chronic pain.[11] Certainly, it is not good medical practice for providers to be arbitrary about patients' spiritual or religious persuasions. In fact, those persuasions may be passively supported as long as they do not interfere with the delivery of medical care necessary for treatment. Many anecdotal reports regarding the efficacy of those modalities have been made, but few scientifically controlled studies have been done to determine efficacy.

Relaxation Therapy

Relaxation therapy is well-established psychogenic modality for managing chronic pain. Jacobson's[12] progressive muscle relaxation techniques have been widely used to manage chronic pain syndromes, particularly myofascial pain syndromes including low back pain.

Hypnosis

Hypnosis has been used with sufficient frequency to warrant investigation. Unfortunately, some providers of hypnotic therapy are not necessarily competent in the method's principles, applications, and nuances.[13] This is precisely the danger of using a modality that has not been rigorously subjected to peer review evaluations. Hypnotherapy or hypnotic relaxation has been used as a sedative for some medical procedures (e.g., colonoscopy).

Chiropractic Therapy

The use of chiropractic therapy is widespread in the United States and is legal. No doubt it has a place in the management of musculoskeletal dysfunction and various myofascial pain syndromes. The modality has continued to develop and can be effective, if properly conducted. Although research into chiropractic is not very widespread, the method is said to be much more effective than other conservative approaches, including bed rest, medication, physical therapy, and massage therapy.

Unfortunately, chiropractic practitioners and medical practitioners have not been able to work together for the good of the patient with chronic musculoskeletal dysfunction. Indeed, inappropriately applied and incompetently administered, chiropractic can be dangerous in some patients and may lead to a worsening of the patient's general condition.

Comfort Measures

The application of comfort measures goes a long way toward making patients feel comfortable and in optimizing their immunosuppressant mechanism to promote rapid healing and recuperation.[14] When properly applied, comfort measures may obviate the need for pharmacologic intervention and may help introduce a soft touch into a medical experience that may appear cold and uncaring.

Transcutaneous Electrical Nerve Stimulation

Initially, transcutaneous electrical nerve stimulation (TENS)[15] was thought of as a primitive alternative therapy modality. Its popularity increased after the publication of the gate-control theory by Melzack and Wall.[16] In fact, a proposed mechanism of action is that electrical stimulation of A-alpha and A-beta fibers suppresses nociception transmitted by A-delta and C fibers. Many published studies show the efficacy of TENS in the management of a large number of pain syndromes,[17] including cancer pain.[18]

Biostimulation Techniques

The various biostimulation techniques include:

- Acupuncture
- Auriculotherapy
- Vibration therapy
- Magnetic field therapy

- Low-power laser therapy
- Movement therapy

A major reason for the popularity of these modalities is that they are usually noninvasive and, in appropriate patients, may be beneficial when used as adjuncts to conventional therapy.

Acupuncture

Acupuncture has been used for more than 2000 years. It is based on various Chinese scientific principles that are not understood or taught in most Western medical systems including the United States. It is clear that acupuncture does control pain in selected patients; however, my impression from observing acupuncture in the former Soviet Union is that patient selection must be meticulous because some patients are more predisposed to benefit from acupuncture than others.

Magnetic Field Therapy

First proposed by Franz Mesmer of Austria, magnetic stimuli and magnetic fields have been used medicinally since the 16th century. In the early 20th century, orthopedic surgeons often used magnetic therapy to correct malunion of long bone fractures. At that time, it was safer to use magnetic therapy than orthopedic surgery for long bone fractures, which were usually associated with osteomyelitis. Recently many claims have been made regarding the efficacy of magnetic field blocks and magnetic fields,[19] but these have not been evaluated scientifically.

To determine the efficacy of magnetic fields, Parris and coauthors[20] investigated the chronic pain animal model (rat) using the sciatic nerve ligation or chronic constructor injury. The study showed that magnetic field therapy reduces hyperalgesia-induced chronic constriction injury of the sciatic nerve in the rat model of chronic pain. These basic science studies are important to help investigate purported mechanisms of analgesia in various alternative modalities. Furthermore, the study suggests that magnetic field therapy may be effective in various forms of neuropathic pain.

Low-power Laser Therapy

Parris and colleagues,[21] using the same animal model described for magnetic field therapy, investigated the effect of low-power laser on neuropathic pain. No biochemical or behavioral changes resulted, illustrating that it is not effective for neuropathic pain; however, low-power laser has been effective for myofascial pain.

S U M M A R Y

As one evaluates new techniques and new drugs, it is also appropriate to evaluate alternative medicine practices, but this must be done scientifically and fairly, not in response to commercial interests but in accordance with scientific principles. To accomplish that goal, the Office of Alternative Medicine has been invaluable not only to the field of pain medicine but also to patients in general. Many aspects of conventional and traditional medicine, if they were subjected to rigorous scientific scrutiny, might be condemned. Nevertheless, the scientific evaluation of alternative medicine may reveal tremendous benefits to patients with chronic pain.

Although practitioners of alternative medicine have no rigid guidelines to follow at present, ideally some regulation will be provided under the leadership of responsible clinical organizations and with general direct, or indirect, governmental oversight.

The future appears bright for alternative medicine, and it is hoped that, in the presence of an unbiased, creative, and honest approach at evaluating alternative medicine modalities, beneficial agents and techniques would be promoted so that patients with chronic pain that is unresponsive to conventional therapeutic modalities may have the option of using approved alternative medicine modalities for pain control.

References

1. Murray RH, Rubel AJ: Physicians and healers: Unwitting partners in health care. *N Engl J Med* 326:61, 1992.
2. Gevitz N, editor: Three perspectives on unorthodox medicine. In *Other healers: Unorthodox medicine in America.* Baltimore, Johns Hopkins University Press, 1988.
3. Cook C, Baisen D: Ancillary use of folk medicine by patients in primary care clinics in southwestern West Virginia. *South Med J* 79:1098, 1986.
4. Superintendent of Documents: GPO Stock No. 052-003-01207-3. Washington, DC, Government Printing Office, 1990.
5. Office of Alternative Medicine Clearing House: Office of Alternative Medicine. Bethesda, Md, National Institutes of Health, 1997.
6. Astin JA: Why patients use alternative medicine: Results of a national study. *JAMA* 279:1548, 1998.
7. Baldwin of Bewdley: Uptake of alternative medicine. *Lancet* 347:972, 1996.
8. Eisenberg DM et al: Unconventional medicine in the United States. Prevalence, costs, and patterns of use. *N Engl J Med* 328:246, 1993.
9. Schorr JA: Music and pattern change in chronic pain. *ANA Adv Nursing Sci* 15:27, 1993.
10. Hanser SB: Using music therapy as distraction during lumbar punctures. *J Pediatr Oncol Nursing* 10:2, 1993.
11. McGuire MB: *Ritual healing in suburban America.* New Brunswick, NJ, Rutgers University Press, 1988.
12. Jacobson E: *Progressive relaxation.* Chicago, University of Chicago Press, 1938.
13. Moret V, Forster A, Laverriere MC et al: Mechanism of analgesia induced by hypnosis and acupuncture: Is there a difference? *Pain* 45:135, 1991.
14. Campion EW: Why unconventional medicine? *N Engl J Med* 328:282, 1993.
15. Whitacre MM: The effect of transcutaneous electrical nerve stimulation on ocular pain. *Ophthalmic Surg* 22:462, 1991.
16. Melzack R, Wall PD: Pain mechanisms: A new theory. *Science* 150:971, 1965.
17. Jensen H, Zesler R, Christensen T: Transcutaneous electrical nerve stimulation (TENS) for painful osteoarthritis of the knee. *Int J Rehab Res* 14:356, 1991.
18. Sotosky JR, Lindsay SM: Use of TENS in arthritis management. *Bull Rheum Dis* 40:3, 1991.
19. Cohen D: Magnetic fields of the human body. *Physics Today* 28:34, 1975.
20. Parris WC, Janicki PK, Johnson BW Jr et al: The behavioral and biochemical effect of pulsating magnetic field (PMFT) on chronic pain produced by chronic constriction injury of sciatic nerve in rat. *Analgesia* 1:57, 1994.
21. Parris WC, Janicki PK, Johnson BW Jr et al: Infrared laser diode irradiation has no behavioral effect or biochemical effect on pain in the sciatic nerve ligation-induced mononeuropathy in rat. *Anesth Prog* 41(4):95, 1994.
22. Waylonis GW, Wilke S, O'Toole D et al: Chronic myofascial pain: Management by low-output helium-neon laser therapy. *Arch Phys Med Rehabil* 69:1017, 1988.

1. Alternative medicine can be defined as

   A. Conventional medicine taught in American schools and hospitals
   B. Unconventional or unorthodox medical interventions not routinely taught in American schools and hospitals
   C. Osteopathic medicine
   D. Allopathic medicine

2. The Office for Alternative Medicine (National Institute of Health) classify the following categories of alternative medical practices except

   A. Herbal medicine
   B. Manual healing methods
   C. Mind-body interventions
   D. Hyperbaric therapy

3. The major reason for the popularity of the following therapies is that they are usually noninvasive and in appropriately selected patients may be beneficial when used as adjuncts to conventional therapies. This is true for all of these except

   A. Acupuncture
   B. Magnetic field therapy
   C. Low-power laser therapy
   D. Myoneural injections

4. Acupuncture has been used more than

   A. 100 years
   B. 500 years
   C. 1000 years
   D. 2000 years

5. In the literature, chronic pain secondary to rheumatoid arthritis has been shown to be controlled by

   A. Music therapy
   B. Aromatherapy
   C. Phototherapy
   D. Sedentary activity

ANSWERS

1. B
2. D
3. D
4. D
5. A

CHAPTER 29

Palliative Medicine

MARK J. STILLMAN

According to the dictionary, *palliation* is defined as the relief of suffering—physical, psychologic, sociologic, or existential—and applies in particular to situations in which cure is no longer a possibility. Palliative medicine is conducted by an integrated, interdisciplinary team of physicians, nurses, social workers, clergy, volunteers, home health aides, and therapists in a fashion similar to interdisciplinary management of chronic (nonmalignant) pain.

BACKGROUND AND TERMINOLOGY

The field of palliative medicine, as defined by the National Health Service of Great Britain, which recognized it as a subspecialty in 1987, is "the study and management of patients with active, progressive, far-advanced disease, for whom the prognosis is limited and the focus of care is the quality of life."[1]

Various terms have been used, some accurately, some not, to describe palliative care services. The distinction among them can be very blurred, particularly in the United States, because different fields of medicine contribute practitioners to palliative medicine. Among oncologists treating cancer, there are gradations in the level of care of patients.

Supportive care refers to symptomatic treatment, often during (curative) antitumor therapy, and should not be considered synonymous with palliative care.[2,3]

Although supportive care is commonly seen on oncology wards, it by no means falls solely within the domain of curative oncology. For example, it is not uncommon to see the use of bisphosphonates in hospice patients to prevent painful bony involvement in such diseases as prostate cancer and multiple myeloma.

Hospice is a term often used interchangeably with palliative medicine. In the United States, hospice is only a subset of the entire subspecialty. The beginnings of palliative medicine, however, can be traced clearly to the hospice movement in Great Britain in the 1960s and the work of Dame Cicely Saunders.

Comprehensive palliative medicine units have developed in academic medical centers for acute symptom management, and these are associated with either on-campus of off-campus residential units and home hospice services.[4] The services offered by these hospital-based palliative medicine units include preventative and symptom-therapy. The units are linked to inpatient and outpatient consultation services for patients with symptom control needs; these patients may be in the curative phase or in palliative symptom-relieving phases of their illness. Table 29–1 outlines services offered by a model palliative medicine department.

GOALS OF PALLIATIVE MEDICINE

Simply stated, the goals of palliative medicine are to relieve the physical, psychologic, social, and spiritual distress of the dying patient and the family and caregivers. The patient and caregivers are treated as a unit by the palliative medicine (e.g., hospice) team, with bereavement care provided after the patient's death. The focus shifts from the disease to the patient and family, from the disease process to the individual.

Physical symptoms routinely addressed by practitioners of palliative medicine include pain, dyspnea, nausea and vomiting, weight loss, fatigue or asthenia, diarrhea, constipation, agitation, and confusion. Discussion of palliative techniques is beyond the scope of this chapter, but the principles of pain treatment follow the guidelines espoused by the Agency for Health Care Policy and Research (AHCPR) and are combined with the practices of multidisciplinary care now commonly applied to nonmalignant pain disorders.[5] The emphasis is on low-tech, user-friendly, patient-controlled analgesia, and therapy follows the five tenets outlined by Twycross[6,7]: (1) by the clock, (2) by mouth (orally), (3) by the analgesic stepladder, (4) frequent reassessment, and (5) the use of adjuvant medications.

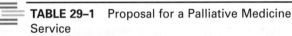

TABLE 29–1 Proposal for a Palliative Medicine Service

Type	Specific Services Offered
Inpatient	Symptom control service (acute care hospital service)
	1. Patients receive "curative" therapy (chemotherapy, radiation therapy, surgery)
	2. Patients with incurable disease
	Palliative care consultation service
	1. Patients receiving treatment with curative intent
	2. Patients with no hope of cure
	Residential hospice for patients not receiving treatment with a curative intent
Outpatient	Palliative care consultation service (clinic)
	1. Patients receiving "curative" therapy
	2. Patients with incurable disease
	Home-based hospice care

ECONOMICS OF PALLIATIVE MEDICINE

In the United States, unlike Great Britain, socialized, state-sponsored medicine has failed to gain a foothold in the financing of medical care for the majority of the population. For people age 65 or older and those with chronic debilitation and special medical needs, Medicare was instituted by Congress in the mid-1960s and stands as the closest example of universal coverage. For people whose incomes fall below the poverty line, each state has insurance known as Medicaid, which provides basic care and medications.

MEDICARE HOSPICE BENEFIT

The hospice agency must forge contractual agreements with the admitting hospital because the hospice agency in any capitated system is responsible for inpatient fees charged by the hospital. Clearly, the hospice with "healthier" patients, whose management can be predominantly home based, in contrast to inpatient, is an agency that can manage to keep out of debt. The problem of deficit spending exists when patients are admitted to hospice care late in the trajectory of their illness. These patients often die quickly and with intensity, sometimes in the hospital, preventing the hospice agency time enough to recoup the expense of its care and labor costs with per diem payments under the Medicare Hospice Benefit.

According to one review of the cost savings in the first decade of the Medicare Hospice Benefit, the National Hospice Organization plotted a trend of diminishing savings with longer lengths of stay. In the first 6 to 7 months before death, home-based hospice care accrued savings compared with inpatient savings under Medicare Part A.[8,9] The cost savings were due to reduced hospitalizations.[10] The longer a patient stayed on hospice, past 6 months, the more costly hospice care was to Medicare. By the end of 1 year, a patient on hospice accrued, at best, 10% savings over conventional medical care provide by Medicare.[9]

CLINICAL BENEFIT OF PALLIATIVE MEDICINE AND HOSPICE

Despite the concerns regarding potential cost savings, or lack thereof, with hospice versus conventional medical care, there is no controversy about the benefits of and satisfaction with the multidisciplinary approach of hospice.[11–14] Physicians and caregivers alike extol the virtues of the hospice approach in patients with terminal illnesses. Early in

the life span of the Medicare Hospice Benefit, rural physicians seemed to be more familiar with and more willing to enlist the help of hospice services than urban physicians.[11] Physicians endorsed hospice services especially for the psychologic support provided to patients and caregivers and for the help received in pain and comfort care and because it enabled patients to die at home. Caregivers pointed to the same benefits.[11]

SUMMARY

Palliative medicine and its most visible ambassador, hospice, are nascent subspecialties in medicine. Like pain medicine, palliative medicine uses an interdisciplinary approach in reaching its goal of comfort and quality of life for patients with incurable disease. The approach leads to patient, caregiver, and physician satisfaction and the promise of cost savings in a cost-conscious medical economic environment.

References

1. Doyle D, Hanks G, MacDonald N: *Oxford textbook of palliative medicine.* Oxford, UK, Oxford University Press, 1993.
2. Kaasa S, Klepp O, Hagen S et al: Treatment intention in hospitalized cancer patients in oncological wards in Norway: A national survey. *Cancer Treat Rev* 22(suppl A):33, 1996.
3. Porzsolt F, Wirth A, Mayer-Steinacker R et al: Quality assurance by specification and achievement in goals in palliative cancer treatment. *Cancer Treat Rev* 22(suppl A):41, 1996.
4. Walsh TD: Continuing care in a medical center: the Cleveland Clinic Foundation Palliative Care Service. *J Pain Symptom Manage* 5:273, 1990.
5. *Clinical practice guideline no. 9: Management of cancer pain.* Rockville, Md, Agency for Health and Human Services, 1994.
6. Twycross RG: Opioid analgesics in cancer pain: Current practice and controversies. *Cancer Surv* 7:29, 1988.
7. Twycross RG: The management of pain in cancer: A guide to drugs and dosages. *Oncology* 2:35, 1988.
8. Kidder D: The effects of hospice coverage on Medicare expenditures. *Health Serv Res* 27:195, 1992.
9. National Hospice Organization Item Code 712901: *An analysis of the cost savings of the Medicare hospice benefit.* Miami, Fla, National Hospice Organization, 1995.
10. Emanuel EJ: Cost savings at the end of life: What does the data show? *JAMA* 275:1907, 1996.
11. Gochman D, Bonham G: Physicians and the hospice decision: Awareness, discussion, reasons and satisfaction. *Hospice J* 4:25, 1988.
12. Forster L, Lynn J: Predicting life span for applicants to inpatient hospice. *Arch Intern Med* 148:2540, 1988.
13. Forster L, Lynn J: The use of physiologic measures and demographic variables to predict longevity among inpatient hospice applicants. *Am J Hospice Care* 6:31, 1989.
14. Stillman M, Syrjala K: Differences in physician access patterns to hospice care. *J Pain Symptom Manage* 17:157, 1999.

Questions • Palliative Medicine

1. Palliative medicine is considered a subspeciality to study and manage patients with aggressive and far advanced diseases for which prognosis is limited and the focus of care is the quality of life. In which country did this concept first start

   A. United States of America
   B. United Kingdom
   C. Frances
   D. Scandinavia

2. Goals of palliative medicine for a dying patient are all of the following except

   A. To relieve physical distress
   B. To relieve psychologic distress
   C. To relieve social and spiritual distress
   D. To cure terminal illness

3. Physical symptoms routinely addressed by practitioners of palliative medicine included

   A. Pain
   B. Weight gain
   C. Confusion
   D. Fatigue

4. Comprehensive palliative medical care units have been developed in academic health care centers for acute management. The services offered by them are all of the following except

   A. Preventative therapy
   B. Symptom therapy
   C. Diet control
   D. Psychotherapy

5. Palliative medicine uses the following approach in reaching its goal of comfort and quality of life in patients with incurable diseases

   A. Unidisciplinary approach
   B. Multidisciplinary approach
   C. Psychologic approach
   D. Medical approach

ANSWERS

1. B
2. D
3. B
4. C
5. B

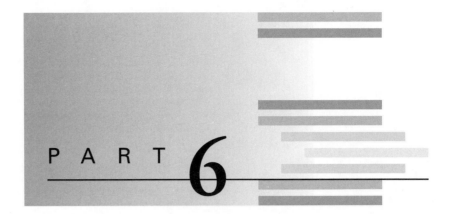

PART 6

Special Situations

CHAPTER 30

Pediatric Pain*

JOELLE F. DESPARMET-SHERIDAN

There is ample proof in the literature that children receive less analgesia than do adults for equivalent surgical procedures. A number of reasons are given for the discrepancy.

The need for analgesics may go unrecognized if the child's pain is not adequately assessed or if he or she cannot voice the pain. Sometimes analgesics are withheld on the grounds that they can do more harm than good in children, an argument used especially with small children. This reflects ignorance of pediatric physiology, pharmacology, psychology, and behavioral reaction to pain and demonstrates the attitude of many adults toward childhood pain. It also explains in part why children as a group, especially younger ones, receive the least adequate relief from pain.

This chapter attempts to establish the reality of pain in children, describes ways to assess it, and outlines the difficulty of doing so in preverbal children. The management of various pediatric pain syndromes is also discussed. The anatomy and physiology of pain and the basic functions and organization of the nervous system are not repeated here because they are well reviewed in the clinical section of this book.

REALITY OF PAIN IN CHILDREN

Perception of Children's Pain by Those Who Surround Them

The perception and treatment of children's pain has been amply studied. A 1988 British poll[1] asked pediatric anesthetists how they treated postoperative pain. When questioned about children of different age groups, only 80% to 85% of the anesthetists replied that babies from birth to 1 month perceive pain. All believed that beyond 1 month of age all children feel pain. It is interesting that 13% stated that newborns cannot feel pain and that 2% did not know.

Most of these anesthetists (more than 80%) never prescribed opioids preoperatively to newborns and infants, and close to 30% still did not prescribe opioids to this age group after major surgery. Although all the anesthetists questioned thought that children between 1 and 12 months perceived pain, more than 10% still refrained from providing them with adequate pain relief after major surgery. The reasons given for this lack of pain treatment were that the dangers of prescribing major analgesics in that age group outweighed the advantages in that particular clinical setting and that safer but less potent drugs were preferable to alleviate pain in children.

Studies reported in 1996 show that caregivers continue to undertreat pain in children. Reasons have ranged from the lack of knowledge or belief in safe doses of analgesics to the lack of will to administer analgesics at prescribed doses.[2,3] These studies show that the evaluation of pain in children is difficult and that pain management depends on the subjective appreciation and emotional involvement of the persons in charge, particularly when the children are prelingual and, therefore, unable to voice whether and to what degree they feel pain. Although children have a remarkable capacity to recover from physically painful events, no data support the belief that they neither feel nor remember pain. Indeed, more and more evidence indicates the contrary.

Development of Pain in the Fetus and the Neonate

Because early studies of neurologic development concluded that the fetus and newborn were incapable of having organized responses to painful stimuli, could not perceive or localize pain,[4,5] and had no memory of pain, the concept that newborns did not require analgesia—even for very painful procedures—was generally accepted.[6,7]

There is a reason to believe that at birth, and even before birth, the human body is able to perceive pain and demonstrate physiologic responses to nociception.[8] Nociceptive nerve endings are present in the skin of newborns[9]; cutaneous sensory perception spreads from the perioral area to the face, hands, feet, and trunk at 7 weeks of gestation and to proximal parts of the limbs by 15 weeks. By 20 weeks, there is sensory perception on all cutaneous and mucous surfaces.[10,11] In addition by that time, synapses between sensory fibers and interneurons in the dorsal horn of the spinal cord are formed.[12,13]

By 30 weeks, all types of cells in the dorsal horn have developed. The fact that myelination of nerves and nerve endings is incomplete at birth is the major argument used to support the lack of pain perception in babies.[14-17] However, myelination starts in nerve tracts in the spinal cord and brainstem at 22 weeks of gestation and is completed in the central nervous system (CNS) by the third trimester.[18] Therefore, the fact that there is incomplete myelination in peripheral nerves only means that conduction is slower, and this is compensated for by the shorter distance the sensory message has to travel in a neonate's body. Different developmental changes are summarized in Figure 30–1.

Physiologically, newborns react to noxious stimuli by demonstrating changes in cardiovascular parameters; transcutaneous PO_2 and palmar sweating[19-22]; and increases in

* Editor's Note: This chapter has not been updated since it was previously published. The author advises the reader to consult other sources to provide the latest information on drugs and techniques.

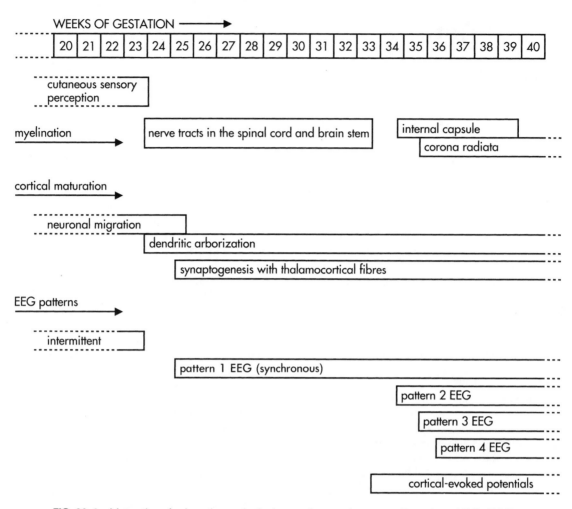

FIG. 30–1 Maturation of pain pathways in the human fetus and neonate. *(From Anand KJS, Phil D, Hickey PR: Pain and its effects on the human neonate and fetus.* N Engl J Med *317:1321, 1986).*

stress hormones such as catecholamines, aldosterone, cortisol, glucagon, and insulin.[23] These changes can be avoided by local anesthesia or sedation.[24] Behavioral changes associated with pain have also been documented in newborns, and they range from motor responses to pinprick with crying and grimacing[25,26] to a number of facial expressions that are a specific reaction to a painful stimulus, such as heel lancing.[27,28]

ASSESSMENT OF PAIN IN CHILDREN

One of the challenges to health care professionals who treat children is to find tools to assess their pain appropriately. Unlike most adults, children lack the cognitive and behavioral competency to understand questions concerning their pain and to describe their pain. Therefore, strategies to evaluate children's pain have been and remain a major issue despite the proliferation of professional literature on the subject.

Although many different tools are used to measure and assess pain, no single one supplies enough information about pain and its different components to be used as the standard measure of pain in children. McGrath and Unruh[29] identified three components of pain and analyzed them accordingly:

- Cognitive or self-report
- Behavioral
- Physiologic

Melzack[30] was concerned with sensation of pain and reactions to pain. There are many ways to view pain; to treat pain adequately, one must consider its many aspects.

Assessment of Pain by Self-Report

The assessment of pain by self-report addresses the cognitive component of pain.

Questions and Answers

The simplest way to assess pain is to ask about it. Self-report has been used and researched mostly in adults[30] because they have the ability and the experience to express their pain verbally. In recent years, however, children have been the object of research aimed at the measurement and assessment of pain.

There are various problems with self-reporting in children. The questioner influences the child's answer, with differences depending on whether the mother or the physician is asking the question. The answer also varies with the type of question, whether it is open-ended or a checklist type.[31]

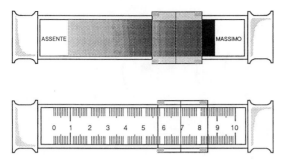

FIG. 30–2 Analogue chromatic continuous scale.

Furthermore, younger children are not always able to express how they feel because they either do not understand the question or do not have the vocabulary to give a meaningful answer.

Another problem is that some children deny pain to avoid additional painful treatment, such as injections and unpleasant-tasting medication. Conversely, children may overestimate the intensity and frequency of occurrence of pain to ensure that they will receive treatment.[32] To minimize these problems, pain scales have been devised that do not require elaborate cognitive skills.

Numerical and Spatial Scales

The easiest scale to use is the *visual analogue scale,* which is similar to the one used for adults. This is a slide ruler, 10 cm long, with "no pain" written at one end and "maximal pain" at the other. The patient slides the cursor along the ruler until it reaches the level that represents the intensity of his or her pain. The other side of the ruler is gradated over 100 mm and gives the investigator a numerical measure of pain.[33] This scale has been modified for smaller children,[34] enabling them to equate pain intensity with colors on the *analogue chromatic continuous scale* (ACCS) (Fig. 30–2). Another variation of these scales is the *pain thermometer.*

The Face Scale

A number of scales use happy-sad faces to measure pain in small children. *McGrath's scale* has drawings of nine faces depicting varying degrees of pain, ranging from no pain to a lot of pain, and children choose the face that best approximates their pain (Fig. 30–3). Beyer developed the *Oucher,* which is used in children aged 3 to 12 years. This up-and-down scale has photographs of a child in six increasing degrees of pain scored from 0 for the comfortable and calm face to 100 for the upset, crying face and withdrawn attitude (Fig. 30–4).

There is a strong correlation between the scores obtained with the ACCS and the Oucher and with behavior scores in children 3 years of age and older.

Assessment of Pain by Self-Representation

The assessment of pain by self-representation requires the child to draw a picture of herself or himself indicating where the pain is and how much it hurts.[35] A similar tool asks the child to show on a printed figure of the body where and how intense the pain is; the child fills in the area that hurts with various colors that represent different intensities of pain for that particular child.[36] This method requires the child to have a certain degree of cognitive development and is limited to use with children older than 6 or 7 years.

Behavioral Assessment

Behavioral assessment studies the reaction to pain or the behavior component of pain. The expression of pain (whether acute or chronic) can be modified by cultural influences, the behavior of others in the environment,[37] and the subjective experience of the individual in pain. Because of this, the thorough evaluation of pain must include a behavioral assessment. In acute pain, vocal and facial expressions of pain are assessed. In persistent or recurrent pain (chronic pain), the way the pain influences normal activity such as school attendance, interaction with family and friends, and participation in group activities and sports, and factors reinforcing the pain behavior are also evaluated.[38]

DIFFERENT PAIN SYNDROMES IN CHILDREN

Recurrent Abdominal Pain

The definition of recurrent abdominal pain in childhood and adolescence is pain with no organic cause occurring on at least three occasions over a 3-month period that is severe enough to alter the child's normal activity. This definition excludes abdominal pain resulting from known medical conditions, such as pain from neurologic disorders, metabolic disease, hematologic disease, gastrointestinal disease, gynecologic conditions, chronic infection, and pain related to congenital anomalies.[39] It also excludes acute pain from acute renal, intestinal, and gynecologic disorders, which can be treated surgically.

Pain for which no organic cause is found is often regarded as psychogenic and can be misdiagnosed or denied by parents or physicians and treated inadequately. Therefore, recurrent abdominal pain would better be considered as psychophysiologic.[40] This implies that it is real pain triggered by stress, depression, or family-related conflicts. These stressors may be associated with physiologic disorders, such as autonomic instability, lactose intolerance, and constipation.

The diagnosis of recurrent abdominal pain is based on the absence of an organic cause. Laboratory tests other than complete blood cell counts, urinalysis, and stool guaiac are usually not necessary if nothing is found on history and physical examination because they rarely reveal a pathologic condition. Symptoms related to a specific psychophysiologic factor in the child's life of family history are, conversely, often present.

Because this type of pain is a multifactorial phenomenon and can be related to stress in the family or school setting, treatment can be difficult to initiate. Treatment includes management of stress factors, if need be, through referral to behavior medicine specialists for relaxation, biofeedback techniques, and ways to change the child's attitude toward stressors.[38]

Headache and Migraine

Headache

Headache is the most common type of pain of which children complain. It can be a benign symptom often accompanying

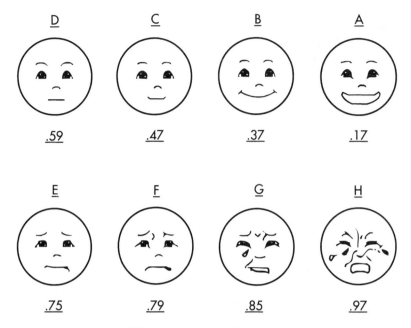

FIG. 30–3 McGrath's face scale.

common illnesses such as colds or viral infections; it can be then treated with minor drugs and disappears as the illness resolves. Headache can also be recurrent and accompany other, more severe, disorders.

One important fact should be kept in mind when treating a child with recurrent headache; meningitis, encephalitis, cerebral abscess, vascular malformations, trauma, tumoral masses of the meninges or cerebral structures, and degenerative cerebral disease with or without intracranial hypertension are all cases of headache.

The diagnosis of benign recurrent headache should not be considered unless a complete history and physical examination, including funduscopy, are normal. Laboratory investigations can be conducted to confirm the absence of a pathologic cause of the headaches if clinically indicated.

Treatment starts by addressing the ailment causing the headache.

Migraine

Migraine in children can be defined as recurrent headache accompanied by three of the following symptoms:

- Recurrent abdominal pain with without nausea or vomiting
- Throbbing pain on one side of the cranium
- Relief of the pain by rest
- A visual, sensory, or motor aura
- A family history of migraine[41,42]

Childhood migraine seems to be a vascular and neurologic disease, as evidenced by the frequent association with electroencephalographic abnormalities.[43,44] Clinically, migraine has various presentations.

Common migraine is the type seen in children before puberty. Most recurrent childhood migraine is of this type.

Other less common types include *classic migraine, ophthalmoplegic migraine,* and *tension headache.*

Prophylactic treatment has classically been based on ergotamine, which causes vasoconstriction of extracranial blood vessels. Drugs such as anticonvulsants, antidepressants, antihypertensives, antihistamines, and calcium channel blockers have been reported as successful long-term preventive treatments. Behavioral treatments have proved effective in treating pediatric migraine. Biofeedback, relaxation, and self-hypnosis are used successfully in many centers.

Recurrent Chest Pain

Chest pain is relatively common in children. It ranks third in frequency after headache and abdominal pain and may be as common as limb pain. It is seen most often between 10 and 21 years of age. There is little information on etiology, evaluation, and treatment of chest pain. Costochondritis, trauma, muscle strain, chest wall syndrome, rib anomalies, and hyperventilation have been cited as causes of the pain. Physical examination rarely finds signs of a patent disorder. One should rely more on the patient's history for some indication, such as a complaint of palpitations or the presence of stressful situations that trigger the pain, suggesting a psychogenic cause. Nonetheless, a physical cause should be sought.

Costochondritis is the most common cause of chest pain in children. It often occurs after an upper respiratory infection, can radiate to the back, and can last from a few days to several months.

Another cause is a stitch—a sharp, crampy pain under the costal margin that occurs while one is walking or running and is caused by stress on the peritoneal ligaments when they are stretched between the fast-moving diaphragm and the abdomen. Asthma and other lung-, diaphragm-, or pleura-related disorders can also cause chest pain.

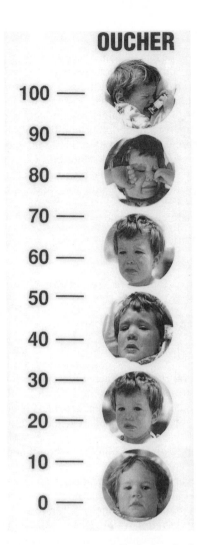

OUCHER

100 —
90 —
80 —
70 —
60 —
50 —
40 —
30 —
20 —
10 —
0 —

FIG. 30–4 The caucasian version of the Oucher. Scale is also available in a 0 = 10 format. Developed and copyrighted by Judith E. Beyer, RN, PhD, 1983.

Identification of the origin of the pain and reassurance of the patient and family are often the most important elements of treatment provided that specific organic causes have been identified.[45]

MEDICALLY CAUSED PAIN

Sickle Cell Anemia

Sickle cell anemia is the most common hemoglobinopathy in the United States. Pain occurs during vaso-occlusive crisis, the frequency of which is unpredictable and ranges from less than one crisis a year to a crisis several times a year or several times a month.[46] Pain occurs when and where there is occlusion of small blood vessels by sickled erythrocytes: affects small bones of the extremities in small children and abdomen, chest, long bones, and lower back in older children.

Hemophilia

Hemophilias are the most common inherited coagulation disorders in children and include deficiencies of factors VIII, IX, and XI. Factor VIII deficiency is the most common hemophilia; factor IX deficiency is less common.

Hematomas can occur at any age, but hemarthroses usually appear when the child starts walking. Bleeding also occurs in deep soft tissues and muscles as well as intracranially.[47] Hemarthrosis is a major problem in severe and moderate hemophilia and leads to permanent damage and pain from synovial and bone changes.

Analgesic therapy is an important part of the management of hemophilia, although it is secondary to replacement therapy.

Diabetes

The epidemiology of *diabetes mellitus* is not well defined because studies do not characterize the disease the same way. The overall prevalence of diabetes mellitus is approximately 1%, and juvenile diabetes accounts for about one fourth of that. Juvenile diabetes is not a painful disease in itself, and children are not seen in pain clinics until they become teenagers, at which time they present with early signs of peripheral diabetic neuropathy.

Juvenile diabetes mellitus is labile, and the first signs of neuropathy are often seen at the time of an acidoketotic crisis. The most frequent complication of diabetes mellitus is symmetrical peripheral neuropathy,[48] but mononeuropathies involving only one peripheral or cranial nerve seem to be more common than previously believed.

Juvenile Rheumatoid Arthritis

Juvenile rheumatoid arthritis is not a rare disease, with 250,000 affected children in the United States. Although the cause is still unclear, the disease is characterized by chronic synovitis with or without extra-articular manifestations.

Juvenile rheumatoid arthritis differs from adult-onset arthritis in that lasting damage to articular cartilage occurs later in the course of the disease, and many children never have permanent joint damage. In rheumatoid factor–positive arthritis, however, joint destruction with stiffness and pain may be present, especially when many joints are involved. Pauciarticular disease (which is not seen in adults) occurs in 30% of juvenile rheumatoid arthritis patients, affects mostly girls, starts before age 4 years, and can be associated with iridocyclitis.

Systemic-onset arthritis occurs in 20% of patients and is characterized by a high intermittent fever and a rash. The evolution of the disease is marked by remissions and exacerbations.

Musculoskeletal Pain

Growing Pains

Under the category of growing pains come deep pains that are often felt by children in the lower limbs bilaterally and for which no organic cause is apparent. This type of pain occurs in school-aged children, in whom stress or emotional factors are sometimes found.[49,50]

Myofascial Pain

Myofascial pain is rare in children before their teenaged years, at which time it is similar to that of adults. Yunus and Masi[51] described a pain syndrome in children (*juvenile primary fibromyalgia syndrome*) that associates depression, sleeping disorders, and problems at school or in the family setting and pain very similar to myofascial pain. This may well be a global pain-dysfunction syndrome combining myofascial pain and behavior modifications resulting from long-standing pain (chronic pain syndrome).

Complex Regional Pain Syndrome (RSD)

Complex regional pain syndrome (CRPS, RSD) is not well understood. Its pathophysiology is the source of great controversy. It was once thought to be sympathetically determined and maintained, but because of the lack of response of some forms of RSD to sympathetic blocks, it is regarded more as a form of receptor sensitization. Although the causal injury is not always recognized, the most widely accepted theory of the pathogenesis of RSD is that following initial tissue and nerve damage or irritation, afferent impulses from injured neurons to the spinal cord increase, causing dysregulation of sympathetic activity at the spinal cord level. This creates a self-perpetuated abnormal reflex arc with peripheral vasomotor and sudomotor changes and pain, which again causes increased impulses, and so on.[52]

RSD is now referred to as *complex regional pain syndrome type I* (CRPS I) and causalgia with its definite nerve injury (CRPS II). Even though the syndrome, response to treatment, and usually outcome differ in children compared with adults, CRPS I does exist in children and is more common than previously thought. It has been reported in children as young as 3 years.[52] CRPS I is characterized by severe pain, often burning in quality, persisting much longer than would be expected after the initial injury.

Sometimes a particular psychologic profile can be seen in children with CRPS I or CRPS II. The children are usually intelligent, driven overachievers who are involved (usually with success) in very competitive activities and who often react to the loss of this activity with depression. Other psychologic issues such as family discord and divorce and enmeshment with one parent are found. School attendance is often an issue.

Cancer Pain

Cancer is the third leading cause of death in the United States in children 1 to 4 years old and second most common cause of death between 5 and 19 years of age. Children with cancer have pain not only from tumor compression of surrounding structures but also from side effects and the required venous access of antimitotic drugs. Repeated small procedures such as bone marrow and organ biopsies are also painful. Fear of treatments and of death can cause depression, thereby worsen the pain experience.

The most common tumors in children are leukemias, lymphomas, brain tumors (posterior fossa), neuroblastomas, hepatoblastomas, and bone sarcomas. Pain can be visceral, resulting from the stretching of abdominal structures by voluminous tumors; it may be present in bones as a consequence of primary tumors, metastatic disease, or bone marrow expansion, as in leukemia; or it may be caused by nerve stretching or headache stemming from increased intracranial pressure. Antimitotic drugs can also cause peripheral neuropathies that can be very painful and difficult to treat.

Acute Pain

Because of widespread fear of overdosing, children have always been and still are grossly undermedicated after painful trauma or major operations. However, pharmacokinetic and pharmacodynamic studies have shown that proper doses of potent analgesics and local anesthetics are no more dangerous in children than they are in adults,[53–58] and thus, there is no reason to withhold these modalities of pain relief, even in small children. On the contrary, increasing evidence shows that pain relief techniques using potent drugs not only are safe for children but also can improve outcome.[59]

Common sources of acute pain for children are:

1. Sports injuries
2. Burns
3. Trauma
4. Preoperative, intraoperative, and postoperative pain

PARENTERAL MEDICATIONS

In the immediate postoperative period when medications cannot be taken orally, the best rout for analgesic administration is intravenously. When intravenous (IV) access is available, there is little, if any, indication for the intramuscular (IM) route in children because it has obvious psychologic disadvantages and no pharmacologic advantage over the IV route.

Drugs can be given as boluses or continuous infusions. Boluses are easy to administer and provide rapid pain relief; however, they have the disadvantage of providing short periods of analgesia sometimes associated with side effects when serum drug concentration peaks, followed by inadequate pain relief while the level decreases until the next injection. Continuous infusions, conversely, avoid this roller coaster of pain relief followed by pain and provide continuous analgesia with low plasma levels of drugs even in newborns and infants.[60–62] Probably the best way to administer drugs is to give a loading dose titrated to provide patient comfort, followed by an infusion. Currently used narcotics are morphine or methadone (which have the same potency but different duration of action) and meperidine.

ORAL MEDICATIONS

Oral analgesics combined with benzodiazepines provide sedation and reduce anxiety preoperatively.[63] Postoperatively, when the oral route can again be used, methadone can be prescribed at a dose one- to two-fold that of the IV route. In any case, pain should be repeatedly evaluated with simple pain and behavior scales, and pain medication should be adapted to the pain scores provided by these scales and by physiologic findings.

REGIONAL ANESTHESIA

Pediatric-size epidural and spinal equipment is available and greatly facilitates regional techniques in children as young as a few months of age.

Although no data support this, spinal anesthesia has had limited indications in children and adolescents because of the incidence of postspinal headache in this age group.

Pharmacokinetic studies have shown that epidural (lumbar or caudal) local anesthetics and narcotics can be used safely in children[64-69] and that bolus injections and continuous infusions provide adequate analgesia and safe plasma concentrations postoperatively. Regional anesthesia can be used intraoperatively to provide analgesia and a certain, often sufficient, degree of muscle relaxation during the operation.

Other blocks are successfully performed in children, including (1) penile blocks for circumcisions,[70,71] (2) ilioinguinal blocks for hernias,[72] (3) intercostal and intrapleural analgesia for thoracic surgery,[73,74] and (4) peripheral nerve blocks (axillary, supraclavicular plexus, peroneal, ankle, and femoral blocks) for limb surgery.[75,76]

FUTURE PROSPECTS

Pediatric Pain Clinics

The need for pain clinics designed specifically to manage acute as well as chronic pain in children is obvious. The pathology, treatments, and outcome of pain syndromes differ in children and adults, and a special type of clinic could address these issues for the pediatric patient.

An ideal pediatric pain treatment center deals with acute and chronic pain in a multidisciplinary way, treating all components in one place. Such a center includes a chronic pain management service to establish a diagnosis and initiate treatment, a department of behavioral medicine to instigate psychologic therapy and behavior modification, and a physical therapy unit and a number of consultants for specialized evaluations and management. The ideal center also has an acute pain service specifically organized to manage pain in the postoperative period on the wards or in the intensive care units. This service is responsible for managing postoperative pain and cancer-induced or medically induced pain and also manages IV and epidural infusions of narcotics and local anesthetics, patient-controlled analgesia, and all techniques for postoperative pain relief.

Education

Health care professionals must be educated about the vast possibilities in the field of pain relief in children. Research in pediatric physiology and pharmacology has provided important information on the need for appropriate analgesia in children to ameliorate outcome.

Research

Although there have been extensive studies in the field of physiology and pharmacology in children, comparatively less clinical research has been conducted on the occurrence and degree of pain that children experience. Large series of children must be studied to determine the best ways to assess pain. Once this is known, the best ways to treat different types of pain will follow. The validity and sensitivity of measures of pain, the effectiveness and safety of one treatment versus another, and the ratio of benefit versus morbidity or cost must be ascertained.

References

1. Purcell-Jones G, Dormon F, Sumner E: Pediatric anesthetists' perception of neonatal and infant pain. *Pain* 33:181, 1988.
2. Romsing J: Assessment of nurses' judgment for analgesic requirements of postoperative pain. *J Clin Pharm Ther* 21:159, 1996.
3. Broome ME, Richtsmeier A, Maikler V et al: Pediatric pain practices: A national survey of health professionals. *J Pain Symptom Manage* 11:312, 1996.
4. Levy DM: The infant's earliest memory of inoculation: A contribution to public health procedures. *J Genet Psychol* 96:37, 1960.
5. Merskey H: On the development of pain. *Pain* 10:116, 1970.
6. Lippmann M, Nelson RJ, Emmanouilides GC et al: Ligation of patent ductus arteriosus in premature infants. *Br J Anaesth* 48:365, 1976.
7. Katz J: The question of circumcision. *Int Surg* 62:490, 1977.
8. Anand KJ, Hickey PR: Pain and its effects in the human neonate and fetus. *N Engl J Med* 317:1321, 1987.
9. Gleiss J, Stuttgen G: Morphologic and functional development of the skin. In Stave U, editor: *Physiology of the neonatal period,* vol 2. New York, Appleton-Century-Crofts, 1970.
10. Humphrey T: Function of the central nervous system during prenatal life. In Stave U, editor: *Perinatal physiology,* vol 2. New York, Plenum Press, 1978.
11. Valman HB, Pearson JF: What the fetus feels. *Br Med J* 280:233, 1980.
12. Tilney F, Rosett J: The value of brain lipoids as an index of brain development. *Bull Neurol Inst* 1:28, 1931.
13. Schulte FJ: Neurophysiological aspects of brain development. In *Mead-Johnson symposium on perinatal and developmental medicine,* vol 6. Evansville, Ind., Mead-Johnson, 1975.
14. Can a fetus feel pain? [editorial]. *Br Med J* 291:1220, 1985.
15. Swafford LE, Allan D: Pain relief in the pediatric patient. *Med Clin North Am* 23:131, 1968.
16. Jackson-Rees G: Anesthesia in the newborn. *Br Med J* 2:1419, 1950.
17. Betts EK, Downes JJ: Anesthetic considerations in newborn surgery. *Semin Anesth* 3:59, 1984.
18. Henderson-Smart DJ, Pettigrew HJ, Campbell DJ: Clinical apnea and brain neural function in preterm infants. *N Engl J Med* 308:353, 1983.
19. Holve RL, Bromberger PJ, Groveman HD et al: Regional anesthesia during newborn circumcision: Effect on infant pain response. *Clin Pediatr (Phila)* 22:813, 1983.
20. Owens ME, Todt EH: Pain in infancy: Neonatal reaction to a heel lance. *Pain* 20:77, 1984.
21. Johnson CC, Strada ME: Acute pain response in infants: A multidimensional description. *Pain* 24:373, 1986.
22. Field T, Goldson E: Pacifying effects of nonnutritive sucking on term and preterm neonates during heelstick procedures. *Pediatrics* 74:1012, 1984.
23. Fiselier T, Monnens L, Moerman E et al: Influence of the stress of venepuncture on basal levels of plasma renin activity in infants and children. *Int J Pediatr Nephrol* 4:181, 1983.
24. Maxwell LG, Yaster M, Welzel RC: Penile nerve block reduces the physiologic stress to newborn circumcision. *Anesthesiology* 65:A432, 1986.
25. Rich EC, Marshall RE, Volpe JJ: The normal neonatal response to pinprick. *Dev Med Child Neurol* 16:432, 1974.
26. Franck LS: A new method to quantitatively describe pain behavior in infants. *Nurs Res* 35:28, 1986.
27. Ekman P, Oster H: Facial expressions of emotion. *Ann Rev Psychol* 30:527, 1979.
28. Izard EC, Huebner RR, Risser D: The young infant's ability to produce discrete emotional expressions. *Dev Psychol* 16:132, 1980.
29. McGrath PJ, Unruh AM: The measurement and assessment of pain. In McGrath PJ, Unruh AM, editors: *Pain in children and adolescents.* New York, Elsevier, 1987.
30. Melzack R, editor: *Pain measurement and assessment.* New York, Raven Press, 1985.
31. Andrasik F, Burke EJ, Attanasio V et al: Child, parent and physician reports of a child's headache pain: relationships prior to and following treatment. *Headache* 25:421, 1985.
32. Ross DM, Ross SA: The importance of type of question, psychological climate and subject set in interviewing children about pain. *Pain* 19:71, 1984.
33. Huskisson EC: Visual analogue scales. In Melzack R, editor: *Pain measurements and assessment.* New York, Raven Press, 1985.

34. Grossi E, Borghi C, Cerchiari EL et al: Analogue chromatic continuous scale (ACCS): A new method for pain assessment. *Clin Exp Rheumatol* 1:337, 1983.

35. Katz ER, Kellerman J, Siegel SE: Behavioral distress in children with cancer undergoing medical procedures: Developmental considerations. *J Consult Clin Psychol* 48:356, 1980.

36. Unruh A, McGrath P, Cunningham SJ et al: Children's drawing of their pain. *Pain* 17:385, 1983.

37. Shaw EG, Routh DK: Effect of mother's presence on children's reactions to aversive procedures. *J Pediatr Psychol* 7:33, 1982.

38. Masek BJ, Russo DC, Varni JW: Behavioral approaches to the management of chronic pain in children. *Pediatr Clin North Am* 31:1113, 1984.

39. Levine M, Rappaport LA: Recurrent abdominal pain in school children: The loneliness of the long-distance physician. *Pediatr Clin North Am* 31:969, 1984.

40. Stone RT, Barbero GJ: Recurrent abdominal pain in childhood. *Pediatrics* 45:732, 1970.

41. Selby G, Lance JW: Observations of 500 cases of migraine and allied vascular headache. *J Neurol Neurosurg Psychiatry* 23:23, 1960.

42. Bille B: The prognosis of migraine in children. *Dan Med Bull* 22:112, 1975.

43. Lai CW, Ziegler DK, Lansky LL et al: Hemiplegic migraine in children: Diagnostic and therapeutic aspects. *J Pediatr* 101:696, 1982.

44. Rossi LN, Vassella F, Bajc O et al: Benign migraine-like syndrome with CSF pleocytosis in children. *Dev Med Child Neurol* 27:192, 1985.

45. Coleman WL: Recurrent chest pain in children. *Pediatr Clin North Am* 31:1007, 1984.

46. Vichinsky EP, Lubin BH: Sickle cell anemia and related hemoglobinopathies. *Pediatr Clin North Am* 27:429, 1980.

47. Nathan DG, Oski FA: *Hematology of infancy and childhood,* ed 2, vol 2. Philadelphia, WB Saunders, 1981.

48. Locke S: The peripheral nervous system in diabetes mellitus. *Diabetes* 13:307, 1984.

49. Oster J, Nielson A: Growing pains: A clinical investigation of a school population. *Acta Pediatr Scand* 61:321, 1972.

50. Naish JM, Apley J: Growing pains: A clinical study of non-arthritic limb pains in children. *Arch Dis Child* 26:134, 1951.

51. Yunus MB, Masi AT: Juvenile primary fibromyalgia syndrome. A clinical study of thirty-three patients and matched normal controls. *Arthritis Rheum* 28:138, 1985.

52. Carron H, McHue F: Reflex sympathetic dystrophy in a ten year old child. *South Med J* 65:631, 1972.

53. Nahata MC, Miser AW, Miser JS et al: Variation in morphine pharmacokinetics in children with cancer. *Dev Pharmacol Ther* 8:182, 1985.

54. Miser AW, Miser JS, Clark BS: Continuous intravenous infusion of morphine sulfate for control of severe pain in children with terminal malignancy. *J Pediatr* 96:930, 1980.

55. Ecoffey C, Desparmet J, Maury M et al: Bupivacaine in children: Pharmacokinetics following caudal anesthesia. *Anesthesiology* 63:447, 1985.

56. Berde CB, Sethna NF, Holzman RS: Pharmacokinetics of methadone in children and adolescents in the perioperative period. *Anesthesiology* 67:A519, 1987.

57. Attia J, Ecoffey C, Sandouk P et al: Epidural morphine in children: Pharmacokinetics and CO_2 sensitivity. *Anesthesiology* 65:590, 1986.

58. Benlabed M, Ecoffey C, Levron JC et al: Analgesia and ventilatory response to CO_2 following epidural sufentanyl in children. *Anesthesiology* 67:948, 1987.

59. Tyler DC: Respiratory effects of pain in a child after thoracotomy. *Anesthesiology* 70:873, 1989.

60. Koren G, Butt W, Chinyanga H et al: Postoperative morphine infusion in newborn infants: Assessment of disposition characteristics and safety. *J Pediatr* 107:963, 1985.

61. Lynn AM, Opheim KE, Tyler DC: Morphine infusion after pediatric cardiac surgery. *Crit Care Med* 12:863, 1984.

62. Bray J: Postoperative analgesia provided by morphine infusion in children. *Anaesthesia* 38:1075, 1983.

63. Brzustowicz RM, Nelson DA, Betts EK et al: Efficacy of oral premedication for pediatric outpatient surgery. *Anesthesiology* 60:475, 1984.

64. Ecoffey C, Debousset AM, Samii K: Lumbar and thoracic epidural anesthesia for urologic and upper abdominal surgery in infants and children. *Anesthesiology* 65:87, 1986.

65. Meignier M, Souron R, Le Neel JC: Postoperative dorsal epidural analgesia in the child with respiratory disabilities. *Anesthesiology* 59:473, 1983.

66. Ecoffey C, Attia J, Samii K: Analgesia and side-effects following epidural morphine in children. *Anesthesiology* 63:A470, 1985.

67. Shapiro LA, Jedeikin RJ, Shalev D et al: Epidural morphine analgesia in children. *Anesthesiology* 61:210, 1984.

68. Broadman LM: "Kiddy" caudals: Experience with 1154 consecutive cases without complications. *Anesth Analg* 66:S18, 1987.

69. Krane EJ, Jacobson LE, Lynn AM et al: Caudal morphine for postoperative analgesia in children: A comparison with caudal bupivacaine and intravenous morphine. *Anesth Analg* 66:647, 1987.

70. Maxwell LG, Yaster M, Wetzel RC et al: Penile nerve block reduces the physiologic stress of newborn circumcision. *Anesthesiology* 65:3A, 1986.

71. Yeoman PM, Cooke R, Hain WR: Penile block for circumcision? A comparison for caudal blockade. *Anaesthesia* 38:862, 1983.

72. Markham SJ, Tomlinson J, Hain WR: Ilioinguinal nerve block in children: A comparison with caudal block for intra and postoperative analgesia. *Anaesthesia* 41:1098, 1986.

73. Rothstein P, Arthur GR, Feldman HS et al: Bupivacaine for intercostal nerve block in children: Blood concentrations and pharmacokinetics. *Anesth Analg* 65:625, 1986.

74. McIlvaine WB, Knox RF, Fennessey PV et al: Continuous infusion of bupivacaine via intrapleural catheter for analgesia after thoracotomy in children. *Anesthesiology* 69:261, 1988.

75. McNicol LR: Lower limb blocks for children: Lateral cutaneous and femoral nerve blocks for postoperative pain relief in paediatric practice. *Anaesthesia* 41:27, 1986.

76. Dalens B: Regional anesthesia in children. *Anesth Analg* 68:654, 1989.

Questions • Pediatric Pain

1. It has been reported that caregivers continue to undertreat pain in children. Reasons include all of the following except

   A. Treatment of children is extremely expensive
   B. Lack of knowledge of the pharmacologic effect of the drugs in children
   C. Belief that safe doses of analgesics are lower in children than adults
   D. Lack of will to administer effective doses in children, even if the caregivers know the effective dose

2. Physiologically, newborns react to noxious stimuli by demonstrating changes in all of the following except

   A. Cardiovascular parameters
   B. Transcutaneous PO_2
   C. Transcutaneous PCO_2
   D. Palmar sweating

3. Of all of the scales described to measure pain in small children, which scale is used best for children from 3 to 12 years of age

   A. McGrath's scale (nine faces depicting varying degrees of pain)
   B. Oucher scale
   C. Visual analog scale (VAS)
   D. McGill's questionnaire

4. Common syndromes in children amenable to pain management are all of the following except

   A. Recurrent abdominal pain
   B. Headaches
   C. Recurrent chest pain
   D. Sickle cell anemia

5. Juvenile primary fibromyalgia syndrome consist of all of these signs and symptoms except

   A. Depression
   B. Pain very similar to myofascial pain
   C. Problems in school or family setting
   D. Sound, deep sleep

ANSWERS

1. A

2. C

3. B

4. D

5. D

CHAPTER 31

Geriatric Pain

DANIEL LYNCH

DEFINITION OF GERIATRIC PAIN

What is chronic geriatric pain? The International Association for the Study of Pain (IASP) has defined pain as, "an unpleasant sensory and emotional experience associated with actual or potential tissue damage, or described in terms of such damage."[1] Similarly, *chronic pain* was described as pain that persisted "past the time of healing" or for more than 3 months. *Chronic geriatric pain* is, therefore, an unpleasant sensory and emotional tissue damage in persons who are either 65 to 79 years old or 80 and older and who have had pain for greater then 3 months.

EPIDEMIOLOGY

The National Long-Term Care Survey

The National Long-Term Care Survey (NLTCS) was taken in 1982, 1984, and 1989 for Medicare-eligible community-dwelling adults age 65 and over. This survey explored the morbidity, mortality, and disability trends of this rapidly growing segment of the population. Based on the NLTCS survey, Manton and colleagues[2] performed multivariant analysis on the NLTCS data, which resulted in extraction of six unique disability profiles from 27 different measures of *functional limitation* (the difficulty in performing personal care and home management tasks).

The scale used to measure the ability to perform physical tasks related to personal care is called activities of daily living (ADLs) and refers to such activities as eating, bathing, and toileting. Instrumental activities of daily living (IADLs) measure more complex tasks, such as managing personal finances, shopping, cooking, and so forth.

Six disability profiles have been classified by Manton's group[2]:

- Type I (unimpaired) persons with a few physical limitations
- Type II (healthy) persons with minimal physical limitations
- Type III (IADL and physically limited)
- Type IV (IADL and cognitively impaired) persons with 42.9% and 47.4%, respectively, of the total number (27) of limitations
- Type V (ADL limited) persons with more ADL limitations but fewer IADL limitations
- Type VI (frail) patients with the most number of limitations

Table 31–1 describes the six disability profiles of 29 common medical illnesses affecting older adults.[2] The first column in Table 31–2 shows the marginal frequency of various medical conditions affecting older adults.

IMPLICATIONS OF AGING ON HEALTH CARE POLICY

The increase of the elderly population globally and, in particular in the United States, has resulted in a shrinking percentage of persons younger than 65 years. This decrease has significant implications for individuals, families, and governments throughout the world. Maintaining quality health care services for older Americans will become increasingly difficult in 2010 as the baby boomers reach age 65. The tax base previously available for funding health care programs will erode dramatically, given current demographic trends and governmental policy.

The implications are that the Medicare Trust Fund, according to the 1998 annual report of the board of trustees for the Federal Hospital Insurance Trust Fund (i.e., Medicare), will be depleted. The 1998 annual report of the board of trustees for the Social Security Trust Fund determined that it, too, would be depleted of funds by the year 2032.

CHRONIC GERIATRIC PAIN

Rheumatologic diseases are by far the most common medical problem affecting older adults (see Table 31–2), even when broken down among the different disability profiles. An exception is the frail (Type VI), in whom the probability of occurrence matches that of circulatory problems. Many other studies have also verified that the predominant cause of pain in older adults is, by far, musculoskeletal (i.e., rheumatoid arthritis, osteoarthritis); the second most common source of pain is cancer.[3-6] Rheumatologic diseases are, therefore, important to the pain practitioner because these diseases are usually amenable to various treatment modalities.

Approximately 80% of all cancer patients suffer from pain, and cancer is the second leading cause of death in older adults next to heart disease.[5] With respect to cancer pain, the pain specialist can have a major impact on quality-of-life concerns. Diseases of the heart have been treated by sympathetic blocks and, more recently, by neuroaugmentation, both of which increase myocardial blood flow, increase exercise

TABLE 31-1 Projections (in Thousands) of American Elderly Population Stratified by Functional Types and Age (1995, 2010, 2025, and 2045)

	1	2	3	4	5	6	7		
Age	Uninpaired	Healthy	IADI, and Physically Limited	IADI, and Cognitively Impaired	ADL Limited	Frail	Institutionalized	Total Age-Specific Population	Population Increase Since 1995 by a Factor of
1995									
65+	25,229 (76.8%)*	2981 (9.1%)*	425 (1.3%)*	422 (1.3%)*	1086 (3.3%)*	803 (2.4%)*	1887 (5.7%)*	32,834	
85+	1636 (45.0%)*	434 (11.9%)*	86 (2.4%)*	112 (3.1%)*	287 (7.9%)*	226 (6.2%)*	857 (23.6%)*	3639	
95+	111 (32.1%)*	28 (8.0%)*	6 (1.7%)*	9 (2.7%)*	37 (10.7%)*	27 (7.7%)*	129 (37.1%)*	347	
2010									
65+	31,950 (73.0%)*	4043 (9.2%)*	618 (1.4%)*	649 (1.5%)*	1678 (3.8%)*	1268 (2.9%)*	3566 (8.1%)*	43,772	1.3
85+	3612 (42.8%)*	945 (11.2%)*	195 (2.3%)*	258 (3.0%)*	675 (8.0%)*	544 (6.4%)*	2215 (26.2%)*	8444	2.3
95+	489 (31.6%)*	106 (6.8%)*	27 (1.8%)*	40 (2.6%)*	145 (9.4%)*	114 (7.4%)*	624 (40.4%)*	1545	4.5
2025									
65+	48,074 (74.7%)*	5764 (9.0%)*	856 (1.3%)*	878 (1.4%)*	2296 (3.6%)*	1730 (2.7%)*	4750 (7.4%)*	64,347	2.0
85+	4210 (41.4%)*	1081 (10.6%)*	229 (2.3%)*	304 (3.0%)*	825 (8.1%)*	663 (6.5%)*	2848 (28.0%)*	10,161	2.8
95+	856 (32.0%)*	176 (6.6%)*	47 (1.8%)*	69 (2.6%)*	248 (9.3%)*	191 (7.1%)*	1090 (40.7%)*	2677	7.7
2045									
65+	52,180 (71.2%)*	7099 (9.7%)*	1069 (1.5%)*	1152 (1.6%)*	3006 (4.1%)*	2259 (3.1%)*	6565 (9.0%)*	73,330	2.2
85+	6625 (42.6%)*	1715 (11.0%)*	357 (2.3%)*	471 (3.0%)*	1240 (8.0%)*	997 (6.4%)*	4133 (26.6%)*	15,538	4.3
95+	1014 (32.0%)*	211 (6.6%)*	56 (1.8%)*	82 (2.6%)*	293 (9.2%)*	228 (7.2%)*	1287 (40.6%)*	3170	9.1

*Percentage of total number of functional type for the specified age.

IADL, instrumental activities of daily living; ADL, activities of daily living.

TABLE 31–2 Relationship of 29 Medical Conditions to Six Disability Profiles Among Medicare Eligible Adults Aged 65+

	Frequency	1 Unimpaired	2 Healthy	3 IADL and Physically Limited	4 IADL and Cognitively Impaired	5 ADL Limited	6 Frail
Rheumatoid arthritis	72.8	97.8	63.0	98.9	44.2	81.6	65.7
Paralysis*	8.5	4.8	1.3	6.2	0.0	10.5	34.9
Permanent stiffness	23.4	33.8	11.6	50.8	8.7	25.0	33.6
Multiple sclerosis	0.6	0.6	0.1	0.6	0.0	1.4	1.4
Cerebral palsy	0.4	0.0	0.1	0.8	0.3	0.3	1.0
Epilepsy	0.8	0.3	0.5	1.5	0.8	0.1	2.3
Parkinson's disease	2.8	4.1	0.9	0.8	2.9	1.0	9.4
Glaucoma	9.2	7.6	5.4	5.0	26.2	5.7	12.3
Diabetes	16.3	20.1	9.5	24.3	17.6	16.1	23.1
Cancer	6.0	5.4	5.2	6.2	4.9	4.1	11.0
Constipation	30.8	39.4	16.6	58.9	29.3	25.7	44.4
Insomnia	39.3	61.2	25.8	85.0	26.4	29.4	41.6
Headache	16.6	31.4	7.8	51.1	15.2	4.0	17.8
Obesity	23.6	37.2	24.5	40.9	0.2	29.8	11.8
Arteriosclerosis	27.8	33.4	13.5	38.5	42.3	17.5	48.8
Mental retardation	1.4	0.0	0.0	0.0	5.6	0.1	4.9
Dementia	7.8	0.3	0.5	0.0	26.9	0.5	34.1
Heart attack	5.8	7.7	2.2	16.1	6.3	4.3	7.5
Other heart problems	29.3	48.2	17.3	60.2	26.4	20.0	32.8
Hypertension	45.6	61.6	38.0	72.3	30.3	48.3	40.8
Stroke	6.6	4.5	1.4	3.5	6.6	4.2	24.9
Circulation trouble	50.2	74.1	27.8	88.7	38.5	46.8	66.4
Pneumonia	5.8	7.4	2.6	11.0	5.9	3.6	10.8
Bronchitis	13.6	25.3	9.3	34.7	7.7	5.8	13.3
Flu	17.8	31.1	14.4	32.3	12.6	12.1	15.2
Emphysema	9.7	14.3	6.9	19.5	9.5	5.1	11.2
Asthma	7.3	13.9	5.1	22.1	2.7	3.1	5.5
Broken hip	2.1	0.6	0.3	0.0	0.0	7.4	4.8
Other broken bone	5.2	5.2	3.1	8.8	0.0	8.9	7.8
Mean age		73.5	75.2	75.5	84.6	80.2	81.2
Female	65.5	78.1	51.3	100.0	53.4	81.6	57.8

*Conditions in *italic* type cause pain as well as disability.
IADL, instrumental activities of daily living; ADL, activities of daily living.

capacity, and reduce symptoms in intractable angina pectoris.[7–10] Other types of pain found commonly in older adults include herpes zoster; postherpetic neuralgia; temporal arteritis; polymyalgia rheumatica; atherosclerotic and diabetic peripheral vascular disease; cervical spondylosis; trigeminal neuralgia; sympathetic dystrophies; and neuropathies from diabetes mellitus, alcohol abuse, and malnutrition.[11,12] Although much work has been published on cancer pain and acute postoperative pain, much less attention has been given to *chronic, nonmalignant geriatric pain.*

PAIN ASSESSMENT

Pain assessment in older adults is usually more difficult than in the young because it is often complicated by poor health, poor memory, psychologic concerns, depression, denial, and distress. Caution in not attributing new pain complaints to preexisting disease processes is mandatory. Most pain complaints in older adults are of organic, not psychiatric, origin.[13]

The optimal geriatric pain assessment incorporates a multidisciplinary team approach to diagnosis and management.[14,15] The multidisciplinary team is composed of a pain specialist, a psychologist or psychiatrist, and a physical therapist, all performing their own independent evaluations of the patient.

The assessment must include a determination of the patient's functional level. This evaluation is very important because functional limitation affects the patient's degree of independence, quality of life, and subsequent need for caregivers.

Once all members of the multidisciplinary team have evaluated the patient, a consensus treatment plan is developed in conference. This plan should include how to decrease pain perception and how to improve patient functioning.

Cognitively Impaired Patients

Assessing pain in the cognitively impaired is often necessary because up to 15% of the geriatric population have mental process deficiencies and up to 50% of nursing home residents have dementia or psychologic illnesses.[16] Intellectual evaluation can be done using the Mini-Mental Status Questionnaire or the Short Mental Status Questionnaire.[17,18] The cognitively impaired do not respond as quickly to pain assessment questionnaires, but if given a simple, easy-to-read intensity scale, such as the Visual Analogue Scale (VAS) or the Numerical Scale Rating (NSR), they do respond appropriately in self-assessment of current pain level.[19]

Furthermore, in assessing elderly pain patients with possible dementia, one must differentiate between pain as a result of pathophysiologic processes and pain symptoms manifesting in an attempt to mask impaired mental processing. Malingering by an elderly patient is an attempt to divert attention away from the possible need of caregivers or institutionalization, which would greatly affect the person's degree of independence.

Affective Dimension

The affective dimension in elderly chronic pain assessment includes determining the degree of anxiety and depression present. Although studies vary, older people generally have lower anxiety levels than their younger counterparts, whereas depression shows no age difference.[20,21]

Pain assessment also includes determining the patient's coping skills to relieve pain and how effective these skills have been.

Psychometric Tools

There are primarily two types of pain assessment tools: unidimensional, single-item scales or multidimensional measures scales. The former includes the VAS, NSR, the Verbal Descriptor Scale (VDS), and the Pain Thermometer. The multidimensional prototype is the McGill Pain Questionnaire (MPQ).

PATHOPHYSIOLOGY OF AGING

The normal aging process involves the steady decline of organ system function and homeostatic controls. This decline is often first observed during periods of maximum stress and is eventually of such magnitude that even a minor stressor eventually overwhelms the body and results in death. No organ system is immune from the ravages of aging, but some systems are much more resilient than others.

Central Nervous System

Neurologic Changes

Central nervous system (CNS) dysfunction is commonly encountered by the clinician; 93% of the older people who depend on others for their care have some type of neurologic problem.[22] Among the disabled, 48% have neurologic disease. Neurologic dysfunction has significant implications for the pain practitioner because pain assessment and efficacy of treatment modalities can be very difficult.

In general, the CNS and peripheral nervous system (PNS) in otherwise healthy people begin to deteriorate as early as 50 years of age, although in many individuals this process does not occur until they are in their 70 or 80s.[23] The precise mechanisms causing this deterioration are unknown, but clearly heredity, concomitant disease, and physical and mental daily activities are important factors in determining the onset of this decline.[24]

Cognitive Function

Many neurologic diseases have a negative effect on cognitive function in older adults. These include:

- *Dementia:* a generalized limitation of cognitive function that is usually progressive but not associated with depressed level of consciousness[25]
- *Alzheimer's disease:* affects aging populations equally and is a slowly progressive disorder of unknown cause that does not have pathognomonic clinical findings
- *Parkinson's disease:* another common ailment of older adults that does not affect cognitive function

Hepatic System

The liver is the major organ system responsible for clearance of drugs from the blood. The aging liver prolongs the clearance of drugs from the blood because of prehepatic, intrahepatic, or posthepatic causes:

- Prehepatic dysfunction includes decreased first-pass and blood extraction, which can be due to decreased gastrointestinal (GI) absorption or decreased portal and arterial blood flow to the liver.
- Intrahepatic dysfunction results from hepatocellular pathologic conditions (i.e., cirrhosis).
- Posthepatic dysfunction is due to either biliary tree or enterohepatic circulation pathologic conditions.

Renal System

The normal aging process includes a decline in renal function. In general, numerous age-related changes in kidney structure and function have been described, but clinical tests suggest that kidney function is well maintained in the "normal" older adult.[26]

TREATMENT MODALITIES

Treatment options for the elderly pain patient include:

- Pharmacotherapy
- Interventional pain management
- Psychologic modalities
- Physical rehabilitation

By far the most commonly employed modality for geriatric pain control is pharmacotherapy.

Drug Therapy

There is scant evidence that pharmacotherapy is the best treatment option; others have considered the multidisciplinary approach to geriatric pain to be the most effective.[14,15] Nonetheless, the first treatment modality usually employed to control geriatric pain is pharmacotherapy.

Pharmacotherapy is relatively simple to implement, and most practitioners are comfortable and have experience in prescribing nonsteroidal anti-inflammatory drugs (NSAIDs), muscle relaxants, and opioids. Unfortunately, too often this option is implemented even though the cause of the pain syndrome has not been elucidated. This results in a "shotgun" approach to prescribing systemic medications, which can then lead to the development of untoward side effects that affect the patient's cognitive, physiologic, and functional status.

In 1998, in an attempt to redress this and other problems in treating these pain patients, the American Geriatric Society (AGS) presented the following guidelines[27,28]:

1. Pain should be an important part of each assessment of older patients; along with efforts to alleviate the underlying cause, pain should be aggressively treated.
2. Pain and its response to treatment should be objectively measured, preferably by a validated pain scale.
3. NSAIDs should be used with caution. In older patients, NSAIDs have significant side effects and are the most common cause of adverse drug reactions.

4. Acetaminophen is the drug of choice for relieving mild to moderate musculoskeletal pain.
5. Opioid analgesic drugs are effective for relieving moderate to severe pain.
6. Nonopioid analgesic medications may be appropriate for some patients with neuropathic pain and other chronic pain syndromes.
7. Nonpharmacologic approaches used alone or in combination with appropriate pharmacologic strategies should be an integral part of care in most cases.
8. Referral to a multidisciplinary pain management center should be considered when pain management efforts do not meet the patient's or the health care provider's goals.
9. Regulatory agencies should review existing policies to enhance access to effective opioid analgesic drugs for older patients in pain.
10. Pain management education should be improved at all levels for all health care professionals

Assuming that the patient in pain is not terminally ill, there is a significant overlap with the many geriatric pain complaints (and pain syndromes) and those of cancer pain patients. In realizing this frequent overlap, it is instructive to follow the World Health Organization (WHO) approach to drug therapy[29]:

- By mouth
- By the clock
- For the individual
- With attention to detail
- By the ladder

The guiding principle of the "analgesic ladder" is that analgesics are selected according to severity of pain. Therefore, the WHO recommends the following:

1. For mild pain, the relatively safe analgesic acetaminophen is an appropriate first choice.
2. For mild to moderate pain or pain uncontrolled with acetaminophen, the application of NSAIDs is appropriate.
3. For pain conditions refractory to NSAID treatment or rated as moderate at outset, a weaker opioid is an appropriate first choice. Other weaker opioids include hydrocodone, propoxyphene, and oxycodone in combination with acetaminophen.
4. For pain refractory to these weaker opioids or for pain initially rated as severe at outset, a pure opioid agonist is selected. Other drugs in this class include hydromorphone, fentanyl, levorphanol, and oxycodone.

Pharmacokinetic and Pharmacodynamic Changes

Many treatment modalities exist for effective geriatric pain control; however, pharmacotherapy remains the mainstay for pain control in older adults. Therefore, it is important to elaborate on those factors that affect the pharmacokinetics and pharmacodynamics of aging.

Pharmacokinetics

Pharmacokinetic principles determine the relationship between dose of drug administered and the concentration of the drug at the receptor site. Pharmacokinetic processes change with aging, especially with respect to the elimination, clearance, and distribution of drugs.

Pharmacodynamics

Pharmacodynamic principles describe the responsiveness of cell receptors at the effector site. They involve clinically observing the patient's response to various plasma concentrations of drug, assuming equilibrium of drug has been established at the receptor site.

Patient Compliance with Medications

The rate of compliance with long-term medication regimens is approximately 50% across most age groups.[30,31] Many reasons have been cited for this low rate, but the major factor predicting compliance is simply the total number of different medications taken; the more medications, the worse the compliance.[31,32]

Modifications to the WHO Recommendations

Because of the tremendous heterogeneity of the elderly population with their varied individual responses to medications and coexisting diseases, the graded use of analgesics must be tailored to each individual. As a result of changing pharmacokinetic, pharmacodynamic, and coexisting diseases in the elderly, the likelihood of adverse drug reactions and toxicity is significantly increased.[33] Along each step on the analgesic ladder the risk-to-benefit ratio must be assessed; for this reason, the newly developed cyclooxygenase-2 (COX-2) inhibitors should be given before either NSAIDs or opioids. Furthermore, if weak opioids are not efficacious in attenuating pain intensity, an analysis of the risk-to-benefit ratio would recommend that therapeutic nerve blocks or low-risk neuroablative pain procedures should be employed before strong opioids.

Acetaminophen

Acetaminophen is an effective, safe analgesic for older patients.

COX-2 Inhibitors

COX-2 inhibitors work by inhibiting an enzyme (COX-2) that is responsible for producing pain and inflammation without affecting cyclooxygenase-1 (COX-1), an enzyme that primarily protects the stomach lining. The inhibition of COX-1 is believed to be the cause of serious GI side effects. These side effects have been associated with the use of NSAIDs, which inhibit COX-1 and COX-2 enzymes.

NSAID Therapy

NSAIDs are currently the most commonly prescribed medications (18%) in older adults for chronic pain complaints and have reportedly resulted in more than 76,000 hospitalizations and 7600 deaths each year in the United States.[33,35] The incidence of these side effects is even higher in older adults, who are already predisposed to GI ulceration by virtue of age alone.[34] NSAIDs can also cause renal and hepatic failure, especially in those older adults who already have marginal renal or hepatic function.[36]

Other common side effects are platelet dysfunction and, possibly, bleeding diathesis. The effect on platelets is irreversible with aspirin but reversible with other NSAIDs.

Not all NSAIDs have the same side-effect profiles, and there is large individual variation in the minimal effective dose, toxic dose, and ceiling dose for each NSAID. Therefore, if an intolerable side effect develops with the use of a particular NSAID, an alternative NSAID should be considered.

The rules for NSAID use are as follows:

1. Select the NSAID according to the needs of the patient.
2. Administer with food (but not COX-2 inhibitors).
3. Give on a time-contingent basis (once a lack of side effects is shown).
4. Give in the lowest effective initial dose (i.e., a 25% to 50% decrease from adult dose).
5. Give with a slower escalation of drug until maximum ceiling dose or side effects are reached.
6. Frequently monitor the patient for side effects.
7. Give with the antiulcer drug misoprostol.

Opioid Therapy

Once again, the risk-to-benefit ratio of using a particular opioid must be assessed for each individual at each point along the pain treatment continuum.

In general, the drug therapy guidelines already advocated for NSAIDs should be applied to opioids with the following modifications:

1. Select the opioid according to the needs of the patient.
2. Use the lowest effective initial dose (i.e., a 25% to 50% decrease in the adult dose).
3. Initially use an opioid with a short half-life.
4. Give on a time-contingent basis (once a lack of side effects is shown).
5. Frequently monitor the patient for side effects, especially during the first six half-lives.
6. Give with a slower escalation of drug.
7. Increase the dose until either uncontrollable side effects are obtained or they are not efficacious. There is no maximum "ceiling dose" reached with opioids, as with NSAIDs.
8. Give with a stool softener.

When opioid therapy is first begun, it is desirable to use drugs with short half-lives, while a therapeutic blood level of drug is being obtained. Consequently, drugs such as hydromorphone and oxycodone, which have minimal active metabolites and relatively short half-lives (i.e., 2 to 3 hours), are more desirable than drugs with variable half-lives, such as methadone (i.e., half-life of 12 to 190 hours) or meperidine with its accumulation of metabolites toxic to kidneys and the CNS.[37]

Once effective pain control with minimal side effects has been established with a short-acting opioid, it is reasonable to employ controlled-release formulations of the opioid. Controlled-release morphine is often the first opioid employed for chronic pain control, but concern about the accumulation of its active metabolites, which have been implicated to cause hyperalgesia, allodynia, myoclonus, and cognitive changes, may limit its use with older adults.[38–40] Conversely, other commercially available long-acting opioid formulations generate metabolites with minimal side effects

along with minimal differences in pharmacokinetics between the young and old (i.e., formulation involving oxycodone and, most recently, hydromorphone).[14,41–44]

Adjuvant Drug Therapy

In general, adjuvant drugs[45]:

- Are used at all stages of the analgesic ladder
- Enhance the analgesic efficacy of opioids
- Treat concurrent symptoms that exacerbate pain
- Provide independent analgesia for specific types of pain

Adjuvant drugs for geriatric management[45,46] span the entire spectrum of drug types and include (but are not limited to):

- Muscle relaxants
- Corticosteroids
- Anticonvulsants
- Antidepressants
- Neuroleptics
- Antihistamines
- Local anesthetics
- Antiarrhythmics
- α_2-Adrenergic agonists
- Psychostimulants
- Calcitonin
- Capsaicin

Interventional Pain Management

Nerve Blocks

Diagnostic nerve blocks not only can help determine the origin of the pain process but also offer the patient a chance to experience what a longer-lasting, neurolytic or neurosurgical procedure would be like. In general, nerve blocks offer the following advantages:

- Diagnostic: aid in determining the etiology of pain
- Prognostic: aid in predicting the outcome of permanent interventions or neuroablative techniques
- Preemptive: aid in preventing painful sequelae of procedures that may cause phantom limb or causalgia
- Therapeutic: aid in treating painful conditions that respond to nerve blocks, as in sympathetically maintained pain

Anatomic Approach for the Diagnostic Nerve Block

Before diagnostic nerve block, the anatomic site of the pain must be grossly localized. In this approach, after injection of a placebo, the sympathetic, sensory, and motor fibers are blocked sequentially; this requires that local anesthetic be injected at points where each injection blocks a specific nerve fiber type. The anatomic approach in determining the etiology of pain varies from the pharmacologic approach, wherein a differential spinal or epidural is performed.[47] The pharmacologic approach is based on the fact that different-sized myelinated nerve fibers are blocked at different concentrations of local anesthetic.[48] The advantage of the anatomic approach is that it can be applied to any anatomic region of the body, whereas a differential epidural-spinal injection can be applied only to painful conditions involving the abdomen, pelvis, or legs.

Visceral pain of the thorax, abdomen, and pelvis is nociceptive, and afferent C fibers travel with the efferent sympathetic C fibers.[49] To rule in this type of pain in the thorax, a dilute thoracic epidural block is employed; for the abdomen, either a celiac plexus block or a splanchnic nerve block is used.[47,50,51] Visceral pain in the pelvis is ruled in by applying a superior hypogastric nerve block.[52] Interpretation of the results of a diagnostic nerve block is as follows:

- If application of a sympathetic or visceral nerve block does not result in pain relief, a somatic nerve block at either the nerve root level or more distally in a nerve plexus or peripheral nerve is needed.[50]
- If the patient receives pain relief from a sympathetic, visceral, or somatic nerve block, longer-lasting pain relief can be obtained with additional nerve blocks using local anesthetic and steroids, neuroablative techniques, chemical neurolysis, or neurosurgery.
- If the patient receives no pain relief from any of these procedures, the origin of pain is central, self-sustaining encephalization or psychogenic or malingering is present.[47,50]
- For painful states that are not psychogenic but central in origin or that have not responded to these treatment modalities, either neuroaugmentation or neuroaxial delivery of medications can be tried.

Chemical Neurolysis

Chemical neurolysis is employed as an adjuvant treatment in providing longer lasting pain relief to the geriatric patient. It works by destroying the nerves that are in contact with the neurolytic solution. It is often used in patients with terminal cancer or certain neuralgias or when neurolysis by other modalities cannot be readily performed.

Radiofrequency Lesioning

Radiofrequency lesioning (radiofrequency thermocoagulation [RFTC]) is a relatively new technique that has enjoyed tremendous success in interventional pain management.[53,54] Like cryoneurolysis, this technique can selectively destroy tissue, thereby removing the pain-generating source. This technique is very attractive in geriatric pain control because it is safe, simple, and effective to use, especially since the introduction of RFTC needles.

The simplicity of RFTC is manifested in the radiofrequency circuit needed for lesioning. This circuit is composed of three basic components: (1) an active RFTC needle electrode fluoroscopically placed at the pain generator site, (2) a dispersing electrode placed some distance away from the active electrode, and (3) a radiofrequency generator source to which the two electrodes are connected. Confirmation of proper needle-tip position of the electrode on the pain-generating site is accomplished grossly by injection of contrast dye through the hollow electrode and, more precisely, by electrical sensory stimulation of the neural tissue to be lesioned. The operator then begins the procedure by applying a 1-MHz frequency to the active electrode tip, which in turn generates an electromagnetic field around the active electrode tip.[53] This alternating electromagnetic field then generates frictional heat in the immediate surrounding tissue, which is conducted back to the electrode tip, where a thermistor then records the temperature.[54]

Lesioning temperatures in excess of 45°C in the brain can cause permanent neural damage, whereas typical peripheral nerve lesioning uses temperatures of 80°C.[55] Factors that affect lesion size include active needle electrode tip size, duration of lesioning, and temperature attained. The time dependence on lesion size is easily eliminated by obtaining thermal equilibrium at the electrode tip with the surrounding tissue; this occurs within 60 seconds.[53] The temperature generated in the tissue is a complex function of impedance, voltage, amperage, frequency, and current density. The radiofrequency operator usually attains a temperature of 80°C by manipulating the voltage on the radiofrequency generator.[53,56]

Cryoanalgesia

Cryoanalgesia is a relatively new technique that allows the pain practitioner to use low temperatures to generate pain relief. Application of this technique is attractive in the older adults because it is relatively simple, safe, and effective with minimal complications compared with other invasive techniques.

This technique is best suited for small, localized lesions, such as neuromas, or entrapment neuropathies of peripheral nerves. Cryolesioning must be preceded by a series of diagnostic nerve blocks using local anesthetics. If good analgesia is subsequently obtained, cyrodenervation may follow. Common indications for cyrolesioning include painful neuromas; intercostal neuralgia; biomechanical pain from facet arthropathy; and ilioinguinal, genitofemoral, and iliohypogastric neuropathy.[57]

Neuroaugmentation

Spinal cord stimulation (SCS) is yet another invasive technique that has enjoyed success in controlling many pain syndromes (Table 31–3).[58,59] SCS is achieved by electrical stimulation of the dorsal columns of the spinal column via electrodes placed percutaneously in the epidural space, which are then attached to a pulse generator.

Proper patient selection for a SCS trial is crucial for good outcomes in older adults. Guidelines for implantation of SCS have been developed by the Health Care and Finance Administration[60] and include:

TABLE 31–3 Indications for Spinal Cord Stimulation

Failed back surgery syndrome
Arachnoiditis
Sympathetically maintain pain
CRPS I
CRPS II
Neuropathic pain syndromes
Radiculopathies
Phantom limb pain
Postherpetic neuralgia
Peripheral neuropathies
Nerve root avulsions
Plexopathies
Cervical
Brachial
Lumbosacral
Spinal cord injury
Angina
Peripheral vascular insufficiency

CRPS, complex regional pain syndrome.

- Patients with chronic, intractable pain
- Failure of other treatment modalities, specifically,
  (1) pharmacotherapy, (2) physical therapy,
  (3) psychologic counseling, and (4) surgery
- Patients who have undergone careful screening and
  diagnosis by a multidisciplinary team
- Ability of the patient or caregiver to properly operate,
  maintain, and answer all questions concerning SCS
- Demonstration of pain relief with a temporarily placed
  SCS electrode
- Patients with demonstrated pathologic conditions
- Patients with no evidence of drug or alcohol addiction

Neuraxial Drug-Delivery Systems

The neuraxial delivery of medication to either the epidural or subarachnoid space is yet another invasive technique that can be used in pain control. Again, patient selection is very important to ensure a successful outcome with this treatment modality in older adults, and age per se is not a contraindication. The selection criteria to consider for this delivery of medications include all the guidelines and contraindications mentioned earlier for implementation of SCS in addition to the following guidelines[59,61,62]:

- Persistence of intractable pain despite aggressive
  administration of systemic opioids and adjuvant drug
  therapy
- Development of intolerable side effects from
  systemically administered opioids that are not
  correctable by ordinary treatment
- Ability of the patient or caregiver (or support system) to
  operate and maintain the delivery system
- Pain syndromes that are not amenable to an SCS trial
  (nociceptive or central neuropathic pain)
- A successful trial of epidurally or intrathecally
  administered medication

The Cognitive-Behavioral Model

The cognitive-behavioral perspective to pain management maintains that pain must be viewed as a complex sensory and emotional experience and not simply viewed in the biomedical model.[63,64] The biomedical model explains pain in a mechanistic approach to the human body in which injured tissue or disease results in painful nociceptive input to the brain.[65] Indeed, the biomedical model fails to explain why some individuals with extensive disease have minimal pain complaints, whereas others with only minimal tissue damage have extensive complaints of pain. This model also fails to explain why patients in pain continue to have persistent pain despite aggressive pharmacotherapy and interventional pain management techniques.

Figure 31–1 illustrates the cognitive-behavioral perspective on pain complaints as applied to chronic geriatric patients.[66] Clearly, many factors contribute to the subjective experience of pain, and this experience of pain is manifested by the patient as verbal descriptors and certain types of pain behavior.

Cognitive-behavioral interventions use cognitive therapy and behavioral therapy in treating geriatric pain patients. Although this technique is equally efficacious in all age groups, individuals with severe depression or major cognitive dysfunction are poor candidates for this modality.[67]

Patients who are screened for this treatment modality are taught a variety of skills that include:

- Relaxation training
- Activity pacing
- Distraction techniques
- Calming self-statements (cognitive restructuring)
- Meditation[66,68]

Relaxation

Relaxation training may help by allowing patients with chronic pain to break the vicious circle between pain and those factors worsening pain: stress, muscular tension, and emotional upheaval.[69–71] The progressive muscle relaxation technique or biofeedback can be employed to teach relaxation techniques.[66,72–74] Both of these techniques must be individually tailored to the patient to maximize the benefit. Two other popular and effective relaxation strategies are music and humor.

Activity-Rest Cycle

Activity-rest cycling is helpful for patients who are either overdoers or underdoers.[66] Overdoers tend to overdo physical activity when they have mild to moderate pain, which in turn results in extended periods of excessive pain with minimal activity. Underdoers associate all types of physical activity with pain and are therefore apt to be sedentary. This technique can help both groups by breaking the cycle of pain with activity. It accomplishes this by making activity level a function of time and not dependent on pain-free episodes.

Attention-Diversion Technique

Attention-diversion strategies may help patients in that they divert attention away from pain and refocus their thoughts on something else. The less time people spend focusing on their pain, the less likely they will feel it.[64,75] Attention-diversion strategies are taught by using one of the following techniques[66,76]:

1. Pleasant imagery involves contemplating a pleasant
   scene in lieu of negative thoughts.
2. Focal point distraction involves focusing attention on
   events, tasks, or objects in the immediate vicinity of the
   patient.
3. The counting method technique involves first employing
   relaxation techniques, then counting back from 100.

Cognitive Restructuring

Cognitive restructuring techniques allow patients to decrease pain by helping them to identify and subsequently correct distorted conceptualizations.[77] For many older pain patients, negative thoughts can begin to feel realistic and cause a worsening of anxiety and depression, which then result in more pain.[78] Cognitive restructuring techniques teach patients to[66]:

- Identify negative, automatic thought processes
- Realize the relationship among thoughts, feelings,
  behaviors, and pain
- Judge the evidence for and against negative thought
  processes
- Formulate a more realistic interpretation of the pain
  experience

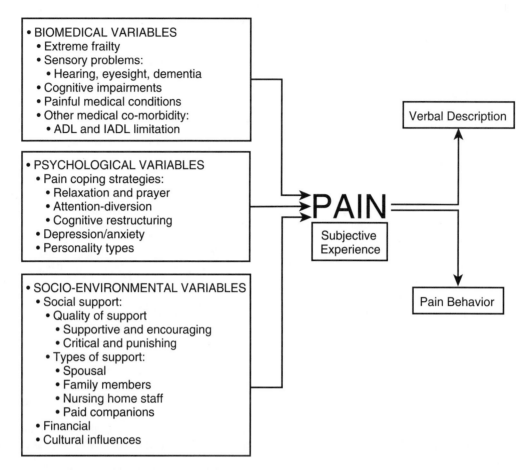

FIG. 31–1 Cognitive-behavioral model for chronic geriatric pain patients. ADL, activities of daily living; IADL, instrumental activities of daily living. *(Modified from Keefe FJ, Beaupre PM, Weiner DK: Pain in older adults: a cognitive-behavioral perspective. In Ferrell B, Ferrell B, editors:* Pain in the elderly. *Seattle, IASP Press, 1996).*

Meditation

Meditation or prayer incorporates many of the aforementioned coping strategies.

Physical Therapy and Rehabilitation

Rehabilitation is an important treatment modality for the older patient in pain. By decreasing pain and improving function, rehabilitation allows the patient to live a more independent life with enhanced dignity. Rehabilitation among chronic geriatric pain patients involves adapting, in an optimal way, to the loss of physical, psychologic, or social skills they once possessed before complaints of chronic pain.

The rehabilitation process of the chronic pain patient proceeds in an orderly fashion with the following objectives[79]:

- Stabilize the primary disorder whenever possible
- Prevent secondary disabilities whenever possible
- Decrease pain perception by employing a multidisciplinary approach
- Treat functional deficits
- Promote adaptation between the person and the disability, the environment and the person, and the family and the person

The Rehabilitation Team

Rehabilitation requires a multidisciplinary approach in assessing and treating the geriatric chronic pain patient.

Potentially Helpful Nondrug Treatment Modalities

Each geriatric chronic pain patient has a unique set of impairments and, most likely, disabilities requiring an individually tailored treatment plan. The physical therapy treatment plan can span the entire spectrum of activities, including different types of exercise programs and a multitude of various assistive aid devices. The services and equipment can be obtained at physician offices, home, a certified outpatient rehabilitation facility, and various types of outpatient settings.

Proposed Pain Treatment Continuum

An enhanced pain treatment continuum is proposed in Box 31–1, which builds on the previous discussions (including pharmacotherapy, interventional pain management, cognitive-behavioral therapy, and rehabilitation) and employs the guidelines recently developed by the American Geriatric Society. The graded approach outlined in Box 31-1 reflects the gradual decline in end-organ function and

---

BOX 31–1 Proposed Pain Treatment Algorithm for the Chronic Geriatric Pain Patient

---

Initial Primary Care Contact and W/U
- Tentative pain syndrome Dx
- Acetaminophen a.t.c.
- Rx COX-2 inhibitors and adjuvants a.t.c.

Referral to Multidisciplinary Pain Clinic
Detailed H & P, Lab, Imaging W/U with Tentative Dx
1. *Diagnostic nerve block if needed*
2. *Rx COX-2 inhibitors and adjuvants a.t.c.*
3. *Rx NSAIDs and misoprostol a.t.c.*
   a. With caution and short term, if possible
4. *Cognitive and behavioral therapies**
   a. *Relaxation training and biofeedback*
   b. *Activity-diversion, cognitive restructuring*
5. *Physical and/or rehabilitation therapies**
   a. *Programmed exercises and assistive aid devices*
   b. *Heat, cold, massage therapy, or TENS therapy*
6. *Weak opioids and adjuvants a.t.c.*
7. *Myoneural injections with L.A. and steroids*
   a. *Later with botulinum toxin (Botox) injections*
8. *Low-risk, therapeutic nerve blocks with L.A. and steroids*
   a. Peripheral nerve and plexus blocks
      (1) Occipital, intercostal, lateral femoral, ilioinguinal, and so on
      (2) Cervical, brachial, lumbar-sacral plexus

   b. Sympathetic ganglia: stellate and lumbar
   c. Epidural steroid injection
      (1) Lysis of epidural adhesions/caudal neuroplasty
   d. Joint injections with L.A. and steroids
      (1) Facets: cervical, thoracic, lumbar
      (2) Sacroiliac and joint capsules
   e. Later with low-risk, neuroablative procedures using cryoneurolysis or RFTC
9. *Correctable surgery if possible*
10. *Strong opioids and adjuvants a.t.c.*
    a. Oral route first; other routes as needed
11. *Medium-risk, therapeutic nerve blocks with L.A. and steroid*
    a. Sphenopalatine ganglia and trigeminal ganglia
    b. Splanchnic/celiac plexus and hypogastric plexus
    c. Dorsal root ganglionotomy
    d. Later with medium-risk, neuroablative procedures using cryoneurolysis or RFTC
12. *Neuroaugmentation*
    a. Both SCS and PNS
13. *Neuraxial medication*
    a. Both epidural and intrathecal systems
14. *Chemical neurolysis*

Major Neurosurgical Neuroablative Procedures
- *Cordotomy, DREZ lesioning, thalamic stimulation, and so on*

---

*Note: Cognitive, behavioral, and rehabilitative therapies should, ideally, be administered concurrently with other treatment modalities, such as pharmacotherapy and interventional pain management.

Rx, prescribed; Dx, diagnosis; TENS, transcutaneous electrical nerve stimulation; NSAID, nonsteroidal anti-inflammatory drugs; DREZ, dorsal root entry zone; a.t.c., around the clock; RFTC, radiofrequency thermocoagulation; COX, cyclooxygenase; W/U, work-up; L.A., local anesthetic; SCS, spinal cord stimulation; PNS, peripheral nerve stimulation; H & P, History and Physical.

---

homeostatic controls that affect older adults. The schema adheres to the maxim of "keep it safe and simple" in which seemingly innocent around-the-clock medications (i.e., NSAIDs) or invasive pain procedures can have a profound impact on patient well-being. Inherent in this schema is a graded safety profile for the analgesics used in chronic geriatric pain; acetaminophen and COX-2 inhibitors are recommended before NSAIDs and opioids are.

The proposed pain treatment continuum (see Box 31–1) attempts to optimize the risk-to-benefit ratio at each step along the continuum, with special attention to the nuances applicable in the elderly population. For example, the pain treatment continuum recommends that COX-2 inhibitors be given before either NSAIDs or opioids because these are inherently safer drugs with similar analgesic properties to NSAIDs. NSAIDs and opioids should be given at the appropriate time sequence, as outlined in the continuum. Furthermore, if weak opioids are not efficacious in attenuating pain intensity, therapeutic nerve blocks or low-risk neuroablative pain procedures should be employed before strong opioids are recommended.

References

1. International Association of the Study of Pain, Subcommittee on Taxonomy: Classification of chronic pain: Descriptions of chronic pain syndromes and definitions of pain terms. *Pain* 3(suppl):S1, 1986.
2. Manton KG: Chronic morbidity and disability in the U.S. elderly populations. In Mostofky DI, Lomranz J, editors: *Handbook of pain and aging.* New York, Plenum Press, 1997.
3. Schick FL, Schick R: Growth of the older population, actual and projected: 1900 to 2050, Table A1-9. In *Statistical handbook on aging Americans.* Phoenix, Ariz, Oryx Press, 1994.
4. Davis MA: Epidemiology of osteoarthritis. *Clin Geriatr Med* 4:241, 1988.
5. Foley K: Pain in the elderly. In Hazzard WR, Bierman EL, Blass JP, editors: *Principles of geriatric medicine and gerontology.* New York, McGraw-Hill, 1994.
6. Ling SM, Bathon JM: Osteoarthritis in older adults. *J Am Geriatr Soc* 46:216, 1998.
7. Mobilia G, Zuin G, Zanco P et al: Effects of spinal cord stimulation on regional myocardial blood flow in patients with refractory angina: A positron emission tomography study. *G Ital Cardiol* 28:1113, 1998.
8. Oosterga M, ten Vaarwerk IA, DeJongste MJ et al: Spinal cord stimulation in refractory angina pectoris: Clinical results and mechanisms. *Z Kardiol* 86(suppl 1):107, 1997.
9. DeJongste MJ, Tenvaarwerk IA, Jessurun GA et al: Efficacy of spinal cord stimulation as adjuvant therapy for intractable angina pectoris: A prospective, randomized clinical study. Working Group on Neurocardiology. *J Am Coll Cardiol* 23:1592, 1994.
10. Hautvast RW, DeJongste MJ, Staal MJ et al: Spinal cord stimulation in chronic intractable angina pectoris: A randomized, controlled efficacy study. *Am Heart J* 136:1114, 1998.
11. Gordon RS: Pain in the elderly: Patterns change with age. *JAMA* 241:2191, 1979.
12. Hewitt DJ, Foley KM: Pain and pain management. In Cassell CK, Cohen HJ, Larson EB, editors: *Geriatric medicine,* ed 3. New York, Springer-Verlag, 1997.

13. Sorkin BA, Rudy TE, Hanlon RB et al: Chronic pain in old and young patients: Differences appear less important than similarities. *J Gerontol* 45:P64, 1990.

14. Melzack R, Wall PD: *The challenge of pain.* London, Penguin Books, 1996.

15. Gibson SJ, Farrell MJ, Katz B: Multidisciplinary management of chronic nonmalignant pain in order adults. In Ferrell BR, Ferrell BA: *Pain in the elderly.* Seattle, IASP Press, 1996.

16. Ferrell B: Overview of aging and pain. In Ferrell BR, Ferrell BA: *Pain in the elderly.* Seattle, IASP Press, 1996.

17. Foltstein MF, Foltstein SE, McHush PR: Mini-Mental State: A practical method of grading the cognitive state of patients for the clinician. *J Psychiatr Res* 12:189, 1975.

18. Pfieffer E: A short portable mental status questionnaire for the assessment of organic brain deficit in elderly patients. *J Am Geriatr Soc* 23:433, 1975.

19. Ferrell BA, Ferrell BR, Rivera L: Pain in cognitively impaired nursing home patients. *J Pain Symptom Manage* 10:591, 1995.

20. McCracken LM, Gross RT: Does anxiety affect coping with chronic pain? *Clin J Pain* 9:253, 1993.

21. Herr KA, Mobily PR, Smith C: Depression and the experiences of chronic back pain: A study of related variables and age differences. *Clin J Pain* 9:104, 1993.

22. Broe GA: The neuroepidemiology of old age. In Tallis R, editor: *The clinical neurology of old age.* Chichester, United Kingdom, Wiley, 1989.

23. Hickey R, Sloan TB: Physiological changes with aging in the central nervous system. In Smith RB, Gurkowski MA, Bracken CA et al, editors: *Anesthesia and pain control in the geriatric patient.* New York, McGraw-Hill, 1995.

24. Samorajski T: How the human brain responds to aging. *J Am Geriatr Soc* 24:4, 1976.

25. Simon RP, Aminoff JJ, Greenberg DA: *Clinical neurology.* Norwalk, Conn, Appleton & Lange, 1989.

26. Beck LH: Changes in renal function with aging. *Clin Geriatr Med* 14:199, 1998.

27. AGS Panel on Chronic Pain in Older Persons: The management of chronic pain in older persons. *Geriatrics* 53(suppl 3):S8, 1998.

28. AGS Panel on Chronic Pain in Older Persons: The management of chronic pain in older persons. *J Am Geriatr Soc* 46:635, 1998.

29. World Health Organization (WHO): *Cancer pain relief and palliative care: Report of a WHO expert committee.* Geneva, WHO 1990.

30. Sackett DL, Snow JC: The magnitude of compliance and noncompliance. In Haynes RB, Taylor DW, Sackett DL, editors: *Compliance in health care.* Baltimore, The Johns Hopkins University Press, 1979.

31. Darnell JC, Murray MD, Martz BL et al: Medication use by ambulatory elderly: An in-home survey. *J Am Geriatr Soc* 34:1, 1986.

32. German PS, Klein LE, McPhee SJ et al: Knowledge of and compliance with drug regimens in the elderly. *J Am Geriatr Soc* 30:568, 1982.

33. Cooner E, Amorosi S: *The study of pain and older Americans.* New York, Louis Harris and Associates, 1997.

34. Hurwitz N: Predisposing factors in adverse reactions to drugs. *Br Med J* 1:536, 1969.

35. Fries JF: NSAID gastropathy: The second most deadly rheumatic disease? Epidemiology and risk appraisal. *J Rheumatol Suppl* 28:6, 1991.

36. Sunshipne A, Olson NA: Non-narcotic analgesics. In Wall PD, Melzack R, editors: *Textbook of pain,* ed 2. New York, Churchill Livingstone, 1989.

37. Portenoy RK: Opioid analgesics. In Portenoy RK, Danner RM, editors: *Pain management: Theory and practice.* Philadelphia, FA Davis, 1996.

38. Sjogren P, Thunedborg LP, Christrup L et al: Is development of hyperalgesia, allodynia and myoclonus related to morphine metabolism during long-term administration? Six case histories. *Acta Anaesthesiol Scand* 42:1070, 1998.

39. Sjogren P, Jensen NH, Jensen TS: Disappearance of morphine-induced hyperalgesia after discontinuing or substituting morphine with other opioid agonists. *Pain* 59:313, 1994.

40. Tisco PJ: Morphine-6-glucuronide concentrations and opioid-related side effects: A survey in cancer patients. *Pain* 61:47, 1995.

41. Ishida T, Oguri K, Yoshimura H: Determination of oxycodone metabolites in urines and feces of several mammalian species. *J Pharmacobiodyn* 5:521, 1982.

42. Bruera E, Sloan P, Mount B et al: A randomized, double-blind double-dummy, crossover trial comparing the safety and efficacy of oral sustained-release hydromorphone with immediate-release hydromorphone in patients with cancer pain: Canadian Palliative Care Clinical Trials Group. *J Clin Oncol* 14:1713, 1996.

43. Hagen NA, Babul N: Comparative clinical efficacy and safety of a novel controlled-release oxycodone formulation and controlled-release hydromorphone in the treatment of cancer pain. *Cancer* 79:1428, 1997.

44. Kaiko RF, Benziger DP, Fitzmartin RD et al: Pharmacokinetic-pharmacodynamic relationships of controlled-release oxycodone. *Clin Pharmacol Ther* 59:52, 1996.

45. Jacox A, Carr DB, Payne R: *Management of cancer pain: Clinical practice guideline no. 9.* AHCPR Publication No. 94-0592. Rockville, Md, Agency for Health Care Policy and Research. U.S. Department of Health and Human Services, Public Health Service, 1994.

46. Popp B, Portenoy R: Management of chronic pain in the elderly: Pharmacology of opioids and other analgesic drugs. In Ferrell BR, Ferrell BA: *Pain in the elderly.* Seattle, IASP Press, 1996.

47. Winnie A: Differential neural blockade for the diagnosis of pain mechanisms. In Waldman S, Winnie A, editors: *Interventional pain management.* London, WB Saunders, 1996.

48. Strichartz GR: Neural physiology and local anesthetic action. In Cousins MJ, Bridenbaugh PO, editors: *Neural blockade in clinical anesthesia and management of pain,* ed 2. Philadelphia, JB Lippincott, 1988.

49. Raj PP: Prognostic and therapeutic local anesthetic blockade. In Cousins MJ, Bridenbaugh PO, editors: *Neural blockade in clinical anesthesia and management of pain,* ed 2. Philadelphia, JB Lippincott, 1988.

50. Strong WE: Diagnostic neural blockade. In Ramamurthy S, Rogers JN, editors: *Decision making in pain management,* St. Louis, Mosby, 1993.

51. Waldman SD, Patt RB: Celiac plexus and splanchnic nerve block. In Waldman S, Winnie A, editors: *Interventional pain management.* London, WB Saunders, 1996.

52. Patt RB, Plancarte R: Superior hypogastric plexus block: A new therapeutic approach for pelvic pain. In Waldman S, Winnie A, editors: *Interventional pain management.* London, WB Saunders, 1996.

53. Kline MT: Radiofrequency techniques in clinical practice. In Waldman S, Winnie A, editors: *Interventional pain management.* London, WB Saunders, 1996.

54. Noe CE, Racz GB: Radiofrequency. In Raj P, editor: *Pain medicine: A comprehensive review.* St. Louis, Mosby, 1996.

55. Brodkey J, Miyazaki Y, Ervin FR: Reversible heat lesions: A method of stereotactic localization. *J Neurosurg* 21:49, 1964.

56. Kline MT: *Stereotactic frequency lesions as part of the management of pain.* Orlando, Fla, Deutsch Press, 1992.

57. Arthur JM, Racz GB: Cryolysis. In Raj P, editor: *Pain medicine: A comprehensive review.* St. Louis, Mosby, 1996.

58. Bedder MD: Spinal cord stimulation and intractable pain: Patient selection. In Waldman S, Winnie A, editors: *Interventional pain management.* London, WB Saunders, 1996.

59. Padfield NL: Invasive procedures: Technical details. In Dolan S, Pateman JA, editors: *Pain clinic manual.* Oxford, Butterworth-Heinemann, 1996.

60. Health Care and Finance Administration: *Guidelines for spinal cord stimulation implantation.* Washington, DC, 1979.

61. Krames opioids for nonmalignant pain syndromes: A U.S. experience. In Waldman S, Winnie A, editors: *Interventional pain management.* London, WB Saunders, 1996.

62. DuPen SL, Williams A et al: Tunneled epidural catheters: Practical considerations and implantation techniques. In Waldman S, Winnie A, editors: *Interventional pain management.* London, WB Saunders, 1996.

63. Tan SY, Leucht CA: Cognitive-behavioral therapy for clinical pain control: A 15-year update and its relationship to hypnosis. *Int J Clin Exp Hypn* 45:396, 1997.

64. Turk DC, Meichenbaum D, Genest M: *Pain and behavioral medicine: A cognitive-behavioral perspective.* New York, Guilford Press, 1983.

65. Hewa S, Hetherington RS: Specialists without spirit: Limitations of the mechanistic biomedical model. *Theor Med* 16:129, 1995.

66. Keefe FJ, Beaupre PM, Weiner DK: Pain in older adults: A cognitive-behavioral perspective. In Ferrell BR, Ferrell BA, editors: *Pain in the elderly.* Seattle, IASP Press, 1996.

67. Puder RS: Age analysis of cognitive-behavioral group therapy for chronic pain outpatients. *Psychol Aging* 3:204, 1988.

68. Ferrell BR: Patient education and nondrug interventions. In Ferrell BR, Ferrell BA, editors: *Pain in the elderly.* Seattle, IASP Press, 1996.

69. Linton SJ, Melin L, Gotestam KG: Behavioral analysis of chronic pain and its management. *Prog Behav Modif* 18:1, 1984.

70. Schwartz L, Slater MA, Birchler GR: Interpersonal stress and pain behaviors in patients with chronic pain. *J Consult Clin Psychol* 62:861, 1994.

71. Dyrehag LE, Widerstrom-Noga EG, Carlsson SG et al: Relations between self-rated musculoskeletal symptoms and signs and psychological distress in chronic neck and shoulder pain. *Scand J Rehabil Med* 30:235, 1998.

72. Graffam S, Johnson A: A comparison of two relaxation strategies for the relief of pain and its distress. *J Pain Symptom Manage* 2:229, 1987.

73. Flor H, Birbaumer N: Comparison of the efficacy of electromyographic biofeedback, cognitive-behavioral therapy, and conservative medical interventions in the treatment of chronic musculoskeletal pain. *J Consult Clin Psychol* 61:653, 1993.

74. McCaul KD, Malott JM: Distraction and coping with pain. *Psychol Bull* 95:516, 1984.

75. Johnson MH, Petrie SM: The effects of distraction of exercise and cold pressor tolerance for chronic low back pain sufferers. *Pain* 69:43, 1997.

76. Jaffe D, Bresler D: Guided imagery: Healing through the mind's eyes. In Gordon J, Jaffe D, Bresler D, editors: *Mind, body, and health.* New York, Human Sciences Press, 1984.

77. Beck A, Rush AJ, Shaw BS: *Cognitive therapy of depression.* New York, Guilford Press, 1979.

78. Gil KM, Williams DA, Thompson RJ: The relationship of negative thoughts to pain and psychological distress. *Behav Ther* 21:349, 1990.

79. Brummel-Smith K: Rehabilitation. In Cassel CK, Cohen HJ, Larson EB, editors: *Geriatric medicine,* ed 3. New York, Springer-Verlag, 1997.

1. An unpleasant sensory and emotional experience associated with actual or potential tissue damage in patients aged 65 years and older who have had pain for greater than 3 months is termed

   A. Adult chronic pain
   B. Chronic geriatric pain
   C. Chronic psychogenic pan
   D. Chronic neuropathic pain

2. Pain assessment in older adults is usually more difficult than in the young because it is often complicated by all of the following except

   A. Good memory
   B. Poor health
   C. Depression
   D. Denial

3. Many neurologic diseases have a negative effect on the cognitive function in older adults. These included all of the following except

   A. Diabetic neuropathy
   B. Dementia
   C. Alzheimer's disease
   D. Parkinson's disease

4. The rate of compliance with long-term medication regimen is 50%. The reason cited for this low rate of compliance is due to

   A. Increasing age
   B. Psychopathology of the patient
   C. Increased number of different medications taken
   D. Increased cost

5. The value of adjuvant drug therapy is all of the following except

   A. Enhance the analgesic efficacy of opioids
   B. Do not treat concurrent symptoms that exacerbate pain
   C. Provide independent analgesia
   D. Are used in all stages of the analgesic ladder

ANSWERS

1. B

2. A

3. A

4. C

5. B

CHAPTER 32

Quality Assurance and Improvement in Pain Practice

MARSHALL BEDDER

The topics of quality assurance and quality improvement in pain medicine encompass multiple regulatory and clinical issues. There is an increased awareness of the importance to adequately treat acute, chronic, and cancer pain in all populations and, thereby, to improve patient satisfaction, outcomes, and costs.

Guidelines for improving care have been formulated and distributed by federal and state agencies and medical societies with variable results.

To implement quality assurance and quality improvement in pain management necessitates attention to the following areas:

1. Accreditation in pain practice
2. Practice guidelines and policy statements
3. Quality indicators

ACCREDITATION IN PAIN PRACTICE

Physicians involved with pain management have traditionally come from the field of anesthesiology. John Bonica[1,2] began the modern era of pain management with the establishment of the first pain center in Tacoma, Washington in 1946. He recognized the importance of a multidisciplinary approach to these difficult patients and developed a world-renowned center at the University of Washington in Seattle, where collaborative treatment of these patients was carried out.

The American Board of Anesthesiology (ABA) mandated pain management as part of the anesthesiology residency program and established pain management as a subspecialty, introducing the certification of additional qualifications in pain management in 1993. Diplomates of the ABA and other selected ABMs must apply for acceptance to the examination and are judged based on additional training or experience in pain management.

The American Academy of Pain Medicine (AAPM), founded in 1983 as the American Academy of Algology, is a multidisciplinary physician organization made up of members "with a sustained interest in pain disorders and their management." Their stated mission is to enhance the practice of pain medicine in the United States by working to promote a socioeconomic and political climate conductive to the effective and efficient practice of pain medicine.

Third-party payers are being confronted by neurologists, neurosurgeons, orthopedic surgeons, and internists that rep-resent themselves as pain practitioners. Many of these physicians have attended only weekend courses or limited seminars yet seek to evaluate and treat complex pain patients. Although such courses can serve as an excellent introduction for already trained pain practitioners, they are not adequate substitutes for a proper fellowship training program or mentored instruction.

Some pain management physicians, from all disciplines, have developed an extremely dubious reputation among insurers in certain parts of the United States because of ineffective and costly care focused mainly around injections. This represents a disservice to the many dedicated professionals who attempt to provide a comprehensive assessment and treatment for pain patients.

The issue of credentials is becoming more important to pain practitioners as hospitals and surgery centers increasingly grant or deny privileges based on board certification in their primary specialty and evidence of fellowship training in their subspecialty along with demonstration of competency for advanced interventional pain techniques. Many centers grant provisional status privileges to protect themselves, focusing on the following:

1. Review of outcome data through peer review and quality improvement
2. Review of variance reports
3. Review of infection rates (where applicable)
4. Actual observation of procedures performed when necessary
5. Documentation of the previous considerations in credential files

The credentialing and privileging system provides the major and perhaps the only way by which a facility or institution can exert some control over the practitioners and the quality of their practices.[3]

PRACTICE GUIDELINES AND POLICY STATEMENTS

Practice guidelines allow physicians and administrators who are unfamiliar with the practice of pain medicine to gain an understanding of how care should generally be delivered. These guidelines can never anticipate every patient circumstance and are acknowledged to be starting points from which one must adapt to suit difficult cases. Clinical practice guidelines can be used by the practitioner and the patient to assist in decisions about appropriate health care in a specific situation.

Clinical Practice Guidelines

The Agency for Health Care Policy and Research (AHCPR) has developed clinical practice guidelines for acute pain management[4] and the management of cancer pain.[5]

AHCPR carries out its mission by conducting and supporting general health services research, including medical effectiveness research; facilitating the development of clinical practice guidelines; and disseminating research findings and guidelines to health care providers, policy-makers, and the public.

The clinical practice guideline on acute pain management used an interdisciplinary expert panel made up of physicians, nurses, a pharmacist, a psychologist, a physical therapist, a patient/consumer, and an ethicist.

The guideline emphasizes:

- A collaborative, interdisciplinary approach to pain control, including all members of the health team and input from the patient and the patient's family, when appropriate
- An individualized proactive pain control plan developed preoperatively by the patient and practitioners (because pain is easier to prevent than to bring under control once it has begun)
- Assessment and frequent reassessment of the patient's pain
- Use of both drug and nondrug therapies to control or prevent pain
- A formal, institutional approach to the management of acute pain, with clear lines of responsibility

The AHCPR clinical practice guideline on the management of cancer pain followed and made reference to the earlier guideline on acute pain management. The guideline makes recommendations about the assessment and management of pain.

The guideline on the management of cancer pain has 10 goals:

1. To inform clinicians and patients and their families that most cancer pain can be relieved by available methods
2. To dispel unfounded fears that addiction results from the appropriate use of medications to control cancer pain
3. To inform clinicians that cancer pain
   - Accompanies both disease and treatment
   - Changes over time
   - May have multiple simultaneous causes
   - If relieved, can affect the patient's physical, psychologic, social, and spiritual well-being
4. To promote prompt and effective assessment, diagnosis, and treatment of pain in patients with cancer
5. To strengthen the ability of patients with cancer and their families to communicate new unrelieved pain to secure prompt evaluation and effective treatment
6. To provide clinicians with a synthesis of the literature and expert opinions for application to the management of cancer pain

7. To familiarize patients and their families with options available for pain relief and to promote their active participation in selecting among these
8. To provide a model for cancer pain management to guide therapy in selected painful, life-threatening conditions such as the acquired immune deficiency syndrome (AIDS)
9. To provide information and guidelines on the use of controlled substances for the treatment of cancer pain that distinguishes the use of these drugs for legitimate purposes from their abuse as illegitimate drugs
10. To identify health policy and research issues that affect cancer pain management

Despite the availability of extensive guidelines, pain management physicians still find themselves confronting the same issues regarding undertreatment of cancer and noncancer chronic pain. Foley[6] has suggested that the undertreatment of pain is only one of the compelling factors that lead patients to request physician-assisted suicide and euthanasia.

Practice guidelines for cancer pain management were developed by the American Society of Anesthesiologists (ASA) Task Force on Pain Management, Cancer Pain Section[7] and a panel of consultants who assessed the scientific evidence as derived from aggregated research literature, with meta-analyses where appropriate. The purpose of these guidelines is to (1) optimize pain control; (2) minimize side effects, adverse outcomes, and costs; (3) enhance functional abilities and physical and psychologic well-being; and (4) enhance the quality of life for cancer patients.

Nine areas were reviewed by the task force:

1. Comprehensive evaluation and assessment of the patient with cancer pain
2. Longitudinal monitoring of pain
3. Involvement of specialists from multiple disciplines
4. Paradigm for the management of cancer pain
5. Management of cancer-related symptoms and adverse effects of pain therapy
6. Recognition, assessment, and management of psychosocial factors
7. Home parenteral therapy
8. End-of-life care
9. Recognition and management of special features of pediatric cancer pain management

These guidelines went further than earlier guidelines in conceptualizing the pharmacologic management of cancer pain as a continuum from indirect drug delivery to direct drug delivery. The World Health Organization (WHO) has recommended an analgesic ladder for the administration of oral analgesics.[7]

Public Policy Statements

The AAPM, American Pain Society (APS), and American Society of Addiction Medicine (ASAM) have all recently issued public policy statements centered on the appropriate use of opioid medications in both cancer and noncancer chronic pain.

One of the most difficult and controversial areas is the prescribing of opioids for chronic noncancer pain. A balance must be struck in using this very appropriate therapy for the correct patient.

QUALITY INDICATORS

Quality initiatives in medicine have been variously called quality assurance, quality assessment, quality improvement, continuous quality improvement (CQI), integrated quality assessment, quality management, quality resource management, total quality control, focused improvement strategies, and total quality management. It has been pointed out that the more names applied to an illness in medicine, the less is really known about it.[8] Part of the problem is that quality is hard to measure, and the definition of quality often depends on the population of patients being cared for.

The problem appears to be that outcomes management and quality management seek to improve the efficiency of health care through different principles that may seem incompatible.[9] Outcomes management developed from the assumption that if physicians knew the outcomes of their actions in health care, they could develop systematic guidelines and standards for what those actions should be. Quality management focuses on achieving better quality and efficiency by improving processes, and although having better outcomes is the ultimate goal, a focus on outcomes alone is inefficient. It has been pointed out that these two systems differ significantly in at least three elements: time frame, principal focus of activity, and philosophy about people. The interrelationship of these two systems—outcomes management and quality management—is shown in Table 32–1.

Stratiegies for Pain Medicine Improvement

The APS has developed quality assurance standards for the relief of acute pain and cancer pain.[10] The standards focus on these types of pain because it was felt that there was a significant scientific consensus regarding treatment methods, particularly the use of analgesic medications. The APS encouraged the examination of the treatment of chronic pain or the outcomes of nonpharmacologic treatment.

The basic standards were to:

- Recognize and treat pain promptly
- Make information about analgesics readily available
- Promise patients attentive analgesic care
- Define explicit policies for the use of advanced analgesic techniques
- Monitor adherence to standards

A system must also be created for process and outcomes measurement and reporting. There are many barriers to the implementation of disease management programs, such as:

TABLE 32–1 Interrelationship of Outcomes Management and Quality Management

	Outcomes Management	Quality Management
Purpose	Define, point to system goal	Reduce variation and complexity in processes of care
Time frame	Months, years, decades	Days, weeks, months
Principal measurement	Patient-reported outcomes	Key quality characteristics of processes
Analogy	Compass	Rudder

1. Limited resources to develop a program
2. Inadequate information systems to identify patients and to measure process and outcomes
3. Disruption of continuity of care
4. Perception of a "cookbook" approach
5. Difficulty in changing practice patterns

S U M M A R Y

Quality outcomes and quality management are important areas in all of modern medicine. Pain medicine is in a phase of rapid growth, which demands attention to the many variables that can ensure quality at all levels. Economic and societal pressures mandate accountability and innovative approaches to ensure superior patient care. Pain medicine will benefit and ultimately will be made more viable if there is a rigorous and systematic approach to the global issues associated with this subspecialty practice.

References

1. Bonica JJ: History of pain concepts and therapies. In *The management of pain*, ed 2, vol I. Philadelphia, Lea & Febiger, 1990.
2. Bonica JJ: Multidisciplinary/interdisciplinary pain programs. In *The management of pain*, ed 2, vol I. Philadelphia, Lea & Febiger, 1990.
3. Zusman J: *Credentialing and privileging systems.* Tampa, ACPE Publication, 1990.
4. Acute Pain Management Guideline Panel: *Acute pain management operative or medical procedures and trauma: Clinical practice guideline.* AHCPR Pub. No. 92-0032. Rockville, Md, Agency for Health Care Policy and Research, Public Health Service, U.S. Department of Health and Human Services, 1992.
5. Jacox A: *Management of cancer pain: Clinical practice guideline no. 9.* AHCPR Pub. No. 94-0592. Rockville, Md, Agency for Health Care Policy and Research, Public Health Service, U.S. Department of Health and Human Services, 1994.
6. Foley KM: Pain, physician-assisted suicide and euthanasia. *Pain Forum* 4:163, 1995.
7. Practice guidelines for cancer pain management: A report by the American Society of Anesthesiologists Task Force on Pain Management, Cancer Pain Section. *Anesthesiology* 84:1243, 1996.
8. Bigelow B, Arndt M: Total quality management: field of dreams? *Health Care Manage Rev* 20:15, 1995.
9. Reinersten JL: Outcomes management and continuous quality improvement: The compass and the rudder. *Qual Rev Bull* 19:5, 1993.
10. Max M: American Pain Society quality assurance standards for relief of acute and cancer pain. *Proceedings of the Sixth World Congress on Pain*, Vol 4. Amsterdam, Elsevier Science Publishers, 1991.

1. The clinical practice guidelines emphasize all of the following except

   A. A collaborative interdisciplinary approach to pain control
   B. An individualized pain control plan
   C. No assessment of a patient's pain
   D. A formal institutional approach for the management of acute pain with clear lines of responsibilities

2. The American Academy of Pain Medicine, the American Pain Society, and the American Society of Addiction Medicine have issued public policy statements on the appropriate use of

   A. Antidepressant medications
   B. Muscle relaxants
   C. Nonsteroidal anti-inflammatory agents
   D. Opioid administration

3. Quality initiatives in medicine have been variously called all of the following except

   A. Quality assurance
   B. Continuous quality improvement
   C. Total quality control
   D. Quality maintenance

4. The American Pain Society developed standards for the relief of acute cancer pain and chronic pain. The basic standards are all of the following except

   A. Recognize and treat all the pain as late as possible
   B. Make information about analgesics readily available
   C. Promise patients attentive analgesic care
   D. Define policies for the use of advanced analgesic techniques

5. There are many barriers to the implementation of pain management programs. These are all of the following except

   A. Limited resources to develop a program
   B. Ease in changing practice patterns
   C. Inadequate information systems to identify and measure processes and outcomes of treatment
   D. Perception of a "cookbook" approach

ANSWERS

1. C
2. D
3. D
4. A
5. B

CHAPTER 33

Economics of Pain Medicine

BENJAMIN W. JOHNSON JR.
AND MARSHALL BEDDER

OVERVIEW

The financiers of today's current dynamic health care environment demand justification from health care providers, such as pain clinicians, for medical decisions and accountability for health care expenditures before they grant approval for reimbursement of services rendered. The basis of accountability is becoming outcome-based efficacy of diagnostic and therapeutic services. The economic analysis of the cost-effectiveness of alternative diagnostic and therapeutic interventions is an important component of the decision-making processes that health care financiers use to decide on the most efficient use of their economic resources.

FUNDAMENTAL PRINCIPALS OF ECONOMICS

As Ridsdale has stated, "Refusal to learn the language of economics and engage in an adult dialogue with those who are responsible for resource allocation may reflect feelings of professional pride and a distaste for money and trade, but it also puts doctors, nurses, and patients at a profound disadvantage."[1]

The discipline of economics involves analyzing the choices that individuals or organizations make in using their limited resources to produce, exchange, and consume goods and services. Microeconomics is the study of decision-making processes of firms and individuals in a market setting.[2]

It is vital for students and practitioners of pain medicine to understand basic economic principles for at least two reasons: (1) the present dynamic environment of modern health care and (2) the unique nature of pain medicine in contrast to other medical specialties.

Medical ethics cannot be disengaged from medical economics because it attempts to provide viable models of the reasoning processes that health care providers exhibit when they are presented with conflicts of interest.[3] As the principal front-line decision makers, in the allocation of resources for the health care system, the physician's decision-making behavior is a logical target for economic analysis.[4]

Scarcity

Because consumers of health care resources (i.e., patients, physicians, and health care providers) usually want more goods and services than they can afford, they must make priority-directed choices.[1]

Similarly, physicians and other health care providers usually desire more health care resources than they may be willing to "pay" for and also must make priority-directed choices.

Choice

Because of the limited resources allocated (scarcity), trade-offs must be made according to the opportunity costs of each choice not selected.[1]

Specialization

The specialization theory addresses the tendency of an individual or organization to focus on tasks for which they are well suited. Specialization creates wealth through such strategies as differentiation, improvements in efficiency, superior product quality, and innovation.

Exchange

The theory of exchange deals with the expected ability of an individual or organization to trade specialized goods. In a large multihospital setting, for example, enterprising individual hospitals can trade or barter their specialized services, such as specialized surgical instruments, state-of-the-art diagnostic and therapeutic services, or specialized transport services, to avoid unnecessary expense and duplication of resources.

Marginal Analysis

The marginal analytic technique is one of the most important tools of economic decision making. Marginal analysis examines the effect of making incremental changes in the current state of affairs.[1]

Weighing the additional incremental benefit (marginal benefit) against the corresponding incremental cost (marginal cost) of alternatives is the foundation of marginal analysis. If the marginal benefits outweigh the marginal costs, the strategy should be undertaken.

Supply and Demand

There is an inverse relationship between the price of a product and the quantity demanded by consumers who are willing and able to purchase the product. The goal of the consumer's decision to buy or not to buy a given product or service is known as *utility*. Utility is defined by economists as the amount of pleasure or satisfaction derived from consuming the good.[1]

The factors that influence the demand of a given product or service include the following:

- Price of the product
- Price of substitute goods (i.e., alternative goods)

- Price of complementary good (i.e., goods whose demand increases concomitantly)
- Consumer's money income
- Consumer's tastes and preferences
- Relationship between the actual price and the expected price

Elasticity

Elasticity describes the relationship of price sensitivity to supply and demand, that is, the relationship between a change in the price of a product and the resulting change in demand. For example, the relationship that describes the effect of a change in price on the demand for a product or service is known as the "price elasticity of demand," and this is the most critical factor of demand.

In an elastic situation, the revenues obtained from the increased demand outweigh the decrease in price. The factors that influence price elasticity are:

- Availability of substitutes
- Importance to the consumer's budget
- Frequency of purchase
- Time

If a change in the price does not result in a change in demand, the ratio of percentage of change in demand to percentage of change in price is less than one. This situation is described as "inelastic," or price insensitive.

One of the most important determinants of price elasticity is the availability of substitute products or services. As the availability of substitute products increases, the customer's tolerance for price increases in a given product decreases and the customer becomes price sensitive (elastic demand). This situation is especially relevant if price is the primary difference between products or is the sole priority of the consumer.

Cross-price Elasticity

When the price of one product influences the price of another, the relationship is known as the "cross-price elasticity of demand." If the cross-price elasticity is positive, that is, if an increase in the price of Product A creates an increase in the demand for Product B, then Product B is a substitute for Product A.

Another important cross-price elasticity concept is the "income elasticity of demand," which describes the relationship between a change in the consumer's income and the resultant purchasing tendencies.

The "Elasticity" of Health

One of the more practical applications of economic theory to health care is the concept of the elasticity of health, which is a ratio containing the change in health in the numerator and the change in medical expenditures in the denominator.

One might speculate that a similar calculation of elasticity could be developed for acute, chronic, or cancer pain, and this relevant elasticity formula might involve the change in length of hospital stay, improvement in pain relief, or quality of life,[5,6] respectively, in the numerator and the change in expenditures in the denominator. From the calculated pain elasticity, the improvement in a given pain outcome measure per dollar of expenditure could be estimated and compared with other inputs of societal health, such as lifestyle and environmental variables.

ECONOMIC MYTHS[2]

The False-Cause Fallacy

The false-cause fallacy assumes that because two events occur together, one event has caused the other. Statistical correlation of two variables is often of no benefit in identifying causation. For cause to be established, there must be a logical theory to explain the effect of one variable on another.

The Fallacy of Composition

The fallacy of composition myth relates to the erroneous assumption that what is true for each separate part of a market is true for the whole or vice versa.

APPLIED ECONOMIC CONCEPTS

The economic principles just presented can be applied practically to health care scenarios, such as pain medicine, as long as a few caveats regarding the status of medical practice within our society are acknowledged.

Healthcare Economics—An Oxymoron?

Controversy exists in both health care and economic literature regarding the applicability of the discipline of economics to health care. To apply economic principles to health care, one must address the relevance of several fundamental economic principles. The assumptions concerning issues such as the rational consumer or profit maximization are presented.

The Concept of the Rational Consumer

The discipline of economics makes a fundamental assumption that the consumer of a good or service is able to obtain enough information about the intended purchase to make a rational decision regarding that purchase in lieu of other possible purchases. Economists assume that consumers are "rational," that is, well-informed individuals who have enough product or service information to make the most appropriate choice.[2] In health care, a considerable knowledge gap exists between the health care provider and the consumer (e.g., physician and patient, pain specialist and "gatekeeper," or pain specialist and hospital administrator).[7] This information asymmetry can keep the consumer from making rational and knowledgeable decisions regarding the purchase of health care goods and services.

The Concept of Profit Maximization

Economists assume that profit maximization guides managerial decision making.[8] In health care organizations, the maximization of profit must be weighed against the ethical concerns regarding the practice of medicine in society.

A theory that challenges the profit maximization theory is the *concept of satisficing behavior*. Satisficing behavior describes decision makers who do not seek or possess the precise knowledge of cost and demand needed for profit maximization; instead, they settle for minimal standards of achievement that are consistent with long-term survival of the organization.

Day and Tinney[9] suggests that the performance of such an organization tends to vector toward profit maximization by following two principles:

1. Successful behavior should be repeated, and unsuccessful behavior should be avoided.
2. If a change in circumstances indicates that previously unsuccessful behavior should be repeated, its use should be approached with caution.

Day also noted that the length of the path toward profit maximization depends on the decision maker's "learning function," that is, the tendency to overreact or under-react to factual input such as losses in profit.[9]

Another perspective on the issue of profit maximization and ethical behavior suggests that decision makers in profit-maximizing firms are motivated to behave responsibly when consumers are willing to pay for such behavior.[10]

The Business of Corporate Health Care

A business firm's basic goal is profit maximization and/or increased wealth of its shareholders, and this is achieved by using such strategies as increasing sales growth and market share. Profit maximization plays a crucial role in the allocation of scarce resources by determining which goods and services will be produced.[11]

However, because the profit-maximizing firm avoids engaging in unprofitable activities that do not positively affect its profitability, governmental regulation is often necessary to enforce a level playing field within the health care market.

Managed care is a business strategy developed by the corporate health care industry to provide incentives for medical practitioners to deliver cost-effective medical care by compensating for reduced reimbursements with an increased patient volume.[12]

One of the financing strategies used by health care financiers in determining the current worth of the "insured lives" of insured individuals is to calculate the net cash flows produced by the average individual who pays premiums to the plan for a given period. This calculation, termed as *securitization* by Reinhardt,[13] is a "present value equivalent" of the anticipated future cash flow, representing the current market value of the covered individual to the insurer. These present value equivalents can then be bought and sold on the open market.

Consumers of medical services may erroneously assume that the reduced premium rates result from economics of scale rather than the more likely reduced benefits package, which may include a restrictive preferred provider network. One unfortunate result of the emphasis of profit maximization in corporate health care management is the stifling effect of cost control and diversion of profits on innovations in medical therapy.

The end result of reduced reimbursement for the clinical activities of academic physicians is a decrease in the speed at which technologic and medical research efforts result in innovations in disease management, which may potentially benefit the health care industry and its consumers.

Decision making is a vital part of any business entity. A modern business trend involves the delegation of tactical decision making into the hands of those expected to have the most ready access to vital information, such as lower and middle-level managers or even line employees.

This strategy allows top-level executives to avoid micromanagement, instead concentrating on developing strategic planning.[12] The strategic corporate decisions to be made include (1) relations with outsiders, (2) allocation of scarce resources within the organization's infrastructure, (3) identification of critical factors needed in decision making, and (4) tactical versus strategic decisions. This *bottom-up philosophy* of medical decision making can adversely affect obtaining authorization for reimbursement for proposed pain treatment.

One potential benefit to the increased scrutiny of the pain management specialty by the corporate health care industry is the expected emphasis on the use of appropriately credentialed pain specialists to evaluate and manage pain disorders. Using properly credentialed pain medicine specialists to perform precision diagnostic and therapeutic procedures and to properly select patients for placement of implantable technology should greatly decrease the financial expenditures for medical services related to pain management.

Cost Considerations in Profit Maximization for the Pain Medicine Practitioner

The accuracy with which a pain specialist determines the true costs involved with a preferred style pain medicine practice and the diligence applied to controlling factors affecting the costs of practice determines the potential for survival of his or her practice entity.

A number of pain medicine practices have closed because the physicians and their support staff failed to seriously consider the economic aspects of medical practice.

In the current health care market, in which physicians are operating in the environment of sharply discounted reimbursement rates with sharply reduced profit margins, the consideration of cost reduction measures becomes tantamount to economic survival.

Another important cost consideration is the calculation of a "break-even" point in regard to the volume of patients, or the number of procedures necessary to ensure adequate revenue generation for economic survival of the corporate entity. The break-even point is defined as the total fixed cost of the practice entity divided by the variable costs (Fig. 33–1) subtracted from the price of the average intervention. Calculation of the break-even point can provide the pain medicine practitioner with valuable information, which can be used in the process of price negotiation with managed care insurers (Table 33–1; Fig. 33–2).

Another helpful calculation that can be determined, if accurate cost data can be obtained, is the average cost curve per patient. If one graphs the total costs per specified time interval against the patient volume over the same time interval, the result should graphically indicate the most economical volume of patients that the present practice arrangement can handle. The current practice can handle from 12 to 30 patients per day at the lowest possible total cost (Fig. 33–3).

The Pain Physician as a Member of Society

The increasing decline of the physician's autonomy and control over the patient is termed *deprofessionalism* by

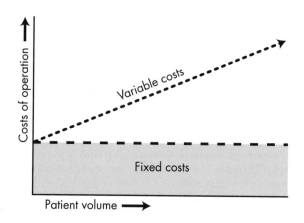

FIG. 33–1 Graph of fixed costs and variable costs.

TABLE 33–1 Break-even Analysis for a Pain Clinic Using a Single Procedure	
Break-even Analysis ($)	
Average price per procedure	500
Average discount or allowance	−50
Net price per procedure	450
Annual fixed cost	500,000
Variable cost per procedure	200
Break-even Calculation ($)	
Net price per procedure	450
Variable cost per procedure	−200
Contribution martin per procedure	250 (A)
Fixed costs	500,000 (B)
Break-even number of procedures (B/A)	2000*

*Assuming 250 working days, in this scenario eight of these procedures per day would be required for the practice to break even.

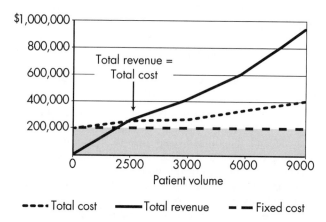

FIG. 33–2 Break-even graph demonstrates the intersection of total revenue and total cost. *(Modified from Hultman JA; Economics 101: Understanding relevant costs for decision making. In Reengineering the medical practice. Reston, Va, St. Anthony Publishing, 1996).*

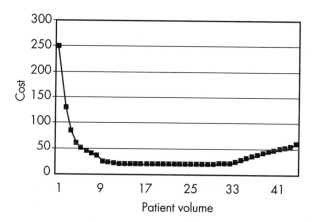

FIG. 33–3 Average cost curve per patient demonstrates the most cost-effective patient volume for the practitioner. *(Modified from Hultman JA; Economics 101: Understanding relevant costs for decision making. In Reengineering the medical practice. Reston, Va, St. Anthony Publishing, 1996).*

medical sociologists.[14] The trend of increasing governmental control of health care, the increasing degree of competition among corporate health care providers, and the greater numbers of savvy health care consumers are changing the philosophy of medical practice from that of a substantive rationality to that of a formal rationality.[11] The result of these trends is transforming the traditional physician-patient relationship to that of a provider-consumer relationship.

Society's perspective of the physician is too often assumed to be the *self-interest model* or the *medical ethics model,* both of which have little concern for the cost-effective medical service. These perceptions coupled with the business executive's perceptions of physicians as poor businessmen leaves physicians at a definite disadvantage at the negotiating table.

Concerns Regarding the Identity of the Purchaser

In contrast to many nonmedical markets, the purchaser of medical services is often the provider (e.g., the physician) not the consumer (e.g., the patient). Thus, one might argue that the physician has a financial motivation in the purchase of treatments. Such suspicions have led to the institution of

regulatory disincentives to discourage overuse of medical services associated with the prescribing physician.

The Mediating Role of Medical Care

Economists perceive that health care has a mediating effect on individual well-being—thus, creating the need for health care financiers to be aware of either overuse or underuse of medical goods and services.

Overuse constitutes use of health care services that is estimated to be greater than necessary. Enthoven[15] suggests that the relationship between resource allocation and improvement in health status (Fig. 33–4) is not a linear relationship; rather, it reveals a decreasing improvement in health status with increasing allocation of health care resources after a plateau phase is reached.[15]

For patients, increasing the consumption of health care goods and services beyond the point of maximum benefit incurs the risk of unnecessary iatrogenic injury as well as the opportunity costs of time and money. For the health care provider, the consumption of health care goods and services by the patient or provider beyond the point of maximum

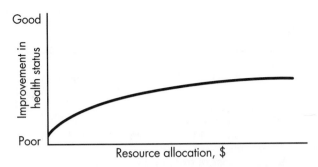

FIG. 33–4 Relationship between health care resource allocation and improvement in health status. This relationship shows the "law of diminishing returns": after a certain level of health care resource allocation, there is a decreasing marginal health improvement. *(Adapted from Macario A: Defining value in health care: outcomes. In Macario A, Lang AD, editors: Health economics and practice management in anesthesia. Int Anesthesiol Clin 33:15–32, 1995.)*

benefit may mar his or her provider profile and hasten the specter of economic credentialing.

If the provider invests the same amount of time and expertise in a more suitable patient, the outcome should be more favorable, producing the following beneficial effects:

- Improving outcome statistics
- Increasing the provider's marketability
- Enhancing advertising effectiveness
- Decreasing the advertising costs (by increasing word-of-mouth advertising)
- More effectively using support staff (e.g., fewer telephone calls or prescriptions)

Underuse of appropriate health care resources implies that the delivery of needed medical care may not be satisfactory for some individuals. The well-described undertreatment of cancer pain and postoperative pain worldwide is an example of the underuse of available medical services and technology.[16–19] The costs of uncontrolled pain are manifested in some of the following ways:

Increased physician visits
Increased telephone call volume
Decreased support staff effectiveness because of increased calls and visits
Increased adjunct medication prescriptions
Lost workdays for transportation of ill patients

Is Health Care an Output or an Input?

Health care can be viewed as an output of physicians, hospitals, and other health care providers and can, therefore, be analyzed in regard to the efficiency of production. On the other hand, health care can be viewed as one of the inputs for the production of "wellness." From this perspective, one must analyze the optimal allocation of resources to produce wellness.

It is vital that both perspectives on health care be used to provide optimal health resources for society.

To determine the most cost-effective combination of inputs for achieving an increase in health (individual or societal), it is necessary to develop a *health production function.* This concept describes the relationship between combinations of inputs and the resulting output. The health production function allows economists to identify the most economically efficient (the least expensive) combination of inputs.

After experts in pain management have identified the best alternative inputs for decreasing the incidence of low back pain, the economist can use optimization tools to determine the best allocation of the society's health resources to achieve the stated objectives.[20]

In consideration of medical service as an output of health care providers, the first step in appropriate therapeutic decision making consists of determining an acceptable output or specific outcome to be achieved. The relatively small number of satisfactorily performed outcome studies regarding the impact of medical treatment of chronic low back pain can hinder the economic analysis of therapeutic interventions.[21]

Economic Models of Physician Decision making

The three economic models proposed by Tussing[22] help the economist analyze physician decision-making behavior:

1. The *agency model* characterizes the physician as a provider of technical expertise, acting exclusively in the best interest of the patient. Maximizing cost-effective treatment of the patient is a priority in this model.
2. The *self-interest model* describes the physician's priority as one of optimizing the combination of personal income and lifestyle.
3. The *medical ethics model* identifies the physician as a health care provider who is motivated to maximize care for the patient without concern for cost.

Using these three models as a starting point, one can surmise that each provider may be a dynamic blend of the three models.

The Unique Nature of Pain Medicine

The most widely accepted definition of pain is "an unpleasant sensory and/or emotional experience based on actual or potential tissue damage, or described in terms of such damage."[23] The experience of pain involves a dynamic mix of both an objective pathologic condition and a behavioral pathologic condition. Quantifying the variable mix of tissue and behavioral pathologic conditions in each patient, as well as acknowledging the various philosophies regarding the proper approach for optimal cost-effective pain management, can render the economic analysis of pain medicine problematic.

In analyzing the various models of effective pain management, Justins[21] observes, "The adoption of the biopsychosocial model rather than the traditional disease model is one of the most important advances in the management of chronic nonmalignant pain; and, when appropriate, has allowed therapy to be directed away from the traditional search for a 'cause and a cure'."

Leaders in the development of pain outcome studies have long documented the treatment efficacy of multidisciplinary pain control centers.[25,26] However, the failure of pain

---

BOX 33–1 Production and Cost in the Long Run*

Production Efficiency†

- Maximum efficiency from given set of inputs
  - Patients
  - Support staff
  - Provider staff
  - Time

Economic efficiency

- Quantity of output at the lowest cost
  - Patient
  - Provider and support staff
  - Payers (e.g., insurance companies)

---

*See Figure 33–3 for a graphic representation of economic efficiency.
†Production efficiency analysis begins with a predetermined set of inputs; economic efficiency analysis attempts to determine the most satisfactory set of inputs.

BOX 33–2 Formula for Cost-Effectiveness Ratio ($\Delta C/\Delta E$)*

$$\Delta C = \Delta C_{Rx} + \Delta C_{se} - \Delta C_{morb} + \Delta_{CR \times \Delta LE}$$

where
  ΔC = net health care costs
  ΔC_{Rx} = all direct medical and health care costs
  ΔC_{morb} = all health care costs associated with iatrgenic effects
  $\Delta_{CR \times \Delta LE}$ = cost of treating disease that occurred because of a patient's increased life span after interventional therapy

$$\Delta E = \Delta\gamma + \Delta\gamma\,morb - \Delta\gamma se$$

where
  ΔE = net health effectiveness (measured in quality adjusted life-years)
  $\Delta\gamma$ = expected number of unadjusted life-years (the difference between age-specific life expectancy with and without the intervention)
  $\Delta\gamma\,morb$ = improvements in the quality of life-years due to alleviation of morbidity
  $\Delta\gamma se$ = change in quality of life-years due to iatrogenesis of intervention

Note: The units of the denominator are quality adjusted life-years (QALYs)

$$QALYs = Ys \times \lambda s$$

where
Ys = the number of years spent at a given health status
λs = health status (range: 0.0–1.0 with 0.0 = mild disability and 1.0 = near death)

Data from Weinstein MC, Stason WB: Foundations of cost-effectiveness analysis for health and medical practices. N Engl J Med 296:716–721, 1997.
*Shows the detailed calculation of net health care costs divided by the net health effectiveness.

---

medicine providers, as a whole, to coordinate their efforts in generating valid outcome studies has, in part, contributed to the reluctance of health care financiers to reimburse for pain treatment as readily as for the medical treatment of other chronic diseases.

Because reimbursement for pain medicine providers can be considered a scarce resource, the science of economics can offer a systematic, disciplined analytic approach to the following questions:

1. How is cost-effectiveness in pain medicine measured?
2. Can the practice of pain medicine be profitable?
3. How is pain medicine valued within the health care industry?

Optimizing the Production of Medical Services

The relationship of production and cost in the delivery of health care services involves two important economic themes (Box 33–1):

1. *Production efficiency* seeks to obtain the maximum output for the costs generated from a given set of inputs.
2. *Economic efficiency* involves the generation of a given quality of output at the lowest cost to patients, provider staff, support staff, or payers.

The combination of services and inputs is both technically and economically efficient if the health care provider's costs are minimized; thus, the provider must be able to monitor the cost of the practice accurately. Therefore, the optimal combination of inputs (health care personnel, time, space, and capital) must be considered in achieving economical efficiency (i.e., output at the lowest cost).

Principles of Cost-effectiveness Analysis

Evaluating the outcome of therapeutic interventions in pain medicine necessitates a satisfactory economic analytic ins-

trument. Although both cost-benefit and cost-effectiveness analyses are amenable to health care economic issues, cost-effectiveness is the preferred tool, because it does not attempt to place a dollar value on the human life. Instead, it presents costs in monetary terms and effectiveness in qualitative measures such as pain-free days, complications avoided, and quality-adjusted life-years (QALYs). A cost-effectiveness ratio is defined as a ratio of net increase in health care costs to net effectiveness in quality of life and enhanced life expectancy (Box 33–2). The lower the ratio, the more favorable is the benefit from a given health care expenditure or intervention.

SUMMARY

As the practice of medicine becomes increasingly business-like, physicians must become more conversant in economics, marketing, strategy, operations, and other unfamiliar disciplines. As they struggle to overcome the traditional adversarial relationship with health care administrators and as they participate in a more synergistic relationship, quality patient care should not be compromised. Pain medicine specialists and their specialty-governing organizations must market their profession intelligently after careful consideration of the milieu existing within the current dynamic health care industry. Conducting more satisfactory outcome studies of therapeutic interventions in pain medicine will help legitimize the indicated treatments and reduce the use of unsatisfactory medical therapy. The identification of outcome-driven alternative inputs for evidence-based decision making in pain medicine will not only prove cost-effective but will also help substantiate the legitimacy of pain medicine as a specialty.

References

1. Ridsdale L, editor: The economic aspects of general practice. In *Evidence-based general practice.* London, WB Saunders 1995.
2. Ruffin RJ, Gregory PR: *Principles of microeconomics,* ed 5. New York, HarperCollins, 1993.
3. Berwick DM, Godfrey AB, Roessner A: *Curing health care: New strategies for quality improvement.* San Francisco, Jossey-Bass, 1990.
4. Orkin FK: Work force planning for anesthesia care. *Int Anesthesiol Clin* 33:69, 1995.
5. Guyatt GH: The philosophy of health-related quality of life translation. *Qual Life Res* 2:461, 1995.
6. Johnson BW: The economics of pain practice. *Curr Rev Pain* 1:324, 1994.
7. Shughart WF II, Chappell WF, Cottle RL: *Modern managerial economics: Economic theory for business decisions.* Cincinnati, Ohio, Southwestern Publishing, 1994.
8. Day RH: Profits, learning, and the convergence of satisficing to marginalism. *Q J Econ* 81:302, 1967.
9. Day RH, Tinney EH: How to co-operate in business without really trying: A learning model of decentralized decision making. *J Political Econ* 67:583, 1969.
10. Navarro P: Why do corporations give to charity? *J Business* 61:65, 1988.
11. Shughart WF II, Chappell WF, Cottle RL: *Modern managerial economics.* Cincinnati, Ohio, Southwestern Publishing, 1994.
12. Ossorio RC, Alper MJ: Fee-for service medicine, preferred provider organizations, and health maintenance organizations. In Gitnick G, Rothenberg F, Weiner JL, editors: *The business of medicine,* New York, Elsevier, 1991.
13. Reinhardt UE: Hippocrates and the securitization of patients. *JAMA* 277:1850, 1997.
14. Cockerham WC: The physician in a changing society. In *Medical sociology.* Englewood Cliffs, NJ, Prentice-Hall, 1992.
15. Enthoven AC: *Health plan: The only practical solution to the soaring cost of medical care.* Reading, Mass, Addison-Wesley, 1980.
16. Flexner JM: Appropriate management of cancer pain: Not the second order of business anymore. In Parris WCV, editor: *Cancer pain management: Principles and practice.* London, Butterworth-Heinemann, 1997.
17. Chrubasik J, Chrubasik S: Meta-analysis on the efficacy of intrathecal and epidural opiates. In Parris WCV, editor: *Cancer pain management: Principles and practice.* London, Butterworth-Heinemann, 1997.
18. Kaiko RF: The use of controlled-released opioids. In Parris WCV, editor: *Cancer pain management: Principles and practice.* London, Butterworth-Heinemann, 1997.
19. Acute Pain Management Guideline Panel: *Acute pain management: Operative or medical procedures and trauma.* AHCPR Pub. No. 92-0032. Rockville, Md, Agency for Health Care Policy and Research, Public Health Services, U.S. Department of Health and Human Services, 1992.
20. Turner JA, Deyo RA, Loeser JD et al: The importance of placebo effects in pain treatment and research. *JAMA* 271:1609, 1994.
21. Justins DM: Basic principles of chronic pain management. In Campbell JN, editor: *Pain 1996: An updated review.* Seattle, IASP Press, 1996.
22. Tussing AD: *Irish medical care resources: An economic analysis.* Paper 126. Dublin, The Economic and Research Institute, 1986.
23. Merskey H: Classification of chronic pain: Descriptions of chronic pain syndromes and definitions of pain terms. *Pain* 33(suppl 3):S1, 1986.
24. Cutler RB, Fishbain DA, Rosomoff HL et al: Does nonsurgical pain center treatment of chronic pain return patients to work? A review and meta-analysis of the literature. *Spine* 19:643, 1994.
25. Rosomoff HL, Rosomoff RS: Comprehensive multidisciplinary pain center approach to the treatment of low back pain. *Neurosurg Clin North Am* 2:877, 1991.

1. Managed care is a business strategy developed by the healthcare industry to provide all of the following except

   A. Incentives for medical practitioners
   B. Delivery of cost-effective medical care
   C. Compensation for reduced reimbursement with increasing patient volume
   D. Prompt approval of the plan of treatment as outlined by the physician

2. The increasing decline of the physician's autonomy and control is called deprofessionalism by sociologists. This trend is facilitated by

   A. Increasing government control of healthcare
   B. Decreasing the degree of competition among healthcare providers
   C. Changing the philosophy of medical practice from that of substantive rationality to that of a formal rationality
   D. Decreasing physician remuneration for patient care

3. There are three economic models that the economist analyze for physician decision-making behavior

   A. The agency model, which characterizes the physician as a provider of technical expertise. Maximizing the cost-effective treatment of the patient is a priority in this model
   B. Self-interest model, which describes the physician priority as optimizing the combination of personal income and lifestyle
   C. Hospital model, which describes the interest of the physician to maximize profits to the hospital with expensive care to the patient
   D. The medical ethics model identifies the physician as a healthcare provider who is motivated for maximizing care without concern for cost

4. As the practice of medicine becomes increasingly business-like, physicians must become more conversant in

   A. Economics
   B. Marketing
   C. Other familiar disciplines
   D. Strategy

5. To legitimize pain medicine, one must do all of the following except

   A. Conduct more satisfactory outcome studies
   B. Reduce the use of more unsatisfactory medical therapy
   C. Do not encourage well-trained pain physicians
   D. Provide adequate information to the third-party payers

ANSWERS

1. D
2. B
3. C
4. C
5. C

CHAPTER 34

Regulatory Issues Affecting Pain Medicine

MICHAEL A. ASHBURN AND STEPHEN P. LONG

The health care system is undergoing rapid change despite the apparent failure of President Clinton's health care reform efforts in the early 1990s.[1] This change is occurring on a state and federal level, as well as in the private sector,[2] and has a direct impact on our ability to care for our patient' needs.

Improvement can be accomplished only if members of the pain management community become involved in developing the health policies that affect them. The pain management community has entered an era of evolution in the health care system that will change the pain management programs that have been created and that may threaten their survival.[3]

POLICY ISSUES AFFECTING PAIN MANAGEMENT

Clinical Practice Guidelines

In the early 1990s, the practice of pain management came under increased scrutiny. To foster continued improvement in acute pain management, the Agency for Health Care Policy and Research (AHCPR) published clinical practice guidelines for the management of acute pain,[4] cancer pain, and acute low back pain. The stated goal of the acute pain guideline was to:

> ... reduce the incidence and severity of patients' acute postoperative or post-traumatic pain, educate patients about the need to communicate unrelieved pain so they can receive prompt evaluation and effective treatment, enhance patient comfort and satisfaction, and... contribute to fewer postoperative complications and, in some cases, shorter stays after surgical procedures.[4]

Other organizations, including the International Association for the Study of Pain (IASP) and the American Society of Anesthesiologists, have also developed pain-related guidelines.[5,6] The impact of these guidelines on the care of patients is questionable.[7]

Payment for Pain Management Services

The increased interest in pain management by government and private organizations is not reflected by an equal desire to pay for such services.[8] Additional difficulties lie in the current methods to determine whether acute pain treatment is appropriate and should be paid for.

Recently, Medicare intermediaries have begun to establish payment guidelines for pain management services. These intermediaries are becoming increasingly resistant to payment for pain-related physician services, especially recurrent nerve block therapy. As a result, some intermediaries are using expert opinion, published practice guidelines, or internal resources to establish payment guidelines that refuse payment for selected services and to limit payment for other services to specific circumstances.

Unfortunately, payment for nonphysician pain management services, such as psychologic services, has also been eliminated or strictly curtailed, despite studies showing that the pain patient population benefits greatly from these services. Often payments for mental health services are made only to a closed provider list, and pain management psychologists are not included.

In the provision of acute care services, health care reform has led to the development of health care alliances and the establishment of bundled fees for hospital-related services.

Growing data support the argument that the pain services provide cost-effective care through the health care organization in which it functions.

Based on recent changes in payment practice, it appears that the pain community will be challenged to document that the services provided add value to the care provided to patients.

Assessment of Patient Outcomes

Considerable interest has developed over the last several years in the development and use of utilization management and critical pathways.[9] Critical pathways describe a course of care for patients with similar problems and treatments.[10] The process of developing a critical pathway is intended to lead to the development of an integrated interdisciplinary plan that will result in cost-effective, high-quality care. Growing data support the view that this model of care does lead to improved outcomes and reduced costs.[11,12]

The AHCPR Acute Pain Management Guidelines advocate that health care institutions develop and implement an institutional plan for pain management.[4] Such an institutional plan is important in establishing an environment conducive to the appropriate management of pain for the hospitalized patient, but evidence is lacking that the presence of such a plan will lead to improved pain management in hospitalized patients.[13]

The current system of acute pain management often does not integrate pain management into the process of care for the perioperative patient. Even with the use of interdisciplinary acute pain management services, a traditional acute pain service provides pain management in consultation with the primary care service by carving out pain management from the remainder of the patient's care.

The development of a critical pathway for the surgical patient must begin with the preoperative assessment and must extend to the moment of discharge. Although acute pain management would be a vital part of such a plan, other elements are equally important, such as:

- A preoperative evaluation clinic provides high-quality, cost-effective care to its patient population.[14]
- The selection of anesthetic agent has a direct impact on postoperative pain control.[15]
- Effective early postoperative pain control may reduce the chances for long-term chronic pain problems.[16]

With the use of a patient-focused approach similar to critical pathway development, pain management is integrated into a global rehabilitation plan for the surgical patient.[17]

Early data indicate that this approach may lead to improved outcomes as well as earlier recovery and faster hospital discharge.[18-24]

Limited data exist on the outcomes associated with the care of individuals with chronic pain.[25] However, such individuals often do not experience long-term pain relief or improved quality of life from single-modality therapy. In addition, growing data support the use of an interdisciplinary approach in which the patient receives care via multiple modalities in a coordinated manner.[26-28]

In selected patient populations, standardized care plans to decrease variability in patient care have been shown to improve clinical outcomes and to decrease the cost of care.[11,12,19,24] This process has several key steps, including:

- Use of evidence-based medicine to guide the selection of treatment options
- Integration of disease-specific practice guidelines into patient care
- Monitoring of health outcomes

When a program is being developed to improve patient care in specific settings, measures of outcome can be effectively based on data specific to that patient population. For the acute care setting, these measures may include:

- Morbidity and mortality
- Incidence and severity of complications
- Length of stay

Generic measures of health attempt to access basic human values that are relevant to everyone's functional status and well-being.[29] Although these measures are not ideal and are usually based on patients' perspective of their health status, they appear to be valuable in monitoring health outcomes in many health care settings.[30,31]

An example of a generic measure of health is the SF 36, developed by the Medical Outcomes Study Group.[29] The SF 36 was designed for tracking populations and has too much imprecision for use in following the outcomes of individual patients (Table 34-1).

The Total Outcomes of Pain Score (TOPS) was developed by adding supplemental questions to the SF 36, then validating it so as to ensure that it is efficient and meets the required reduced variance and can be used for tracking individual chronic pain patients. The added scales are:

- Pain symptoms
- Functional limitations
- Perceived family/social disability
- Real family/social disability
- Formal work disability
- Patient satisfaction

Clinicians and researchers will continue to develop the skills necessary to integrate measurement of quality,[32] outcomes,[33] patient satisfaction, and cost effectiveness[34,35] into clinical practice.

TABLE 34-1 Summary Information on Short-Form Health Survey-36 (SF 36) Scales

Scale	Definition of Lowest Possible Score	Definition of Highest Possible Score
Physical functioning (PF)	Is limited in performing all physical activities, including bathing or dressing owing to poor health	Performs all types of physical activities, including the most vigorous, without limitations due to health
Role, physical (RP)	Has problems with work or other daily activities as a result of poor physical health	Has no problems with work or other daily activities as a result of physical health
Bodily pain (BP)	Experiences severe and extremely limiting pain	Has no pain or limitations due to pain
General health (GH)	Evaluates personal health as poor and believes that it is likely to become worse	Evaluates personal health as excellent
Vitality (VY)	Feels tired and worn out all of the time	Feels full of pep and energy all of the time
Social functioning (SF)	Experiences extreme and frequent interference with normal social activities owing to physical and emotional problems	Performs normal social activities without interference caused by physical or emotional problems
Role, emotional functioning (REF	Has trouble with work or other daily activities resulting from emotional problems	Has no problems with work of other daily activities as a result of emotional problems
Mental health (MH)	Feels nervous and depressed all of the time	Feels peaceful, happy, and calm all of the time

Data from Ware JE: Measuring patient function and well-being: Some lessons from the Medical Outcomes Study. In Heitgoff K, Lohr K, eds: Effectiveness and outcomes in health care: Proceedings of an invitational conference by the Institute of Medicine, Division of Health Care Services. Washington, DC, National Academy Press, 1990, pp 107–119.

FEDERAL POLICY ISSUES

Medicare

Changes to Medicare reimbursement in 1997 improved the financial viability of the Medicare program. However, it is expected that the Medicare program will enter yet another era of financial instability beginning in the year 2010, when the first members of the "Baby Boomer" generation enter into retirement. This crisis is expected to worsen until 2030.

Because the *Balanced Budget Act* of 1997 has taken the immediate financial crisis away, further efforts to fundamentally change the Medicare program are not expected for several years. However, the Health Care Financing Administration (HCFA) has received several mandates for modification of the program that will require significant publication of regulations over the next several years.

The Balanced Budget Act of 1997

President Clinton signed into law major changes in the Medicare program that were included in the Balanced Budget Act of 1997. These changes were intended to curb Medicare spending, which now accounts for more that 11% of the federal budget.

Beginning in 1998, the Act required payments to physicians to be based on the 1997 primary care services conversion factor, which will then be adjusted by the use of an adjusted Medicare economic index (MEI). In addition, the Act delayed implementation of the resource-based practice expense methodology by 1 year, then required the implementation of this payment system over 4 years.

In the short term, $390 million will be moved from the practice expense component for procedural services to the practice expense component for office visit services, effective in 1998.

For hospital services the new law slows the rate of increase of the prospective payment rates for inpatient care by:

1. Establishment of no increase in the rates for 1998
2. An increase of 1.9 percentage points below market basket (an established measure of the inflation rate for the cost of inpatient health care services) in 1999
3. 1.8 percentage points below market basket in 2000
4. 1.1 percentage points below market basket in 2001 and 2002

The law also required the establishment of a prospective payment system for hospital-based outpatient services to be implemented in 1999.

Direct graduate medical education (DGME) and indirect medical education (IME) will be carved out over the next 5 years from the rate that Medicare pays for Medicare managed care programs. This money will then be directly paid to teaching hospitals according to a formula based on the number of Medicare managed care patients admitted to each hospital for care.

Finally, the new law created a 17-member National Bipartisan Commission on the Future of Medicare to develop recommendations for future changes to maintain the program's long-term solvency. Unfortunately, this commission was unable to develop recommendations that were acceptable to the required supermajority of members, and the commission dissolved without making formal recommendations to Congress.

Quality and Patient's Bill of Rights

President Clinton established an advisory committee that recommended a "patient's bill of rights" in spring 1998. In addition, a coalition of nonprofit managed health organizations, in cooperation with several patient advocacy groups and provider organizations, prepared a model "quality" initiative that includes several provisions intended to protect a patient's rights.

ADMINITRATION OF CONTROLLED SUBSTANCES

Federal Regulation

Federal control over the use of controlled substances comes from two sets of law, which are implemented through federal regulation.

The *Food, Drug, and Cosmetic Act,* administered by the Food and Drug Administration (FDA), is responsible for ensuring the availability of safe and effective drugs and medical devices.

The *Controlled Substances Act* (CSA), administered by the Department of Justice, establishes federal law regarding the administration of controlled substances.

To educate the physician on issues regarding the administration of controlled substances, the Drug Enforcement Administration (DEA) published the *Physician's Manual: An Informational Outline of the Controlled Substances Act of 1970.*[36]

State Regulation

State law regarding the administration of opioids has presented barriers to the use of these drugs for pain management in many states throughout the United States.

Many states have begun a thoughtful review of state policy affecting pain management. This has resulted in the revision of state law governing the administration of controlled substances as well as the formation of consensus statements on this and other topics.[37]

State Policy Issues

Public policy with regard to the oversight of health insurance has traditionally been administered at the state level. However, the *Employee Retirement Income Security Act* (ERISA) established federal control over self-insured health plans.

Intractable Pain Bills

Increasing attention is being given to the role of opioids for the management of chronic noncancer pain. Although it has long been recognized that opioids are the cornerstone of drug therapy for acute and cancer pain, there have been strong barriers to the use of opioids for the treatment of chronic noncancer pain.[38] Opioids are often avoided in this patient population because of concerns over potential addiction, although these fears appear to be unfounded.[39,40]

Barriers continue to exist that prevent access to appropriate pain management, including:

- Poor integration of pain education into the training of physicians and other health care providers
- Unavailability of well-trained pain management physicians in some areas of the country
- Legal barriers (or fear of existing laws) regarding the administration of potent opioids
- Reimbursement issues for professional and facility services for pain care

Some of these can be effectively addressed through legislation at the state level; however, other issues must be addressed at the federal level, and still other issues involve changes in attitudes, beliefs, or practices that cannot be legislated. In addition, although there may be a temptation to turn to the legislative process to force change, such efforts can have unintended consequences.

The Virginia Experience

In 1994, Virginia was one of the first states to address the topics of acute, chronic, and cancer pain through a comprehensive task force, incorporating opinions from multiple areas of representation from both legal and health care arenas.

The group consisted of several elected officials, lay members, and physicians. They assimilated information and heard testimony from nationally recognized clinicians and researchers, conducted site visits to pain facilities, hosted a national pain symposium, and received input from insurance carriers and state regulatory agencies. As a result of the success of their efforts, many states are modeling their pain commissions and task forces after the Virginia experience.

S U M M A R Y

Individuals experiencing pain should receive the best possible care to relieve their suffering. Interdisciplinary pain programs have had a significant impact on improving care to those suffering from pain and should have the opportunity to continue serving individuals experiencing pain. In addition, individuals who experience trauma and surgery continue to experience pain and will require the care that acute pain services provide. Likewise, as the population ages and the number of patients with cancer increases, this very deserving group will continue to use significantly more resources for the humane treatment of their pain and suffering.

Health care providers who attempt to be rigid and resistant to change rarely stop change. They do, however, often end up left in the wake of that change. It is vital that pain management providers continue to strive to meet the needs of the people they serve, and in doing so they will remain a vital part of the health care system. This will require them to improve their efforts at impacting the direction of health care policy development. It is imperative that organized efforts on the part of all pain care providers occur at the local and state level. The federal government has traditionally deferred specifics of health care policy to the individual state legislatures. However, the recent trend has been for more national intervention into direct day-to-day operational and policy issues. This will mandate more focus toward Washington and the development of federal policy that impacts the care of the patient with pain.

References

1. Etheredge L, Jones SB, Lewin L: What is driving health system change? *Health Affairs* 15:93, 1996.
2. Bodenheimer T: The HMO backlash: Righteous or reactionary? *N Engl J Med* 335:1601, 1996.
3. Andreopoulos S: The folly of teaching-hospital mergers. *N Engl J Med* 336:61, 1997.
4. Acute Pain Management Guideline Panel: *Acute pain management: Operative or medical procedures and trauma*. Clinical practice guideline. Rockville, Md: Agency for Health Care Policy and Research, Public Health Service, U.S. Department of Health and Human Services, 1992.
5. Ready LB: Practice guidelines for acute pain management in the perioperative setting: A report of the American Society of Anesthesiologists Task Force on Pain Management (Acute Pain Section). *Anesthesiology* 82:1071, 1995.
6. Task Force on Acute Pain: *Management of acute pain: A practical guide*. Seattle, IASP Publications, 1992.
7. Lomas J, Anderson GM, Domnick-Pierre K et al: Do practice guidelines guide practice? The effect of a consensus statement on the practice of physicians. *N Engl J Med* 321:1306, 1989.
8. Ferrell BR, Griffith H: Cost issues related to pain management: Report from the Cancer Pain Panel of the Agency for Health Care Policy and Research. *J Pain Symptom Manage* 9:221, 1994.
9. Forman HP, McClennan BL: Meeting of managerial science with medicine: The pace quickens. *JAMA* 276:1599, 1996.
10. Crummer MB, Carter V: Critical pathways: The pivotal tool. *J Cardiovasc Nurs* 7:30, 1993.
11. Rich MW, Beckham V, Wittenberg C et al: A multidisciplinary intervention to prevent the readmission of elderly patients with congestive heart failure. *N Engl J Med* 333:1190, 1995.
12. Ransom SB, McNeeley SG, Yono A et al: Implementation of a clinical pathway for cesarean section. *Am J Managed Care* 2:1374, 1996.
13. Blumenthal D, Epstein AM: Quality of health care. Part 6: The role of physicians in the future of quality management. *N Engl J Med* 335:1328, 1996.
14. Fischer SP: Development and effectiveness of an anesthesia preoperative evaluation clinic in a teaching hospital. *Anesthesiology* 85:196, 1996.
15. Rockeman MG: Prophylactic use of epidural mepivacaine/morphine, systemic diclofenac, and metamizole reduces postoperative morphine consumption after major abdominal surgery. *Anesthesiology* 84:1027, 1996.
16. Katz J, Jackson M, Kavanagh BP et al: Acute pain after thoracic surgery predicts long-term post-thoracotomy pain. *Clin J Pain* 12:50, 1996.
17. Brown DL: Providing perioperative analgesia care: A special unit or a special program? *Reg Anesth* 21:105, 1996.
18. Liu SS, Carpenter RL, Mackey DC et al: Effects of perioperative analgesia technique on rate of recovery after colon surgery. *Anesthesiology* 83:757, 1995.
19. Cheng DC, Karski J, Peniston C et al: Early tracheal extubation after coronary artery bypass graft surgery reduces costs and improves resource use: A prospective, randomized, controlled trial. *Anesthesiology* 85:1300, 1996.
20. Collier PE: Are one-day admissions for carotid endarterectomy feasible? *Am J Surg* 170:140, 1995.
21. Engelman RM, Rousou JA, Flack JE 3rd et al: Fast-track recovery of the coronary bypass patient. *Ann Thorac Surg* 58:1742, 1994.
22. Moniche S: Convalescence and hospital stay after colonic surgery with balance analgesia, early oral feeding, and enforced mobilization. *Eur J Surg* 161:283, 1995.
23. Pedersen SH, Douville LM, Eberlein TJ: Accelerated surgical stay programs. A mechanism to reduce health care costs. *Ann Surg* 219:374, 1994.
24. Weingarten S, Riedinger M, Conner L et al: Hip replacement and hip hemiarthroplasty surgery: Potential opportunities to shorten lengths of hospital stay. *Am J Med* 97:208, 1994.
25. Feine JS, Lund JP: An assessment of the efficiency of physical therapy and physical modalities for the control of chronic musculoskeletal pain. *Pain* 71:5, 1997.

26. Turk D: Interdisciplinary approach to pain management: Philosophy, operations, and efficacy. In Ashburn M, Rice L, editors: *The management of pain.* New York, Churchill Livingstone, 1998.

27. Hubbard JE, Tracy J, Morgan SF et al: Outcome measures of a chronic pain program: A prospective statistical study. *Clin J Pain* 12:330, 1996.

28. Fricton JR, Dall'Arancio D: Interdisciplinary management of myofascial pain of the masticatory muscles. In Friction J, Dubner R, editors: *Orofacial pain and temporomandibular disorders.* New York, Raven Press, 1995.

29. Ware JE: Measuring patient function and well being: Some lessons from the Medical Outcomes Study. In Heitgoff G, Lohr KN, editors: *Effectiveness and outcomes in health care: Proceedings of an invitational conference by the Institute of Medicine, Division of Health Care Services.* Washington DC, National Academy Press, 1990.

30. Tarlov AR, Ware JE Jr, Greenfield S et al: The Medical Outcomes Study: An application of methods for monitoring the results of medical care. *JAMA* 262:925, 1989.

31. Lepläge A, Hunt S: The problem of quality of life in medicine. *JAMA* 278:47, 1997.

32. Brook RH, McGlynn EA, Cleary PD: Quality of health care. Part 2: Measuring quality of care. *N Engl J Med* 335:966, 1996.

33. Chassin MR: Quality of health care. Part 3: Improving the quality of care. *N Engl J Med* 335:1060, 1996.

34. Smith JM: Effectively costing out options. *JAMA* 276:1180, 1996.

35. Russell LB, Gold MR, Siegel JE et al: The role of cost-effectiveness analysis in health and medicine. Panel on Cost-Effectiveness in Health and Medicine. *JAMA* 276:1172, 1996.

36. Drug Enforcement Administration: *Physician's manual: An information outline of the Controlled Substances Act of 1970.* Washington, DC, U.S. Department of Justice, 1990.

37. Koontz W: Guidelines for the use of opioids in the management of chronic, non-cancer pain. *Va Med Q* 125:11, 1998.

38. Portenoy RK: Opioid therapy for chronic nonmalignant pain: A review of the critical issues. *J Pain Symptom Manage* 11:203, 1996.

39. Perry S, Heidrich G: Management of pain during debridement: A survey of U.S. burn units. *Pain* 13:267, 1982.

40. Porter J, Jick H: Addiction rare in patients treated with narcotics. *N Engl J Med* 302:123, 1980.

1. The development of a critical pathway for the surgical patient must begin

    A. With postoperative assessment
    B. At the time of discharge
    C. In the operating room
    D. With preoperative assessment extending to the time of discharge

2. In an acute care setting, the outcome measures required are

    A. Morbidity and mortality
    B. Incidence and severity of complications
    C. Effectiveness of surgery
    D. Length of stay

3. The Balanced Budget Act of 1997 was intended to

    A. Curb Medicare spending
    B. Increase Medicare spending
    C. Have no effect on Medicare spending
    D. Abolish Medicare spending

4. Federal control over the use of controlled substances come from one of the following

    A. Balanced Budget Act of 1997
    B. Food and Drug Cosmetic Act administered by the Food and Drug Administration
    C. Judicial branch of the government
    D. Executive branch of the government

5. Public policy with regard to the oversight of health insurance has traditionally been administered at

    A. The federal level
    B. The state level
    C. The county level
    D. The city level

ANSWERS

1. D

2. C

3. A

4. B

5. B

CHAPTER 35

Pain Medicine and the Legal System

GEORGE E. PARSONS AND
WILLIAM T. ROBINSON III

Encounters between the medical profession and the legal system often result in an atmosphere of hostility, confrontation, resentment, and mutual distrust (characteristic of the East-West confrontations of the 1960s). To modify this situation and reduce natural hostilities, the parties involved must learn to view each encounter on a case-by-case basis. To do this effectively, the professionals in a legal-medical dispute must define, recognize, and respect the other's role and what is expected of them. The pain doctor, for example, is responsible for developing a treatment program and coordinating diagnostics and medical services for a patient. He or she is, therefore, responsible to the patient first, no matter what the purpose of a particular examination. Doctors should not be so interested in the legal implications. The doctor's approach, rather, should be objective: to examine, assess, diagnose, and treat. On the other hand, the lawyer generally enters the medical arena as an advocate for a patient, insurance company, or agency. The lawyer's purpose is to litigate or resolve issues. These matters often do not directly concern doctors, who are often seen as the lawyer's professional tool (i.e., they provide evidence that lawyers need to establish cause, condition, loss, and permanency between the patient and the legal arena). Thus, the role of the lawyer is often to coordinate services or information.

One analogy of the respective roles of doctors and lawyers compares the lawyer to a yard master on the railroad, who controls the scheduling of trains and is mindful of all the auxiliary services needed to run the train; whereas the doctor is the railroad engineer, who runs the train and is concerned with its daily functioning and its successful arrival at its destination. The lawyer, therefore, must be aware not only of the condition of the patient while under the doctor's care, but of all the million and one issues associated with daily living, such as how the patient relates to others, his or her economic stability, and family concerns, to name just a few. Doctors, although concerned with such issues, must not let them dictate patient care. To this end, the lawyer can, therefore, be very instrumental in helping set up financial assistance, gaining approval for medical care and placement, and perhaps reducing psychologic dependency and subsequent anxiety and depression so often seen in patients.

One should remember that a number of patients cannot work because of their pain, are, thus, without benefits or support, and have actually been forced to seek out legal representation.

MEDICAL RECORDS

The *catch* to this holistic approach of professional cooperation is that doctors must accept lawyers as legitimately and professionally concerned for patients and present written or oral information that fosters, not hinders, the relationship. Such cooperation begins with the initial consultation, including the doctor's handwritten notes, and continues until the patient is discharged. Even then, the doctor may be asked to testify with a reasonable degree of medical certainty about treatment and events that occurred years in the past.

Medical files play an important role in any legal case because they represent observations, opinions, and suggestions and are generally the first item lawyers attempt to obtain and review. In most jurisdictions, this requires a medical authorization signed by the patient.

In recording patient histories, doctors are strongly recommended to ask the patient to provide information about the cause of the pain. For instance, was this pain the result of an accident? How or where did it first occur? What was the nature of the activity when the pain began? Did the pain come on suddenly or develop over time? Had this pain or condition ever been present in the past?

Attention to prior pain or symptoms is of potential significance in the legal-medical process. Lack of prior pain or symptoms is typically used by the plaintiff's attorney to support the required causal relationship between a compensable condition and a legally significant event. On the other hand, the existence of prior pain or symptoms is typically used by the defense attorney to undermine the plaintiff's claim.

It is important that:

1. The doctor determines the residual effects of a patient's condition, both physical and psychologic. It is recommended that the doctor be specific and find out how much or how frequently the patient can lift; how long the patient can stand, sit, or walk; if the patient can bend, stoop, crawl, climb, reach, feel, see, taste, and smell; if the patient can get along with others, remember items, take care of daily activities, handle responsibilities, or be independent.
2. The doctor determines the permanency of the patient's condition. This can be done by ascertaining the activity level before the onset of pain, either by using the American Medical Association (AMA) *Guidelines to Impairment* (which every doctor should have in the office) or by measuring functional or psychologic loss.

3. Just because a patient is involved in litigation or some type of legal claim and has obtained the services of an attorney, it does not necessarily mean that the patient is not interested in treatment or that he or she will not get better until litigation is resolved. In contemporary American society, a patient's opportunity for good medical care is often tied to some legal or claims-related process. Unless the doctor acknowledges this reality and professionally cooperates with the patient or the patient's legal representative, the patient may often be denied the opportunity for good medical care.

MEDICAL-LEGAL COOPERATION

Doctors are encouraged to approach each situation on a case-by-case basis. A doctor's policy of not assisting patients in legal matters, either by not writing reports or by not providing testimony in depositions or in court appearances, may reduce greatly that doctor's interaction with lawyers but, on the other hand, skews that doctor's patient load. Realistically, such a closed-door approach by a doctor does not stop lawyers from seeking and obtaining consultations or written progress notes and medical records.

In medical-legal matters, the basic difficulty for doctors is that their training has typically been limited to the medical care and treatment of patients. Doctors are usually not sensitive to patients' social or economic needs or, more directly, are not aware of how their medical opinions or statements are interpreted by professionals outside the medical community. Doctors typically do not realize that their opinions can result in favorable or unfavorable socioeconomic decisions for their patients outside the medical arena.

Any doctor is well advised to maintain the highest professional and ethical standards at all times. Although flexibility and cooperation are essential to a good professional working relationship, every doctor must expect every lawyer to approach each legal-medical matter ethically and professionally. The doctor will get the respect that he or she demands. The destruction or strategic "loss" of medical records or file materials is absolutely wrong, and the suggestion of such should be resisted without exception. In addition to being ethically wrong, the destruction or strategic loss of medical records or file materials may well result in significant legal liability for the doctor as well as the lawyer.

Although the negative must be reviewed and emphasized, most lawyers, like most doctors, approach a legal-medical matter ethically and professionally. The American system of dispute resolution is rooted in an adversary system. Adversary does not mean hostile or argumentative but rather indicates respect for the right of parties in a dispute to present their respective positions in the best possible light for a particular decision maker, be that decision maker a judge, a workers' compensation hearing officer, or an administrative law judge in a Social Security case. It is important that the doctor cooperate with a patient's legal representative to the extent ethically permissible. Each doctor must determine the extent to which he or she will play an advocacy role in the patient's legal matters. Again, the doctor must make such determinations on a case-by-case basis.

FORMULATION AND COMPILATION OF EVIDENCE

The first encounter between doctors and lawyers on a legal-medical matter is usually the point at which medical records and documentation complied in the ordinary course of medical practice constitute evidence. Although such evidence could be considered hearsay, it is admissible and significant in the legal process because the law presumes that a patient in pain is truthful because of the patient's perceived interest in getting better. Such evidence is typically recorded before the legal process even begins and is not tainted by the possibility of strategic legal considerations.

The experienced doctor is sensitive to the potential legal significance of medical records. In legal-medical matters, accuracy and thoroughness in record keeping are critically important for the doctor as well as the patient. Obviously, the patient has a vested interest in having accurate medical record to substantiate a legitimate legal claim if necessary. However, the doctor, too, has a vested interest in such medical records. The doctor's interests are first of all related to the doctor's own potential liability as a practicing physician in contemporary society, in which malpractice litigation is not an infrequent problem. Moreover, a doctor's professional reputation and effectiveness as a witness is enhanced if that doctor's testimony in a deposition or court case is accurately rooted in correct medical data recorded in the clinical record of the patient.

In most cases, there is a dichotomy between the written medical materials or progress notes developed during examination and treatment and the lawyer's need to use such medical information strategically to serve the socioeconomic interests of the lawyer's client (the doctor's patient).

NEED FOR BEHAVIORAL OBSERVATIONS

The doctor should respond to these competing interests by being as objective as possible. It is better for the doctor to report actual behavior and test findings and quote the patient's own comments and response to treatment. Such observations in the medical record should be tied to date, time, and circumstances. Lawyers prefer that doctors present documentation enhanced by concrete examples of behavior. If, as is the general rule at the time of examination, a patient is asked to cite restrictions or changes in daily-life activities, then the doctor has in the chart a factual basis to support the conclusions and opinions he or she later offers in testimony.

The doctor's recorded observations about the patient's behavior can have "nuclear" significance in the legal arena. A casual comment that is only part of a larger clinical picture may be taken out of context by the lawyer to advance the interests of his or her client or undermine the doctor's testimony at a later proceeding. Although there is absolutely no way to protect the patient or the doctor in this regard, accurate, factual record keeping affords the doctor more opportunity for amplification later in the case when more medical data and clinical progress can be evaluated and factored into a clinical observation or legal opinion. Problems in this area often result when clerical office personnel record statements from the patient in the medical chart. The doctor should always maintain supervisory and critical control of the chart in this regard.

Occasionally, a lawyer may tell a doctor that his or her testimony will damage the client's case. This conclusion is more likely to be drawn by a plaintiff's attorney who sees the case as "a loser." Doctors do not win or lose cases. Quality care and treatment are the major concerns.

Consideration should be given to how much discretion should properly be vested in the role of clerical personnel. It should be remembered that in court, the doctors' testimony is measured against the medical chart as if the doctor made every entry about the particular patient. To the extent then that any part of record charting is delegated, it should be done under clear and specific office or institutional policies that ensure a high standard of completeness and accuracy.

THE MEDICAL REPORT

Not infrequently, a doctor's first encounter with the lawyer is a written request for a copy of the doctor's medical records on a patient and a medical report setting out the course of treatment and the doctor's opinions. The law is clear throughout the United Sates that the medical chart belongs to the patient. Attempts to deny or forestall a request for the medical chart only results in aggravation and, sometimes, needless legal expense for the doctor. The medical report is not legally required but it is typically provided.

Typically, the next procedural step for the doctor is to write a medical report on that patient. The medical report can be helpful in the most damaging step in the legal-medical maze. Usually this report is written without the guidance of the patient's lawyer and without recognition of the potential legal dangers involved.

Too often, the responsibility for compiling the report is delegated to office personnel. Such an approach is short-sighted and often backfires on the doctor. Although clerical personnel can be helpful in pulling together information from the chart, the doctor should personally review the chart and dictate the report to ensure that it is accurate and does not understate or overstate the doctor's opinions. Again, in the hands of a skillful cross-examining lawyer, an unartfully or inaccurately drawn report can be a sharp sword on which the doctor is verbally impaled.

It should be noted that the clerical costs associated with providing medical records to the requesting lawyer are fully reimbursable to the doctor. As for a medical report, which typically takes time from the doctor's clinical practice, it is standard for the doctor to receive a fee for providing such a report card and, especially in larger metropolitan areas, it is not untypical for the doctor to require payment for the report in advance.

The accuracy of the medical report is directly dependent on the accuracy and completeness of the medical chart. The medical report should indicate history, treatment, diagnosis, causation, and prognosis. The medical report is a good way of summarizing medical observations, findings, and conclusions and should follow a normal consultation format. Rather than setting out recommendations, the medical report should be limited to facts and data gleaned from the medical chart and the doctor's opinion and prognosis. The legal system requires that such opinions be offered within the realm of reasonable medical certainty or probability. Every doctor is advised to consult with a respected lawyer with litigation expertise to learn the meaning of *reasonable medical certainty* or *reasonable medical probability* because these terms may be used in the legal jurisdiction where the doctor practices medicine. Most jurisdictions define the terms as meaning "more likely than not."

TESTIMONY UNDER OATH

The typical dispute resolution format of the legal medical process can be compared to a baseball diamond: first base is examination/treatment; second base is the accumulation of medical records; third base is the medical report; and home plate is the doctor's testimony, either by deposition or in person at the trial.

Testimony under oath causes doctors anxiety, fear, and aggravation. Some doctors attempt to avoid giving testimony and approach this responsibility with an uncooperative attitude. Testimony from a doctor taking such an approach can be damaging to the patient's case and can result in friction and frustration for all the parties. On the other hand, doctors who approach this responsibility knowledgeably and with a positive attitude can assist the patient in the legal process and, at the same time, receive reasonable compensation for the services that are provided.

Sworn testimony is a method of introducing facts and opinions into evidence and may be obtained and recorded by deposition or by personal appearance in court. Depositions may be used for discovery or to later present testimony at trial.

For the lawyer, stage presentation is very important. Therefore, a good lawyer meets with a doctor before the court appearance to review the medical chart and, just as important, information that the lawyer obtained from other sources. Every doctor faced with the prospect of testifying should welcome and, in fact, insist on an opportunity to learn what pertinent information the attorney has about the particular case.

Lawyers do have to contend with rules and regulations that may appear foreign to doctors but are, nonetheless, important to the trial and, therefore, must be observed and respected. Rules of evidence are an example. It is important that the doctor concentrate on the substance of the medical testimony and not be concerned with the lawyer's maneuvers with objections or interruptions.

During the doctor's testimony, which is done under oath and recorded for future reference, lawyers object to content, inferences, and perhaps methods of questioning or response. In a courtroom situation, the objection receives a response from the judge or referee, who states "sustained" or "overruled." Some lawyers may use the objection to upset the witness or disrupt the flow of testimony. Again, it is important that the doctor witness not openly react but rather allow the opposing attorneys and the judge to resolve the situation. A lawyer who gets overruled on a frequent basis will appear to be losing.

The Deposition

The deposition is certainly *show time*. For the most part, the plaintiff's lawyer wants to make the client look deserving, whereas the defense attorney attempts to undermine, challenge credibility, or lessen the chance for the plaintiff to succeed. The treating physician is almost always the first witness approached by the plaintiff's attorney, both in case preparation and in the presentation of court testimony. Direct testimony comes before cross examination. Direct testimony begins with witness identification and professional qualifications. Some doctors submit 30 or more typewritten pages detailing medical practice experience, educational institutions attended, hospitals where clinical programs were successfully completed, hospitals where staff privileges are enjoyed, and an itemization of professional publications. Such a lengthy recitation of facts can be tedious for the doctor witness; however, the impressive list of credentials and professional experience makes an impression on the judge or jury who decide the case. The opposing attorney tries to stipulate, or agree that the doctor is qualified, but the attorney using the doctor as a witness takes the time to impress everyone in the courtroom with the professional credibility of the doctor witness.

Once the qualifications of the doctor witness have been established in question-and-answer format, the lawyer generally asks if the doctor is familiar with the patient and how the doctor's professional relationship with the patient began and developed. The doctor then may verbally review, step-by-step, the clinical course taken with the patient and indicate differential diagnoses and, when appropriate, the final diagnoses. Typically, the doctor witness is requested to provide a prognosis, explaining residual functional impairment, if any.

Again, it is important for the doctor to understand that the lawyer is attempting to depict the doctor as qualified, knowledgeable, compassionate, thorough, flexible, hard working, and, most of all, credible. Negative impressions are the goal of the opposing counsel on cross examination. Most appear to have taken a graduate course in Machiavellian studies and to have graduated magna cum laude.

For the experienced, well-prepared doctor witness, testimony under oath is a challenging opportunity with a number of positive characteristics or advantages. Objectively, a doctor's testimony may have little to do with his or her ability as a doctor but may have a great deal to do with his or her quality of patient care and education of the public about medicine and doctors' efforts to assist others in society by means other than medical treatment.

When medical testimony is given in the courtroom, the judge immediately rules on objections and determines what is or what is not admissible as evidence. When medical testimony is given by deposition, objections are made but not ruled on by the judge until some later date. The decision maker or judge is not present; therefore, the objection is made but has no bearing on the doctor's testimony. The doctor witness should not testify any differently in a deposition than in the courtroom. So as a rule, the doctor should not change a thing but should continue to testify as if there had been no objection. If the objection is upheld at some later date, then the doctor's testimony may be edited at that time. If the deposition is recorded stenographically, less attention must be paid to personal appearance and the physical circumstances surrounding the deposition.

Preparing the Testimony

In preparing for any testimony, a doctor is well advised to thoroughly review the patient's file and include all materials that have been accumulated, used, and relied on to administer treatment to and reach conclusions about the patient. The doctor can be questioned about medical records and opinions from other doctors and medical providers that are in the file and that have been used for treatment. It is advisable then, in preparation for giving testimony, that a doctor witness take the time to call other physicians or medical providers who may have participated in the patient's clinical course, especially when that physician or medical provider's findings and opinions have been relied on by the doctor witness. Contradictions between different doctor witnesses can develop if doctors and medical providers do not communicate with each other in advance of testimony.

Clinical notes and records represent a doctor's professional findings and observations and are designed to be meaningful to that doctor and other medical professionals who may refer to the chart later for diagnosis or treatment.

Charges and Rates

Once medical testimony has been given by the doctor witness, the doctor's role in the legal dispute is usually finished. If the testimony has been given at trial, the doctor should immediately leave. For the doctor to hang around the courtroom or the administrative hearing may indicate to the judge, jury, or hearing officer that the doctor witness is too much of an advocate or has too much of an interest in the outcome of the proceedings. Having given the testimony as requested, all that remains for the doctor is to be fairly compensated for giving the testimony. Payment for the doctor's testimony may never be contingent on the outcome of the legal proceedings. The doctor should understand that he or she is being paid for the time. Doctors are encouraged to check with other doctors who regularly testify in their particular market or geographic areas to determine standard charges and rates for such services.

In many cases, during the course of the doctor's testimony, the opposing lawyer asks the amount of the doctor's charges for medical reports and for giving testimony. Many doctors are confused about the purpose of questions about the costs of the medical treatment that has been provided to the patient. In the legal system such medical expenses represent damages and must be proved to be recoverable. It is, therefore, necessary for the doctor to make available a written statement for past fees charged for care and treatment of the patient.

Independent Medical Examinations

From time to time, in the ordinary course of medical practice, doctors are regularly requested to perform independent medical examinations for other physicians. For the most part, such requests generally involve providing a second opinion concerning diagnosis, treatment, and prognosis. In the medical arena, this is seen as a resource document designed to assist and enlighten fellow professionals and to meet insurance requirements. Most doctors are comfortable giving such second opinions.

In the legal community, an independent medical examination generally has a much broader scope and significance than a second medical opinion. An independent medical examination can be used to validate a condition, a cause, or a particular type of treatment. It may also produce opposite or counter-opinions to that of the attending physician, thus creating an issue of confidence and/or credibility.

To a litigation lawyer, every case must be prepared as if it is to be tried. Such a lawyer has two primary tasks: (1) to find evidence to support or establish his or her case and (2) to undermine or distort the opinions of professional witnesses and thereby raise doubts about the validity, credibility, and reliability of the evidence. The independent medical examination is a tool that lawyers use to accomplish these tasks. It is also important that doctors understand that the opinions expressed in an independent medical examination may also be used to support or deny medical treatment.

Independent medical examinations are also used to neutralize, rather than defeat, an opposing party's case or claim. An independent medical examination may reduce the ultimate finding of permanent impairment or residual disability and thereby lessen the amount of the award or verdict. Of course, it is always possible that the independent medical examination will strongly support and verify a condition and its cause and be in total agreement with the treatment physician. When such a finding occurs, most attorneys would be recommended to settle or cave in. Settlement often is related more to the potential verdict than it is to the substantive evidence pointing in one direction. Although the independent medical examination may not be the deciding factor with regard to a settlement, it certainly strongly influences the attorney to prolong the case.

It may surprise a doctor to learn that the selection of certain doctors to perform an independent medical examination is determined by whether the lawyers represent plaintiffs or defendants. From the defense side, the lawyer typically looks for a doctor who will find, as a result of the injury in question, that "the patient is better than God made him." The plaintiff's lawyer typically looks for a doctor who will consistently offer the opinion that this patient is one "whose chances for recovery are slim or none." To someone unfamiliar with the system, it may often appear that the findings of the independent medical examination are too often consistent with the interests of the party paying for the independent medical examination. Realistically, however, good lawyers do not seek precooked opinions but rather opinions that have credibility. On the other hand, many claims for bodily injury involve gray areas of interpretation and, like people in other walks of life, doctors tend to base their conclusions on either a conservative or liberal philosophical outlook. As one would expect, defense lawyers look for doctors with a more conservative philosophy, and plaintiff lawyers look for doctors with a more liberal philosophy. The conservative doctor usually concludes that the claimant does not have objective findings to support the claimant's subjective complaints, whereas the more liberal doctor usually finds that the claimant's subjective complaints are consistent with the test data and clinical findings.

A contractual agreement usually precedes the independent medical examination. This contract or letter hopefully avoids any future disputes about payment. Asking for a reasonable amount of money up front as a retainer is acceptable to the legal community and is generally expected.

Consistency, both in defense and plaintiff's work, certainly adds to the reputation for objectivity of the physician performing an independent medical examination. A word to the wise, request for payments for legal services rendered by the doctor should be the same for both plaintiff's or defense attorneys and not based on which party has more financial support; if not, the doctor will give the appearance of subjectivity and favoritism.

In addition to a contractual agreement for payment, it is also helpful that the attorney provide the doctor performing the independent medical examination with all relevant and necessary medical information in advance. Without such information, the doctor's objectivity and accuracy can be compromised, and the doctor's opinion may be successfully challenged later in the legal proceedings. It is also advisable that the doctor freely communicate with the lawyer who arranged the independent medical examination to ensure that all relevant and material information is available to the doctor and is consistent with the doctor's findings. Such an approach can also make the independent medical examination a more efficient procedure, thereby reducing the costs to the responsible party.

Good attorneys show initiative and thoroughly prepare pertinent material for the doctor performing the independent medical examination. On the other hand, it is frustrating and counterproductive if the doctor does not take the time to thoroughly review the materials provided and incorporate the information into his or her report. Although the compensation for an independent medical examination is typically generous, a doctor should not accept such a responsibility unless he or she is prepared to take sufficient time to conduct the examination correctly. An improper or inadequate independent medical examination not only can damage the case of the party who has arranged for it to be performed but also can damage the credibility and reputation of the doctor who is unable to withstand the challenges presented by an efficient cross examination. Like death and taxes, cross examination is always around the corner in litigation. Moreover, the doctor who performs an independent medical examination must be able to confidently stand behind the opinion rendered and not be persuaded by an overly enthused lawyer whose advocacy clouds or compromises the doctor's ethical standards.

A litigation lawyer views the independent medical examination as a positive tool to balance the case at hand; it provides another opinion that is hopefully not swayed by the partiality that typically exists between a treating physician and a patient. To the practicing physician, the independent medical examination can be an interesting professional exercise for which the compensation is excellent and the performance of which can offer opportunities for learning beyond those offered in the daily practice of medicine.

SUMMARY

Before concluding, there are a few additional points that may be useful to the reader. First of all, a doctor should not be rushed or hurried in carrying out responsibilities as a doctor witness. A doctor's testimony is more credible and persuasive if the doctor's is confident and deliberate. The doctor's confidence is enhanced if the doctor takes enough time to thoroughly prepare and cooperates with the lawyer who has requested the doctor's professional assistance. The doctor should be, and should appear to be, objective, not a hired gun. A doctor should be careful with attempts at humor; embarrassment may be the only result. A doctor should avoid appearing to be an advocate; that is the lawyer's job. At all times, a doctor witness must keep personal emotions under control. If a mistake is made, the doctor should admit it. On the other hand, the doctor should not be too quick to concede a point to the cross-examining lawyer when a good explanation would help the patient and enhance the doctor's credibility. It is okay to be imperfect, to have a sense of humor, or even to ask an attorney to repeat a question. Lastly, silence can be as effective a tool of communication as speech but must be used effectively and goes hand in hand with being a good listener.

By their natures, the practices of law and medicine always interrelate with some degree of tension. On the other hand, professionalism and mutual respect can foster effective communication and positive results in the best interests of their patient/client. Hopefully, this chapter has offered some insight into the potential for an effective working relationship between doctors and lawyers. This brief treatment of such a complex subject only scratches the surface.

True, doctors and lawyers disagree on many points regarding the purpose and intent of their professional roles. However, as a diversion for normal professional duties and as a method of educating the public about the treatment and care of pain patients, the involvement of the doctor with lawyers, courts, and testimony can be personally exhilarating and professionally rewarding.

Questions • Pain Medicine and the Legal System

1. The first item the lawyers attempt to obtain for review

   A. Patient's medical bills
   B. Patient's place of residence
   C. Patient's relatives
   D. Patient's medical files

2. The medical report requested by a lawyer should contain all of the following except

   A. The patient's diagnosis
   B. The patient's course of treatment
   C. The doctor's opinions
   D. The cost of treatment

3. In preparing for any testimony, a doctor is well advised to do all of the following except

   A. Thoroughly review a patient's file
   B. Include in the testimony materials relied on to direct treatment
   C. Include in the testimony materials to reach conclusions
   D. Discard the referral letter received by the physician

4. In the legal community an independent medical examination when compared to a second medical opinion generally has

   A. Lesser significance
   B. Greater significance
   C. Equal significance
   D. No significance

5. As an expert witness a doctor should be all of the following except

   A. Credible
   B. Evasive
   C. Confident
   D. Deliberate

ANSWERS

1. D
2. D
3. D
4. B
5. B

CHAPTER 36

Ethical Issues in Pain Management

R. G. ADDISON

Ethics can best be described as proper conduct in human relationships. Clinical medicine ethics embodies the highest principles of clinical medicine and forms the basis of the highest standards of clinical pain ethics.

The foundation of consensual ethical values, as described by Josephson Institute of Ethics, that helps form an ethical society is honesty, integrity, respect, caring, fairness, keeping of promises, pursuit of excellence, civic duty, accountability, and loyalty.

The American Medical Association publishes a *Code of Medical Ethics,* which includes fundamental elements of the patient-physician relationship and principles of medical ethics involving professional responsibility and obligations of physicians.

Moral considerations become the professional elements of responsibility and accountability in medical ethics. The Hippocratic oath has, as one of its foundations, "The good of the patient" and determines the credibility of a morally sound decision.

Ethics as it relates to health care providers sometimes is confused by quality of care. Ethical dilemmas specific to medical ethics for the delivery of health care for those in pain include:

1. The issue of rigidity in medication delivery versus the pain medication needs of the individual. An ethical principle should be not to prescribe the same treatment for all people in pain
2. The need to consider emotional and/or social aspects of people complaining of pain
3. The biopsychosocioeconomic impact of chronic pain

The best tenet of ethical conduct for the pain therapist must include the development and maintenance of a deeply ingrained commitment to the best interest of the patient. Ethical conduct should be no different than the principles espoused in the Ten Commandments and/or the Golden Rule. It is important to bridge the gap existing between law, religion, economics, and ethics.

Some controversial ethical issues need to be studied, including cancer pain, pain involving AIDS, euthanasia, acute pain, chronic pain syndrome, and administration of placebos.

Concepts such as patients' rights, autonomy, and best interests need to be an integral part of pain management, especially as it deals with chronicity, sensitivity to the many ways that chronic pain affects the patient, the ways it affects the family and social relationships, and the impact it makes on the system of health and social welfare care.

Some ethical and bioethical problems are constantly present, including:

- Ways to care for indigent patients who seek treatment
- Ways to adjust quality of care in the present managed-care society
- Relationship between the caregiver and the patient
- Dealing with patients who refuse to participate in adequate health care
- The personal skills and technical capability of the health caregiver
- The dilemma of spiraling costs

Good clinical care and good clinical ethics go hand in hand, and both standards must be equally high. Another issue involves regulations placed on caregivers by the laws of the land. The patient is, today, a consumer who demands that the physician be proficient in the basic skills of his or her specialty including history taking, physical diagnosis, analysis of clinical data, and clinical decision making. Equally important is the ability to communicate findings to the patient and appropriate colleagues; to be a friend, advisor, advocate, educator, and student; and to guide the patient through the medical bureaucracy.

Trust between the patient and doctor has to be earned. There is a need to retain and revitalize the doctor-patient relationship. Medicine is inherently a moral enterprise that depends greatly on the integrity of the individual professional facing the daily needs of the patient.

The patient should be the absolute center of medical concerns, which is more and more difficult in the present managed-care society. The health care professional must be aware of the issues that enable him or her to select, initiate, and ethically terminate treatment. This can be accomplished by setting appropriate goals that take into account the patient's autonomy, the professional effectiveness, and commitment to proper care for people in pain.

Physicians must continue to remind themselves of the need for confidential trust and truth. Although physicians will continue to be challenged by rising costs, ability to pay, stress, and personal physical and outside pressures, they must revitalize the patient-doctor relationship and return to the basic tenets of the moral code of ethics of the medical profession.

Those committed to the care of patients should continue to refine their commitment to ethical principles. The various pain organizations should refresh awareness of ethics, continue to review complaints of patients, and suggest revisions to the code of ethics when appropriate. Although enforcement is always difficult, ethical opinions need to be developed. It behooves all physicians to be aware of their specialty's position related to ethical matters and conduct.

Suggested Reading

1. American Medical Association: *Code of medical ethics, current opinion.* Chicago, American Medical Association, 1992.
2. Callahan D, Bok S, editors: *Hastings Center, project on the teaching of ethics: Summary recommendations.* New York, Plenum Press, 1980.
3. Hass JF: Ethics in rehabilitation medicine. *Arch Phys Med Rehabil* 67:270, 1986.
4. Josephson M: *Making ethical decisions.* Los Angeles, Josephson Institute of Ethics, 1992.

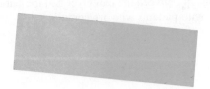

Questions • Ethical Issues in Pain Management

1. Medical ethics can best be described as

   A. Proper conduct in patient relations
   B. Proper care of the patient
   C. Proper appearance of the physician when first encountering the patient
   D. Proper documentation of the examination of the patient

2. Ethical dilemmas for the delivery of healthcare include

   A. The issue of rigidity in medication delivery versus the pain medication needs of the individual
   B. The need to consider the emotional or social aspect of the pain patient
   C. Biopsychosocialeconomic impact of chronic pain
   D. Patient's relationship with his or her close relatives

3. Some ethical and bioethical problems include all of the following except

   A. Ways to care for indigent patients who seek treatment
   B. Relationship between the caregiver and the patient
   C. Dealing with patients who are compliant
   D. Dilemma of spiraling cost

4. Trust between the patient and the doctor

   A. Has to be earned
   B. Is easy to obtain
   C. Is difficult to obtain
   D. Is not important

5. A code of medical ethics that includes fundamental elements of the patient-physician relationship and principles of medical ethics involving professional responsibility and obligations of physicians is published by

   A. American Board of Specialties
   B. American Medical Association
   C. International Association for the Study of Pain
   D. Office of Human and Health Services

ANSWERS

1. A
2. D
3. C
4. A
5. B

Test Bank I

For the following questions, choose one correct answer.

1. In which of the following ancient countries was pain considered the result of spirits of the dead entering an individual's body through an ear or nostril?

   A. India
   B. Egypt
   C. Greece
   D. China

2. The site of substance P in the peripheral tissues is

   A. Plasma
   B. Vascular endothelium
   C. Nerve terminals
   D. Mast cells

3. Within the medical history, limitations of activity created by painful disorders are often recorded as part of the

   A. Chief complaint
   B. Systems review
   C. Past medical history
   D. Social occupational history

4. A history of being "allergic" to a specific analgesic medication should be checked to determine whether the symptoms that occurred following ingestion represented

   A. An unexpected bitter taste
   B. A common unpleasant side effect
   C. Reduced efficacy of the medicine
   D. A potentially serious adverse reaction

5. A WBC differential has all of the following components EXCEPT

   A. Basophils
   B. Neutrophils
   C. Eosinophils
   D. Microphils

6. Magnetic resonance imaging is not the study of choice in which disease state of the brain?

   A. Neoplasm
   B. Inflammation
   C. Acute hemorrhage
   D. Demyelinating disease

7. The most significant difference between the active and passive phenomena measured during electrodiagnostic testing is that

   A. The former are associated with spontaneous or evoked changes in electrical potential difference
   B. The latter are only created by passive stretching of nerve roots
   C. The former may be used to diagnose severe active joint disease
   D. Measurements of the latter may be made on neural, but not nonneural, tissue

8. The principle of modified differential spinal block is to observe changes in the patient's pain

   A. At the onset of the block
   B. During the effect of the block
   C. At the recovery of the block
   D. After the recovery of the block

9. In chronic pain therapy the best route of drug administration is

   A. Intraspinal
   B. Intravenous (IV)
   C. Oral
   D. Transdermal

10. The mechanism of benzodiazepine is through binding with a specific receptor that is complexed to

    A. Dopamine receptor
    B. $GABA_A$ receptor
    C. Opiate receptor
    D. α-Adrenergic receptor

11. Landmarks for caudal block are all of the following EXCEPT

    A. Posterior superior iliac spine
    B. Anterior superior iliac spine
    C. Sacral cornu
    D. Sacral hiatus

12. A successful brachial plexus block by the interscalene approach will provide analgesia of all of the following EXCEPT

A. Shoulder
B. Inner aspect of the upper arm and elbow
C. Forearm
D. Hand

13. The celiac plexus is located just anterior to the crux of the diaphragm and extends several centimeters

A. Anterolaterally around the aorta
B. Posterolaterally around the aorta
C. Anteromedial to lumbar sympathetic ganglia
D. Posteromedial to lumbar sympathetic ganglia

14. A 30-year-old man had low back pain that radiated to the lateral aspect of his right leg. The pain was precipitated by the patient lifting a heavy object 3 days before onset. Which of the following statements is true?

A. An electromyogram (EMG) should be performed to localize the involved nerve root
B. A computed tomography (CT) scan is of no value because the injury is recent
C. Physical examination will show decreased knee jerk
D. The patient will probably have a good response to an epidural steroid injection

15. Segmental epidural analgesia mandates placement of an epidural catheter at sites adjacent to dermatomes covering the field of pain. This reduces dose requirements while increasing the specificity of spinal analgesia. Suggested interspaces for thoracic surgery are

A. T9 to T11
B. T2 to T8
C. C6 to T1
D. T12 to L2

16. Behavioral abnormalities that may interfere with the patient's ability to assess pain relief during preimplementation trials include

A. Preexisting chemical dependence on opioid analgesics
B. Preexisting psychiatric disease
C. Compliance of the patient
D. Patient desire for sedation and anxiolysis associated with systemic opioids

17. In terms of neurolytic activity, 40% ethanol is equal to approximately

A. 3% phenol in saline
B. 3% phenol in glycerin
C. 6% phenol in glycerin
D. 6% phenol + 3% chloroprocaine

18. Heat develops in tissue during radiofrequency thermocoagulation by

A. Convection
B. Conduction
C. Friction
D. The tip of the probe heat

19. There is controversy as to the mechanisms of faction of IV local anesthetic agents. Earlier theories suggested peripheral site of action at the arteriolar and capillary endothelia. The later theory suggests central nervous system (CNS) activity because

A. Spinal electrogram of deafferentation is changed with IV local anesthetics
B. IV local anesthetics affects the low-frequency discharge activity in the CNS
C. IV local anesthetic causes numbness in the periphery
D. Patient experiences hypotension with the use of IV local anesthetics

20. If trigeminal neuralgia fails to respond to oral medication, the most appropriate next step is to

A. Refer the patient for psychologic counseling and biofeedback
B. Inject the trigger zone with local anesthetic
C. Prescribe a combination of tricyclic mood elevators and phenothiazines
D. Refer the patient for rhizolysis of the nerve root or ganglion

21. The major factor in successful spinal cord stimulation is

A. Electrode positioning
B. Electrode combination
C. Size of electrode
D. Amount of current passed between electrodes

22. A process in which electrically charged molecules (ions) are driven into the tissue with an electrical field is known as

A. Vibration
B. Compression
C. Biofeedback
D. Iontophoresis

23. The standard practice of providing analgesia during labor is

A. Paracervical block
B. Continuous lumbar epidural analgesia
C. Patient-controlled analgesia
D. Spinal block

24. A specific nonarteriosclerotic lesion involving arteries, veins, and nerves that often leads to gangrene and is confined to medium-sized arteries of the distal leg or the arm is due to

A. Thromboangiitis obliterans
B. Thrombophlebitis
C. Diabetic gangrene
D. Frostbite

25. Side effects of methysergide include which of the following?

A. Anemia
B. Hyperglycemia
C. Retroperitoneal fibrosis
D. Photosensitivity

26. Glossopharyngeal neuralgia

    A. Can be diagnosed by finding trigger points
    B. Affects the abdominal viscera
    C. Is rarely seen in multiple sclerosis
    D. Occurs about as often as trigeminal neuralgia

27. The primary neurotransmitter at the preganglionic-postganglionic synapses in both divisions of the autonomic nervous system (ANS) is

    A. Serotonin
    B. Acetylcholine
    C. Vasoactive intestinal peptide
    D. Norepinephrine

28. Sympathomimetics, or adrenergic agonists, include all the following EXCEPT

    A. Phenylephrine
    B. Ritalin
    C. Methamphetamine
    D. Phentolamine

29. One of the reasons for failure of surgical sympathectomy has been

    A. Reinnervation of contralateral sympathetic chain
    B. Permanent destruction of the cut sympathetic chain
    C. Inability of myelinated A fibers to take over the function of sympathetic fibers
    D. Increased vascularity of the region effected by sympathectomy

30. Phantom limb sensation was first described in 1551 by

    A. Weir Mitchell
    B. Ambroise Paré
    C. Hippocrates
    D. Damas

31. Newborns respond to pain by demonstrating changes in the following EXCEPT

    A. Blood pressure and heart rate
    B. Transcutaneous PO_2
    C. Stress hormones
    D. Urine output

32. The percentage of school-aged children who complain of nonorganic abdominal pain is

    A. 0% to 5%
    B. 10% to 15%
    C. 15% to 20%
    D. 20% to 25%

33. The mechanism of action of IV regional bretylium is

    A. Accumulation and blockade of norepinephrine release from adrenergic nerves
    B. Depletion and release of norepinephrine from adrenergic nerves
    C. Blockade of the action of prostaglandins
    D. Reduction in the accumulation of substance P

34. The cell body of the neospinothalamic tract is located in which lamina?

    A. II
    B. III
    C. IV
    D. V

35. Second-order neurons of the nociceptive afferents are located in the

    A. Afferent axons
    B. Dorsal root ganglion
    C. Dorsal horn of the spinal cord
    D. Sympathetic ganglion

36. A commonly used drug for epidural steroid injection has the following ingredients EXCEPT

    A. Methylprednisolone acetate
    B. PEG 3350
    C. Myristyl-gamma picolinium chloride
    D. Benzyl alcohol

37. Which of the following symptoms is associated with pain and should be documented in the medical history?

    A. Paresthesias
    B. Hypesthesia
    C. Weakness
    D. Loss of vibration sense

38. Baclofen acts on what type of receptor?

    A. Opiate
    B. $GABA_B$
    C. α-Adrenergic
    D. Benzodiazepine

39. The mechanism of antipsychotic action of neuroleptics is due to the blockade of which type of receptor?

    A. Adrenergic
    B. Dopamine
    C. Opiate
    D. Serotonin

40. The most appropriate diagnostic nerve block for pain in the upper abdominal viscera is

    A. Intercostal block
    B. Lumbar sympathetic block
    C. Celiac plexus block
    D. Hypogastric plexus block

41. A facet joint injection of local anesthetic and steroids results in prolonged pain relief of 6 months or more in what percentage of patients?

    A. 30%
    B. 50%
    C. 70%
    D. 90%

42. Seizures produced by local anesthetics appear to arise from what area of the brain?

    A. Thalamus
    B. Geniculate bodies
    C. Reticular activating system
    D. Amygdala

43. Appropriate treatment of atypical facial pain includes which of the following?

    A. Antidepressants
    B. Anticonvulsants
    C. Antiemetics
    D. Cranial nerves V and IX section

44. Prohormone dynorphin (Pro enk B) is a natural ligand of which receptor type?

    A. μ
    B. κ
    C. δ
    D. ε

45. Which of the following is not a guiding principle of physical medicine and rehabilitation?

    A. Pain control
    B. Functional restoration
    C. Return to work and leisure activities
    D. Patient dependence on prolonged physical therapy

46. Areas innervated by the maxillary nerve include all of the following EXCEPT the

    A. Maxilla
    B. Skin over the middle third of the face
    C. Teeth of the upper jaw
    D. Tongue

47. All of the following statements are true of red blood cell (RBC) indexes EXCEPT

    A. They define the size and hemoglobin content of the RBCs
    B. They have replaced the need for examination of the peripheral blood smear in the diagnosis of anemia
    C. Microcytic indexes with anemia may result from iron deficiency
    D. Macrocytic indexes may result from folate deficiency

48. A celiac plexus block is effective in reducing pain originating from all of the following organs EXCEPT

    A. Pancreas
    B. Transverse portion of the large colon
    C. Gallbladder
    D. Descending portion of the pelvic colon

49. Which of the following is not a characteristic of central pain?

    A. Hyperesthesia
    B. Spontaneous pain
    C. Hypertrophia
    D. Hyperpathia

50. Which of the following statements regarding endometriosis is not true?

    A. It is a common cause of pelvic pain
    B. It is hormonally maintained and hormonally responsive
    C. A diagnosis can only be made with laparoscopic histopathologic confirmation
    D. A moderate to severe condition may be associated with an absence of painful sequelae

51. A patient complains of morning stiffness and pain in multiple joints, including the joints of the hand. Subcutaneous nodules are present over the extensor surfaces, and diagnostic tests indicate abnormal amounts of HLA-DR4. The most likely diagnosis is

    A. Osteoarthritis
    B. Rheumatoid arthritis
    C. Gout
    D. Degenerative arthritis

52. Skeletal pain generally emanates primarily from

    A. C fibers
    B. Joints
    C. Bones
    D. Surrounding soft tissue

53. The most common side effect from a lumbar sympathetic block is

    A. Dizziness
    B. Backache
    C. Nausea
    D. Hypotension

54. The most accurate pain assessment tools for preverbal children are

    A. Spatial scales
    B. Facial scales
    C. Numerical scales
    D. Physiologic measurements

55. Which of the following conditions mimics thalamic pain syndrome?

    A. Wallenberg's syndrome
    B. Syringomyelia
    C. Lateral medullary syndrome
    D. Parietal cortical lesion

56. A steady state of blood-drug concentration is achieved only after how many half lives?

    A. 1
    B. 3
    C. 5
    D. 7

57. Mydriasis, tachypnea, tachycardia, delirium, and a modest decrease in pain can be produced by agonists of which receptor type?

A. μ
B. κ
C. δ
D. σ

58. Transcutaneous electrical nerve stimulation relieves pain by

A. Depleting neurotransmitters in nociceptors
B. Stimulating C fibers directly
C. Activating inhibitory neurons
D. Destroying nociceptors

59. The peripheral theory of phantom limb pain suggests that pain is caused by

A. Spontaneous firing of neuromas
B. Early discharges from C fibers
C. Decreased sympathetic afferent activity
D. Late discharges from A delta fibers

60. What is the medium diameter efferent fiber to the muscle spindles?

A. A alpha
B. A beta
C. A delta
D. C

61. A lateral femoral cutaneous block is indicated for which of the following conditions?

A. Meralgia paresthetica
B. Femoral neuralgia
C. Saphenous neuralgia
D. Groin pain

62. Posttraumatic facial neuralgia is characterized by

A. Absence of sensory deficits
B. Trigger zones
C. Symptoms outside the trigeminal nerve distribution
D. Burning discomfort

63. Which of the following tests is confirmatory in the diagnosis of carpal tunnel syndrome?

A. Thermography
B. Somatosensory evoked potentials
C. Electromyography
D. Magnetic resonance imaging (MRI)

64. Which of the following medications does not relieve central pain?

A. Phenobarbital
B. Morphine sulphate
C. Carbamazepine
D. Amitriptyline

65. All of the following are contraindications to performing an MRI EXCEPT

A. Cerebral aneurysm clips
B. Cardiac pacemakers
C. Mechanical ventilation
D. Lack of patient cooperation

66. Which of the following interventions is not appropriate for treating acute disk herniation?

A. Muscle relaxation by cyclobenzaprine
B. Nonsteroidal anti-inflammatory drugs (NSAIDs)
C. Gentle limbering exercises
D. Cervical laminectomy and fusion

67. Stump pain occurs in what percentage of amputees?

A. 10%
B. 25%
C. 50%
D. 75%

68. Which of the following is used to assess reduction of range of motion associated with painful neuromuscular disorders?

A. Goniometry
B. Electromyography
C. Posturography
D. Inclinometry

69. Posterior rhizotomy is most effective in treating which of the following conditions?

A. Intractable chest wall pain
B. Sciatica after laminectomy
C. Pelvic pain and dyspareunia
D. Lumbar plexalgia secondary to metastatic lumbar vertebral lesion

70. The goals of treatment for rheumatoid arthritis include all of the following EXCEPT

A. Relief of pain
B. Reduction of inflammation
C. Preservation of function
D. Immobilization and bed rest

71. The credit of classifying the humors into phlegmatic, sanguine, choleric, and melancholic is given to which of the following?

A. Asclepias
B. Galen
C. Plato
D. Hippocrates

72. The most commonly used assessment tools for chronic pain are based on

A. Health care staff observations
B. Patient medication usage
C. Patient self-reporting
D. Psychiatric assessment

73. A standard laboratory "database" includes all of the following EXCEPT

    A. Urinalysis
    B. Complete blood count
    C. Serum protein electrophoresis
    D. Sedimentation rate

74. Painful paresthesias of the hands occurring at night may be associated with

    A. Slow nerve conductors across the ulnar groove
    B. Prolonged distal latencies at the wrist
    C. Reduced electromyographic amplitude
    D. Reduced somatosensory evoked response amplitude

75. When prescribing sublingual or buccal route of administration, the best drug (55%) for absorption is

    A. Methadone
    B. Fentanyl
    C. Morphine
    D. Buprenorphine

For questions 76 to 100 choose from the following

    A. **1, 2, and 3**
    B. **1 and 3**
    C. **2 and 4**
    D. **4**
    E. **All of the above**

76. Which of the following groups of patients are at risk for inadequate measurement?

    1. Elderly
    2. Pediatric
    3. Burn patients
    4. Low back pain patients

77. Which of the following statements about medical thermography is(are) true?

    1. It may be used as a graphic representation of a patient's pain
    2. Thermal asymmetry of more than 0.6°C is typically abnormal
    3. Proximal changes occur before distal changes
    4. Skin temperature continually fluctuates in response to physiologic and environmental conditions

78. The following symptoms of depression are observed in chronic pain patients

    1. Sleep disturbance
    2. Appetite disturbance
    3. Suicidal ideation
    4. Poor concentration and memory disturbance

79. Which of the following opioids are naturally occurring?

    1. Morphine
    2. Hydromorphone
    3. Codeine
    4. Methadone

80. Which of the following statements about ethanol are true?

    1. The minimum concentration of ethanol required for neurolysis is 10%
    2. Ethanol and local anesthetics are sometimes used together
    3. Ethanol is sometimes mixed with glycerin
    4. Alcohol spreads rapidly from the injection site

81. Which of the following types of cryoprobes are currently in clinical use?

    1. Gas expansion
    2. Helium gas
    3. Change of phase
    4. Joule-Thompson

82. A 7 year old involved in a multitrauma is evaluated by the pain management team. Appropriate options to be considered, dependent on the injuries sustained, might include

    1. Epidural analgesia
    2. Patient-controlled analgesia (PCA)
    3. Brachial plexus catheter
    4. Interpleural catheter

83. Injury of the long thoracic nerve will result in a deficit of the ipsilateral

    1. Scapula
    2. Chest wall sensation between T4 to T6
    3. Sensation of the underneath side of the upper arm
    4. Decreased respiratory effect secondary to block of the intercostalis muscles

84. Rational use of opioids in postoperative pain includes the following

    1. They should be used in the treatment of moderately severe to severe postoperative pain
    2. Meperidine should never be used because of accumulation of normeperidine
    3. The oral route should be used as soon as the patient tolerates oral intake
    4. They should not be withheld even with respiratory rates of less than 8 breaths/minute

85. Which of the following statement(s) is(are) true of symptoms of allodynia present in central pain?

    1. The appearance of symptoms may be delayed after the introduction of the eliciting stimulus
    2. The symptoms may be produced by nonpainful stimuli
    3. The symptoms may be excruciating
    4. The symptoms can be produced by mild stimuli

86. Which of the following medications is(are) appropriate for treatment of diabetic peripheral neuropathy?

    1. Carbamazepine
    2. Amitriptyline
    3. Desipramine
    4. Phenytoin

87. Which of the following neurolytic processes is(are) associated with neuritis or neuroma function?

1. Radiofrequency
2. Phenol neurolysis
3. Alcohol neurolysis
4. Cryoneurolysis

88. Which of the following statement(s) regarding opioid-mediated side effects is(are) true?

1. They can be managed symptomatically (e.g., laxatives, antiemetics, amphetamines)
2. They can be managed with a trial of a nonopioid adjuvant drug
3. They occur frequently, but with the exception of constipation, most usually recede after a short period
4. They may serve as a rationale to institute treatment with a different opioid or a more invasive approach

89. When implanting a drug-delivery system, the patient should be placed in which of the following positions?

1. Lateral
2. Sitting
3. Prone
4. Supine

90. Which of the following factors affect the measurement of oncologic pain?

1. Type of pain
2. Age of patient
3. Physical strength of patient
4. Pain rating scale used

91. The McGill Pain Questionnaire is designed to measure which of the following components of pain?

1. Societal
2. Sensory
3. Quantitative
4. Evaluative

92. Which of the following is(are) characteristic of myofascial trigger points?

1. A firm tense band in the involved muscle
2. A "jump sign" when the muscle band is snapped briskly
3. A predictable referred pain pattern
4. A pain reference zone that may exhibit autonomic changes

93. Selective tissue conductance is most appropriate in the assessment of which of the following conditions?

1. Sudomotor dysfunction
2. Sympathetically mediated pain
3. Postherpetic neuralgia
4. Ulnar neuropathy

94. Contact thermography

1. Is more reliable than infrared thermography
2. Is best performed at normal room temperatures
3. Can picture the entire body
4. Is less expensive than infrared thermography

95. The following therapeutic approaches are useful in treating chronic pain patients

1. Cognitive-behavioral
2. Contingency management or operant approaches
3. Hypnosis
4. Psychoanalytic therapy

96. Which of the following local anesthetics exist as chiral forms?

1. Bupivacaine
2. Mepivacaine
3. Etidocaine
4. Prilocaine

97. Patients with chronic back pain may respond to epidural steroid injections if

1. A local anesthetic is added to the steroid
2. They have a symptom-free interval
3. Three epidural steroid injections are given
4. Their new radiculopathy involves a nerve root different from the one they had before

98. Procedural complications related to the use of neurolytics include

1. Systemic toxic reactions caused by accidental intravascular injection
2. Hypotension secondary to sympathetic block
3. Intense pruritus in the facial area
4. High-output renal failure

99. Which of the following are indications for percutaneous cryoneurolysis?

1. Treatment of neuromas
2. Treatment of flexion contractures
3. Treatment of chest wall pain
4. Treatment of nerve entrapment pain

100. Which of the following premonitory symptoms and/or auras is(are) associated with migraine headaches?

1. Visual disturbances
2. Photophobia
3. Sonophobia
4. Nausea and vomiting

Answers

1. B	26. E	51. D	76. E
2. C	27. B	52. B	77. B
3. D	28. D	53. B	78. E
4. B	29. A	54. D	79. B
5. D	30. B	55. B	80. C
6. D	31. D	56. C	81. E
7. A	32. B	57. D	82. E
8. C	33. A	58. C	83. A
9. C	34. D	59. D	84. B
10. B	35. C	60. C	85. E
11. B	36. D	61. A	86. E
12. B	37. A	62. A	87. A
13. A	38. B	63. C	88. E
14. D	39. B	64. C	89. B
15. B	40. C	65. C	90. B
16. C	41. A	66. D	91. C
17. B	42. D	67. C	92. E
18. C	43. D	68. D	93. A
19. A	44. B	69. D	94. D
20. D	45. D	70. D	95. A
21. A	46. D	71. B	96. E
22. D	47. B	72. C	97. C
23. B	48. D	73. C	98. B
24. A	49. D	74. B	99. E
25. C	50. C	75. D	100. E

Test Bank II

For the following questions, choose one correct answer.

1. The mean conduction velocity of A-delta afferents that transmit nociceptive impulse is

   A. Greater than 15 m/second
   B. Greater than 8 m/second
   C. Greater than 3 m/second
   D. Less than 3 m/second

2. Within the medical history, limitations of activity created by painful disorders are often recorded as part of the

   A. Chief complaint
   B. Systems review
   C. Past medical history
   D. Social occupational history

3. Which of the following is least true of laboratory tests?

   A. They may be used as a confirmation of the working diagnosis
   B. They may aid in following the course of the disease
   C. They may help prevent iatrogenic complications
   D. They should be performed before the development of the initial differential diagnosis

4. On T1-weighted scans the cerebrospinal fluid (CSF) appears

   A. Black
   B. Gray
   C. White
   D. Blue

5. Myelography is the most useful method to evaluate which suspected disease state of the spine?

   A. Herniated nucleus pulposus with radiculopathy
   B. Osteophyte encroachment of neural foramen
   C. Vertebral body metastatic disease
   D. Spinal trauma with fracture of the posterior elements

6. Single-fiber electromyographic (EMG) recordings are helpful in assessing

   A. Sensory nerve fibers affected by ABC syndrome
   B. Jitter that occurs in some myopathies
   C. Postherpetic neuralgia
   D. Trigeminal neuralgia

7. Differential epidural block is inherently appealing because it

   A. Avoids lumbar puncture headache
   B. Takes longer time than differential spinal block
   C. Can be done by a small-gauge needle
   D. Must be done as an outpatient

8. The time required for drug to blood concentration to be alleved by a factor of two is called in pharmacokinetic terms

   A. Clearance
   B. Volume of distribution
   C. Half-life
   D. Redistribution

9. Side effects of neuroleptics include all of the following EXCEPT

   A. Dystonia
   B. Akathisia
   C. Drug-induced parkinsonism
   D. Muscular flaccidity

10. Areas innervated by glossopharyngeal nerve are all of the following EXCEPT

    A. Palatine tonsils
    B. Posterior one third of the tongue
    C. Pharyngeal wall
    D. Epiglottis

11. Cervical epidural anesthesia is indicated for pain relief and surgery for

    A. Carotid endarterectomy
    B. Cholecystitis
    C. Hysterectomy
    D. Knee replacement

12. The intercostal nerve block is commonly done at all of the following EXCEPT

    A. At the angle of the rib posteriorly
    B. At the posterior axillary line
    C. At the midaxillary line
    D. At the head of the rib posteriorly

13. For patients with a large abdominal mass and difficulty in lying prone, this approach is indicated for celiac plexus block

    A. Lateral approach
    B. Anterior approach
    C. Sitting approach
    D. Surgical open approach

14. The polyethylene glycol in depot steroids

    A. Does not cause degenerative lesions in nerves of experimental animals
    B. Is present in methylprednisolone but not triamcinolone
    C. Is not concentrated enough in the commercial preparation to block nerve transmission
    D. Does not cause arachnoiditis when injected intrathecally

15. The diagnosis of facet syndrome is made by all of the following EXCEPT

    A. History
    B. Physical examination
    C. Radiographic evaluation
    D. Blood chemistry

16. In comparison with each drug infused alone, combinations of local anesthetics and opioids provide pain relief

    A. Of lesser magnitude
    B. Of greater magnitude
    C. With more side effects
    D. With lesser reliability

17. Contraindications of implantation of a drug-delivery system include all of the following EXCEPT

    A. Sepsis
    B. Coagulopathy
    C. Bipolar personality
    D. Cancer pain

18. What degree of nerve injury is produced with a cryolesion?

    A. First
    B. Second
    C. Third
    D. Fourth

19. Which of the following sensations is essential for a successful acupuncture treatment?

    A. Cun
    B. Techi
    C. Suan
    D. Ma

20. The side effects of intravenous (IV) local anesthetics are related to central nervous system (CNS) toxicity. Early signs are all of the following EXCEPT

    A. Metallic taste
    B. Tinnitus
    C. Agitation
    D. Increased appetite

21. Mesencephalotomy is a

    A. Procedure done in the midmenstrual cycle
    B. Lesion in the middle of the cerebral hemispheres
    C. Stereotactic lesion not often used today
    D. Special procedure with limited pain treatment

22. Spinal cord stimulation has been demonstrated to be somewhat effective in which of the following disease states?

    A. Spasmodic torticollis
    B. Mixed-migraine headaches
    C. Temporal arteritis
    D. Cluster headaches

23. The contraindication for heat therapy is

    A. Pain
    B. Muscle spasm
    C. Edema
    D. Bursitis

24. Respiratory depression from epidural opioids is characterized by

    A. A respiratory rate that is an adequate indicator of ventilatory status
    B. A pattern of respiratory depression that is slow and progressive rather than sudden apnea
    C. Sedation that is not a significant indicator in its development
    D. Increased incidence unrelated to the vertebral level of opioid injection

25. The most appropriate method of providing analgesia for labor by patient-controlled analgesia (PCA) technique is the following EXCEPT

    A. Drugs 0.125% bupivacaine + 1 ì/ml fentanyl
    B. Lockout dose of 4 ml at 10 min
    C. Basal infusion at 6 ml/hour
    D. Hourly limit of 4 ml

26. Patients with sickle cell disease can experience episodic painful crises, which are characterized by

    A. Hypothermia
    B. Normoxemia
    C. Acidosis
    D. Dehydration

27. The most important assessment procedure to include in a headache evaluation is

A. A magnetic resonance imaging (MRI)
B. A computed tomography (CT) scan
C. An erythrocyte sedimentation rate
D. A targeted history

28. In a patient complaining of pain in the neck and right arm, laminectomy is indicated if the patient has

A. Facet arthropathy
B. Arachnoiditis
C. Spinal cord compression
D. Brachial plexus entrapment

29. In appropriately selected patients, epidural steroid injection is effective in

A. 15% of patients
B. 33% of patients
C. 66% of patients
D. 99% of patients

30. Trigger points

A. Are exquisitely tender points within muscle only
B. Feel like firm nodules or bands within muscle
C. Have direct cortical projections and pain is well localized
D. Show distinct laboratory findings

31. Laparoscopy detects the presence of all of the following conditions EXCEPT

A. Endometriosis
B. Ovarian cyst
C. Uterine malformations
D. Pelvic venous congestion

32. Brain and brainstem lesions that produce central pain are most commonly the result of

A. Vascular incidents
B. Trauma
C. Multiple sclerosis
D. Neoplasm

33. Cholinergic receptors are divided into the following two categories

A. Nicotinic and adrenergic
B. Adrenergic and muscarinic
C. Cholinergic and adrenergic
D. Nicotinic and muscarinic

34. In reflex sympathetic dystrophy (RSD) there is

A. Correlation between pain and known dermatomal distribution
B. Abnormality in EMG studies
C. Abnormality in peripheral angiograms
D. Abnormality in triple-phase bone scan

35. Phantom limb pain is usually described as all of the following EXCEPT

A. Burning, aching, shooting
B. Cold and pull
C. Sharp, shocklike
D. Knifelike

36. The dose of ketorolac which is comparable to 0.1 mg/kg of morphine in children is

A. 0.3 mg/kg
B. 0.6 mg/kg
C. 0.9 mg/kg
D. 1.2 mg/kg

37. In the first month after amputation, the percentage of patients who experience phantom limb pain is

A. 9% to 23%
B. 40% to 63%
C. 70% to 75%
D. 85% to 97%

38. At what age do the spinal cord and dorsal sac rise from the newborn level to the adult level?

A. 1 month
B. 3 months
C. 6 months
D. 12 months

39. Classic hemophilia A is associated with a deficiency of which factor?

A. V
B. VIII
C. IX
D. X

40. The hypogastric plexus is composed of what type of fibers?

A. Postganglionic sympathetic
B. Postganglionic parasympathetic
C. Visceral efferent
D. A delta

41. Which of the following nerve blocks is least helpful in diagnosing sympathetically mediated pelvic pain?

A. Differential spinal
B. Pudendal nerve
C. Superior hypogastric plexus
D. Differential epidural

42. Which of the following statements concerning skeletal pain is not true?

A. Neoplasms in bone are usually metastatic
B. The pain fibers are of A delta and C fiber origin
C. Pain fibers accompany epiphysial vessels
D. It is accompanied by effusion if joints are involved

43. A brachial plexus block is indicated for all of the following conditions EXCEPT

    A. Sympathetic independent pain resulting from RSD
    B. Brachial plexalgia
    C. Angina pectoris
    D. Raynaud's disease

44. Which of the following local anesthetics has a low potency and short duration of effect?

    A. Mepivacaine
    B. Procaine
    C. Prilocaine
    D. Lidocaine

45. The most commonly used route of administration for postoperative pain relief in children is

    A. Subcutaneous
    B. Intramuscular
    C. IV
    D. Rectal

46. Lesions producing central pain occur most commonly in the

    A. Spinal cord
    B. Brainstem
    C. Brain
    D. Frontal cortex

47. The sciatic nerve block originally described by Labat is performed via which approach?

    A. Posterior
    B. Anterior
    C. Lateral
    D. Supine sciatic

48. A diminished triceps jerk indicates a lesion of which nerve root?

    A. C4
    B. C5
    C. C6
    D. C7

49. In most studies, the incidence of chronic pain without an obvious pathologic condition is

    A. Less than 25%
    B. 33% to 50%
    C. 55% to 75%
    D. 80% to 95%

50. All of the following medications are anticonvulsants EXCEPT

    A. Phenytoin
    B. Carbamazepine
    C. Clonazepam
    D. Diazepam

51. Which of the following statements regarding the superior hypogastric plexus block is not true?

    A. It is most appropriate for pelvic pain of visceral origin
    B. It is associated with few side effects
    C. It must be performed with the assistance of fluoroscopy
    D. It is most appropriate for upper abdominal pain

52. Which of the following does not generally provoke visceral pain?

    A. Ischemia of visceral muscle
    B. Dividing the transverse colon
    C. Stretching of Glisson's capsule
    D. Distention of hollow viscera

53. The rootlets of the glossopharyngeal nerve originate in a groove on the lateral aspect of the medulla. It exits the skull via the

    A. Foramen lacerum
    B. Foramen ovale
    C. Foramen rotundum
    D. Jugular foramen

54. The apophysial joint is formed by all of the following EXCEPT

    A. Superior articular facet of the lower vertebra
    B. Inferior articular facet of the upper vertebra
    C. Synovium and fibrous joint capsule
    D. Ligamentum flavum

55. The acupuncture point located between the first and second metatarsal bones in the web is called

    A. Lieh Chuch
    B. Ho Ku
    C. Chih Tse
    D. Chien chen

56. Waddell's signs of a nonorganic basis of low back pain are all of the following EXCEPT

    A. Positive simulation as with skin rolling
    B. Pain increase with light axial loading
    C. Nonanatomic regional hypesthesia
    D. Positive straight leg raising (SLR) at 30 degrees

57. The lesser splanchnic nerve is formed by which of the following sympathetic nerves?

    A. T5 to T7
    B. T8 to T9
    C. T10 to T11
    D. T12

58. The zygapophyseal joint syndrome is characterized by all of the following features EXCEPT

    A. Unilateral back pain
    B. Radiation of midlumbar pain to the buttocks and back of the thigh
    C. Aggravation of pain with flexion
    D. Tenderness over the facet joint

59. Which of the following regional anesthesia techniques is not commonly used with children because of its side effects?

A. Epidural block
B. Subarachnoid block
C. Caudal block
D. Brachial plexus block

60. If symptoms persist after appropriate management of acute cervical disk herniation, the next step is to perform

A. Cervical laminectomy and fusion
B. Cervical epidural injection
C. Chemonucleolysis
D. Cervical facet injection

For questions 61 to 100, choose from the following

A. **1, 2, and 3**
B. **1 and 3**
C. **2 and 4**
D. **4**
E. **All of the above**

61. A terminal patient is experiencing intractable cancer pain that is well localized to one side of the pelvis. Which of the following invasive procedures would be most appropriate for treating the pain?

1. Percutaneous cordotomy
2. Midline myelotomy
3. Epidural block
4. Subarachnoid phenol saddle block

62. The following are methods of achieving hypnotic pain control

1. Alter the perception of pain
2. Substitute the painful sensation with a different or less painful sensation
3. Move the pain to another area of the body
4. Distortion of time

63. Which of the following factors explains the relatively rapid onset of alfentanil as compared with other opioids?

1. Alfentanil is far more lipid-soluble than most opioids, including fentanyl and morphine
2. Alfentanil has a far greater unionized fraction than morphine in plasma
3. Alfentanil has a long elimination half-life relative to other opioids such as sufentanil or fentanyl, allowing it to quickly accumulate high blood concentrations
4. Alfentanil has a very small volume of distribution compared with most of the other opioids

64. Which of the following local anesthetic(s) will most likely produce an allergic reaction?

1. Prilocaine
2. Ropivacaine
3. Etidocaine
4. Benzocaine

65. Radiofrequency thermocoagulation has been successfully used for

1. Dorsal root entry zone lesions
2. Cordotomy
3. Peripheral nerve block
4. Celiac plexus block

66. A patient with a flail chest and lower-extremity fractures is consulted by the trauma team to provide pain management. The most appropriate plan would be

1. Small IV doses of opiates
2. Lumbar epidural with a hydrophilic opiate to promote cephalad distribution to thoracic dermatomes
3. Thoracic epidural with opiate and local anesthetic
4. Thoracic epidural with local anesthetic alone and systemic PCA

67. Intermittent epidural morphine injections for hospitalized wards are acceptable because

1. Respiratory depression is extremely rare, predictable, and easily treated
2. The incidence of urinary retention is not higher than intermittent intramuscular (IM) injections
3. Nurses do not mind giving epidural injections
4. There is low incidence of respiratory depression, and catheter-related problems are minimal

68. Which of the following statements is(are) true concerning thermography?

1. It is useful in localizing trigger points in myofascial pain syndrome
2. It uses infrared radiation from the body for diagnostic purposes
3. It is useful for revealing dysfunction in microcirculation
4. It is usually associated with abnormal laboratory studies

69. Which of the following statements concerning osteoarthritis is(are) true?

1. A history of episodic locking, giving way, and associated effusion is common
2. It usually develops in joints injured by inflammatory or intra-articular derangement
3. Non-weight-bearing radiographs should be taken to confirm the diagnosis
4. Pain is relieved by unloading of the joint

70. Visceral afferents reach the spinal cord through which of the following nerve pathways?

1. Sympathetic
2. Parasympathetic
3. Splanchnic
4. Ventral roots

71. Which of the following medications should not be used in Crohn's disease?

   1. Systemic corticosteroids
   2. Azathioprine
   3. Sulfasalazine
   4. Meperidine

72. Which of the following is(are) the most common causative organism(s) implicated in the genesis of pelvic inflammatory disease?

   1. *Neisseria gonorrhoeae*
   2. *Staphylococcus epidermitis*
   3. *Chlamydia trachomatis*
   4. Herpes simplex virus

73. Which of the following statement(s) is(are) true regarding neuropathic cancer pain syndromes?

   1. They are often due to antitumor treatment directed at the cancer
   2. They may need to be treated with adjuvant analgesics
   3. They are characteristically less opioid-responsive than is nociceptive pain
   4. They are characteristically unresponsive to treatment with the opioids

74. In the comparison of biofeedback with relaxation training, which of the following statements apply?

   1. Patients usually favor the instrumentation and technology associated with biofeedback
   2. Biofeedback and relaxation training are equally effective in the management of chronic pain
   3. Research shows that relaxation training is more cost effective and practical than biofeedback
   4. Biofeedback and relaxation are usually used as conjunctive treatments

75. The presence of positive sharp waves during needle electromyography of a patient who describes debilitating pain and weakness of the limb while being tested is significant because

   1. This waveform is only found in patients with muscular dystrophy and never in pain syndromes
   2. This type of activity is an objective sign of denervation or reinnervation
   3. This pattern is an integral component of Waddell's signs of nonorganic pain behavior
   4. This pattern cannot be created fictitiously, even during reduced voluntary motor effort

76. Which of the following electrodiagnostic studies is typically used to assess radicular pain involving the spine and related extremities?

   1. Selective tissue conductance tests
   2. Nerve conduction velocity studies
   3. Somatosensory evoked potentials
   4. Needle EMG recordings

77. Which of the following complications is(are) associated with radiofrequency thermocoagulation?

   1. Neuropathic pain
   2. Carcinogenesis at lesion site
   3. Nociceptive pain
   4. Infection at lesion site

78. Fibromyalgia differs from myofascial syndrome in that it is characterized by

   1. Tender points that do not necessarily exhibit the "jump sign"
   2. A greater number of tender points than myofascial syndrome
   3. Frequent depression with a disturbed sleep pattern
   4. Lack of response to trigger point injections and/or antidepressants

79. Which of the following solutions is(are) used for neurolysis?

   1. Hypertonic saline
   2. Phenol
   3. Ethanol
   4. Distilled water

80. Which of the following advantages is(are) associated with a Type II (tunneled epidural catheter) drug-delivery system?

   1. Ease of insertion
   2. Ability to implant in outpatient settings
   3. Ease of removal
   4. Decreased risk of infection relative to Type I delivery systems

81. Which of the following implantable drug-delivery systems would be appropriate for a patient with a life expectancy of a few days to several weeks?

   1. Simple epidural catheter
   2. Reservoir/port
   3. Tunneled epidural catheter
   4. Implantable continuous infusion

82. The faces pain diagrams are appropriate for use with which of the following types of patients?

   1. The elderly
   2. Children
   3. Individuals with mental retardation
   4. Postoperative patients on a ventilator

83. Which of the following procedures is(are) important when performing a cryolesion?

   1. Assuring close proximity of the cryoprobe to the site to be frozen by creating motor stimulation
   2. Infiltrating the nerve or site to be frozen with local anesthetic before lesioning
   3. Bending the cryoprobe to achieve the proper angle and proximity to the site to be frozen
   4. Using an IV cannula to help position the cryoprobe and provide extra insulation against inadvertent tissue freezing

84. Which of the following statements regarding phenol and alcohol are true?

   1. They are biotransformed by liver enzymes
   2. They are excreted from the body essentially unchanged via the kidneys
   3. They act by highly selective mechanisms
   4. They cannot be used in patients with pancreatic cancer

85. During a lumbar facet radiofrequency denervation procedure, stimulation at 5 Hz before lesion formation produces neuromuscular activity in a lower extremity. The next action should be

   1. Abandon the procedure
   2. Insert 2% lidocaine
   3. Reposition the probe
   4. Produce a large lesion

86. One advantage of interpleural analgesia over epidural analgesia in the trauma patient is

   1. Improved respiratory parameters with interpleural analgesia
   2. Decreased risk of infection with interpleural catheters
   3. Lower plasma local anesthetic concentrations after a bolus injection through an interpleural catheter
   4. The ability to concomitantly administer systemic opiates with an interpleural technique

87. Preemptive analgesia refers to

   1. Prevention of neuroplasticity changes in the peripheral or CNS after injury
   2. Prevention of pain that can be accomplished by regional nerve blockade or analgesic agents before surgical trauma
   3. The effectiveness of preincisional lidocaine in decreasing the pain after herniorrhaphy
   4. Equal doses of morphine prescribed before or after the injury

88. Which of the following statement(s) regarding tension-type headaches is(are) true?

   1. It was previously referred to as muscle contraction headache
   2. It is characterized as bandlike pressure or pain
   3. It may be associated with cervical spine symptoms
   4. It has a rapid onset-to-peak

89. Cryotherapy is useful in myofascial pain syndromes because it can

   1. Act by direct and indirect mechanism to relieve pain
   2. Stimulate A delta fibers and reduce C fiber activity
   3. Directly reduce pain to the affected area
   4. Increase blood flow to the muscle

90. Which of the following pain management techniques is(are) most appropriate for patients with hepatic carcinoma?

   1. Chemotherapy
   2. Celiac plexus block
   3. Abdominal surgery
   4. Segmental analgesia

91. Which of the following statement(s) regarding the use of parenteral opioids for treating cancer pain is(are) true?

   1. They are usually more effective than treatment with oral anesthetics
   2. They are usually administered by the IV rather than subcutaneous route
   3. They are indicated based on the presence of severe pain
   4. They are most commonly instituted because of gastrointestinal disturbance

92. Which of the following statements is(are) true regarding subarachnoid neurolysis?

   1. The patient should be tilted 45 degrees posteriorly when it is performed with alcohol
   2. It usually requires radiologic guidance
   3. The patient does not need to lie on the painful side when it is performed with phenol
   4. It is safest when performed in the thoracic region

93. Which of the following complications is(are) associated with tunneled epidural catheters?

   1. Infection
   2. Dislodged catheter
   3. Broken catheter
   4. Low-pressure headache

94. If stimulation at 75 Hz produces no pain during a lumbar facet radiofrequency procedure, which of the following actions should be taken?

   1. Form a lesion
   2. Stimulate at 4 Hz
   3. Inject 2% lidocaine
   4. Reposition the probe

95. Data from which of the following pain assessments can be analyzed using parametric statistics?

   1. 11-point visual analogue scale
   2. Pain behavior assessment
   3. Category scale
   4. Visual analogue scale (VAS)

96. Which of the following complications is(are) associated with percutaneous cryoneurolysis?

   1. Motor nerve damage
   2. Frostbite of the skin
   3. Vascular damage
   4. Neuroma formation

97. Which of the following electrophysiologic techniques is most appropriate for assessing chronic ocular or periorbital pain?

    1. Electroculography
    2. Electronystagmography
    3. Electroretinography
    4. Needle electromyography

98. When a pain patient is referred to a psychologist for evaluation, a standard assessment battery generally includes

    1. A clinical interview
    2. A structured pain inventory
    3. Objective psychometric testing
    4. Projective techniques

99. Which of the following opioids are partial agonists?

    1. Heroin
    2. Nalbuphine
    3. Oxycodone
    4. Buprenorphine

100. Which of the following statements is(are) correct regarding the use of hypnosis with chronic pain?

    1. The hypnotic analgesia received is mediated by the endorphin system
    2. It can provide a cure for chronic pain
    3. It is beneficial in treating psychogenic pain of organic pathology
    4. It focuses on the subjective component of pain

Answers

1. C	26. B	51. D	76. C
2. D	27. D	52. B	77. B
3. D	28. C	53. D	78. A
4. A	29. C	54. D	79. E
5. B	30. B	55. B	80. E
6. B	31. D	56. D	81. B
7. A	32. A	57. C	82. E
8. C	33. D	58. C	83. D
9. D	34. D	59. B	84. B
10. D	35. B	60. B	85. B
11. A	36. C	61. E	86. D
12. D	37. B	62. E	87. A
13. B	38. D	63. D	88. A
14. C	39. A	64. D	89. B
15. D	40. A	65. A	90. C
16. B	41. B	66. D	91. D
17. D	42. D	67. D	92. D
18. A	43. C	68. C	93. A
19. B	44. B	69. C	94. D
20. D	45. C	70. E	95. D
21. C	46. B	71. D	96. A
22. A	47. A	72. B	97. B
23. C	48. D	73. A	98. A
24. B	49. B	74. C	99. D
25. D	50. D	75. C	100. D

Index

A

Abdominal nerve, cryoneurolysis of, 297
Abdominal pain
  celiac plexus block for, 260
  diagnosis of, 194–195
  imaging for, 194–195
  in pregnancy, 52–53
  visceral, 98–99
Abdominal viscera, innervation of, 251–252
Abortive therapy for migraine, 28
Abscess, epidural, 221
Abuse
  emotional, 323
  physical, 323
  sexual, 323
  substance, 322
Accessory nerve, cryoneurolysis of, 297
Accessory nerve block, 233–234
Accreditation, 373
Accreditation Council for Graduate
    Education, 7
Acetaminophen
  in elderly, 364
  in hemophilia, 31
  in pregnancy, 50, 55
Acoustic nerve, 134
Acquired immunodeficiency syndrome,
    neuroablation in, 106
Acrocyanosis, 30
Active movement testing, 161
Active range of motion, 330
Activities of daily living, 163
Activity-rest cycle, 367
Acupuncture, 343
Acute disk syndrome, 68
Acute pain
  cancer-related, 111
  category of, 19
  in child, 356
  definition of, 320
Acute pancreatitis, 101
Addiction
  patient history of, 129
  in psychologic evaluation, 154
Adhesive arachnoiditis, 221
Adjuvant therapy
  for cancer pain, 114
  for elderly, 365
Adnexal disorder, 102
Adson test, 144
Affective dimension in elderly, 363
Afferent fiber
  in complex regional pain syndrome, 82
  termination zones of, 10, 12
  visceral, 96–97
Age, headache and, 25
Agency for Health Care Policy and Research,
    45, 374
Alcoholic neuropathy, 78
Algorithm
  for elderly, 369

Algorithm—cont'd
  pain scale selection, 179
  for trauma pain, 39
Alkaloid, ergot, 28
Allergic reaction, 129
Alpha-adrenergic blocker, 88–89
Alternative medicine, 340–343
  classification of, 340, 341
  definition of, 340
  modalities of, 342–343
  office of, 340–341
  prevalence of, 340
  scope of, 341–342
Alveolar injury, 35
American Academy of Pediatrics, 51
American Board of Anesthesiology, 7
American Board of Medical Specialists, 7
American Medical Association, 168
American Pain Society, 8
American Society of Regional Anesthesia, 7–8
Amitriptyline
  for cancer pain, 115
  dosage of, 207
  in fibromyalgia, 73
  pregnancy and, 51
Amplitude in electromyography, 184
Amputation, 36
Analgesia. *See also specific drug*
  antidepressants interacting with, 209
  epidural. *See* Epidural *entries*
  parenteral
    for cancer pain, 113
    home care and, 336
  patient-controlled
    for cancer pain, 114
    epidural, 274
    for surgery, 43–44
  postoperative, 43–47
  regional
    for cancer pain, 115–116
    for trauma, 37–38
    for trigeminal neuralgia, 79
Ancient culture, pain in, 3–4
Anesthesia. *See also specific drug*
  epidural. *See* Epidural *entries*
  local. *See* Local anesthetic
  spinal, 212–215
  for trigeminal neuralgia, 79
Angiography in headache examination, 27
Ankle
  examination of, 140–141
  nerve testing of, 187
  peroneal nerve block and, 246–247
Antalgic gait, 131
Anterior percutaneous splanchnic nerve block,
    104
Anterolateral quadrant of spinal cord, 13
Anticonvulsant
  for cancer pain, 115
  for neuropathic pain, 87–88
  in pregnancy, 52

Antidepressant, 206, 207
  analgesic interactions with, 209
  for cancer pain, 115
  for migraine, 28
  for neuropathic pain, 87
  in pregnancy, 51–52
Antiepileptic drug for neuropathic pain, 87–88
Anti-inflammatory drug, 205–206
  nonsteroidal
    for cancer pain, 113
    in elderly, 364–365
    hemophilia and, 31
    pregnancy and, 49–50, 55
    in sickle cell disease, 31
Anxiety disorder, 322
Anxiolytic drug, 206–207
Aortic dissection, 98
Apley's test, 140
Arachnoiditis
  adhesive, 221
  epidural steroid and, 287
Arc, reflex, referred pain and, 97–98
Arterial occlusion, acute, 29
Arteriography, 194
  in headache examination, 27
Arteriosclerosis obliterans, 30–31
Arthritis, rheumatoid, 31–32
  skeletal pain from, 73–74
Arthrography, 194
  facet, 293
Articular facet, 291
Articular nerve, 71
Artificial synapse in complex regional pain
    syndrome, 82
Ascending spinal nociceptive pathway, 10, 13
Aseptic meningitis
  epidural block causing, 221–222
  epidural steroid and, 287
Aspirin, pregnancy and, 49
Assessment
  in child, 352–353
  in elderly, 362–363
  in home care, 335
  psychologic, 152–160. *See also* Psychologic
    evaluation
  regulatory issues and, 385–386
Association of Anesthesiology Pain Program
    Directors, 7
Atrophy, back pain and, 68
Attention-diversion technique, 367
Auditory nerve, function of, 134
Aura, migraine, 25
Auriculotemporal nerve block, 229–230
Autoimmune disorder, 150
Axial loading, 144
Axillary brachial plexus block, 238
Axis, 322
Axon
  nociceptors and, 10
  pseudomotor, 185
Axonotmesis, 186

B

Back pain
  epidural block causing, 221
  epidural steroid injection for, 280–287, 282
    for back pain, 69, 70, 280–282
    cervical, 285–286
    lumbar, 284–285
    mechanism of action of, 282–283
    for neuropathic pain, 89
    safety of, 286–287
    technique of, 283–284
  in pregnancy, 53–55
Baclofen
  for cancer pain, 115
  for neuropathic pain, 88
  for trigeminal neuralgia, 29, 79
Bacteremia in trauma patient, 39–40
Balanced Budget Act of 1997, 386–387
Beck Depression Inventory, 156
Behavioral approach to exercise, 331
Behavioral assessment, 176–177
  in child, 353
Behavioral therapy, 318–319, 321
Benefit, hospice, 346
Benzodiazepine, 207–208
  for cancer pain, 115
  in pregnancy, 51
Beta blocker
  for migraine, 28
  pregnancy and, 52
Biliary pain, 100
Bill of rights, patient's, 387
Biochemical profile, 148
Biofeedback, 320
  for migraine, 28
Biopsychosocial model, 320–321
Biostimulation, 342–343
Bleeding disorder, 31
Block
  ganglionic
    for cancer pain, 115–116
    for complex regional pain syndrome, 85
    for migraine, 28
  nerve. See Nerve block
  neurolytic, 90
  sequential differential spinal, 195–196
Blockade, facet arthrography with, 293
Blood cell count, 147–148
Blood flow measurement, 270
Blood supply in subarachnoid block, 212
Blunt injury, abdominal, 37
Body mechanics, 163
Bone
  pain pathophysiology in, 71
  scintigraphy of, 194
  subarachnoid block and, 212
Brachial plexopathy, 190
Brachial plexus
  continuous infusion of, 275–276
  injury to, 36
  pain management of, 38
Brachial plexus block
  axillary, 238
  differential, 198
  infraclavicular, 237–238
  interscalene, 236
  supraclavicular, 236
Brain
  central pain from lesion of, 77
  deep stimulation of, 311
Brainstem
  central pain from lesion of, 77
  somatosensory evoked potentials in, 190
Breakthrough cancer pain, 110

Breast-feeding
  drugs in pregnancy, 49
  opioids and, 51
Bretylium, 85
Brisk reflex, 132
Bupivacaine in pregnancy, 51
Buprenorphine, 43
Bupropion, 206
Bursitis
  subacromial, 137
  trochanteric, 138
Butyrophenone, 208

C

Caffeine in pregnancy, 52
Calcitonin, 88
Calcium channel blocker, 28
Calculus, renal or ureteric, 101
Cancer. See also Tumor
  gynecologic, 102
  neuroablation for, 105–106
  pancreatic, 101
    celiac plexus block for, 260
Cancer pain, 110–118
  assessment of, 112–113
  of back, 68
  in child, 356
  opioid tolerance and, 113
  pathophysiology of, 110–111
  postsurgical, 112
  rating scale of, 178
  subarachnoid infusion for, 275
  treatment of, 113–116
Capsaicin, 88
Carbamazepine
  in pregnancy, 51–52
  for trigeminal neuralgia, 29, 79
Carcinoma, renal cell, 101
Cardiac pain, 98
Cardiovascular complications of epidural block, 220–221
Cardiovascular effect of epidural block, 217, 220
Catecholamine drug, 205
Category, of pain, 18–20
Catheter
  for celiac plexus block, 264
  epidural, 272
  for epidural analgesia, 40
  femoral nerve, 277
  for intercostal nerve block, 37
  intrathecal implantation and, 307
  sciatic nerve, 277
Caudal epidural block, 219–220
Causalgia, 36
Celiac nerve block
  complications of, 105
  efficacy of, 105–106
  for visceral pain, 105
Celiac plexus splanchnic nerve block, 259–264
  anatomy in, 259–260
  anterior approach to, 264
  for cancer pain, 114
  catheter placement for, 264
  indications for, 260
  technique of, 260–264
Cell body, preganglionic, 250
Central nerve block
  epidural, 216–222. See also Epidural block
  subarachnoid, 212–215
Central nervous system
  in complex regional pain syndrome, 83

Central nervous system—cont'd
  in elderly, 363
  epidural block complications and, 220
Central pain, 77–78
  differential nerve block for, 196
  neuropathic, 19
Cerebral circulation, local anesthetic in, 89
Cerebral hemisphere, 190
Cerebral nociceptive processing, 14
Cerebrospinal fluid, 212–213
Cervical compression test, 144
Cervical decompression test, 144
Cervical epidural block, 217
Cervical epidural steroid injection, 285–286
Cervical facet
  denervation of, 300
  radiofrequency lesioning of, 293–294
Cervical facet syndrome, 291
Cervical ganglion rhizotomy, 301
Cervical pain, nonorganic, 145
Cervical plexus block, 234–236
Cervical spine
  in headache examination, 26
  range of motion of, 135
Chemical neurolysis in elderly, 366
Chemical sympathectomy, 85
Chemonociceptive receptor, 71
Chemotherapy-related pain, 111
Chest pain
  in child, 354–355
  diagnosis of, 194–195
  visceral, 98
Chest wall injury, 35
Child
  assessment of pain in, 352–353
  fetus and neonate, 351–352
  medically caused, 355–356
  pain scale for, 178
  pain syndromes in, 353–355
  perception of pain of, 351
  trauma in, 36
  treatment of, 356–357
Childbirth pain, 3; see also Obstetrics
Chinese culture, 3
Chiropractic therapy, 342
Chlorpromazine, 208
Cholecystitis, 100–101
Christian view of pain of, 3
Chronic pain
  cancer-related, 110–118
  category of, 19–20
  classification of, 18, 19
  coccygodynia, 119
  definition of, 320
  in elderly, 360, 362
  headache causing, 25
  neuropathic, 77–94. See also Neuropathic pain
  nociceptive, 61–76. See also Nociceptive pain
  orofacial, 120
  psychiatric nomenclature and, 321–325
  subarachnoid infusion for, 275
  thoracic, 120–121
  in trauma patient, 35, 37
  visceral, 95–109. See also Visceral pain
Chronic pain syndrome, 59–123
Chronic pancreatitis, 101
Chronic vasospastic disease, 30–31
Cingulotomy, 309
Clavicle, fracture of, 36
Clinic, pediatric, 357
Clonazepam, 115
Clonidine, 88
Cluster headache, 28–29
Coccygodynia, 119

Cognitive factor, 324
Cognitive restructuring, 367–368
Cognitive therapy, 318–319, 321
Cognitive-behavior model, 365
Cognitively impaired patient, 362–363
Cold injury, 30
Cold therapy, 328
    in functional evaluation, 161
Collagen vascular disease, test for, 150
Comfort measures, 342
Committee, residency review, 7
Compartment block, psoas, 242
Compartment syndrome, 71
Complete blood cell count, 147–148
Complex regional pain syndrome, 82–86
    in child, 356
Compliance by elderly, 364
Compression, nerve root and spinal cord, 61–65
Compression fracture, vertebral, 37
Compression test, 140
    cervical, 144
Computed tomography
    for back pain, 195
    diagnostic, 192–193
    in headache examination, 27
    in neuroablation, 104–105
Conduction, nerve, physiology of, 183
Congenital disorder, test for, 150
Congestion, pelvic, 102
Consumer, 379
Continuous infusion, 272–278
    epidural, 272–275
    peripheral, 276–277
    subarachnoid, 275–276
    sympathetic, 277–278
Controlled substance, 387–388
Contusion, pulmonary, 35
Convergence, viscerosomatic or viscerovisceral, 97
Convergence-facilitation theory of referred pain, 97
Coordination examination, 144
Coping Strategies Questionnaire, 157
Coping strategy, 324–325
Cordotomy, 313
Core curriculum, 8
Coronary arteriography, 194
Corticosteroid. See also Steroid
    for cancer pain, 115
    pregnancy and, 51
Cost, 379
    of home care, 335
Cost-effectiveness, 382
Costochondritis, 121
Cox-2 inhibitor in elderly, 364
Cranial nerve
    examination of, 133–134
    in headache examination, 26
    pain related to, 79
C-reactive protein, 149
Crisis, sickle cell, 31
Cross-price elasticity, 378
Cruciate ligament testing, 142
Crush injury, 38
Cryoneurolysis, 294–302
    abdominal, 297
    contraindications to, 295
    of extremity, 297–298
    of head and neck, 295–297
    lesion characteristics, 295
    patient selection for, 294–295
    pelvic, 297
    spinal, 297
    technique of, 295

Cryotherapy for myofascial pain, 72
Culture, ancient, 3–4
Curriculum, core, 8
Cutaneous nerve, lateral femoral, 297–298
Cutaneous pain, scars causing, 121
Cycle, activity-rest, 367

D
Database, laboratory, 147–150
Decompression
    for neck and shoulder pain, 64
    for trigeminal neuralgia, 79, 91, 311
Decompression test, cervical, 144
Deep brain stimulation, 311
Deep cervical plexus block, 234–235
Deep peroneal nerve block, 246–247
Deep somatic pain, 95
Deep splanchnic nerve block, 104
Degenerative disease
    cervical nerve compression and, 62
    of temporomandibular joint, 37
    test for, 149
Dejerne-Roussy syndrome, 77
Delivery
    implanted drug, 337–338
    of infant, 274–275. See also Obstetrics
Denervation
    radiofrequency, 266–267
    spinal nerve, 314
Dental pain, 120
Deposition, legal, 393–394
Depression, 323–324
    testing for, 156
Dermatome
    cervical nerve compression and, 62–65
    in physical examination, 132–134
Desipramine
    for cancer pain, 115
    dosage of, 207
Desmopressin in hemophilia, 31
Dextroamphetamine, 115
Diabetes mellitus
    in child, 355–356
Diabetic peripheral neuropathy, 78
Diagnostic and Statistical Manual of Mental Disorders, 322
    classification system of, 17–18
    pain disorders in, 17–18
Diagnostic test, 144
Diagnostic testing, 182–201
    electromyography, 182–189. See also Electromyography
    evoked potentials, 189–192
    neural blockade in, 195–198
    radiology in, 192–195
Diarrhea, celiac nerve block and, 105
Diary, pain, 177
Diazepam in pregnancy, 51
Differential nerve block, 195–198
Digital nerve block, 240
Digital nerve cryoneurolysis, 297
Digital substraction angiography, 27
Director of pain fellowship program, 7–8
Disability, perceived, 156
Disability evaluation
    conceptualization of, 167–168
    as medical versus legal process, 169
    objective determination in, 169–170
    of physical capacities, 170
    reporting of, 170
    systems of, 168–169
Discipline, medical, 17

Disk. See Intervertebral disk
Dissection
    aortic, 98
    radical neck, 112
Distraction test, cervical, 144
Dorsal column fiber, postsynaptic, 14
Dorsal horn neuron, spinal cord, 10
Dorsal rhizotomy, 314
Dorsal root entry zone lesion, 313–314
Dorsal root ganglionotomy, 301
Doxepin
    for cancer pain, 115
    dosage of, 207
Drawer sign test, 142
Drawing, pain, 177, 178
DREZ procedure, 313–314
Drop arm test, 137
Drug abuse, 322
    patient history of, 129
Drug history in psychologic evaluation, 154
Drug therapy, 205–211
    antidepressant, 206, 207
        analgesic interactions with, 209
    anti-inflammatory, 205–206
    anxiolytic, 206–207
    for back pain, 69
    benzodiazepines, 207–208
    catecholamines, 205
    for central pain, 78
    for child, 356–357
    for complex regional pain syndrome, 84
    for differential nerve block, 195–196
    for elderly, 363–365
    implanted, 337–338
    indolamines, 205
    for intravenous regional sympathetic block, 267
    muscle relaxants, 208–209
    for neuropathic pain, 87–91
    opioids, 208
    in pain assessment, 177
    pain pathways and, 205
    for phantom limb pain, 81
    for sympathetic infusion, 277
    unusual, 208
DSM-IV, 322
    classification system of, 17–18
    pain disorders in, 17–18
Duodenal pain, 99
Dysfunction, perceived, 156
Dystrophy, reflex sympathetic, 38

E
Economics
    of pain medicine, 377–384
        principles of, 377–378
    of palliative medicine, 346
    payment for services, 385
Education, 7, 8
    in pediatric pain management, 357
Elasticity in economics, 378
Elbow
    examination of, 137–138
    nerve block at, 239
Elderly, 178, 360–369. See also Geriatric pain
Electrical nerve stimulation. See Stimulation, nerve
Electrode in nerve conduction, 183
Electroencephalography, 27
Electromyography, 182–189
    basic, 183–185
    clinical correlations of, 185–187

Electromyography—cont'd
  F-wave, 185
  history of, 182
  Hoffman reflex, 185
  physiology of, 182–183
  quantitative sensory testing, 185–187
  usefulness of, 187, 189
Embolism, pulmonary, 98
Emory Pain Estimate Model, 18
Emotional abuse, 323
Endocrine disorder, 150
Endometriosis, 102
Entrapment, post-thoracotomy nerve fiber, 121
Entry zone lesion, dorsal root, 313–314
Environmental factor in headache, 25
Eosinophil count, 148
Epicondylitis, test for, 138
Epidural analgesia
  for phantom limb pain, 36
  post-thoracotomy, 47
  in surgery, 44–45, 46
  for trauma pain, 37, 39
Epidural block
  anatomy in, 216–217
  caudal, 219–220
  cervical, 217–218
  complications of, 220–222
  differential, 197
  history of, 216
  lumbar, 218–219
  physiologic effects of, 217
  thoracic, 218
Epidural hemorrhage, intrathecal implantation
    and, 307
Epidural infusion
  continuous, 272–275
  home care and, 336
Epidural steroid injection, 280–287
  for back pain, 69, 70, 280–282
  cervical, 285–286
  lumbar, 284–285
  mechanism of action of, 282–283
  for neuropathic pain, 89
  safety of, 286–287
  technique of, 283–284
Equipment
  for cryoneurolysis, 295, 298
  for radiofrequency lesioning, 298
  for subarchnoid block, 213
Ergot alkaloid
  for migraine, 28
  in pregnancy, 52
Erythrocyte sedimentation rate, 149
Erythromelalgia, 30
Esophageal pain, 98
Ethical issues, 398–400
Etiologic pain category, 20
Evaluation
  functional, 161–166
    initial, 161
    occupational therapy in, 163–165
    of treatment, 161–163
  physical, 131–146. See also Physical
      examination
  psychologic, 152–160. See also Psychologic
      evaluation
Event-related potentials, 192
Evoked potentials
  equipment for, 189
  general principles of, 189
  in headache examination, 27
  motor, 191–192
  somatosensory, 189–191
Examination, physical, 131–146. See also
    Physical examination

Examination room, 131–132
Exchange, theory of, 377
Exercise
  in functional evaluation, 162
  resistive, 330
  therapeutic, 329–330
External fixation, 37
Exteroceptive sensation, 133
Extremity
  continuous infusion and, 277
  cryoneurolysis of, 297–298
  differential diagnosis of pain in, 84
  imaging of, 195
  nerve testing of, 187–188, 188
  phantom limb pain and, 80–81
  range of motion of, 135–136
  somatic nerve block of, 236–248. See also
      Somatic nerve block
  somatosensory evoked potentials in,
      189–190, 190
  trauma to, 36, 37

F

Fabere test, 138
Face pain scale, 353, 351
Facet denervation
  cervical, 300
  lumbar, 300–302
  thoracic, 300
Facet joint, 71–72
Facet neurolysis, 291–302
  anatomy in, 291
  arthrography and, 293
  cervical, 291
  cryoneurolysis, 294–302
  lumbar, 292
  radiofrequency lesioning, 293–294,
      298–302
  thoracic, 291–292
Facet syndrome, 68
Facial nerve, 133–134
Facial pain
  atypical, 80
  cancer-related, 111
  diagnosis of, 194
  imaging for, 194
  post-traumatic, 80
  trigeminal neuralgia, 29
Facial trauma, 37
Factitious disorder, 322
Failed back surgery syndrome, 195
Family assessment, 335
Family therapy, 319
Federal policy issues, 384–387
Feigning, testing for, 156
Fellowship, pain, 7
Femoral nerve
  catheterization of, 277
  cryoneurolysis of, 297–298
Femoral nerve block, 243
Fentanyl
  in patient-controlled analgesia, 43
  in pregnancy, 50–51
Fetal hydantoin syndrome, 52
Fetus, pain in, 351–352
Fiber
  afferent
    termination zones of, 10, 12
    visceral, 96–97
  postsynaptic dorsal column, 14
  steroid injection and, 282
Fibromyalgia, 73
Fibrosis, 282

Fibrositis, 73
Financial issues
  economics of pain medicine, 377–384
  payment for services, 385
Finger examination, 138
Fixation, external, 37
Flow chart for trauma pain, 39
Fluid, cerebrospinal, 212–213
Fluoxetine, 206, 207
Fluphenazine, 207
Fluvoxamine, 206
Foot
  anatomy of, 142, 143
  examination of, 141–144
Fossa, popliteal, 245–246
Fracture
  of clavicle, 36
  rib, 35
  scintigraphy of, 194
  sternal, 36
Freezing. See Cryoneurolysis
Frozen shoulder, 137
Functional evaluation, 161–166
  initial, 161
  occupational therapy in, 163–165
  of treatment, 161–163
Functional limitation, 167
F-wave, 185

G

Gabapentin for cancer pain, 115
Gait examination, 131
Ganglion, paravertebral sympathetic, 250–251
Ganglion block
  for cancer pain, 115–116
  for complex regional pain syndrome, 85
  gasserian, 223–224
  impar, 269–270
  sphenopalatine, for migraine, 28
  stellate, 254–258
    anatomy of, 254
    anterior approach for, 255, 257
    indications for, 254–255
    posterior approach for, 257–258
    technique of, 255
Ganglion rhizotomy
  cervical, 301
  lumbar, 301
  thoracic, 301
Ganglionotomy, dorsal root, 301
Gasserian ganglion, 29
Gasserian ganglion block, 223–224
Gastrointestinal disorder, pelvic pain from,
    102
Gastrointestinal effect of epidural block, 217
Gate control theory, 320–321
  back pain and, 70
  in complex regional pain syndrome, 82–83
  phantom limb pain and, 81
Genetic disease, 150
Genicular neuralgia, 313
Genitofemoral nerve block, 242–243
Genitofemoral nerve cryoneurolysis, 297
Genitourinary pain, 101
Geriatric pain, 178, 360–369
  assessment of, 362–363
  chronic, 360, 362
  definition of, 360
  epidemiology of, 360
  health policy and, 360
  pathophysiology of, 363
  treatment of, 363–369
Glossopharyngeal nerve, 134

Glossopharyngeal nerve block, 231–232
Glossopharyngeal neuralgia, 79, 312–313
Glycerol injection for trigeminal neuralgia, 29
Gower's sign, 140
Greater occipital nerve block, 230–231
Greater occipital nerve cryoneurolysis, 297
Greater palatine nerve block, 228–229
Greek culture, 3
Grinding test, 140
Group therapy, 319
Growing pains, 356
Guanethidine, 85
Guidelines, practice, 45, 373–374
Gynecologic cancer, 102

H

Haloperidol, 207, 208
Handbook of Cancer Pain Management, 8
Handicap. *See* Disability
Hardening, work, 165
Head and neck
    cryoneurolysis of, 295–297
    radiofrequency lesioning of, 300
    somatic nerve block of, 223–236
        auriculotemporal, 229–230
        cervical plexus, 234–236
        glossopharyngeal, 231–232
        greater occipital, 230–231
        greater palatine, 228–229
        infraorbital, 227–228
        laryngeal, 232–233
        mandibular, 229
        maxillary, 226–227
        mental, 230
        ophthalmic, 224–225
        spinal accessory, 233–234
        supraorbital and supratrochlear, 225–226
        trigeminal nerve/gasserian ganglion,
            223–224
        vagus, 232
Head injury
    epidural analgesia in, 40
    pain management in, 38
Headache, 25–29
    cancer-related, 111
    in child, 353–354
    cluster, 28–29
    diagnosis of, 27, 194
    imaging for, 194
    migraine, 27–28
    patient history of, 25–26
    physical examination for, 26
    postdural puncture, 221
    post-traumatic, 37
    tension-type, 27
    trigeminal neuralgia, 29
Healing, functional evaluation of, 163–164
Health policy, elderly and, 360
Health services, home, 334
Healthcare economics, 378–382
Heartburn, 98
Heat
    for myofascial pain, 72
    radiofrequency lesioning and, 298
Heat therapy, 327–328
    in functional evaluation, 161
Hematocrit, 148
Hematologic complications of epidural block,
    221
Hematoma, epidural, 221
Hemisphere, cerebral, somatosensory evoked
    potentials in, 190
Hemoglobin A, 31

Hemoglobin testing, 148
Hemophilia, 31
    in child, 355
Hemorrhage in intrathecal implantation, 307
Hepatic system in elderly, 363
Herniated disk, 67, 68
    in pregnancy, 55
Herpes zoster, 79–80
Hip examination, 138
Hip pain in pregnancy, 53
History, patient
    in functional evaluation, 161
    in psychologic evaluation, 153–154
    taking of, 127–129
Hoffman reflex, 185
Home care, 334–338
    assessment in, 335
    components of, 335
    cost of, 335
    epidural infusion in, 336
    goals of, 334
    guidelines for, 335
    history of, 334
    implanted delivery systems and, 337–338
    outcomes of, 335–336
    parenteral infusion in, 336
    types of, 334
Hoover test, 144
Hopping test, 144
Hospice, 5, 345
H-reflex, 185
Human immunodeficiency virus infection, 106
H-wave stimulation, 72
Hydantoin syndrome, fetal, 52
Hydromorphone, 43
Hyperbaric solution, 215
Hyperesthesia, 83
Hypnosis, 319–320, 342
Hypobaric solution, 215
Hypogastric plexus block
    for cancer pain, 116
    superior, 267–269
Hypoglossal nerve, 134
Hypophysectomy, 309
Hypotension
    celiac nerve block and, 105
    neurolytic block and, 264
Hypothalamotomy, 310

I

Ibuprofen in pregnancy, 50
Iliohypogastric nerve block, 242
Iliohypogastric nerve cryoneurolysis, 297
Ilioinguinal nerve block, 242
Ilioinguinal nerve cryoneurolysis, 297
Iliotibial band syndrome, 138
Imaging
    arteriography, 194
    arthrography, 194
    in celiac plexus block, 263–264
    computed tomography, 192–193
        for back pain, 195
        diagnostic, 192–193
        in headache examination, 27
        in neuroablation, 104–105
    for low back pain, 67
    magnetic resonance imaging, 193
        for back pain, 195
        diagnostic, 193
        in headache examination, 27
    myelography, 194
    plain x-ray film, 192
    regional, 194–195

Imaging—cont'd
    skeletal scintigraphy, 194
    venography, 194
Imipramine
    for cancer pain, 115
    dosage of, 207
Immune effects of epidural block, 221
Immunosuppression in rheumatic arthritis, 31
Impar block, ganglion, 266–270
Impingement syndrome, 137
Implantation, intrathecal, 303–307
Implanted drug delivery, 337–338
Incidental cancer pain, 110
Index
    pain assessment, 155
    pain disability, 156
Indolamine, 205
Infarction, myocardial, 98
Inflammation
    in complex regional pain syndrome, 83–84
    of liver or spleen, 100
    mediastinal, visceral pain from, 98
    pelvic pain from, 101–102
    skeletal pain from, 73–74
    test for, 149
Informed consent for nerve block, 255
Infraclavicular brachial plexus block, 237–238
Infraorbital nerve block, 227–228
Infraorbital nerve cryoneurolysis, 295–296
Infusate, 307
Infusion
    continuous, 272–278
        epidural, 272–275
        peripheral, 276–277
        subarachnoid, 275–276
        sympathetic, 277–278
    home care and, 336
    intercostal nerve block and, 37
    intravenous regional, 89
    intraventricular opioid, 310–311
    surgery and, 44
Infusion pump, implantable, 303–307
Inguinal paravascular nerve block, 242
Injection, intraspinal, 258
Inkblot test, 155
Innervation, of heart, 99
Insertional muscle activity, 186
Inspection in functional evaluation, 161
Intercostal nerve block, 37
Interdigital nerve cryoneurolysis, 298
Interference patterns in electromyography, 184
Intermittent epidural morphine injection, 44
International Association for the Study of Pain
    education and, 8
    pain classification of, 18, 20
International Classification of Diseases, 17
Interpleural approach to sympathetic nerve
    block, 259
Interscalene brachial plexus block, 236
Interspace in subarachnoid block, 214
Interventional technique
    continuous, 272–278
        epidural infusion, 272–275
        peripheral infusion, 276–277
        subarachnoid, 275–276
        sympathetic, 277–278
    facet neurolysis, 291–302. *See also* Facet
        neurolysis
    intrathecal implantation, 303–307
    nerve block. *See* Nerve block
Intervertebral disk
    acute disk syndrome and, 68
    fibrosis and, 282
    herniated, 67, 68
    low back pain and, 67

Intervertebral disk—cont'd
  mechanical tension and, 282
  pathophysiology of, 71
  vascular abnormality and, 281
Interview in psychologic evaluation, 152–154
Intestinal pain, 101
Intra-abdominal injury, 37
Intra-abdominal tumor, 105
Intra-articular derangement, 74
Intra-articular morphine injection, 45
Intractable pain legislation, 387–388
Intrafascicular injection of local anesthetic, 89
Intramuscular mechanoreceptor, 71
Intrapleural analgesia for cancer pain, 116
Intrapleural approach to sympathetic
    denervation, 259
Intraspinal injection in stellate ganglion block,
    258
Intraspinal opioid, 44
Intraspinal therapy for cancer pain, 115
Intrathecal hemorrhage, 307
Intrathecal implantation, 303–307
Intravenous regional block
  for complex regional pain syndrome, 85
  sympathetic, 267
  for upper extremity, 240–241
Intravenous regional infusion for neuropathic
    pain, 89
Intraventricular infusion, opioid, 310–311
Inventory
  Millon behavioral health, 155
  Minnesota multiphasic personality, 155
  multidimensional pain, 156–157
  personality assessment, 155
Iontophoresis for myofascial pain, 72
Ischemia
  muscle, 71
  myocardial, 100
  test for, 149
Isobaric solution in subarachnoid block, 215
Isometheptene mucate, 28

J
Jannetta's procedure, 29
Jaw opening test, 144
Joint
  bleeding into, 31
  examination of, 137
  facet, 71–72
  in functional evaluation, 161, 162
  inflammation of, 74
  rheumatic arthritis of, 30–31
  temporomandibular, facial trauma and, 37
  zygapophyseal, 68
Joint capsule, 291
Joint Commission on Accreditation of
    Healthcare Organizations, 334
Juvenile rheumatoid arthritis, 356

K
Kappis splanchnic nerve block, 103
Ketorolac, 50
Knee examination, 138–140

L
Labor pain, 274–275. See also Obstetrics
Laboratory test, 147–151, 177–178
Laminae, Rexed, 10
Laminectomy, lumbar, 68

Laparotomy, injection during, 104
Large intestinal pain, 101
Laryngeal nerve, stellate ganglion block and, 257
Laryngeal nerve block, 232–233
Lasègue's sign, 139
Lateral epicondylitis test, 138
Lateral femoral cutaneous nerve, 297–298
Lateral medullary syndrome, 77
Leg length discrepancy, 138
Legal issue
  behavioral observation and, 392–393
  compilation of evidence and, 392
  disability evaluation as, 169
  medical records, 391–392
  medical report, 393
  medical-legal cooperation, 392
  opioids and, 208
  testimony under oath, 393–395
Legislation, 387–388
Leukocyte count, 147–148
Lidocaine
  for migraine, 28
  for neuropathic pain, 88
  pregnancy and, 51
Ligament
  examination of, 141, 142
  round, 52
  subarachnoid block and, 212
Limb. See Extremity
Limitation, functional, 167
Lipophilic opioid, 274
Lithium for cluster headache, 29
Livedo reticularis, 30
Liver, in elderly, 363
Liver pain, 100
Local anesthetic
  for cancer pain, 115
  epidural infusion and, 272–273
  for labor pain, 274–275
  in patient-controlled analgesia, 274
  pregnancy and, 51
  in subarachnoid block, 212–215
  toxicity of, 89
Long-term morbidity, trauma causing, 36–37
Low back pain, 66–70
  imaging for, 195
Lower extremity
  continuous infusion and, 277
  cryoneurolysis of, 297–298
  differential diagnosis of pain in, 84
  nerve testing of, 188
  somatic nerve block of, 241–248
    femoral, 243
    genitofemoral, 242–243
    ilioinguinal and iliohypogastric, 242
    inguinal paravascular, 242
    obturator, 243
    paravertebral, 241–242
    peripheral, 242
    peroneal, 246–247
    popliteal fossa, 245–246
    psoas compartment, 242
    sacral plexus, 244–245
    saphenous, 243–244
    sural, 247
    tibial, 247
  somatosensory evoked potentials in, 190
Low-power laser therapy, 343
Loxapine, equivalent dose of, 207
Lumbar epidural block, 218–219
Lumbar epidural steroid injection, 284–285
Lumbar facet
  denervation of, 300–302
  radiofrequency lesioning of, 294
Lumbar facet syndrome, 292

Lumbar ganglion rhizotomy, 301
Lumbar nerve block, 265–266
Lumbar placement for post-thoracotomy
    analgesia, 47
Lumbar puncture in headache examination, 27
Lumbar spinal
  stenosis of, 190
Lumbar spine
  laminectomy of, 68
  range of motion of, 135, 136
Lumbar sympathectomy, 301–302
Lumbar sympathetic block, 265–266
Lung
  causes of pain of, 98
  trauma to, 35
Lymphocyte, 148

M
Magnetic field therapy, 343
Magnetic resonance imaging
  for back pain, 195
  diagnostic, 193
  in headache examination, 27
Malingering, testing for, 156
Mandibular nerve block, 229
Mandibular nerve cryoneurolysis, 295–297
Manipulation, 331
Manual technique, 330–331
Maprotiline, 115
Massage, 330
Mastectomy, pain after, 112
Masticatory muscle pain, 120
Maxillary nerve block, 226–227
McGill Pain Questionnaire, 152, 174–176
McGrath's scale, 353
McMurray test, 140
Mechanical tension, vertebral, 282
Mechanoreceptor, intramuscular, 71
Median nerve
  cryoneurolysis of, 297
  testing of, 186
Median nerve block, 239
Mediastinal disease, 98
Mediating role of medical care, 380–381
Medical disease
  acute vascular, 29–30
  chronic vasospastic, 30–31
  headache and facial pain, 25–29
  hemophilia, 31
  pancreatitis, 32
  rheumatoid arthritis, 31–32
  sickle cell disease, 31
Medical history. See Patient history
Medical Outcomes Survey, 157
Medical process, disability evaluation as, 169
Medical record, 391–392
Medical report, 393
Medicare, 386
Medicare hospice benefit, 346
Meditation, 368
Medullary syndrome, lateral, 77
Meninges, subarachnoid block and, 212
Meningitis
  epidural block causing, 221–222
  epidural steroid and, 27
Meniscus, 141
Menstruation, migraine and, 26
Mental nerve block, 230
Mental nerve cryoneurolysis, 297
Mental status in psychologic evaluation, 154
Meperidine
  breast-feeding and, 51
  in patient-controlled analgesia, 43

Metabolic disorder, 150
Metacarpophalangeal joint, 138
Metastasis, back pain from, 68
Metatarsalgia, 141
Methadone
  in patient-controlled analgesia, 43
  in pregnancy, 50–51
Methylphenidate, 115
Methylprednisolone
  for cancer pain, 115
  toxicity of, 287
Methysergide, 28
Mexiletine
  for neuropathic pain, 88
  pregnancy and, 51
Microvascular decompression for trigeminal
    neuralgia, 29, 79, 91, 311
Midbrain spinothalamic tractotomy, 310
Midline myelotomy, 313
Migraine
  characteristics of, 27–28
  in child, 353–354
  in pregnancy, 55
  treatment of, 28–29
Migram test, 144
Millon Behavioral Health Inventory, 155
Minnesota Multiphasic Personality Inventory,
    155
Mirtazapine, 206, 207
Mittelschmerz, 101
Mnemonic, VINDICATE PS, 149
Mobility in functional evaluation, 161, 162
Mobilization, 330
Model, economic, 381–382
Model, Emory pain estimate, 20
Modified differential spinal block, 196–197
Molindone, 207
Monocyte, 148
Mononeuropathy, 186
Mood disorder, 322
Mood state, 154, 155–156
Morphine
  epidural infusion with, 274
  intra-articular injection of, 45
  in patient-controlled analgesia, 43
  in pregnancy, 51
  surgery and, 44–45
Morton's neuroma, 141
Motor evoked potentials, 191–192
Motor function
  in functional evaluation, 161
  in headache examination, 26
  in nerve root compression, 62
Multiaxial Assessment of Pain, 20–21
Multidimensional Pain Inventory, 21,
    156–157
Multidimensional pain scale, 176, 177
Multidisciplinary treatment model, 320–321
Multiple sclerosis, 190
Muscle, potentials of, 182–183
Muscle disorder, electromyography for, 187
Muscle relaxant, 208–209
  for back pain, 69
Muscle spasm, pelvic, 102
Musculoskeletal pain, 71–74
  in child, 356
  of neck and shoulder, 61
  temporomandibular joint and, 120
  thoracic, 120–121
Musculoskeletal system, 356
  examination of, 135–144
    ankle, 140–141
    coordination of motion, 144
    elbow, 137–138
    fingers, 138

Musculoskeletal system—cont'd
    foot, 141–144
    hip, 138
    joints, 137
    knee, 138–140
    range of motion, 135–137
    reproduction of pain in, 144
    shoulder, 137
    thumb, 138
    wrist, 138
  pregnancy and, 52–53
  radiographic evaluation of, 192
Music therapy, 342
Myelography, 194
Myelotomy, midline, 313
Myocardial infarction, 98
Myocardial ischemia, 100
Myofascial pain, 72–73
  characteristics of, 121
  in child, 356
  complex regional pain syndrome vs, 83–84
  trauma causing, 37
  trigger points for, 121
Myofascial technique, 330
Myotome, 62–65
Myth, economic, 378

N
Nalbuphine, 43
Narcotic, 208
  for back pain, 69
  for cancer pain, 113–114, 115
  in epidural infusion, 273
  intraventricular infusion of, 310–311
  legal issues of, 208
  for neuropathic pain, 88
  in pregnancy, 50–51
  in sickle cell disease, 31
  tolerance to, 112
Neck dissection, radical, 112
Neck pain, 61–66
  compression causing, 61–65
  imaging for, 195
  management of, 65–66
  neurogenic, 61
Needle
  in electromyography, 183
  in epidural block
    caudal, 220
    cervical, 217
    lumbar, 218–219
    thoracic, 218
  in neurolytic block, 264
  for subarachnoid block, 213
Nefazodone, 206, 207
Neglect, 323
Neonate, pain in, 351–352
Neoplasm, test for, 149
Nerve, articular, 71
Nerve block
  for back pain, 69
  central
    epidural, 216–222. See also Epidural
      block
    subarachnoid, 212–215
  for complex regional pain syndrome, 84–85
  differential, 195–198
  in elderly, 365–367
  intercostal, 37
  for neuropathic pain, 89
  for phantom limb pain, 81
  somatic, 223–248. See also Somatic nerve
    block

Nerve block—cont'd
  sympathetic, 250–270. See also Sympathetic
    nerve block
  for trigeminal neuralgia, 29, 79
Nerve conduction
  physiology of, 183
  steroid injection and, 282
Nerve fiber
  entrapment of, 121
  steroid injection and, 282
  termination zones of, 12
Nerve injury
  causalgia and, 36
  celiac nerve block and, 105
  diagnostic testing for, 186
  in extremity trauma, 38
  iatrogenic, 89
Nerve pain
  peripheral, 78–80
  spinal, 78
Nerve root compression, 61–65
Nerve root injury, 222
Nerve stimulation. See Stimulation, nerve
Neuralgia
  genicular, 313
  glossopharyngeal, 79, 312–313
  occipital, 313
  postherpetic, 80
  postsympathectomy, 91
  post-traumatic facial, 80
  trigeminal, 29, 81
    neurolysis for, 91
    surgery for, 311
Neuraxial drug delivery system, 367
Neuroablation for visceral pain, 102–107
  alternatives to, 103–105
  changing trends in, 107
  complications of, 105
  difficulty with, 103
  efficacy of, 105–106
  history of, 103
  technique of, 106–107
Neuroaugmentation in elderly, 366–367
Neurochemistry of pain, 205
Neuroendocrine factor in fibromyalgia, 73
Neurogenic pain
  musculoskeletal, 121
  of neck and shoulder, 61
Neurolysis
  celiac, 107
  in elderly, 366
  facet, 291–302. See also Facet neurolysis
  stellate ganglion block and, 257, 258
  for trigeminal neuralgia, 91
Neurolytic block
  complications of, 264
  indications for, 264
  for neuropathic pain, 90
Neuroma
  formation of, 83
  Morton's, 141
  post-thoracotomy, 121
Neuromodulation, for central pain, 78
Neuron, 10
Neuropathic pain, 77–94
  of central nervous system, 77–78
  complex regional pain syndrome and, 82–86
  definition of, 19
  drugs for, 87–91
  outcome studies on, 86
  of peripheral nervous system, 78–80
  phantom, 80–82
Neuropathy
  peripheral, 78–80
  testing for, 186

Neurostimulation. *See* Stimulation, nerve
Neurosurgery. *See* Surgery
Neurotmesis, 186
Neurotoxicity
    of epidural steroid, 286–287
    of nerve block, 89
Neutrophil count, 148
Newborn, pain in, 351–352
Nifedipine for cancer pain, 115
Nociceptive pain, 18–19, 61–76
    low back, 66–70
    musculoskeletal,71–74
    neck and shoulder, 61–66
Nociceptive pathway, ascending spinal, 10, 13
Nociceptive processing, cerebral, 14
Nociceptor
    associated axons and, 10
    visceral, 96
Nomenclature, psychiatric, 321–325
Nonmalignant pain, 320
Non-nociceptive pain, 19
Nonorganic pain, 145
Nonsteroidal antiinflammatory drug
    avoided in hemophilia, 31
    for cancer pain, 113
    in elderly, 364–365
    in pregnancy, 55
    pregnancy and, 49–50
    in sickle cell disease, 31
Nontraumatic neuropathy, 186
Normeperidine, breast-feeding and, 51
Nortriptyline
    for cancer pain, 115
    dosage of, 207
Nucleus caudalis, 312
Nucleus pulposus herniation in pregnancy, 55
Numbness, 68
Numerical pain scale, 173–174, 353

O

Ober's test, 138
Observation in pain assessment, 176–177
Obstetrics, 49–58
    abdominal pain in, 52–53
    anticonvulsants in, 52
    antidepressants in, 51–52
    back pain and, 53–55
    benzodiazepines in, 51
    beta blockers in, 52
    breast-feeding and, 49
    caffeine in, 52
    drugs in pregnancy and, 49
    ergot alkaloids in, 52
    local anesthetics in, 51
    migraine and, 55
    nonsteroidal antiinflammatory drugs in, 49–50
    opioids in, 50–51
    pelvic pain and, 53–55
    sickle cell disease and, 55–56
    steroids in, 51
    sumatriptan in, 52
Obturator nerve block, 243
Occipital nerve block, 230–231
Occipital nerve cryoneurolysis, 297
Occipital neuralgia, 313
Occupational therapy, 163–165
Oculomotor nerve, 133
Olfactory nerve, 133
Operant intervention, 318, 321
Ophthalmic nerve block, 224–225
Opioid, 208
    for cancer pain, 113–114, 115
    in elderly, 365

Opioid—cont'd
    in epidural infusion, 273
    intraventricular infusion of, 310–311
    legal issues of, 208
    for neuropathic pain, 88
    in pregnancy, 50–51
    tolerance to, 112
Optic nerve, 133
Oral analgesia
    for cancer pain, 113
    for child, 357
Orofacial pain, 120
Orthopedic injury, 37
Oswesty Low Back Disability Questionnaire, 156
Outcomes survey, 157
Outpatient celiac neurolysis, 107
Ovarian remnant syndrome, 102
Oxygen
    for cluster headache, 28
    for migraine, 28
Oxymorphone, 43

P

Pain, 10
    ancient cultures and, 3–4
    classification of, 18–22
    definition of, 320
    disease and, 4
    future and, 5
    hospice movement and, 5
    institutions about, 5
    pathways of, 10–14
        ascending spinal nociceptive, 10, 13
        cerebral nociceptive processing, 14
        nociceptors, 10
        postsynaptic dorsal column fibers, 14
        spinal cord dorsal horn neurons, 10
        spinomesencephalic tract, 14
        spinoreticular tract, 13
        spinothalamic tract, 13
    religion and, 3
    in sickle cell disease, 31
    theories of, 4
    in 20th century, 4–5
Pain Assessment Index, 155
Pain clinic, pediatric, 357
Pain Cognition Questionnaire, 157
Pain diary, 177
Pain Disability Index, 156
Pain drawing, 177, 178
Pain fellowship, 7
Pain fellowship program director, 7–8
Pain institution, 5
Pain management, certification in, 7
Pain medicine as specialty, 8
Pain scale, 173–179
    algorithm for, 179
    for cancer pain, 178
    for child, 353
    for children, 178
    for elderly, 178
    instrument selection for, 177
    laboratory methods of, 177–178
    numerical, 173–174
    patient-controlled analgesia and, 43–44
    for psychiatric pain, 178
    psychologic assessment in, 176–177
    self-reporting, 174–176
    single dimension, 174
    verbal descriptor, 173
    visual analog, 174
Pain society, 8

Pain-prone issue, 321
Palatine nerve block, 228–229
Palliative medicine, 345–346
Pancreatic cancer
    celiac plexus block for, 260
    neuroablation for, 105
Pancreatitis, 32
    acute and chronic, 101
    neuroablation in, 106
Paradigm for trauma pain, 39–40
Paraspinous muscle pain, 71
Parasympathetic innervation of heart, 99
Paravascular inguinal nerve block, 242
Paravertebral cause of low back pain, 63
Paravertebral nerve block, 241–242
Paravertebral sympathetic ganglion, 250–251
Parenteral analgesia
    for cancer pain, 112
    for child, 356–357
    home care and, 336
Paroxetine, 206
    for cancer pain, 115
    dosage of, 206, 207
Partial disability, 169
Passive physical therapy, 329–331
Patellar femoral grinding test, 140
Pathology in disability, 167
Pathway, pain, 10–14
Patient history
    in functional evaluation, 161
    in psychologic evaluation, 153–154
    taking of, 127–129
Patient self-reporting pain scale, 174–176
Patient-controlled analgesia, 43–44
    for cancer pain, 114
    epidural, 274
Patient's bill of rights, 387
Patrick test, 139
Pediatric patient, 351–359. *See also* Child
Pelvic innervation, 253
Pelvic nerve cryoneurolysis, 297
Pelvic pain
    causes of, 101–102
    in pregnancy, 53–55
Penetrating injury, abdominal, 37
Pentazocine, 43
Perceived disability, 156
Perception of child's pain, 351
Percutaneous nerve block, splanchnic, 104, 106–107
Percutaneous sympathectomy, 301
    radiofrequency, 301–302
Periarticular soft tissue disorder, 74
Pericarditis, 98
Periosteal pain, 71
Peripheral infusion, continuous, 276–277
Peripheral nerve block, 242
Peripheral nerve disorder, 190
Peripheral nerve stimulation, 90
Peripheral nerve testing, 186–187
Peripheral nervous system pain, 78–80
    cancer-related, 111
Peripheral neuropathic pain category, 19
Peripheral vascular disorder, 30
Permanent disability, 169
Peroneal nerve block, 246–247
Peroneal nerve cryoneurolysis, 298
Perphenazine, 207
Personality disorder, 324
Personality test, 155
Phalen's maneuver, 138
Phantom pain, 36, 80–81
    cancer-related, 112
Pharmacodynamics in elderly, 364

Pharmacokinetics in elderly, 364
Pharmacologic therapy. *See* Drug therapy
Phenothiazine, 115
Phenytoin
    for cancer pain, 115
    for trigeminal neuralgia, 79
Phospholipase A$_2$, 281
Phrenic nerve, 257
Physical abuse, 323
Physical capacities evaluation, 170
Physical examination, 131–146
    diagnostic tests and, 144
    of gait, 131
    general description in, 131
    independent, 394–395
    of musculoskeletal system, 135–144
        ankle, 140–141
        coordination of motion, 144
        elbow, 137–138
        fingers, 138
        foot, 141–144
        hip, 138
        joints, 137
        knee, 138–140
        range of motion, 135–137
        reproduction of pain in, 144
        shoulder, 137
        thumb, 138
        wrist, 138
    of reflexes, 132
    room for, 131–132
    sensory-dermatomal, 132–134
    trophic, 134
    validation tests and, 144–145
    vital signs in, 131
Physical therapy, 327–331
    behavioral approach to, 331
    for complex regional pain syndrome, 85
    for elderly, 368
    electrical stimulation, 328–329. *See also*
        Stimulation
    for myofascial pain, 73
    for neck and shoulder pain, 65–66
    passive, 329–331
    for phantom limb pain, 81
    temperature modalities in, 327–328
Physician, 379–380
    economics of decision making, 381
Pillow test, 145
Platelet count, 148
Pleurisy, 98
Plexopathy
    brachial, 190
    testing for, 187
Plexus, brachial
    injury to, 36
    pain management of, 38
Plexus block
    brachial, 236–237
    for cancer pain, 116
    differential, 198
    hypogastric, 267–269
    sacral, 244–245
Plexus infusion, brachial, 275–276
Pneumomediastinum, 98
Pneumothorax
    intrapleural sympathetic denervation and, 259
    stellate ganglion block and, 258
Policy issues, 385–387
Policy statement, 374–375
Polyethylene glycol, 287
Polyneuropathy, 78
    testing for, 186
Pontine spinothalamic tractotomy, 310
Popliteal fossa block, 245–246

Positioning for subarachnoid block, 213
Postcholecystectomy pain, 101
Postdural puncture headache, 221
Posterior fossa microvascular decompression, 79
Posterior tibial nerve block, 247
Posterior tibial nerve testing, 187
Postherpetic neuralgia, 80
Postoperative analgesia, 43–47
Postsurgical pain, cancer-related, 111, 112
Postsympathectomy neuralgia, 91
Postsynaptic dorsal column fiber, 16
Post-thoracotomy analgesia, epidural, 47
Post-thoracotomy pain, 121
Post-traumatic facial neuralgia, 80
Post-traumatic headache, 37
Postural back pain, 68
Practice guidelines, 45, 373–375
Precrural celiac nerve block, 104
Preemptive analgesia, 43
Preganglionic nerve, 259
Pregnancy, 49–58
    abdominal pain in, 52–53
    anticonvulsants in, 52
    antidepressants in, 51–52
    back pain and, 53–55
    benzodiazepines in, 51
    beta blockers in, 52
    breast-feeding and, 49
    caffeine in, 52
    drugs in pregnancy and, 49
    ergot alkaloids in, 52
    local anesthetics in, 51
    migraine and, 26, 55
    nonsteroidal antiinflammatory drugs in,
        49–50
    opioids in, 50–51
    pelvic pain and, 53–55
    sickle cell disease and, 55–56
    steroids in, 51
    sumatriptan in, 52
Premonitory symptom of migraine, 25
Preventive therapy for neuropathic pain, 86
Program director, pain fellowship, 7–8
Prone position for subarachnoid block, 214
Prophylaxis for tension headache, 27
Proprioception, 133
Prostaglandin, 49–50
Protriptyline, 207
Pseudomotor axon reflex test, 185
Psoas compartment block, 242
Psychiatric disorder
    patient history of, 129
    testing for, 155–157
Psychiatric nomenclature, 321–325
Psychogenic disorder, test for, 150
Psychogenic pain, 19, 321
    differential nerve block for, 196
    rating scale of, 178
    test for, 145
Psychologic evaluation, 152–159, 176–177
    clinical interview in, 152
    interview in, 152–154
    for malingering, 156
    of mood state, 155–155
    perceived disability in, 155–157
    personality testing in, 155
    psychophysiologic assessment in, 157
Psychologic factors in phantom limb pain, 81
Psychologic history, 154
Psychologic reflex, 132
Psychologic rehabilitation for back pain, 70
Psychologic risk factor, 322–325
Psychologic technique, 318–326
    biofeedback, 320
    cognitive-behavioral, 318–319

Psychologic technique—cont'd
    family therapy, 319
    group therapy, 319
    hypnosis, 319–320
    multidisciplinary model of, 320–321
    nomenclature and, 321–325
    operant, 318
    pain definition and, 320
    psychogenic issues and, 321
    relaxation, 320
Psychometric tools for elderly, 363
Psychophysiologic assessment, 157
Public policy statement, 374–375
Pulmonary arteriography, 194
Pulmonary contusion, 35
Pulmonary embolism, 98
Pulvinotomy, 309–310

Q
Quadrant of spinal cord, 13
Quality improvement
    in home care, 335–336, 373–376
Quantitative sensory testing, 185
Questionnaire
    coping strategies, 157
    McGill pain, 152, 174–176
    Oswesty, 156
    pain cognition, 157
    Roland and Morris, 156
Questions for history taking, 127–128

R
Radial nerve
    cryoneurolysis of, 297
    testing of, 187
Radial nerve block, 239
Radical neck dissection, 112
Radiculopathy
    epidural steroid injection for, 89
    somatosensory evoked potentials in, 190
    testing for, 187
Radiofrequency denervation, 257, 266–267
Radiofrequency lesioning, 298–302
    of cervical facets, 293–294
    in elderly, 366
    of head and neck, 300
    lesion characteristics, 298–299
    percutaneous sympathectomy, 301–302
    principles of, 28
    spinal, 300–301
    technique of, 299–300
    of thoracic facets, 294
    for trigeminal neuralgia, 91
Radiographic evaluation
    arteriography, 194
    arthrography, 194
    computed tomography, 192–193
    in headache examination, 27
    for low back pain, 67
    magnetic resonance imaging, 193
    myelography, 194
    in neuroablation, 106
    plain x-ray film, 192
    regional, 194–195
    skeletal scintigraphy, 194
    venography, 194
Radiosurgery for trigeminal neuralgia, 311
Ramus communicans, 301
Range of motion, 329–330
    in physical examination, 135–137
Ratio, cost-effectiveness, 382

Raynaud's disease, 30
  complex regional pain syndrome vs, 84
Raynaud's phenomenon, 30
Receptor in musculoskeletal pain, 71
Record, medical, 391–392
Recurrent laryngeal nerve, 257
Recurrent laryngeal nerve block, 232–233
Referred pain
  classification of, 19
  of neck and shoulder, 61
  visceral, 97–98
Reflex
  back pain and, 68
  in headache examination, 26
  nerve root compression and, 62
  in physical examination, 132
  pseudomotor axon reflex test, 185
Reflex arc theory of referred pain, 97–98
Reflex sympathetic dystrophy, 38
Regional analgesia
  for cancer pain, 115–116
  for child, 357
  for trauma, 39–40
  for trigeminal neuralgia, 79
Regional diagnosis, 194–195
Regional infusion, intravenous, 89
Regional pain syndrome, complex, 82–86
  central nervous system abnormality in, 83
  in child, 356
  clinical features of, 83–84
  mechanism of, 82
  peripheral nerve abnormality in, 82–83
  peripheral tissue abnormality in, 82
  treatment of, 84–86
Regulatory issues, 385–388
Rehabilitation for back pain, 70
Relaxant, muscle, 208–209
  for back pain, 69
Relaxation technique, 320
  for elderly, 367
Relaxation therapy, 342
Religion and pain, 3
Remnant, ovarian, 102
Renal calculus, 101
Renal system in elderly, 363
Renal tumor, 101
Report
  disability evaluation, 170
  medical, 393
Reproducibility of pain, 144
Research in pediatric pain management, 357
Residency review committee, 7
Resistive exercise, 330
Respiratory effects
  of epidural block, 217
  of nerve block, 89
Restructuring
  cognitive, 367–368
Retroaortic splanchnic nerve block, 103
Retrobulbar block, 224–225
Retrocrural celiac nerve block, 104
Reverse Phalen's maneuver, 138
Review committee, residency, 7
Rexed laminae, 10
Rheumatoid arthritis, 31–32
  in child, 356
  skeletal pain from, 73–74
Rhizotomy
  cervical ganglion, 301
  dorsal, 314
  subtemporal sensory, 311
  trigeminal, 300, 312
Rib fracture, 35
Risk factor, psychologic, 322–325
Roland and Morris Disability Questionnaire, 156

Root, dorsal, ganglionotomy, 301
Rorschach inkblot test, 155
Rotator cuff, drop arm test for, 137
Round ligament, 52

S
Sacral plexus block, 244–245
Sacroiliac joint in pregnancy, 55
Safety of epidural steroid injection, 286–287
Salicylate, pregnancy and, 50
Saphenous nerve block, 243–244
Saphenous nerve cryoneurolysis, 298
Scale, pain, 173–179
  for child, 353, 354
Scapulocostal syndrome, 137
Scar
  nerve fiber entrapped in, 121
  painful, 121
Scarcity, 377
Sciatic nerve block, 244–245
Sciatic nerve catheterization, 277
Scintigraphy, 194
Sclerotome, 62–65
Screening for intrathecal implantation, 304–305
Secondary gain, test for, 150
Securitization, 379
Sedative hypnotic, for back pain, 69
Self-reporting pain scale, 174–176
Self-representation of pain, 353
Sensation
  examination of, 132–133
  exteroceptive, 133
Sensory dysfunction, 62
Sensory fiber, visceral, 96–97
Sensory rhizotomy, subtemporal, 311
Sensory-dermatomal examination, 132–137
Sequential differential spinal block, 195–196
Sertraline, 206, 207
Sexual abuse, 323
Sexual dysfunction, 154
Shoulder
  examination of, 137
  frozen, 137
Shoulder pain, 61–66
  compression causing, 61–65
  management of, 65–66
  neurogenic, 61
Sickle cell disease, 31
  in child, 355
  pregnancy and, 55–56
Sickness Impact Profile, 155, 156
Single dimension pain scale, 173, 174
Sitting position for subarachnoid block, 213–214
Skeletal pain, 73–74
Skeletal scintigraphy, 194
Skin
  nerve fiber termination in, 10, 11
  in trophic examination, 134
Sleep disturbance, in psychologic evaluation, 154
Small intestinal pain, 101
Snapping hip syndrome, 138
Social Security disability program, 168
Soft tissue disorder
  of neck and shoulder, 61
  periarticular, 74
  trauma, 36
Soft tissue in functional evaluation, 162
Somatic nerve block
  of head and neck, 223–236
    auriculotemporal, 229–230
    cervical plexus, 234–236
    glossopharyngeal, 231–232
    greater occipital, 230–231

Somatic nerve block—cont'd
    greater palatine, 228–229
    infraorbital, 227–228
    laryngeal, 232–233
    mandibular, 229
    maxillary, 226–227
    mental, 230
    ophthalmic, 224–225
    spinal accessory, 233–234
    supraorbital and supratrochlear, 225–226
    trigeminal nerve/gasserian ganglion, 223–224
    vagus, 232
  for lower extremity, 241–248
    femoral, 243
    genitofemoral, 242–243
    ilioinguinal and iliohypogastric, 242
    inguinal paravascular, 242
    obturator, 243
    paravertebral, 241–242
    peripheral, 242
    peroneal, 246–247
    popliteal fossa, 245–246
    psoas compartment, 242
    sacral plexus, 244–245
    saphenous, 243–244
    sural, 247
    tibial, 247
  of upper extremity, 236–241
    axillary brachial plexus, 238
    digital, 240
    at elbow, 239
    infraclavicular brachial plexus, 237–238
    interscalene brachial plexus, 236–237
    intravenous, 240–241
    suprascapular nerve, 238–239
    at wrist, 239
Somatic pain
  differential nerve block for, 196
  superficial and deep, 95
Somatoform disorder, 323
Somatosensory evoked potentials, 189–191
Spasm, pelvic muscle, 102
Spastic reflex, 132
Spatial pain scale, 353
Specialization, 377
Specialty, pain medicine as, 8
Sphenopalatine ganglion block, 28
Spielberger State-Trait Anxiety Inventory, 156
Spinal accessory nerve
  cryoneurolysis of, 297
  function of, 134
Spinal accessory nerve block, 233–234
Spinal anatomy, 67–68
Spinal block
  modified, 196–197
  sequential differential, 195–196
  subarachnoid, 212–215
Spinal cord
  anterolateral quadrant of, 13
  compression of, 61–65
  dorsal horn neurons of, 10
  stimulation of, 90
  stretching tests of, 144
  subarachnoid block and, 212
  surgery of, 313
Spinal cord lesion
  central pain from, 77
  epidural block causing, 222
  somatosensory evoked potentials in, 190
Spinal nerve
  cryoneurolysis of, 297
  denervation of, 314
  subarachnoid block and, 212
Spinal nerve pain, 78

Spinal nociceptive pathway, ascending, 10, 13
Spinal stenosis, 190
Spine
    compression fracture of, 37
    in headache examination, 26
    radiofrequency lesioning of, 300–301
Spinomesencephalic tract, 14
Spinoreticular tract, 13
Spinothalamic tract, 13
Spinothalamic tractotomy, 310
Splanchnic nerve block
    complications of, 105
    efficacy of, 105–106
    retroaortic, 103
Spleen pain, 100
Spontaneous muscle activity, 183
Spontaneous pain, central, 77
Sprout growth of nerve, 83
State policy, 387
Statement, policy, 374–375
Stellate ganglion block, 254–258
    anatomy of, 254
    anterior approach for, 255, 257
    for cancer pain, 115–116
    indications for, 254–255
    posterior approach for, 257–258
    technique of, 255
Stellate ganglion infusion, 277–278
Stellate ganglionotomy, 301
Stenosis, spinal, 190
Sternal fracture, 36
Steroid
    epidural injection of, 280–287
        for back pain, 69, 70, 280–282
        cervical, 285–286
        lumbar, 284–285
        mechanism of action of, 282–283
        for neuropathic pain, 89
        safety of, 286–287
        technique of, 283–284
    in pregnancy, 51
Stimulation, nerve, 342
    back pain and, 70
    for complex regional pain syndrome, 85–86
    deep brain, 311
    electrical, 312
    in functional evaluation, 162
    indications for, 329
    for myofascial pain, 72
    for neuropathic pain, 90
    physiologic effects of, 328–329
    in pregnancy, 55, 56
Stomach pain, 99
Straight leg raising test, 138, 139, 140
Strain, foot, 141–142
Strengthening exercise, 162–163
Stretching, 329
    in functional evaluation, 162–163
Stretching test, spinal cord, 144
Structured Interview of Reported Symptoms, 156
Stump pain, 83
Subacromial bursitis, 137
Subarachnoid block, 212–215
    anatomy in, 212
    cerebrospinal fluid and, 212–213
    complications of, 215
    spread of anesthetic and, 214–215
    technique of, 213–214
Subarachnoid infusion, continuous, 275–276
Subdural injection, 221
Subjective pain report, 157
Substance abuse, 129, 322
Subtemporal sensory rhizotomy, 311
Sudomotor disorder, 83
Sufentanil, 43

Sumatriptan, 52
Superficial cervical plexus block, 235–236
Superficial peroneal nerve block, 246–247
Superficial somatic pain, 95
Superior gluteal nerve cryoneurolysis, 298
Superior hypogastric plexus block, 267–269
Superior laryngeal nerve block, 232
Supply and demand, 377–378
Supportive care, 345–346
Supraclavicular brachial plexus block, 236
Supraorbital nerve block, 225–226
Supraorbital nerve cryoneurolysis, 295
Suprascapular nerve block, 238–239
Suprascapular nerve cryoneurolysis, 297
Supratemporal nerve block, 225–226
Sural nerve block, 247
Surface temperature monitoring, 270
Surgery, 43–48, 309–317
    for back pain, 69
    for cancer pain, 114–115
    for central pain, 78
    cingulotomy, 309
    for coccygodynia, 119
    combined procedures, 309–310
    for complex regional pain syndrome, 85
    cordotomy, 313
    decompression, 65
    deep brain stimulation and, 311
    dorsal rhizotomy, 314
    dorsal root entry zone lesion, 313–314
    epidural injection for, 44–45
    epidural vs parenteral opioids for, 46
    for genicular neuralgia, 311
    for glossopharyngeal neuralgia, 312–313
    hypophysectomy, 309
    hypothalamotomy, 310
    intra-articular morphine in, 45
    for intrathecal implantation, 306
    midline myelotomy, 313
    nerve block during, 104
    for neuropathic pain, 90–91
    for occipital neuralgia, 313
    opioid infusion and, 310–311
    opioid injection and, 43
    patient-controlled analgesia in, 43–44
    for phantom limb pain, 82
    pontine spinothalamic tractotomy, 310
    practice guidelines for, 45
    preemptive analgesia in, 43
    pulvinotomy, 309–310
    in rheumatic arthritis, 31
    for spinal cord compression, 65
    spinal nerve denervation, 314
    sympathectomy, 314
    thalamotomy, 309
    transdermal fentanyl for, 45
    for trigeminal neuralgia, 79, 311–312
Survey, medical outcomes, 157
Sweat test, 270
Sympathectomy, 314
    for complex regional pain syndrome, 85
    lumbar, 301–302
    neuralgia after, 94
    percutaneous, 301
Sympathetic afferent, 82
Sympathetic dystrophy, reflex, 38
Sympathetic infusion, continuous, 277–278
Sympathetic nerve block, 250–270
    anatomy in, 250–254
    celiac plexus splanchnic, 259–264
    completeness of, 270
    for complex regional pain syndrome, 85
    ganglion impar, 269–270
    history of, 250
    interpleural approach to, 259

Sympathetic nerve block—cont'd
    intravenous regional, 267
    lumbar, 265–266
    neurolytic, 264
    radiofrequency denervation, 266–267
    stellate ganglion, 254–258
    superior hypogastric plexus, 267–269
    thoracic, 259
Sympathetic neuroablation, 102–107
Sympathetic pain
    differential nerve block for, 196
    of neck and shoulder, 61
Sympathic innervation of heart, 99
Symptom checklist-90, 155
Synapse in complex regional pain syndrome, 82
Synaptic transmitter, 206
Synovial joint, 71–72

T
Tarsal tunnel syndrome, 141
Taxonomy, 17–22
    in *Diagnostic and Statistical Manual of Mental Disorders,* 17–18
    international, 17
    medical disciplines and, 17
    need for, 17
    pain classifications, 18–20
Temperature
    in radiofrequency lesioning, 298
    surface, 270
Temporal acute pain category, 19
Temporary disability, 169
Temporomandibular joint
    disorder of, 120
    facial trauma and, 37
    jaw opening test of, 144
Tendon pain, 71
Tennis elbow, test for, 138
TENS. *See* Transcutaneous electrical nerve stimulation
Tension, mechanical, 282
Tension-type headache, 27
    migraine with, 28–29
Terminology, derivation of, 3–4
Test instrument, selection of, 177
Testimony, 393–395
Thalamic pain syndrome, 77
Thalamotomy, 309
Therapeutic exercise, 329–330
    in functional evaluation, 162–163
Thioridazine, 207, 208
Thiothixene, 207
Thoracic disorder, 192
Thoracic epidural block, 218
Thoracic facet
    denervation of, 300
    radiofrequency lesioning of, 294
Thoracic facet syndrome, 291–292
Thoracic ganglion rhizotomy, 301
Thoracic injury, 35
Thoracic nerve block, 259
Thoracic outlet syndrome, 190
Thoracic pain
    musculoskeletal, 120–121
    visceral, 98
Thoracic surgery, 47
Thoracic sympathectomy, 301
Thoracolumbar spine, 135, 136
Thoracostomy tube, 37
Thoracotomy
    cancer-related, 112
    pain after, 121
Thromboangiitis obliterans, 30

Thrombosis, venous, 29–30
Thumb examination, 138
Tibial nerve block, 247
Tibial nerve testing, 187
Tietze's syndrome, 121
Time-related pain category, 19
Tocainide, 115
Tolerance, evaluation of, 161
Tomography, diagnostic, 192–193
Total disability, 169
Toxicity
    of epidural steroid, 286–287
    of nerve block, 89
Trace reflex, 132
Traction, 331
Tractotomy
    spinothalamic, 310
    trigeminal, 312
Transaortic nerve block, 104
Transcrural celiac nerve block, 104
Transcutaneous electrical nerve stimulation, 342
    back pain and, 70
    for complex regional pain syndrome, 85–86
    in functional evaluation, 162
    for myofascial pain, 72
    for neuropathic pain, 90
    in pregnancy, 55, 56
Transdermal administration
    for cancer pain, 114
    of fentanyl, 45
Transition, work, 165
Transmission pathway, pain, 205
Transmitter, synaptic, 206
Trauma, 35–42
    chest wall, 35
    delayed sequelae of, 36–37
    epidural analgesia for, 38
    epidural block causing, 222
    of extremity, 38
    head injury, 38
    intra-abdominal, 38
    nonthoracic, 36
    pain management in, 37–40
    test for, 150
    thoracic, 36, 37
Tricyclic antidepressant, 207, 209
    for neuropathic pain, 87
Trifluoperazine, 207
Trigeminal nerve
    branches of, 224
    function of, 133
    somatosensory evoked potentials in, 190
Trigeminal nerve/gasserian ganglion block,
        223–224
Trigeminal neuralgia, 29, 79
    neurolysis for, 91
    surgery for, 311
Trigeminal rhizotomy, 300, 312
Trigeminal tractotomy, 312
Trigger
    of myofascial pain, 72, 121
    for temporomandibular joint pain, 120
    for tension headache, 27
Trochanteric bursitis, 138
Trophic examination, 134

Tube, thoracostomy, 37
Tumor. See also Cancer
    back pain from, 68
    intra-abdominal, neuroablation for, 105
    mediastinal, 98
    pain related to, 111
    renal, 101
    test for, 149

U
Ulnar nerve
    cryoneurolysis of, 297
    testing of, 186–187
Ulnar nerve block, 239
Upper extremity
    cryoneurolysis of, 297
    imaging of, 195
    nerve testing of, 187
    neurogenic pain of, 61
    somatic nerve block of, 236–241
        axillary brachial plexus, 238
        digital, 240
        at elbow, 239
        infraclavicular brachial plexus, 237–238
        interscalene brachial plexus, 236–237
        intravenous, 240–241
        suprascapular nerve, 238–239
        at wrist, 239
    somatosensory evoked potentials in, 189–190
Uremic neuropathy, 78
Ureteral pain, 101
Ureteric calculus, 101
Urinalysis, 148–149
Urologic disorder, pelvic pain from, 102
Uterus, 52–53
Utility, 377

V
Vagus nerve, 134
Vagus nerve block, 232
Validation test, 144–145
Valproate
    for cancer pain, 115
    in pregnancy, 52
Valsalva test, 144
Vascular disease
    acute, 29–30
    disk degeneration and, 281
    test for, 150
Vasoconstriction, 82
Vasodilation, 802
Vasomotor disorder, 83
Vasoocclusion in sickle cell disease, 31
    in pregnancy, 55–56
Vasospastic disease, 30–31
Venlafaxine
    for cancer pain, 115
    dosage of, 206, 207
Venography, 194
Venous thrombosis, acute, 29–30
Verbal descriptor pain scale, 173

Vertebra. See also Intervertebral disk
    back pain and, 281
    compression fracture of, 37
    low back pain and, 66, 67
    painful conditions of, 121
Veteran's Administration benefits, 168
Vibratory stimulation, for myofascial pain, 72
VINDICATE PS, 149
Viral infection
    herpes zoster, 79–80
    test for, 149
Viscera, sympathetic innervation of, 251–252
Visceral pain, 95–109
    abdominal, 98–99
    cancer, 111
    initiation of, 95–96
    neuroablation for, 102–107
        alternatives to, 103–105
        changing trends in, 107
        complications of, 105
        difficulty with, 103
        efficacy of, 105–106
        history of, 103
        technique of, 106–107
    pelvic, 101–102
    phases of, 95
    referral of, 97–98
    thoracic, 98
Viscerosomatic convergence, 97
Viscerovisceral convergence, 97
Visual analog scale, 174
    patient-controlled analgesia and, 43–44
Visual inspection, 161
Vital signs, 131
Vocational rehabilitation, 70
Voluntary muscle activity, 183–184

W
Waddell's sign, 145
Wallenberg's syndrome, 77
Waveform, 184
Weakness, back pain and, 68
Whiplash, trauma causing, 37
White blood cell, 147–148
Wisconsin Cancer Pain Initiative, 8
Work capacity, evaluation of, 164–165
Work hardening, 165
Workers' compensation, 168–169
World Health Organization, 17
World Society of Pain Clinicians, 8
Wrist
    examination of, 138
    nerve block at, 239

Y
Yergason test, 137

Z
Zygapophyseal joint, 68